Practical Immunodermatology

Xing-Hua Gao • Hong-Duo Chen
Editors

Practical Immunodermatology

Springer

Editors
Xing-Hua Gao
Dermatology
The first affiliated Hospital China Medical University
Shenyang
China

Hong-Duo Chen
Dermatology
The first affiliated Hospital China Medical University
Shenyang
China

ISBN 978-94-024-0900-0 ISBN 978-94-024-0902-4 (eBook)
DOI 10.1007/978-94-024-0902-4

Library of Congress Control Number: 2016960305

Printed on acid-free paper

This Springer imprint is published by Springer Nature
The registered company is Springer Science+Business Media B.V. Dordrecht
The registered company address is Van Godewijckstraat 30, 3311 GX Dordrecht, The Netherlands

Contents

Part I

The Fundamentals of Human Immune System

1.1 An Overview to the Fundamental Concepts in Immunology

Immunology refers to the study of the structure and function of human immune system and the mechanism under which the body fights against infection. We live in an environment surrounded by invading pathogens, but we are rarely infected by these pathogens because of our immune system. Immunology describes the underlying process and battling between pathogens and the immune system, leading to either the clearance of pathogens and thus the cure of pathogen-induced diseases or the persistent invasion of microorganisms with a possible overreactive immune injury to the body. Immunology shares a close connection with cellular biology, molecular biology, genetics, etc., turning this branch of science into one of the most cutting-edge and fundamental discipline in both life sciences and medical sciences.

Immunology is a relatively complex and newly growing science. Over 2000 years ago, it was discovered that people who survived infection during pandemic may exhibit resistibility against such infection during their second challenge, which may be referred to as "immunity." Edward Jenner is always considered as the founder of modern immunology. He introduced the term "vaccination" by demonstrating that smallpox may be prevented by inoculating with cowpox in the eighteenth century. After almost two centuries of this elegant work, smallpox vaccination became universal, and in 1979 the World Health Organization announced its complete eradication. Disease is mainly caused by infectious agents that were defined as microorganisms by Robert Koch in the nineteenth century. We now classify infectious microorganism into four categories: viruses, bacteria, fungi, and parasites. In the 1880s, Louis Pasteur devised a vaccine against cholera in chickens and a rabies vaccine against bitten by a rabid dog. In the early 1890s, Emil von Behring and Shibasaburo Kitasato led to the first discovery of antibodies in the serum of animals immunized with diphtheria or tetanus that could confer short-lived protection against the effects of diphtheria or tetanus toxins in people.

A complete functional immune system includes immune organs, immune cells, and immune molecules (Table 1). The immune system not only can recognize and clear pathogens but also may recognize mutated cells, senescent cells, and other toxic components. The three main functions of the immune system are immune defense, immune surveillance, and immune homeostasis. Immune defense prevents foreign pathogens from entering the body and clears pathogens and other toxic substances that are already inside of the body. Immune surveillance discovers and clears "nonself" components such as tumor cells, senescent cells, and apoptotic cells from the body. Immune homeostasis maintains the balance of the microenvironment by immunotolerance and immunoregulation.

Immune response is the process of the immune system to recognize and clear "nonself" substances from the system which may be divided into innate immunity and adaptive immunity (Table 2). Innate immunity, or the innate immune response, is the first barrier against microorganisms. It involves nonspecific cells such as monocytes/macrophages, dendritic cells, granulocytes, etc., that recognize pathogen-associated molecule patterns (PAMPs) through

Table 1 Components of the immune system

Lymphoid organs		Immunocytes		
Central	Peripheral	Innate immunity	Adaptive immunity	Immune molecules
Bone marrow	Lymph nodes	Monocyte/macrophage	T cell	Complement
Thymus	Spleen	Granulocyte	B cell	Antibody
	Mucosal-associated lymphoid tissue (MALT)	Dendritic cell		Cytokine
		Mast cell		CD molecule
		NK cells		Cell adhesion molecule (CAM)
		Innate lymphoid cell (ILC)		Major histocompatibility complex (MHC)
		Innate-like lymphocyte (ILL)		

Table 2 Distinctive features of innate and adaptive immunity

	Innate immunity	Adaptive immunity
Specificity	Nonspecific	Specific
Production of receptors	Germline-encoded	Somatic recombination of gene segments
Diversity of receptors	Limited	Diversified
Memory	No memory	Memory
Cells	Innate immunocytes	T and B lymphocytes
Molecules	Complements, etc.	Antibodies

their pattern recognition receptors (PRRs). Innate immune response is an immediate response that combats a wide range of pathogens without lasting for a long time. Adaptive immunity, or the adaptive immune response, is a specific immune response of T and B cells to induce a series of functional effects against a particular pathogen after self-activation, proliferation, and differentiation upon encountering this "nonself" antigen. In many cases, an adaptive immune response also results in the phenomenon known as immunological memory, which confers lifelong protective immunity to reinfection with the same pathogen. Innate immunity and adaptive immunity always coordinate with each other, and innate immune response is often the prerequisite to initiate an adaptive immune response.

On one side, the immune system provides defense against foreign pathogens; however, on the other side, when the equilibrium of the immune system is broken, it often results in either over-activation or over-inhibition of the immune responses that leads to serious immunopathology. For example, immune cells may attack self tissues and organs, which results in autoimmune diseases; severe inflammatory process induced by immune responses often results in hypersensitivity; immune responses against harmless antigens often result in allergy; defective immune responses often result in persistent infections; and tolerized immune responses often result in the progression of tumors.

1 Components of the Immune System

Haoyu Sun, Rui Sun, and Zhigang Tian

Contents

H. Sun, R. Sun
Institute of Immunology, School of Life Sciences and Medical Center, University of Science and Technology of China, Hefei, China

Z. Tian (✉)
Institute of Immunology, School of Life Sciences and Medical Center, University of Science and Technology of China, Hefei, China
e-mail: tzg@ustc.edu.cn

1.1 Immune Organs

Immune system is mainly composed of immune organs, tissues, cells, and molecules, all of which interact with each other to perform immune functions. Immune tissues may also be referred to as the lymphoid tissues or lymphoid organs, which are divided broadly into central lymphoid organs and peripheral lymphoid organs.

1.1.1 Central Lymphoid Organs

The central lymphoid organs, including the bone marrow and thymus, are also known as the primary lymphoid organs. They are the major sites of origination, differentiation, development, and maturation of immune cells.

1.1.1.1 Bone Marrow

All the cellular components of the blood, including the red blood cells, the platelets, and the white blood cells, are derived from the hematopoietic stem cells (HSCs) of bone marrow. Hematopoietic stem cells, the precursor cells with high self-renewal capacity and pluripotent differentiation potential, give rise to all different types of blood cells. The process of blood cells undergoing cell growth, division, and differentiation in the bone marrow is referred to as hematopoiesis. Immune responses depend on the activities of the white blood cells or leukocytes that are originated from the bone marrow, making it very important for the differentiation and maturation of B cells and natural killer (NK) cells. When the function of the bone marrow is either deficient or impaired, hematopoiesis, cellular immunity, and humoral immunity may all be severely damaged. For example, large amount of radiation exposure causes inhibition or loss of hematopoietic and immune functions, which may only be restored when the normal bone marrow is implanted.

X.-H. Gao, H.-D. Chen (eds.), *Practical Immunodermatology*, DOI 10.1007/978-94-024-0902-4_1

1.1.1.2 Thymus

Thymus is the site of differentiation, development, and maturation of T cells. The size of the thymus decreases during aging, while lipid tissues substitute medulla and cortex, leading to the alterations in the thymus microenvironment, which in turn reduces T-cell development and maturation, resulting in the loss of the immune functions in the elderly. The thymocytes and the thymus stromal cells (TSCs) are the two major cell types located in the thymus. The thymocytes are T cells at different stages, while thymus stromal cells include thymus epithelial cells, macrophages, dendritic cells, and fibroblasts. Thymus is structurally composed of cortex and medulla (Fig. 1.1). The major cell types in the cortex include immature T cells, thymus epithelial cells, macrophages, and dendritic cells, while the medulla mainly includes medullary thymus epithelial cells and mature thymocytes, monocytes/macrophages, and dendritic cells. Cortex is divided into outer cortex and inner cortex. Thymus epithelial cells of the outer cortex wrap around the thymocytes and are therefore described as the thymic nursing cells. They can produce hormones and cytokines that stimulate the differentiation and development of thymocytes. In addition to its importance in T-cell differentiation and maturation, thymus also plays key roles in the immune regulation and immune tolerance.

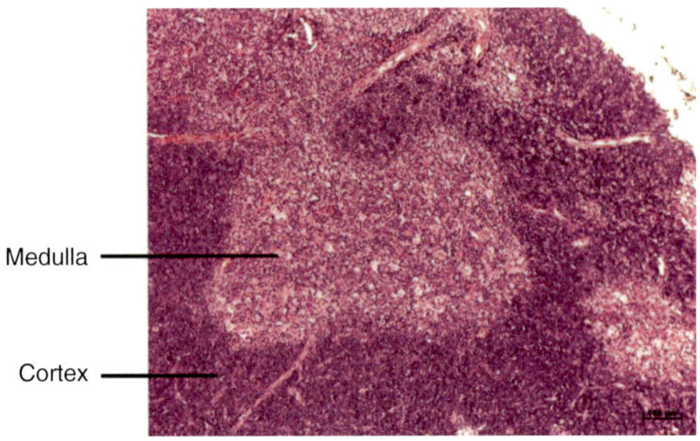

Fig. 1.1 Morphology of the thymus. This photomicrograph shows a portion of a thymic lobule from a hematoxylin-eosin-stained section, illustrating the dense outer cortex and pale inner medulla (Photograph courtesy of Dr. Tian, Zhigang)

1.1.2 Peripheral Lymphoid Organs

Peripheral lymphoid organs, including the lymph nodes, the spleen, and the mucosal immune system (MIS), are also known as the secondary lymphoid organs. They are the residing sites of mature T cells and B cells and the major sites of immune responses.

1.1.2.1 Lymph Nodes

The lymph nodes are the most highly organized peripheral lymphoid organs and the primary residing sites for both T and B cells. They locate at the point where the lymphatic vessels converge, and are the major sites for antigen recognition and the induction of adaptive immune responses. They participate in the lymphoid recirculation and serve as filters of lymph fluid. The lymph node can be divided into two parts: the cortex and the medulla. The cortex subdivides into the outer cortex and the paracortex, and the latter is also referred to as the deep cortex. The outer cortex, also referred to as the B-cell zone, is made up by follicles in which B cells are localized. T cells are more diffusely distributed in the surrounding paracortical areas, also referred to as the T-cell zone (Fig. 1.2). The activation of B cells requires both the binding between the antigen and B-cell receptor (BCR), and the cooperation of helper T (Th) cells. The structure of the lymph node ensures the proper encountering of the helper T cells and antigens when naïve B cells pass through the T-cell zone before entering the follicles, where they become activated. B cells aggregate into primary lymphoid follicle or the

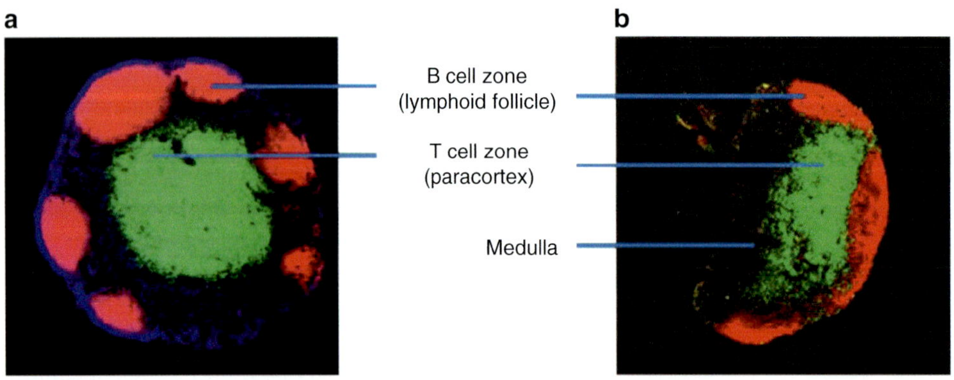

Fig. 1.2 Morphology of the lymph node. In this immunofluorescence-stained section of a lymph node, the B cells located in the follicles are stained in *red*; the T cells in the paracortex are stained in *green*. (**a**) is a transverse section through a lymph node; (**b**) is a longitudinal section through a lymph node (Photograph courtesy of Dr. Tian, Zhigang)

lymph nodule that contains naïve B cells without the presence of the germinal center (GC). The germinal center forms inside of the lymphoid follicle after antigen stimulation, giving rise to the secondary lymphoid follicle, which contains large number of proliferated and differentiated B lymphoblast cells that may eventually differentiate into plasma cells to produce antibodies. The medulla is composed of medullary cord and medullary sinus. Medullary cord comprises of a dense aggregation of lymphocytes (mainly B cells), plasma cells, and some T cells and macrophages, while medullary sinus is rich in macrophages and is more capable at trapping and cleaning pathogens.

1.1.2.2 Spleen

The spleen is located behind the stomach and is the largest peripheral lymphoid organ in the human system. It is the hematopoietic organ during embryonic stage that contains vast blood sinuses. Spleen is the residing site of both T and B cells, in which B cells and T cells comprise around 60 % and 40 % of all immune cell population, respectively. Unlike lymph node, which is the major site of immune responses against lymph fluid-derived antigens, the spleen is the major site of immune responses against blood-derived antigens. Spleen is also important in the formation of bioactive substances and is acting as a filter of blood. Like the other secondary lymphoid organs, spleen also comprises of two parts: the white pulp and the red pulp (Fig. 1.3). The white pulp is a dense lymphoid tissue, composed of periarteriolar lymphoid sheath (PALS), splenic nodule, and the marginal zone. PALS is often mentioned as the T-cell zone, because it mainly composes of T cells along with few dendritic cells and macrophages. The splenic nodule, on the other hand, is often described as the B-cell zone, because it contains large amount of B cells along with few macrophages and follicular dendritic cells (FDCs). It forms germinal center after antigen stimulation and becomes a secondary lymphoid follicle. The marginal zone surrounds the follicle and is the residing site for a resident, non-circulating population of B cells known as marginal zone B cells. The red pulp, mainly composed of splenic cord and splenic sinus, is the site for the disposal of red blood cells. Splenic cord comprises of B cells, plasma cells, macrophages, and dendritic cells.

1.1.2.3 Mucosal Immune System

Mucosal surfaces are protected by the mucosal immune system (MIS), also known as the mucosal-associated lymphoid tissues (MALTs). Mucosal surfaces are the barriers through which most pathogens enter the body, and they are therefore exposed to a variety of potential antigens from the air, food, and the natural microbial flora of the body. MIS comprises of the gut, the nasal and respiratory tract, the urogenital tract, and other mucosa. Gut-associated lymphoid tissue (GALT) includes the tonsils, adenoids, appendix, and Peyer's patches in the small intestine, which all collect antigens from the epithelial surfaces of the gastrointestinal tract. Being distinct from the other tissues, antigen collection in Peyer's patches is achieved by specialized epithelial cells called microfold cells (M cells) (Fig. 1.4). More diffused aggregates of lymphocytes are present in the respiratory tract: the nasal-associated lymphoid tissue (NALT) and the bronchus-associated lymphoid tissue (BALT) [1–5].

1.2 Immunocytes

Immunocytes are a major component of the immune system and refer to cells participating in an immune response. They include T and B cells involved in the adaptive immunity, and natural killer (NK) cells, monocytes/macrophages, dendritic cells (DCs), polymorphonuclear leukocytes (PMNs) (neutrophils, eosinophils, and basophils), mast cells, innate-like lymphocytes (ILLs), and innate lymphoid cells (ILCs) involved in the innate immunity.

The cells of the immune system derive from pluripotent hematopoietic stem cells (HSCs) in the bone marrow. HSCs give rise to two types of stem cells: a common myeloid

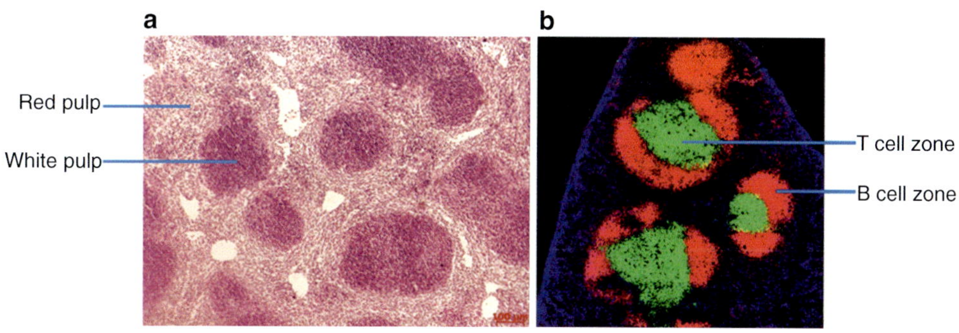

Fig. 1.3 Morphology of the spleen. (**a**) shows a portion of a spleen from a hematoxylin-eosin-stained section, illustrating the dense white pulp and pale red pulp; (**b**) shows a portion of a spleen from an immunofluorescence-stained section, in which B cells are stained in *red* and T cells are stained in *green* (Photograph courtesy of Dr. Tian, Zhigang)

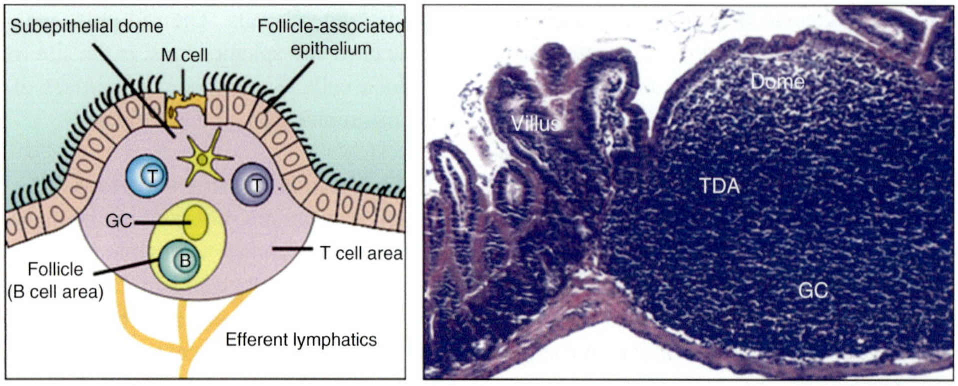

Fig. 1.4 Organization of a Peyer's patch in the gut mucosa. As the diagram on the *left* shows, a Peyer's patch contains numerous B-cell follicles with germinal centers (GCs). T cells occupy the areas between follicles – the T-cell dependent areas (TDAs). The surface epithelium refers to the follicle-associated epithelium (FAE). The layer between the surface epithelium and the follicle is known as the subepithelial dome, and is rich in DCs, T cells, and B cells. A Peyer's patch has no afferent lymphatics, and antigens entered directly from the gut across a specialized epithelium made up of the so-called microfold (M) cells. The hematoxylin-eosin-stained section on the *right* shows a section through a Peyer's patch in the gut wall of the mouse. The Peyer's patch can be seen lying beneath the epithelial tissues (Photograph courtesy of Dr. Tian, Zhigang)

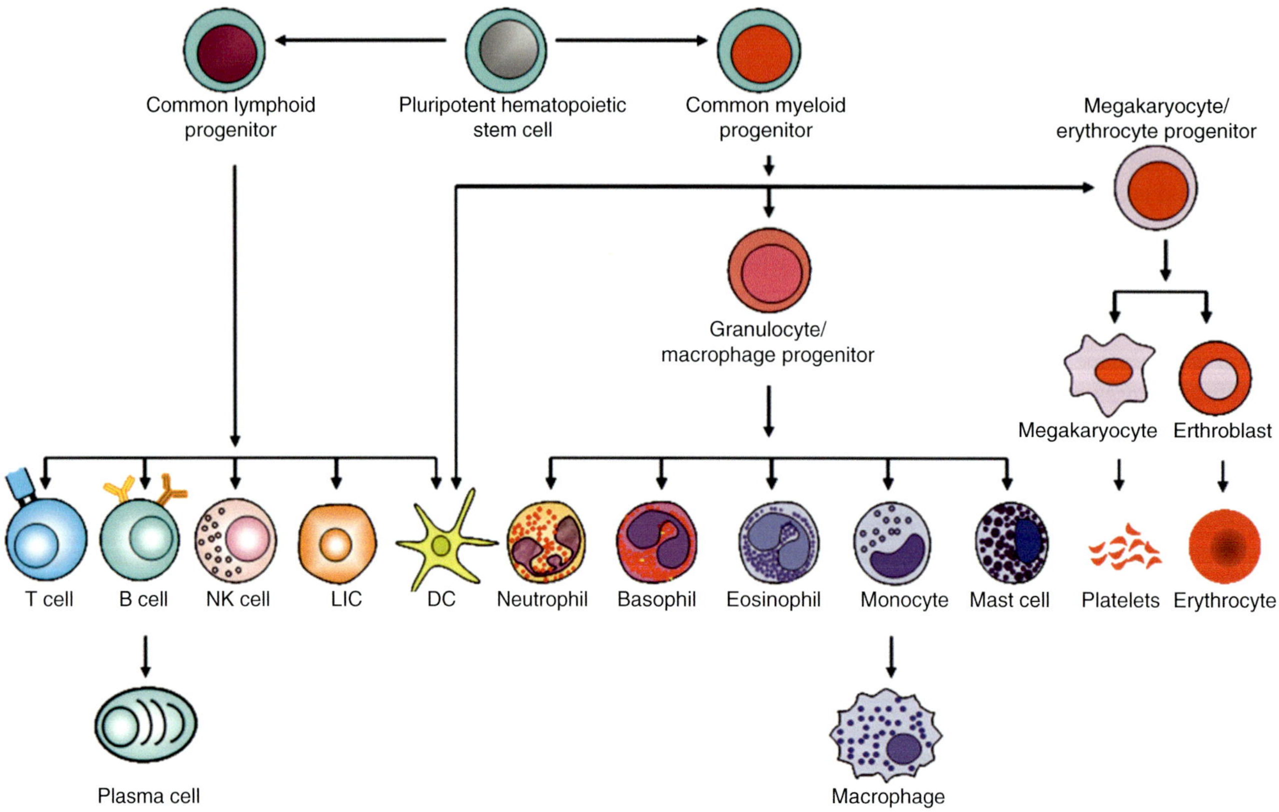

Fig. 1.5 The immunocytes arise from pluripotent hematopoietic stem cells in the bone marrow. *ILC* innate lymphoid cell, *DC* dendritic cell

progenitor (CMP) and a common lymphoid progenitor (CLP). CMP develops into different types of leukocytes, including monocytes/macrophages, granulocytes, mast cells, erythrocytes that carry oxygen, and megakaryocytes that give rise to platelets. CLP develops into different types of lymphocytes, including αβT cells (conventional T cells) and B-2 cells (conventional B cells) of the adaptive immune system, and innate lymphoid cells (ILCs), natural killer (NK) cells, γδT cells, NKT cells, marginal zone (MZ) B cells, and B-1 cells of the innate immune system. The immature dendritic cells arise from both myeloid and lymphoid progenitors in the bone marrow, and develop into mature dendritic cells after encountering potential pathogens (Fig. 1.5). Different membrane proteins expressed by distinct immunocytes are closely associated with the differentiation, maturation, activation, and functions of these cells [1–4].

1.2.1 Immunocytes in Innate Immunity

Immunocytes in innate immunity include monocytes/macrophages, granulocytes (basophils, eosinophils, and neutrophils), dendritic cells, mast cells, ILLs, and ILCs. Macrophages, granulocytes, and dendritic cells are the three major classes of phagocytic cells in the innate immune system, and are collectively termed as phagocytes.

1.2.1.1 Monocyte/Macrophage

The first major class of phagocytes is the monocytes/macrophages. As the main phagocyte population residing in the normal tissues, monocytes are immature form of macrophages that circulate in the blood and continuously migrate into tissues throughout the body where they differentiate and become resident macrophages. Macrophages residing in different tissues are often termed with distinct names. For example, macrophages in the neural tissues are termed as microglial cells, whereas those in the liver are termed as Kupffer cells. They are relatively long-lived cells that play several different roles in the innate and adaptive immune response. Macrophages play an important role in the innate immune response where they engulf and kill invading microorganisms, providing the first line of defense against pathogens. They also present antigens of pathogens and infected cells targeted by the adaptive immune response. Macrophages also participate in the immune responses by assisting the induction of inflammation. They can activate and recruit other immune cells by producing cytokines and chemokines, and can also act as general scavenger cells to clear dead cells and cell debris [1–4, 6]. Two subpopulations of macrophages (M1 and M2) have been identified based on their distinct profiles of chemokine production and iron/glucose metabolism [7–10].

M1 macrophage The "classically activated" proinflammatory (M1) macrophages exhibit a killing/inhibitory capacity [11, 12]. M1-produced NO is an important effector molecule with microbicidal activity and cell proliferation inhibitory capacity [13]. These cells are the key effector cells for the elimination of pathogens, virus-infected cells, and cancer cells [14].

M2 macrophage The "alternatively activated" anti-inflammatory (M2) macrophages can modify their metabolic functions through a heal/growth-promoting setting. M2-produced ornithine can promote cell proliferation and cell repairing through polyamine and collagen synthesis, fibrosis, and other tissue-remodeling machineries [12]. M2 macrophages can also promote tumor growth [10].

1.2.1.2 Granulocyte

Granulocytes are the second major class of phagocytes, and are named for their densely staining granules in the cytoplasm. Granulocytes are also named as polymorphonuclear leukocytes (PMNs) because of their irregularly shaped nuclei. Three subtypes of granulocytes, namely neutrophils, eosinophils, and basophils, can be distinguished from each other depending on the staining properties of their granules.

Neutrophil Neutrophils are short-lived cells that may only survive for several days, and are abundant in blood but absent in healthy tissues. Neutrophils have the strongest phagocytic activity and are the first cells leaving the blood to migrate to the site of infection or inflammation. Neutrophils are very important in innate immunity; their number increases rapidly during infection or inflammation. They catch a variety of microorganisms and destroy them in intracellular vesicles using degradative enzymes and antimicrobial substances stored in the cytoplasmic granules [15, 16].

Eosinophil and Basophil Eosinophils and basophils are less in number compared to neutrophils; they also possess granules containing a variety of enzymes and toxic proteins that are being released upon cell activation. Eosinophils and basophils participate in the defense against parasites and show rather damaging effects in allergic inflammatory reactions [17, 18].

1.2.1.3 Dendritic Cell

The third major class of phagocytes in innate immunity is dendritic cells (DCs) residing in tissues throughout the whole body. DCs are named for their long fingerlike dendrites. They emerge from the bone marrow and migrate to peripheral tissues either directly or through blood, where they ingest foreign substances by phagocytosis, and large amount of extracellular fluid along with its contents by macropinocytosis, a form of endocytosis. Upon encountering pathogens, DCs migrate to lymphoid tissues for maturation and activate antigen-specific T cells by presenting antigens derived from pathogens, which in turn leads to the activation of antigen receptors on T cells. Thus, DCs are also known as antigen-presenting cells (APCs). Although macrophages can also work as APCs, only DCs are specialized in the initiation of an adaptive immune response. There are two main functional classes of DCs: conventional dendritic cells (cDCs) and plasmacytoid dendritic cells (pDCs).

Conventional dendritic cells cDCs are found mostly under surface epithelia and in most organs such as heart and kidneys. Their main function is to proceed with the ingested microbes in order to generate antigen peptides that can activate T cells and induce an adaptive immune response. Thus, cDCs act as a bridge between the innate and the adaptive immune systems [16].

Plasmacytoid dendritic cell Being less important in activating naïve T cells, the pDCs are the major producers of interferons, particularly in response to viral infections. Therefore, pDCs are often considered as part of innate immunity. pDCs express costimulatory molecules and adhesion molecules, and also act as antigen-presenting cells.

Langerhans cell Langerhans cells are immature cDCs residing in the skin. They contain large granules and are actively phagocytic. During skin infection, they capture antigens of invading pathogens and migrate to the regional lymph nodes. They lose their ability to take up antigens rapidly and increase the synthesis of MHC molecules instead, followed by their differentiation into mature DCs. These mature DCs express costimulatory molecules and adhesion molecules and present antigens to activate naive T cells [1–4].

1.2.1.4 Mast Cell

Mast cells derive from HSCs in the bone marrow, but differentiate and mature in the tissues. They contain granules that are rich in acidic proteoglycans, which are released upon cell activation. Mast cells often reside near surfaces that are easily exposed to pathogens and allergens, such as the mucosal tissues and connective tissues surrounding the blood vessels. They are important in inducing inflammation, orchestrating allergic reactions, protecting the internal surfaces of the body against pathogens, and responding against parasitic worms [19–23].

1.2.1.5 Natural Killer Cell

Natural killer (NK) cells are large granular lymphocytes that lack the expression of T-cell receptor (CD3 negative). Many scholars have recently suggested that NK cells may be classified into a newly characterized family: the ILC1. NK cells are not antigen-specific and may carry out their effector functions without prior sensitization, and are therefore considered as part of the innate immunity. They play a central role in the control of viral infections and kill target cells by releasing cytotoxic granules such as granzymes and perforins. NK cells were initially identified through their ability to mediate cellular cytotoxicity against tumor cells. Activation of NK cells in response to type I interferons (IFNs) reported by subsequent studies also identified them as a component of the innate immune response. The cytotoxicity of NK cells is strictly regulated by the complex repertoires of activating and inhibitory receptors to ensure proper activation against pathogens while preventing inadvertent attacks to normal cells. Activation of NK cells is solely dependent on the balance between signals induced by the activating and the inhibitory receptors [24]. When NK cells are in contact with normal cells, major histocompatibility complex (MHC) class I molecules on the normal cells bind to their recognized inhibitory receptors on NK cells, which induces an inhibitory signal to override any other activation signals and keeps NK cells calm. However, when NK cells are engaged with abnormal or stressed cells, with either altered or lost MHC class I molecules, NK cells would be fully activated due to the absence or weakening of MHC class I-induced inhibitory signal. The activating and inhibitory receptors on NK cells fall into two large families: the killer lectin-like receptors (KLRs) composed of receptors homologous to C-type lectins and the killer immunoglobulin-like receptors (KIRs) composed of receptors with immunoglobulin-like domains. Both KLRs and KIRs are able to sense the level of MHC class I expression on target cells. In addition to KLRs and KIRs, NK cells also express natural cytotoxicity receptors (NCRs) that recognize ligands on infected cells directly, including NKp30, NKp44, NKp46, and NKG2D [25–30].

1.2.1.6 Innate-Like Lymphocyte

Innate-like lymphocytes (ILLs) are cells that behave closely to the cells of the innate immunity due to the lack of clonal expansion upon recognizing their antigens. Yet, they are part of the adaptive immune system, because they express RAG-1 and RAG-2, and undergo the process of gene rearrangement. Their antigen receptors encoded by very few common gene rearrangements result in a very limited diversity; their receptors are therefore relatively invariant, and they only present in certain locations within the body. Several types of ILLs have been identified, including B-1 cells, marginal zone (MZ) B cells, natural killer T (NKT) cells, $\gamma\delta$T cells, etc.

B-1 cell B-1 cells (Neonatal B cells) are a subset of B cells that arises early in embryonic development. They constitute around 5–10% of all B cells and participate in the innate immunity. They can be divided into two distinct subsets: B-1a cells with higher CD5 expression that arise early in embryonic liver, and B-1b cells with lower CD5 expression that arise in fetal liver and bone marrow. They may self-renew in tissues outside of the bone marrow, and they are dominant in the peritoneal and pleural membrane with a small extent found in the spleen. B-1 cells mainly respond to polysaccharide antigens and produce IgM without the help from T cells. This B-cell population promotes the clearance of autoantigens released during apoptosis without generating T-cell responses [31–33]. They have also been claimed to make a significant contribution to IgA-producing plasma cells in the lamina propria of gut [34, 35].

Marginal zone B cell Marginal zone (MZ) B cells are a unique subset of B cells. MZ B cells reside in the marginal sinus of the white pulp in the spleen, and are rare at birth but accumulate with age. MZ B cells do not recirculate and replicate autonomously. They express low level of CD23 (the low-affinity receptor of IgE), and high level of both MHC class I-like molecule CD1 and two receptors for the C3 fragment of complement, CR1 (CD35) and CR2 (CD21). MZ B cells have restricted antigen specificities, biased toward self antigens and common bacterial antigens. They may not require the help from T cells to become activated and might be responsible for most physiological TI-2 responses [1–4].

Natural killer T cell Natural killer T (NKT) cells are also known as invariant NKT (iNKT) cells. They are present in both thymus and peripheral lymphoid organs such as the mucosal immune system. These cells possess an invariant T-cell receptor α chain, paired with one of three different β chains, and are able to recognize glycolipid antigens presented to them by the MHC-like molecule CD1. NKT cells respond to antigen stimulation mainly by rapid secretion of cytokines, including IL-4, IL-10, and IFN-γ. It is thought that NKT cells may have a regulatory function [1–4].

γδT cell γδT cells are a minor subset of T cells that reside within epithelia, and they are named for the composition of their antigen receptors: a γ chain and a δ chain. γδT cells are divided into two distinct subsets: one resides in the lymphoid tissues with highly diversified T-cell receptors, while another uncirculated subset resides in the skin, intraepithelial and female reproductive tract with very limited diversity of T-cell receptors. γδT cells do not recognize MHC-peptide complexes as conventional T cells; they recognize molecules that are being expressed in infected epithelia directly and therefore may respond rapidly to many different cell types [1–4].

1.2.1.7 Innate Lymphoid Cell

Innate lymphoid cells (ILCs) are a family of developmentally related cells involved in immune response, tissue development, and tissue remodeling. ILCs are defined by three main features: the absence of RAG-dependent rearranged antigen receptors; the lack of myeloid cells and dendritic cell-associated phenotypic markers; and their lymphoid morphology [36, 37]. ILCs include NK cells, lymphoid tissue-inducer (LTi) cells that are essential in the formation of lymph nodes during embryogenesis, and cells producing IL-5, IL-13, IL-17, and/or IL-22. These ILC subsets are developmentally related, and they require the expression of transcription repressor Id2 and cytokine signals through the common γ-chain of the IL-2 receptor. The functional differentiation of ILC subsets is orchestrated by distinct transcription factors. ILCs play an important role in protective immunity, and they can be categorized into three groups based on the cytokines they produce and the transcription factors regulating their development and function [36–39].

Group 1 ILC (ILC1) Group 1 ILCs are defined by the production of signature cytokine IFN-γ and the inability to produce Th2-type and Th17-type cytokines [37, 40–42].

Group 2 ILC (ILC2) Group 2 ILCs require IL-7 for development and produce Th2-type cytokines in response to stimulations of IL-25, IL-33, and thymic stromal lymphopoietin (TSLP) [43, 44]. They play important roles in the immune response against helminth infections [37, 44].

Group 3 ILC (ILC3) Group 3 ILCs are defined by their capacity to produce cytokine IL-17A and/or IL-22. The development and function of group 3 ILCs depend on the transcription factor RORγt [44]. They provide "help" to MZ B cells [37, 45].

1.2.2 Lymphocytes in Adaptive Immunity

Lymphocytes in the adaptive immunity include T cells and B cells. T cells and B cells are antigen-specific. They recognize different antigens by highly variable antigen receptors and diverse antigen-binding sites, and therefore are considered as part of the adaptive immunity. These lymphocytes are naïve lymphocytes before antigen priming and become activated after antigen encountering and differentiate into fully functional lymphocytes known as effector lymphocytes. Naïve lymphocytes may differentiate directly into memory cells upon antigen stimulation, while effector lymphocytes may also differentiate into memory lymphocytes. Memory lymphocytes are long-lived cells that proliferate and differentiate into effector cells rapidly upon second challenge. Although T and B cells are both part of the adaptive immunity, they possess distinctive types of antigen receptors and thus perform different roles in the immune system [1–4].

1.2.2.1 T Cell

T cells are thymus-dependent lymphocytes, also known as T lymphocytes. HSCs and lymphoid progenitor cells migrate to the thymus through blood circulation, where they further differentiate and develop into mature T cells. These mature T cells migrate to the peripheral lymphoid organs through blood circulation and reside in the thymus-dependent area for antigen stimulations. T cells go through several stages during development: lymphoid progenitor cell, pro-T cell, pre-T cell, immature T cell, and mature T cell. The developmental stages of T cell may also be divided into double negative (DN) stage, double positive (DP) stage, and single positive (SP) stage based on the expression of CD4 and CD8. Single positive cells become mature T cells after negative selection and migrate to peripheral lymphoid organs. These mature T cells that have not yet encountered their specific antigens are generally referred to as naïve T cells. Each T cell bears around 30,000 identical antigen recognition receptors on its surface, known as T-cell receptors (TCRs). The TCR consists of α and β polypeptide chains linked by a disulfide bond. The α:β heterodimers contribute to antigen recognition by most T cells. Naïve T cells become activated after specific binding between peptide:MHC complex and TCR complemented by costimulatory signals, followed by differentiation into different types of effector T cells and memory T cells. Effector T cells may be classified into three major types based on their functions: the cytotoxic T lymphocytes (CTLs), helper T (Th) cells, and regulatory T (Treg) cells [1–4].

$CD8^+$ T cell T cells expressing CD8 molecules are generally referred to as $CD8^+$ T cells. Activated $CD8^+$ T cells, known as cytotoxic T cells, or cytotoxic T lymphocytes (CTLs), target and kill cells infected by pathogens and viruses. They specifically recognize peptide:MHC class I complex and kill the target cells through either the secretion of perforin, granzyme, granulysin, and lymphotoxin A (LTa) or the Fas/FasL pathway.

$CD4^+$ T cell $CD4^+$ T cells are generally referred to as the helper T (Th) cells because they assist in both the activation of antigen-stimulated B cells that differentiate and produce antibodies, and the activation of macrophages that kill the engulfed pathogens. The differentiation of naïve $CD4^+$ T cells into different subsets of helper T cells requires antigen stimulation and coordinated action of cytokines provided by the stimulatory microenvironment, which in turn activate specific transcriptional pathways inducing the expression of different molecules responsible for different effector functions. Helper T cells may be subdivided into Th1, Th2, Th17, Tfh, Th9, Th22, Treg, etc. (Table 1.1) [46–50].

Th1 cell IL-12 and IFN-γ guide the differentiation of $CD4^+$ T cells into Th1 cells with the induction of lineage-specific transcription factor T-bet. Th1 cells mainly produce Th1-type cytokines such as IL-2, IFN-γ, TNF-α/β, etc.

Th2 cell IL-4 guides the differentiation of $CD4^+$ T cells into Th2 cells, with the induction of lineage-specific transcription factor GATA3. Th2 cells mainly produce Th2-type cytokines such as IL-4, IL-5, IL-6, IL-10, IL-13, IL-25, etc.

Th17 cell Th17 subset is named for its production of the proinflammatory cytokine IL-17. Combination of TGF-β and IL-6 guides the differentiation of $CD4^+$ T cells into Th17 cells, with the induction of lineage-specific transcription factor RORγt that can be amplified by IL-23. Th17 cells mainly produce IL-17, IL-6, IL-21, IL-22, IL-26, TNF-α, CXCL8, etc. [49, 51–53].

Tfh cell T follicular helper (Tfh) cells reside in the B-cell follicles of the peripheral lymphoid organs, and they help B cells to induce humoral immune response. IL-6 and IL-21 guide the differentiation of $CD4^+$ T cells into Tfh cells with the induction of lineage-specific transcription factor Bcl6. Typical characteristics of Tfh cells include the expression of ICOS and CXCR5 and the production of IL-21 [47, 54–56].

Th9 cell Th9 subset is named for its preferential production of cytokine IL-9 [57–60]. TGF-β and IL-4 guide the differentiation of $CD4^+$ T cells into Th9 cells, which can be enhanced by IL-1, with the induction of lineage-specific transcription factor PU.1. Th9 cells mainly produce IL-9 and IL-10 [3, 58, 61–65].

Th22 cell Th22 subset resides in the skin and produce IL-22 without the production of IFN-γ, IL-4, and IL-17 [66, 67]. IL-6 and TNF-α guide the differentiation of $CD4^+$ T cells into Th22 cells, with the induction of lineage-specific transcription factor AHR (aryl hydrocarbon receptor) [67–69]. Th22 cells mainly produce IL-22 and TNF-α [49, 68, 70].

Regulatory T cells There are three types of regulatory T cells: Tr1 cells, Th3 cells, and $Foxp3^+$ Treg cells. $Foxp3^+$ Treg cells are the predominant regulatory T cells that include natural regulatory T (nTreg) cells and induced regulatory T (iTreg) cells. nTreg cells develop in the thymus, while iTreg cells form in the periphery from naïve CD4 T cells in the presence of TGF-β [71–77]. Treg cells are often marked as $CD4^+CD25^+Foxp3^+$ T cells, and they may suppress immune

Table 1.1 Characteristics of the Th cell lineages derived from $CD4^+$ T cells

Lineage	Cytokine-induced differentiation	Transcription factor	Cytokine production
Th1 cell	IL-12, IFN-γ	T-bet	IFN-γ, IL-2, TNF-β/α
Th2 cell	IL-4	GATA-3	IL-4, IL-5, IL-6, IL-10, IL-13, IL-25
Th17 cell	TGF-β, IL-6 IL-21, IL-23	RORγt	IL-17A/F, IL-6, IL-21 IL-22, IL-26, TNF-α
Tfh cell	IL-6, IL-21	Bcl-6	IL-21, IL-10
Th9 cell	TGF-β, IL-4	PU.1, IRF4	IL-9, IL-10
Th22 cell	IL-6, TNF-α	AHR	IL-22, TNF-α
Treg cell	TGF-β, IL-10	FoxP3	TGF-β, IL-10, IL-35

responses by either directly suppressing the activation of target cells or indirectly through the secretion of TGF-β and IL-10 [71, 77, 78]. T regulatory type 1 (Tr1) cells are characterized by the ability to secrete high levels of IL-10 and minimal amount of IL-4 and IL-17 [79–82]. They also secrete TGF-β, variable amount of IL-15, GM-CSF, and IFN-γ, and low levels of IL-2 [80, 82]. Tr1 cells suppress T cell and APC responses primarily via the secretion of IL-10 and TGF-β [79, 82–86]. They can also inhibit T-cell responses via CTLA-4/PD-1-mediated cell contact-dependent mechanisms or by disrupting the metabolic state of effector T cells via the production of ectoenzymes CD39 and CD73 [87–89]. In addition, Tr1 cells can release granzyme B and perforin to kill myeloid cells [90, 91]. Th3 cells produce large amounts of TGF-β and IL-10, inhibit the proliferation and function of Th1 and Th2 cells, and promote the production of IgA antibodies. Th3 cells play an important role in local mucosal immunity and induction of oral tolerance.

Memory T cell Memory T cells are long-lived cells with a particular set of cell surface proteins (CD45RA−CD45RO$^+$) that derive from effector T cells and respond to the same specific antigens upon second challenge. A memory lymphocyte re-encountering antigen gives rise to two sets of progenies with the capability of terminal differentiation and self-renewal, respectively [92]. The survival of memory T cells requires stimulation by cytokines IL-7 and IL-15. The circulating memory T cells are generally divided into effector memory T (TEM) cells and central memory T (TCM) cells. TEM cells circulate to nonlymphoid tissues, whereas TCM cells home to secondary lymphoid organs. TEM cells are labeled as CCR7−, whereas TCM cells are labeled as CCR7$^+$ in both humans and mice, based on the expression of CCR7 [93]. Tissue-resident memory T (TRM) cells are also CCR7−, which functions in the first line defense and are retained within peripheral tissues [94, 95]. Locally produced IL-15 and TGF-β in the skin, combined with the expression of CCR10 and absence of KLRG1, seem to be important in the formation and maintenance of skin tissue-resident T-cell pool [95–97]. Although the function of each distinct memory lymphocyte subset remains to be determined, it seems clear that the relative importance of each subset varies depending on the specific pathogen and the route and site of infection [98].

1.2.2.2 B Cell

B cells (also known as B-2 cells) lack the expression of CD5 and are the major cells that produce antibodies to participate in the humoral immune response. B cells develop in the bone marrow through several stages: pro-B cell, pre-B cell, immature B cell, and mature B cell. Mature B cells are also referred to as naïve B cells that express both mIgM and mIgD. Naïve B cells proliferate and differentiate into their effector form, plasma cells, after the binding of the antigens to their B-cell receptors (BCRs), giving them the ability to produce antibodies, which are the secreted form of BCRs that possess the same antigen specificity as the surface proteins. Therefore, the antigens that initially activate B cells become the targets of the antibody attack. B cells gradually differentiate into plasma cells after antigen stimulation and produce antibodies with the help of Th cells. Some of the high-affinity B cells differentiate into memory B cells after first immune response and may activate and differentiate into plasma cells rapidly upon second challenge. The main functions of B cells include the production of antibodies, the induction of humoral immune responses, the presentation of soluble antigens, and the immune regulation by secreting cytokines.

Regulatory B cell B cells that can negatively regulate the immune response by producing regulatory cytokines or directly interacting via cell-to-cell contact are defined as regulatory B (Breg) cells. The regulatory functions of Breg cells have been demonstrated in mouse models or patients of inflammation, cancer, transplantation, and particularly in autoimmunity. Breg cells may be further classified into three subtypes: Br1 cells expressing IL-10, Br3 cells expressing TGF-β, and B-Foxp3 cells expressing Foxp3, among which the Br1 subset seems to be the predominant. The activation of Breg cells involves TLRs. Activated Breg cells facilitate the recruitment of Treg cells, and then disappear once Treg cells become operational. Breg cells play an important role in both autoimmune and allergic diseases [33, 99, 100].

1.3 Immune Molecules

1.3.1 Complement

Complement system or complement is a group of soluble proteins present in blood and other body fluids. The complement system is composed of more than 30 different plasma proteins that are mainly produced by the liver. These proteins circulate in their inactive forms until their encounter with pathogens. Complements are activated either directly by pathogens or indirectly by pathogen-bound antibodies, leading to a cascade of cleavage reactions occurring on the surface of pathogens that generate active components with various effector functions (Fig. 3.3). The process during which the pathogens are coated by antibodies and/or complement fragments so that they are easily taken up and destroyed by phagocytic cells is known as opsonization. These opsonized microbes are recognized and bound by specific complement receptors on phagocytes, followed by phagocytosis. The three pathways involved in the complement activation are the classical pathway that can be triggered directly by pathogens or indirectly by pathogen-bound antibodies; the alternate pathway that can be triggered by the pattern recognition receptors MBL and ficolins; and the lectin pathway that can be triggered by lectin-type proteins that recognize and bind to carbohydrates on pathogen surfaces, providing an amplification loop for the other two pathways and is augmented by properdin. All the three pathways lead to the final outcome of pathogen clearance, either directly or indirectly by facilitating phagocytosis and inducing inflammatory responses against infections. The activity of complement components is modulated by complement regulatory proteins, which can prevent tissue damage caused by inadvertent binding of activated complement components to host cells or spontaneous activation of complement components in the plasma [1–4, 101–105].

1.3.2 Antibody

Antibodies, also known as immunoglobulins (Ig), are circulating proteins produced in human system that react with foreign materials known as antigens. B cells produce two forms of antibodies: the membrane-bound form on the surface of B cells and the secreted form reside in the circulation, tissues, and mucosal sites. The two forms have identical structures, except that the membrane-bound antibody has a hydrophobic carboxy terminus that anchors the molecule in the membrane, while the secreted antibody has a hydrophilic carboxy terminus that allows secretion. Membrane-bound antibodies, also known as B-cell receptors (BCRs), mediate antigen-triggered activation of B cells. Secreted antibodies mediate humoral immune responses to eliminate the bound antigens through various effector mechanisms including neutralization, complement activation, opsonization, and destruction of antibody-coated pathogens through Fc receptors (Fig. 3.3) [1–4].

An antibody molecule is composed of four polypeptide chains, comprising of two identical heavy chains (H chains) and two identical light chains (L chains), giving rise to two identical antigen-binding sites and thus the ability to bind simultaneously to two identical structures. They form a flexible Y-shaped structure in which the two arms of the Y-end are called the variable (V) regions that determine the specificity of the antibody and are involved in antigen binding, and the stem of the Y is called the constant (C) region, which interacts with effector cells and molecules. There are two types of light chains, termed λ and k, and five types of heavy chains, termed μ, δ, γ, α, and ε. The types of heavy chain give rise to the five classes, or isotypes, of immunoglobulins: IgM, IgD, IgG, IgA, and IgE, which determine the functional activity of an antibody. The V domains of the heavy and light chains make up the V region, whereas the C domains of the heavy and light chains make up the C region. The Y-shaped immunoglobulin molecule can be dissected by partial digestion with proteases. Papain cleaves immunoglobulin into three pieces, two Fab fragments and one Fc fragment. Pepsin cleaves immunoglobulin to yield one F(ab')2 fragment and many small pieces of Fc fragments. The Fab fragments are identical and contain antigen-binding activity, while the Fc fragment contains no antigen-binding activity and is easily crystallized [106, 107].

The hypervariable regions HV1, HV2, and HV3 are identified in both the VH and VL domains, and the regions between the hypervariable regions are termed the framework regions, designated FR1, FR2, FR3, and FR4. The hypervariable loops are brought together when the VH and VL domains are paired and create a single hypervariable site for the binding of the antigen. The six hypervariable loops form a surface complementary to the antigen, commonly termed as the complementary-determining regions (CDRs), and the shapes of the surfaces are determined by the amino acid sequences of the CDRs. The structure recognized by an antibody is located on the surface of the protein and is called an antigenic determinant (AD) or epitope. An antigenic determinant composed of discontinuous segments of amino acid sequence and being brought together by protein folding is termed as conformational or discontinuous epitope, while an antigenic determinant composed of a single segment of polypeptide chain is termed as continuous or linear epitope. The interaction between antigens and antibodies also requires assistance from electrostatic forces, hydrogen bonds, van der Waals forces, and hydrophobic forces [108–110].

1.3.3 Cytokine

Cytokines are a broad category of small soluble polypeptide proteins released by immune cells and tissue cells that are important in cell signaling and regulation of cell growth, differentiation, and effector functions, making them essential in the regulation of immune responses. Cytokines are small proteins that range from 8 to 30 kD with short half-lives; they are soluble, inducible, and bioreactive under very low concentrations, and can only work within limited distance due to the required binding between the cytokines and their cell surface receptors. Cytokines may act in three manners: autocrine, paracrine, and endocrine. Autocrine is a form in which the cell secretes a cytokine that binds to the autocrine receptor on the same cell, leading to the change in that cell. Paracrine is a form of cell-cell communication in which the cytokine produced by a cell affects only the nearby cell and induces change in that cell. Endocrine refers to the direct secretion of cytokine into the circulatory system to be carried toward a distant target cell. Several properties are unique to cytokines: (1) a cytokine may affect different cells with different effects, referred to as pleiotropism; (2) two or more cytokines may possess the same or similar biological effects, referred to as redundancy; (3) a cytokine may enhance the activity and function of another cytokine, referred to as synergy; (4) a cytokine may inhibit the activity and function of another cytokine, referred to as antagonism; (5) immune cells may interact with each other by producing different kinds of cytokines that in turn form a complex cytokine network, which is very important in terms of immune regulation and homeostasis. Cytokines are broadly classified into six categories: interleukin (IL) is named for molecules secreted by, and acting on, leukocytes; colony-stimulating factors (CSF) include granulocyte macrophage-CSF (GM-CSF), macrophage-CSF (M-CSF), granulocyte-CSF (G-CSF), EPO, SCF, TPO, etc. that stimulate the proliferation and differentiation of pluripotent hematopoietic stem cells and progenitor cells; interferon (IFN) is named after its ability to interfere with virus replication, and can be divided into two types – type I interferon (IFN-α, IFN-β) and type II interferon (IFN-γ); tumor necrosis factor (TNF) is named after its ability to induce necrosis of the tumor tissues and is further divided into TNF-α and TNF-β; growth factor (GF) generally refers to a broad category of cytokines that may promote growth and differentiation, including transforming growth factor-β (TGF-β), VEGF, EGF, FGF, NGF, PDGF, etc.; and finally chemokine, the chemoattractant cytokine secreted by different types of cells that may induce direct chemotaxis effects in a variety of responsive cells. Chemokines fall mostly into two groups: the CC chemokines with two adjacent cysteines near the amino terminus, or the CXC chemokines with two cysteines separated by a single amino acid [111–115]. Cytokines are very important in regulating the development, differentiation, and function of immune cells in both central lymphoid organs and peripheral lymphoid organs; they are also essential in regulating immune responses through antibacterial effects, antiviral effects, antitumor effects, and the induction of apoptosis [116]. Similar to the other immune molecules involved in immune responses, cytokines also possess a dual character; they participate positively in immune responses by providing antibacterial effects, antiviral effects, antitumor effects, and induction of apoptosis; however, on the other side, they are the cause of a variety of diseases under certain circumstances [1–4].

1.3.4 CD Molecule and Cell Adhesion Molecule

Human leukocyte differentiation antigen (HLDA) refers to the markers expressed on cell surface during different stages along the differentiation of hematopoietic stem cells, the differentiation of different cell lineages, and the maturation process. The cluster of differentiation (CD) is a worldwide nomenclature used for the identification of cell surface molecules; cell surface molecules with the same human leukocyte differentiation antigen are assigned one CD number. HLDA is divided into three categories based on their functions: the receptors, the costimulatory/inhibitory molecules, and the cell adhesion molecules.

Cell adhesion molecules (CAMs) are proteins located on the cell surface involved in the cell-cell or cell-extracellular matrix (ECM) interactions, a process known as cell adhesion. Cell adhesion molecules help the cells to get adhered to each other and to their surroundings through the binding between receptors and ligands. They participate in the recognition, activation and signal transduction, proliferation and differentiation, extension, and movement [117]. Cell adhesion molecules are classified into four broad categories based on their structural properties: the immunoglobulin superfamily (IgSF), the intergrin family, the selectin family, and the cadherin family. Immunoglobulin superfamily is the largest and most diverse group of immune cell surface molecules that are involved in the recognition, binding, adhesion, and signal transduction of cells. Integrins are transmembrane receptors composed of an α chain and a β chain that induce cell-ECM interaction and adherence by binding to intercellular adhesion molecules (ICAMs). Selectins are single-chain transmembrane glycoproteins with a distal lectin-like domain that induce the adherence between leukocytes and endothelial cells, and include L-selecitn, P-selectin, and E-selectin [118]. Cell adhesion molecules participate in the interactions between immune cells, the recruitment of lymphocytes, and the adherence between leukocytes and endothelial cells during inflammation [1–4].

1.3.5 Major Histocompatibility Complex

The major histocompatibility complex (MHC) is a group of genes in all vertebrates that determines the compatibility of donors for organ transplantation and controls a major part of the immune system. MHC genes in humans are called human leukocyte antigen (HLA) genes, and in the mouse, they are known as H-2 genes [119]. MHC is a very complex structure; it is both polygenic and polymorphic. Each individual possesses at least three different MHC class I molecules and three (or four) MHC class II molecules on his/her cell, in addition to the multiple variants of each gene within the population as a whole, giving rise to a huge diversity among human beings [120]. In humans, MHC molecules are encoded by several genes clustered in the same region on chromosome 6, while in mice, they locate on chromosome 17. There are three major classes of MHC genes: class I, class II, and class III. Due to the discovery of large amount of non-classical MHC genes, MHC genes are often classified into two major categories: the first one include classical MHC class I and class II genes, which are highly polymorphic, important for antigen presentation, and participate in the activation and differentiation of T cells; the second one include MHC genes that are related to immune functions, including the traditional MHC class III genes and some newly found ones, which also participate in antigen processing and regulation of adaptive immune responses, however, they show limited or no polymorphism.

MHC class I and II molecules differ in both structure and expression pattern on the tissues. Although their overall structures are closely related, they show differences in their subunit composition. Both classes possess two paired domains resembling immunoglobulin domains, and two domains that fold together to create an elongated cleft in the extracellular surface, which is the site of peptide binding. MHC class I molecules consist of two polypeptide chains: an α chain that spans the membrane and folds into three α domains: $\alpha 1$, $\alpha 2$, and $\alpha 3$; and β_2-microglobulin, a noncovalently associated smaller chain that does not span the membrane. The folding of $\alpha 1$ and $\alpha 2$ creates a peptide-binding cleft that closes at both ends and binds short peptides of eight to ten amino acids [121, 122]. MHC class II molecules consist of two glycoprotein chains: an α chain and a β chain that both span the membrane. Each chain has two domains, among which $\alpha 1$ and $\beta 1$ domains fold into the peptide-binding cleft that opens at both ends and binds unconstrained length of peptides [123, 124].

MHC class I and II molecules trap peptides from different sources and present them to different functional classes of T cells, implying their distinct distributions among cells. MHC class I molecules trap peptides derived from proteins synthesized in the cytosol such as viral proteins and bind to the peptide fragments of viral proteins in ER followed by transportation to the cell surface. On the cell surface, MHC class I molecules bearing viral peptides are preferentially recognized by $CD8^+$ cytotoxic T cells, leading to the killing of the infected cell. Because viruses can infect any nucleated cells, almost all such cells express MHC class I molecules. In contrast, MHC class II molecules trap peptides derived from proteins in intracellular vesicles either formed through bacterial infection or antigen internalization, and bind to peptide fragments in intracellular vesicles followed by transportation to the cell surface. On the cell surface, MHC class II molecules bearing pathogen-derived peptides are recognized by $CD4^+$ T cells, leading to the activation of other effector cells of the immune system. Thus, MHC class II molecules are normally found on antigen-presenting cells such as B cells, dendritic cells, and macrophages [2].

MHC molecules are essential in the activation of both $CD4^+$ and $CD8^+$ T cells. The interactions between CD4 and CD8 molecules on the T cells and the MHC molecules on the target cells are required for proper antigen presentation. CD4 and CD8 are known as coreceptors, T cells bearing receptors specifically for MHC class I molecules always express CD8 coreceptors, whereas T cells bearing receptors specifically for MHC class II molecules always express CD4 coreceptors, ensuring proper interactions between T-cell receptors and peptide:MHC complexes, a process known as MHC restriction [1–4].

1.4 Signaling Pathways Involved in the Immune System

Recognition of microbial pathogens is essential to the initiation of innate immune responses such as inflammation. It is mediated by germline-encoded pattern recognition receptors (PRRs) that recognize universal molecular structures of pathogens, known as pathogen-associated molecular patterns (PAMPs) [2, 125, 126]. Upon PAMP-PRR recognition, PRRs trigger a series of signaling cascades that execute defensive responses essential to the clearance of infectious microbes. In addition, PRR signaling pathway simultaneously induces the maturation of DCs, which are responsible for the induction of adaptive immunity.

1.4.1 Signal Transduction in Innate Immunity

The PRRs of the innate immune system are divided into four distinct classes: Toll-like receptors (TLRs), the nucleotide-binding, oligomerization domain (NOD)-like receptors (NLRs), retinoic acid-inducible gene (RIG)-I-like receptors (RLRs), and C-type lectin receptors (CLRs).

1.4.1.1 TLR Signaling Pathways

Toll-like receptors (TLRs) were the first PRRs being identified. TLRs are type I transmembrane proteins comprising of an ectodomain with leucin-rich repeats (LRRs) that mediate the recognition of PAMPs, a transmembrane region, and cytosolic Toll-IL-1 receptor (TIR) domains that activate downstream signaling pathways. Ten functional TLRs have been identified in human, and they play important roles in the recognition and response to microbial pathogens [125].

Cellular localization of TLRs TLRs are expressed either on the cell surface or within intracellular vesicles. Among all identified TLRs, TLR1, TLR2, TLR4, TLR5, and TLR6, which mainly recognize microbial membrane components, are localized on the cell surface, whereas TLR3, TLR7, TLR8, and TLR9, which recognize nucleic acids, are localized within intracellular vesicles [127]. TLR11 and TLR13 are also expressed in intracellular compartments [125, 127, 128].

Recognition by TLRs TLRs may recognize components derived from distinct PAMPs, including those from viruses, bacteria, fungi, and parasites. For example, lipoproteins are recognized by TLR1, TLR2, and TLR6; double-stranded (ds) RNAs are recognized by TLR3; lipopolysaccharides (LPS) are recognized by TLR4; flagellins are recognized by TLR5; single-stranded (ss) RNAs are recognized by TLR7 and TLR8; and DNAs are recognized by TLR9 [125, 129].

Downstream signaling pathways Upon PAMPs recognition, TLRs recruit a specific set of adaptor proteins and initiate downstream signaling cascades. Engagement with PAMPs induces conformational change in TLRs, allowing homophilic or heterophilic interactions of TLRs and the recruitment of adaptor proteins. The specific response of each TLR depends on the recruitment of a single, or a combination of, TIR domain-containing adaptor proteins [125, 130].

MyD88-dependent pathway MyD88 (myeloid differentiation primary response protein 88) is utilized by all TLRs with an exception of TLR3. TLR2 and TLR4 use TIRAP (TIR domain-containing adaptor protein) as a supplementary adaptor to recruit MyD88. They transmit signals that initiate the activation of NFkB and MAP kinase and induce the secretion of inflammatory cytokines [126].

TRIF-dependent pathway TLR3 and TLR4 use TRIF (TIR domain-containing adaptor protein inducing IFN-β) to activate an alternative pathway. TRAM (TRIF-related adaptor molecule) acts as a bridge between TLR4 and TRIF. They transmit signals that lead to the activation of NFkB and IRF3, and induce the secretion of type I interferons and inflammatory cytokines [126].

TLR4 is the only TLR that recruits four adaptor proteins and activates both the "MyD88-dependent" and "TRIF-dependent" pathways [127]. TLR4 initially recruits TIRAP and MyD88, in which TIRAP localizes to the plasma membrane via its interaction with PIP2 and serves to bridge the interaction between MyD88 and TLR4 upon LPS engagement [131]. MyD88 then recruits IRAKs (interleukin receptor-associated kinases), TRAF6 (TNFR-associated factor 6), and the TAK1 (TGF-β activated kinase 1) complex, leading to the early-phase activation of NFkB and MAP kinase pathways. TLR4 is subsequently endocytosed and delivered to intracellular vesicles to form a complex with TRAM and TRIF, which then recruits TRAF3 and protein kinases TBK1 and IKKi that catalyze the phosphorylation of IRF3, leading to the expression of type I IFN [131]. TRAM-TRIF also recruits TRAF6 and TAK1 to mediate late-phase activation of NFkB and MAP kinase pathways [126].

1.4.1.2 NLR Signaling Pathways

Nucelotide-binding, oligomerization domain (NOD)-like receptors (NLRs) are a family of innate immune receptors that act as intracellular sensors of bacterial infections and use LRR scaffold domains to detect pathogen products. They are generally composed of three domains: a LRR domain near the carboxy terminus that works in the recognition of PAMPs and DAMPs (danger-associated molecular patterns) and in autoregulation; a NBD (nucleotide-binding domain) or NACHT (nucleotide-binding domain or NAIP, CIITA, HET-E, and TP1) domain that binds nucleotides and is possibly involved in the induction of conformational change and self-oligomerization necessary for NLR functions; and CARDs (caspase activation and recruitment domains) and PYDs (the pyrin domains) at the N terminus that are involved in the homeotypic protein interactions and allow the recruitment of downstream effector molecules. Subfamilies of NLRs can be distinguished on the basis of their protein domains found near the amino terminus [132–134].

NOD1 and NOD2 γ-glutamyl diaminopimelic acid (iE-DAP)-sensed NOD1 and muramyl dipeptide (MDP)-recognized NOD2 are derived either from extracellular, intracytosolic, intravesicular bacteria, or viral ssRNA [135, 136]. NOD1/NOD2 recruits CARD-containing serine-threonine kinase RIPK2 (also known as RICK and RIP2) upon recognition of its ligand. RIPK2 activates kinase TAK1, which in turn mediates activation of NFkB and MAP kinase pathways, inducing the expression of genes associated with inflammatory cytokines. In addition, recognition of *H. pylori* by NOD1 and recognition of ssRNA by NOD2 stimulate the transcription of type I IFN via IRF7 and IRF3, respectively [137–139]. NOD1 and NOD2 may also recruit ATG16L to the site of bacterial phagocytosis to initiate autophagy [133, 140, 141].

NALPs Another large subfamily of NLRs is known as the NALP family (also called the NLRP family), with a PYD or CARD at the amino terminus. NALP proteins sense cellular damage and activate the processing of proinflammatory cytokines. In contrast to the NOD proteins, several members of the NLR family may form multiprotein complexes, namely "inflammasomes." Inflammasomes require two signals for their biological functions: signal 1 is often provided by TLR and NFkB signaling and initiates transcription activation of inflammasome components, whereas signal 2 initiates inflammasome assembly. Inflammasomes are assembled through homophilic CARD-CARD and PYD-PYD interactions between NLRs, ASC (apoptosis-associated speck-like protein containing a CARD), and procaspase-1 [142, 143]. Inflammasomes result in the activation of caspase-1, which subsequently induces the secretion of potent proinflammatory cytokines and pyroptosis, a form of cell death. Inflammasome-mediated process is important in microbial infection and in regulating both metabolic process and mucosal immune response. NALP3, the best characterized NALP, is an important sensor of cellular damage and stress. The LRR domain of NALP3 associates with cytoplasmic proteins under normal physiological conditions; however, when cells are microbial infected or under stress, NALP3 senses either direct microbial molecules or indirect signals associated with cellular perturbations such as increased ROS production, release of lysosomal proteases into the cytoplasm, and potassium efflux from damaged cells, contributing to the dissociation of cytoplasmic proteins from NALP3. NALP3 dimerization recruits complex of the adaptor protein ASC and caspase-1, resulting in the formation of inflammasome that leads to the activation of caspase-1, which in turn cleaves pro-IL-1 and pro-IL-18 into mature IL-1 and IL-18 [144, 145]. In the case of NLRC4, recognition of cytoplasmic flagellin leads to pyroptosis via an ASC-independent mechanism. NLRC4 also induces processing of pro-IL-1β and pro-IL-18 via ASC-dependent mechanism [133, 140, 141].

1.4.1.3 RLR Signaling Pathways

RIG-I-like receptors (RLRs) are a family of DExD/H box RNA helicases that function as cytoplasmic sensors of PAMPs within viral RNA. RLRs are broadly expressed in most tissues where they signal innate immune activation in a variety of cell types. RLR expression is typically maintained at low levels in resting cells but is greatly upregulated under IFN exposure and after viral infections. RLRs trigger the activation of downstream transcription factor to drive the production of type I IFN and the expression of antiviral genes. They are type I transmembrane proteins that include three members: RIG-I (retinoic acid-inducible gene I), MDA5 (melanoma differentiation-associated factor 5), and LGP2 (laboratory of genetics and physiology 2), among which RIG-I and MDA5 share a number of structural similarities including the organization of three distinct domains: an N-terminal region consisting of tandem CARD, a central DExD/H box RNA helicase domain with the capacity of hydrolyzing ATP and binding and possibly unwinding RNA, and a C-terminal repressor domain (RD) embedded within the C-terminal domain (CTD) that is involved in the autoregulation in case of RIG-I [146–148]. LGP2 that lacks the N-terminal CARDs is likely to function as a regulator of RIG-I and MDA5 [147, 149].

Downstream signaling pathways RLRs are essential in the sensing of RNA viruses to initiate and modulate antiviral immunity. RLRs detect viral RNA ligands or processed self-RNA in the cytoplasm to trigger innate immunity and impart gene expressions that may control infections. In the resting state, RIG-I is held in a "closed" conformation that holds the CARDs unavailable for signaling. During viral infections, RIG-I binds to 5′-triphosphate RNA containing poly-U/UC motif and assumes an "open" conformation that releases the CARDs [149–151]. These interactions trigger a signaling cascade that leads to the production of IFN and the expression of proteins associated with direct antiviral and immune-modulating activities [149].

1.4.1.4 CLR Signaling Pathways

C-type lectin receptors (CLRs) comprise of a heterogeneous group of transmembrane proteins. Many of these proteins are expressed in myeloid cells and signal in response to pathogen-derived or self-ligands to initiate or regulate cell activation. Thus, C-type lectin family encompasses upward of 1000 members with diverse functions including cell adhesion, regulation of natural killer function, complement activation, tissue remodeling, platelet activation, endocytosis, phagocytosis, and innate immunity [152–154].

CLR signaling and endocytosis Mannose receptor, DEC-205, and langerin are CLRs with endocytic activities and bind to bacteria, fungi, and viruses. They mediate the internalization of their ligands, followed by direct cargo into intracellular compartment, where the antigens are being processed and presented. However, there is limited evidence to date that signals from these receptors alone are adequate to induce microbicidal effector functions in myeloid cells or to induce gene transcription that is typical to innate immunity [154].

CLR signaling and gene expression Most CLR signals are transmitted by tyrosine-based signaling motifs. CLRs that bear either hemITAM (immunoreceptor tyrosine-based activation motif) or ITIM (immunoreceptor tyrosine-based inhibition motif) are considered as type II transmembrane proteins. Phosphorylation of the two tyrosines located within the hemITAM or ITAM by kinases of the Src family generates a docking site for the tandem SH2 domains of Syk and allows for stable recruitment and activation of Syk kinase. Binding of Syk to proteins with ITAM causes a conformational change that leads to the activation of Syk and the phosphorylation of various substrates (including Syk itself), which in turn initiate downstream signaling cascade. Syk acts as a key element in the subsequent activation of NFkB, MAP kinase, and NFAT signaling pathways, which all cooperatively regulate the expression of innate response genes. In addition, Syk also regulates the production of reactive oxygen species that may contribute, among others, to the activation of NALP3 inflammasomes. Many CLRs also use tyrosine-based motifs to signal for endocytosis and to regulate antigen processing. A separate subgroup of CLRs antagonizes Syk activity by means of ITIM in which they recruit phosphatases SHP-1, SHP-2, and SHIP. CLRs with ITIM can raise the threshold of myeloid cell activation [154–157].

1.4.2 Signal Transduction in Adaptive Immunity

The ability of T and B cells to recognize and respond to specific antigens is critical in adaptive immunity. T-cell receptor (TCR) and B-cell receptor (BCR) are composed of antigen-binding chains – the α and β chains in TCR and the heavy and light immunoglobulin chains in BCR. These variable antigen-binding chains possess precise specificity for each antigen without intrinsic signaling capacity. Fully functional antigen receptor complexes are associated with invariant accessory proteins that may initiate signaling, and assembly of these accessory proteins is essential for the transportation of receptors to the cell surface.

1.4.2.1 TCR Signaling Pathways

TCR-CD3 complex and TCR coreceptor T-cell receptor (TCR) is composed of antigen-binding chains TCRα and TCRβ; however, the intracytoplasmic region of the TCR chain is too short to transduce signals alone. The functional TCR complex is composed of the antigen-binding TCRα:β heterodimer associated with the CD3 complex consisting of four signaling chains: a CD3γ chain, a CD3δ chain, two CD3ε chains, and a homodimer of CD3ζchains. Each CD3 chain comprises of an extracellular immunoglobulin-like domain and an ITAM except for ζ chain, which has only one short extracellular domain and three ITAM. Signaling from TCR is initiated by tyrosine phosphorylation of ITAM within the cytoplasmic region of CD3γ, δ, ε, and ζ chains. Engagement of coreceptors with TCR complex enhances the phosphorylation of ITAM (Fig. 1.6) [1–4, 158].

Signal transduction by TCR Antigen recognition by TCR and its coreceptors results in Src-family kinase-mediated phosphorylation of ITAM. Phosphorylated ITAM of the CD3ζ chain forms a recognition unit that recruits a member of the TPK family, tyrosine kinase ZAP-70 (ζ-associated protein of 70 kD). Activation of ZAP-70 results in the phosphorylation of scaffold proteins LAT and SLP-76, which then recruit the most important signaling protein, phospholipase PLC-γ. Activation of PLC-γ requires costimulatory molecule CD28 in order to generate second messenger diacylglycerol (DAG) and inositol trisphosphate (IP3). DAG is involved in the activation of protein kinase C-γ (PKC-γ) and small G protein Ras. PKC-γ activates transcription factors NFkB and AP-1, while activation of Ras stimulates mitogen-activated protein kinase (MAPK) and induces expression of AP-1. IP3 plays an important role in inducing changes in the intracellular calcium concentration. Entrance of $Ca2^{+}$ activates transcription factor NFAT. Activation of all three transcription factors AP-1, NFAT, and NFkB induces the transcription of IL-2, which is necessary for proliferation and differentiation of activated T cells [1–4, 158].

Costimulatory signal for T-cell activation Antigen-presenting cells that activate naïve T cells bear costimulatory molecules on their cell surface. These molecules interact with costimulatory receptors on naïve T cells, providing the second signal required for T-cell activation. CD28 is a costimulatory receptor that presents on the surface of all naïve T cells, and its ligands B7.1 (CD80) and B7.2 (CD86) are expressed only on specialized antigen-presenting cells such as dendritic cells. Only a combination of antigen stimulation and costimulatory signal may activate T cells. Engagement of CD28 with B7.1 and B7.2 induces CD28 tyrosine phosphorylation. Activating members of the CD28 family provides costimulatory signal that amplifies the signal of TCR and are important in ensuring appropriate activation of naïve T cells by target cells (Fig. 1.6) [1–4, 158].

1.4.2.2 BCR Signaling Pathways

BCR complex and BCR coreceptor B-cell receptor (BCR) is composed of heavy and light immunoglobulin chains and recognizes antigens without generating signals by itself. The BCR complex is composed of cell surface immunoglobulin with invariant signaling proteins Igα (CD79α) and Igβ (CD79β), each of which comprises of a single ITAM in the cytosolic tail. Igα and Igβ form a disulfide-linked heterodimer that associates with the heavy chains. The BCR coreceptors including CD19, CD21 (also known as complement receptor 2, CR2), and CD81 contribute to the enhancement of antigen-dependent signaling of BCR by simultaneously binding to their ligands and clustering with the antigen receptor. CD21 alone does not transduce signals; however, it can deliver signals into cells by cross-linking with CD19, which contains several constitutive tyrosine residues that can recruit signaling molecules such as Lyn and Fyn. CD81 mainly functions in connecting CD19 and CD21, and in stabilizing the complex (Fig. 1.6).

Signal transduction by BCR Signal transduction of BCR is similar to that of TCR with the exception of some components unique to B cell. Three protein tyrosine kinases of the Src family, namely Fyn, Blk, and Lyn, may phosphorylate ITAM. These kinases associate with BCRs in resting cells by low-affinity interaction with unphosphorylated ITAM in Igα and Igβ chains, and they become cross-linked upon binding of a multivalent antigen to the BCR, followed by their activation and phosphorylation of the tyrosine residues in ITAM. The phosphorylated ITAM then recruits another tyrosine kinase Syk, and activation of Syk results in the phosphorylation of scaffold protein BLNK, which then recruits a variety of SH2-containing proteins, including enzymes and adaptor proteins, to form several distinct multiprotein signaling complexes. A key B cell specific signaling protein is Bruton's tyrosine kinase (Btk) that may hydrolyze PIP2 to form DAG and IP3. Similar to signal transduction of TCR, signaling by calcium and DAG leads to the activation of downstream transcription factors. BCR coreceptors serve to strengthen signals derived from antigen recognition. BCR and CD21 are cross-linked by antigens, leading to the phosphorylation of CD21. CD21 is cross-linked with CD19, which in turn induces the phosphorylation of cytoplasmic tail of CD19 through BCR-associated tyrosine kinases, leading to the binding of the Src family kinases. Ligation of these coreceptors increases BCR signaling by 1000–10,000 folds through the enhancement of signal transduction of BCR and

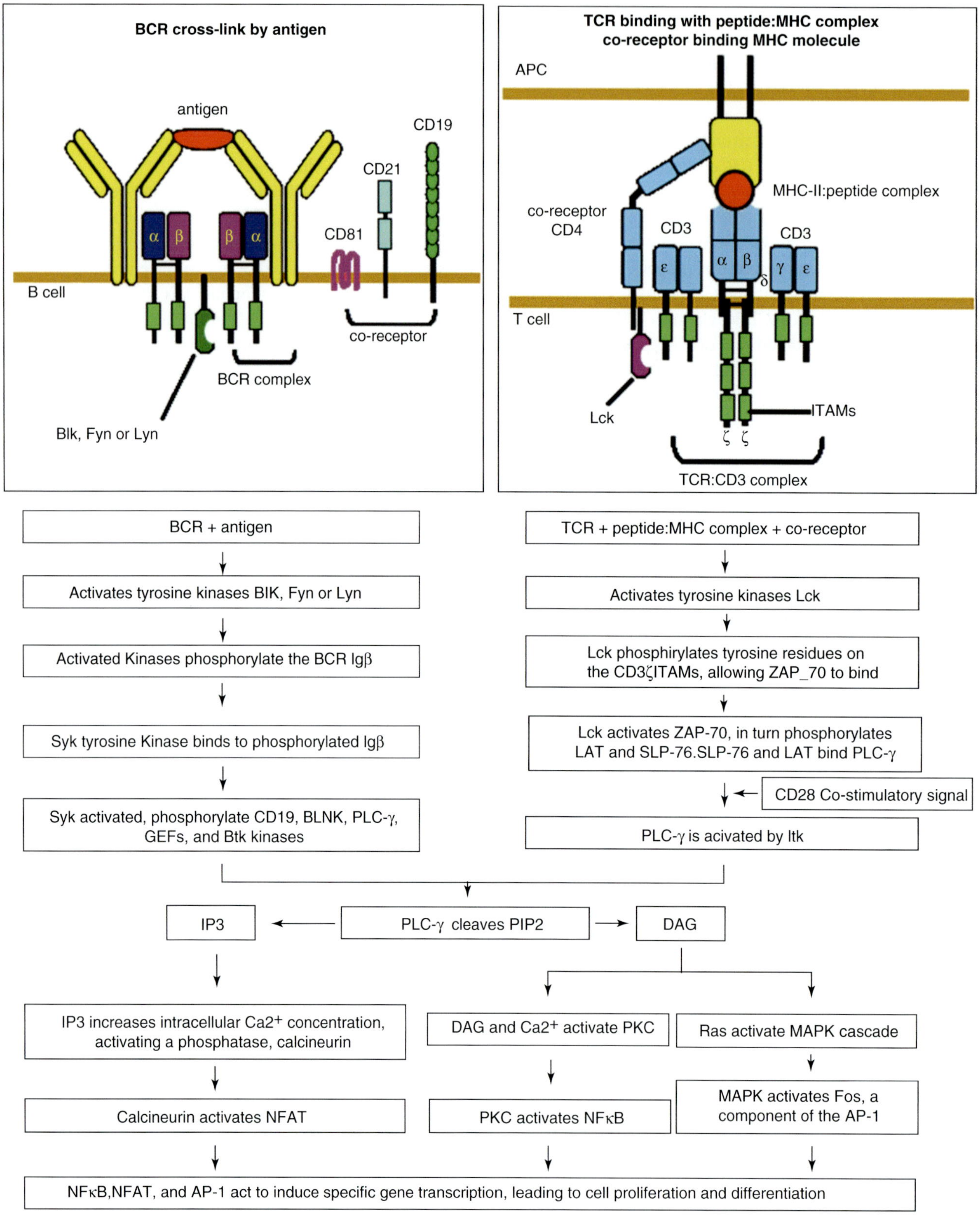

Fig. 1.6 Simplified outline of the intracellular signaling pathways initiated by the B-cell receptor complex and its coreceptors, as well as the T-cell receptor complex and its coreceptors

sensitivity of B cells to antigens, and also by reducing the threshold of BCR activation. Some inhibitory receptors are also present on lymphocytes, and they may attenuate or completely block signals from activating receptors. Regulated expression of activating and inhibitory receptors and their ligands generates a sophisticated level of control in the immune response (Fig. 1.6) [1–4].

References

1. Paul WE. Fundamental immunology. 7th ed. Philadelphia: Wolters Kluwer Health: Lippincot Williams & Wilkins; 2012.
2. Murphy K. Janeway's immunology. 8th ed. New York: Garland Science; 2011.
3. Abbas AK, Lichtman AH, Pillai S. Cellular and molecular immunology. 6th ed. Philadelphia: Saunders; 2010.
4. Parslow TG, Stites DP, Terry AI, Imboden JB. Medical immunology. 10th ed. New York: McGraw-Hill/Appleton & Lange; 2001.
5. Smith PD, MacDonald TT, Blumberg RS. Principles of mucosal immunology. New York: Garland Science; 2013.
6. Aderem A, Underhill DM. Mechanisms of phagocytosis in macrophages. Annu Rev Immunol. 1999;17:593–623.
7. Mantovani A, Sica A, Sozzani S, Allavena P, Vecchi A, Locati M. The chemokine system in diverse forms of macrophage activation and polarization. Trends Immunol. 2004;25(12):677–86.
8. Biswas SK, Mantovani A. Orchestration of metabolism by macrophages. Cell Metab. 2012;15(4):432–7.
9. Rodriguez-Prados JC, Traves PG, Cuenca J, Rico D, Aragones J, Martin-Sanz P, et al. Substrate fate in activated macrophages: a comparison between innate, classic, and alternative activation. J Immunol. 2010;185(1):605–14.
10. Italiani P, Boraschi D. From monocytes to M1/M2 macrophages: phenotypical vs. functional differentiation. Front Immunol. 2014;5:514.
11. Mills CD. M1 and M2 macrophages: oracles of health and disease. Crit Rev Immunol. 2012;32(6):463–88.
12. Mills CD, Kincaid K, Alt JM, Heilman MJ, Hill AM. M-1/M-2 macrophages and the Th1/Th2 paradigm. J Immunol. 2000; 164(12):6166–73.
13. MacMicking J, Xie QW, Nathan C. Nitric oxide and macrophage function. Annu Rev Immunol. 1997;15:323–50.
14. Gordon S, Taylor PR. Monocyte and macrophage heterogeneity. Nat Rev Immunol. 2005;5(12):953–64.
15. Urban CF, Lourido S, Zychlinsky A. How do microbes evade neutrophil killing? Cell Microbiol. 2006;8(11):1687–96.
16. Savina A, Amigorena S. Phagocytosis and antigen presentation in dendritic cells. Immunol Rev. 2007;219:143–56.
17. Zucker-Franklin D. Eosinophil function and disorders. Adv Intern Med. 1974;19:1–25.
18. Rothenberg ME, Hogan SP. The eosinophil. Annu Rev Immunol. 2006;24:147–74.
19. Metcalfe DD, Baram D, Mekori YA. Mast cells. Physiol Rev. 1997;77(4):1033–79.
20. Gurish MF, Austen KF. Developmental origin and functional specialization of mast cell subsets. Immunity. 2012;37(1):25–33.
21. Galli SJ, Nakae S, Tsai M. Mast cells in the development of adaptive immune responses. Nat Immunol. 2005;6(2):135–42.
22. Marshall JS. Mast-cell responses to pathogens. Nat Rev Immunol. 2004;4(10):787–99.
23. Wernersson S, Pejler G. Mast cell secretory granules: armed for battle. Nat Rev Immunol. 2014;14(7):478–94.
24. Sun H, Sun C, Xiao W. Expression regulation of co-inhibitory molecules on human natural killer cells in response to cytokine stimulations. Cytokine. 2014;65(1):33–41.
25. Cooper MA, Fehniger TA, Caligiuri MA. The biology of human natural killer-cell subsets. Trends Immunol. 2001;22(11):633–40.
26. Altfeld M, Fadda L, Frleta D, Bhardwaj N. DCs and NK cells: critical effectors in the immune response to HIV-1. Nat Rev Immunol. 2011;11(3):176–86.
27. O'Leary JG, Goodarzi M, Drayton DL, von Andrian UH. T cell- and B cell-independent adaptive immunity mediated by natural killer cells. Nat Immunol. 2006;7(5):507–16.
28. Paust S, Gill HS, Wang BZ, Flynn MP, Moseman EA, Senman B, et al. Critical role for the chemokine receptor CXCR6 in NK cell-mediated antigen-specific memory of haptens and viruses. Nat Immunol. 2010;11(12):1127–35.
29. Jost S, Altfeld M. Control of human viral infections by natural killer cells. Annu Rev Immunol. 2013;31:163–94.
30. Tian Z, Gershwin ME, Zhang C. Regulatory NK cells in autoimmune disease. J Autoimmun. 2012;39(3):206–15.
31. Klinker MW, Lundy SK. Multiple mechanisms of immune suppression by B lymphocytes. Mol Med. 2012;18:123–37.
32. Shaw PX, Horkko S, Chang MK, Curtiss LK, Palinski W, Silverman GJ, et al. Natural antibodies with the T15 idiotype may act in atherosclerosis, apoptotic clearance, and protective immunity. J Clin Invest. 2000;105(12):1731–40.
33. Berthelot JM, Jamin C, Amrouche K, Le Goff B, Maugars Y, Youinou P. Regulatory B cells play a key role in immune system balance. Joint Bone Spine. 2013;80(1):18–22.
34. Roy B, Shukla S, Lyszkiewicz M, Krey M, Viegas N, Duber S, et al. Somatic hypermutation in peritoneal B1b cells. Mol Immunol. 2009;46(8-9):1613–9.
35. Fettke F, Schumacher A, Costa SD, Zenclussen AC. B cells: the old new players in reproductive immunology. Front Immunol. 2014;5:285.
36. Spits H, Artis D, Colonna M, Diefenbach A, Di Santo JP, Eberl G, et al. Innate lymphoid cells – a proposal for uniform nomenclature. Nat Rev Immunol. 2013;13(2):145–9.
37. Klose CS, Flach M, Mohle L, Rogell L, Hoyler T, Ebert K, et al. Differentiation of type 1 ILCs from a common progenitor to all helper-like innate lymphoid cell lineages. Cell. 2014;157(2):340–56.
38. Gasteiger G, Rudensky AY. Interactions between innate and adaptive lymphocytes. Nat Rev Immunol. 2014;14(9):631–9.
39. Spits H, Di Santo JP. The expanding family of innate lymphoid cells: regulators and effectors of immunity and tissue remodeling. Nat Immunol. 2011;12(1):21–7.
40. Hoyler T, Klose CS, Souabni A, Turqueti-Neves A, Pfeifer D, Rawlins EL, et al. The transcription factor GATA-3 controls cell fate and maintenance of type 2 innate lymphoid cells. Immunity. 2012;37(4):634–48.
41. Mjosberg J, Bernink J, Golebski K, Karrich JJ, Peters CP, Blom B, et al. The transcription factor GATA3 is essential for the function of human type 2 innate lymphoid cells. Immunity. 2012;37(4):649–59.
42. Yagi R, Zhong C, Northrup DL, Yu F, Bouladoux N, Spencer S, et al. The transcription factor GATA3 is critical for the development of all IL-7Ralpha-expressing innate lymphoid cells. Immunity. 2014;40(3):378–88.
43. Moro K, Yamada T, Tanabe M, Takeuchi T, Ikawa T, Kawamoto H, et al. Innate production of T(H)2 cytokines by adipose tissue-associated c-Kit(+)Sca-1(+) lymphoid cells. Nature. 2010;463(7280): 540–4.
44. Neill DR, Wong SH, Bellosi A, Flynn RJ, Daly M, Langford TK, et al. Nuocytes represent a new innate effector leukocyte that mediates type-2 immunity. Nature. 2010;464(7293):1367–70.

45. Magri G, Miyajima M, Bascones S, Mortha A, Puga I, Cassis L, et al. Innate lymphoid cells integrate stromal and immunological signals to enhance antibody production by splenic marginal zone B cells. Nat Immunol. 2014;15(4):354–64.
46. Debock I, Flamand V. Unbalanced neonatal CD4(+) T-cell immunity. Front Immunol. 2014;5:393.
47. Ma CS, Suryani S, Avery DT, Chan A, Nanan R, Santner-Nanan B, et al. Early commitment of naive human CD4(+) T cells to the T follicular helper (T(FH)) cell lineage is induced by IL-12. Immunol Cell Biol. 2009;87(8):590–600.
48. Kaplan MH. Th9 cells: differentiation and disease. Immunol Rev. 2013;252(1):104–15.
49. Akdis M, Palomares O, van de Veen W, van Splunter M, Akdis CA. TH17 and TH22 cells: a confusion of antimicrobial response with tissue inflammation versus protection. J Allergy Clin Immunol. 2012;129(6):1438–49; quiz50-1.
50. Murphy KM, Reiner SL. The lineage decisions of helper T cells. Nat Rev Immunol. 2002;2(12):933–44.
51. Annunziato F, Cosmi L, Liotta F, Maggi E, Romagnani S. Human Th17 cells: are they different from murine Th17 cells? Eur J Immunol. 2009;39(3):637–40.
52. Basu R, Hatton RD, Weaver CT. The Th17 family: flexibility follows function. Immunol Rev. 2013;252(1):89–103.
53. Weaver CT, Hatton RD, Mangan PR, Harrington LE. IL-17 family cytokines and the expanding diversity of effector T cell lineages. Annu Rev Immunol. 2007;25:821–52.
54. Schmitt N, Ueno H. Human T follicular helper cells: development and subsets. Adv Exp Med Biol. 2013;785:87–94.
55. Chen M, Guo Z, Ju W, Ryffel B, He X, Zheng SG. The development and function of follicular helper T cells in immune responses. Cell Mol Immunol. 2012;9(5):375–9.
56. Crotty S. Follicular helper CD4 T cells (TFH). Annu Rev Immunol. 2011;29:621–63.
57. Licona-Limon P, Henao-Mejia J, Temann AU, Gagliani N, Licona-Limon I, Ishigame H, et al. Th9 cells drive host immunity against gastrointestinal worm infection. Immunity. 2013;39(4):744–57.
58. Veldhoen M, Uyttenhove C, van Snick J, Helmby H, Westendorf A, Buer J, et al. Transforming growth factor-beta 'reprograms' the differentiation of T helper 2 cells and promotes an interleukin 9-producing subset. Nat Immunol. 2008;9(12):1341–6.
59. Staudt V, Bothur E, Klein M, Lingnau K, Reuter S, Grebe N, et al. Interferon-regulatory factor 4 is essential for the developmental program of T helper 9 cells. Immunity. 2010;33(2):192–202.
60. Bouchery T, Kyle R, Ronchese F, Le Gros G. The differentiation of CD4(+) T-helper cell subsets in the context of helminth parasite infection. Front Immunol. 2014;5:487.
61. Dardalhon V, Awasthi A, Kwon H, Galileos G, Gao W, Sobel RA, et al. IL-4 inhibits TGF-beta-induced Foxp3+ T cells, and together with TGF-beta, generates IL-9+ IL-10+ Foxp3(-) effector T cells. Nat Immunol. 2008;9(12):1347–55.
62. Schmitt E, Beuscher HU, Huels C, Monteyne P, van Brandwijk R, van Snick J, et al. IL-1 serves as a secondary signal for IL-9 expression. J Immunol. 1991;147(11):3848–54.
63. Schmitt E, Germann T, Goedert S, Hoehn P, Huels C, Koelsch S, et al. IL-9 production of naive CD4+ T cells depends on IL-2, is synergistically enhanced by a combination of TGF-beta and IL-4, and is inhibited by IFN-gamma. J Immunol. 1994;153(9):3989–96.
64. Uyttenhove C, Brombacher F, Van Snick J. TGF-beta interactions with IL-1 family members trigger IL-4-independent IL-9 production by mouse CD4(+) T cells. Eur J Immunol. 2010;40(8):2230–5.
65. Schmitt E, Klein M, Bopp T. Th9 cells, new players in adaptive immunity. Trends Immunol. 2014;35(2):61–8.
66. Duhen T, Geiger R, Jarrossay D, Lanzavecchia A, Sallusto F. Production of interleukin 22 but not interleukin 17 by a subset of human skin-homing memory T cells. Nat Immunol. 2009;10(8):857–63.
67. Trifari S, Kaplan CD, Tran EH, Crellin NK, Spits H. Identification of a human helper T cell population that has abundant production of interleukin 22 and is distinct from T(H)-17, T(H)1 and T(H)2 cells. Nat Immunol. 2009;10(8):864–71.
68. Fujita H. The role of IL-22 and Th22 cells in human skin diseases. J Dermatol Sci. 2013;72(1):3–8.
69. Ramirez JM, Brembilla NC, Sorg O, Chicheportiche R, Matthes T, Dayer JM, et al. Activation of the aryl hydrocarbon receptor reveals distinct requirements for IL-22 and IL-17 production by human T helper cells. Eur J Immunol. 2010;40(9):2450–9.
70. Hao JQ. Targeting interleukin-22 in psoriasis. Inflammation. 2014;37(1):94–9.
71. Abdoli R, Najafian N. T helper cells fate mapping by co-stimulatory molecules and its functions in allograft rejection and tolerance. Int J Organ Transplant Med. 2014;5(3):97–110.
72. Chen W, Jin W, Hardegen N, Lei KJ, Li L, Marinos N, et al. Conversion of peripheral CD4+CD25- naive T cells to CD4+CD25+ regulatory T cells by TGF-beta induction of transcription factor Foxp3. J Exp Med. 2003;198(12):1875–86.
73. Shevach EM. Regulatory T, cells in autoimmmunity*. Annu Rev Immunol. 2000;18:423–49.
74. Takahashi T, Tagami T, Yamazaki S, Uede T, Shimizu J, Sakaguchi N, et al. Immunologic self-tolerance maintained by CD25(+)CD4(+) regulatory T cells constitutively expressing cytotoxic T lymphocyte-associated antigen 4. J Exp Med. 2000;192(2):303–10.
75. Hori S, Nomura T, Sakaguchi S. Control of regulatory T cell development by the transcription factor Foxp3. Science. 2003;299(5609):1057–61.
76. Fontenot JD, Gavin MA, Rudensky AY. Foxp3 programs the development and function of CD4+CD25+ regulatory T cells. Nat Immunol. 2003;4(4):330–6.
77. Ohl K, Tenbrock K. Regulatory T cells in systemic lupus erythematosus. Eur J Immunol. 2014;45(2):344–55.
78. Lin S, Yang X, Liang D, Zheng SG. Treg cells: a potential regulator for IL-22 expression? Int J Clin Exp Pathol. 2014;7(2):474–80.
79. Bacchetta R, Bigler M, Touraine JL, Parkman R, Tovo PA, Abrams J, et al. High levels of interleukin 10 production in vivo are associated with tolerance in SCID patients transplanted with HLA mismatched hematopoietic stem cells. J Exp Med. 1994;179(2): 493–502.
80. Bacchetta R, de Waal Malefijt R, Yssel H, Abrams J, de Vries JE, Spits H, et al. Host-reactive CD4+ and CD8+ T cell clones isolated from a human chimera produce IL-5, IL-2, IFN-gamma and granulocyte/macrophage-colony-stimulating factor but not IL-4. J Immunol. 1990;144(3):902–8.
81. Gagliani N, Magnani CF, Huber S, Gianolini ME, Pala M, Licona-Limon P, et al. Coexpression of CD49b and LAG-3 identifies human and mouse T regulatory type 1 cells. Nat Med. 2013;19(6):739–46.
82. Groux H, O'Garra A, Bigler M, Rouleau M, Antonenko S, de Vries JE, et al. A CD4+ T-cell subset inhibits antigen-specific T-cell responses and prevents colitis. Nature. 1997;389(6652):737–42.
83. Barrat FJ, Cua DJ, Boonstra A, Richards DF, Crain C, Savelkoul HF, et al. In vitro generation of interleukin 10-producing regulatory CD4(+) T cells is induced by immunosuppressive drugs and inhibited by T helper type 1 (Th1)- and Th2-inducing cytokines. J Exp Med. 2002;195(5):603–16.
84. Veldman C, Hohne A, Dieckmann D, Schuler G, Hertl M. Type I regulatory T cells specific for desmoglein 3 are more frequently detected in healthy individuals than in patients with pemphigus vulgaris. J Immunol. 2004;172(10):6468–75.
85. Brun V, Bastian H, Neveu V, Foussat A. Clinical grade production of IL-10 producing regulatory Tr1 lymphocytes for cell therapy of chronic inflammatory diseases. Int Immunopharmacol. 2009;9(5): 609–13.
86. Brun V, Neveu V, Pers YM, Fabre S, Quatannens B, Bastian H, et al. Isolation of functional autologous collagen-II specific IL-10

producing Tr1 cell clones from rheumatoid arthritis blood. Int Immunopharmacol. 2011;11(8):1074–8.
87. Akdis M. T-cell tolerance to inhaled allergens: mechanisms and therapeutic approaches. Expert Opin Biol Ther. 2008;8(6): 769–77.
88. Bergmann C, Strauss L, Zeidler R, Lang S, Whiteside TL. Expansion and characteristics of human T regulatory type 1 cells in co-cultures simulating tumor microenvironment. Cancer Immunol Immunother. 2007;56(9):1429–42.
89. Mandapathil M, Szczepanski MJ, Szajnik M, Ren J, Jackson EK, Johnson JT, et al. Adenosine and prostaglandin E2 cooperate in the suppression of immune responses mediated by adaptive regulatory T cells. J Biol Chem. 2010;285(36):27571–80.
90. Magnani CF, Alberigo G, Bacchetta R, Serafini G, Andreani M, Roncarolo MG, et al. Killing of myeloid APCs via HLA class I, CD2 and CD226 defines a novel mechanism of suppression by human Tr1 cells. Eur J Immunol. 2011;41(6):1652–62.
91. Roncarolo MG, Gregori S, Bacchetta R, Battaglia M. Tr1 cells and the counter-regulation of immunity: natural mechanisms and therapeutic applications. Curr Top Microbiol Immunol. 2014;380: 39–68.
92. Fearon DT, Manders P, Wagner SD. Arrested differentiation, the self-renewing memory lymphocyte, and vaccination. Science. 2001;293(5528):248–50.
93. Sallusto F, Lenig D, Forster R, Lipp M, Lanzavecchia A. Two subsets of memory T lymphocytes with distinct homing potentials and effector functions. Nature. 1999;401(6754):708–12.
94. Clark RA, Watanabe R, Teague JE, Schlapbach C, Tawa MC, Adams N, et al. Skin effector memory T cells do not recirculate and provide immune protection in alemtuzumab-treated CTCL patients. Sci Transl Med. 2012;4(117):117ra7.
95. Eyerich S, Zielinski CE. Defining Th-cell subsets in a classical and tissue-specific manner: examples from the skin. Eur J Immunol. 2014;44(12):3475–83.
96. Mackay LK, Rahimpour A, Ma JZ, Collins N, Stock AT, Hafon ML, et al. The developmental pathway for CD103(+)CD8+ tissue-resident memory T cells of skin. Nat Immunol. 2013;14(12):1294–301.
97. Xia M, Hu S, Fu Y, Jin W, Yi Q, Matsui Y, et al. CCR10 regulates balanced maintenance and function of resident regulatory and effector T cells to promote immune homeostasis in the skin. J Allergy Clin Immunol. 2014;134(3):634–44 e10.
98. Chang JT, Wherry EJ, Goldrath AW. Molecular regulation of effector and memory T cell differentiation. Nat Immunol. 2014;15(12):1104–15.
99. Yang M, Rui K, Wang S, Lu L. Regulatory B cells in autoimmune diseases. Cell Mol Immunol. 2013;10(2):122–32.
100. Rosser EC, Blair PA, Mauri C. Cellular targets of regulatory B cell-mediated suppression. Mol Immunol. 2014;62(2):296–304.
101. Cooper NR. The classical complement pathway: activation and regulation of the first complement component. Adv Immunol. 1985;37:151–216.
102. Lu J, Teh C, Kishore U, Reid KB. Collectins and ficolins: sugar pattern recognition molecules of the mammalian innate immune system. Biochim Biophys Acta. 2002;1572(2-3):387–400.
103. Frank MM, Fries LF. The role of complement in inflammation and phagocytosis. Immunol Today. 1991;12(9):322–6.
104. Carroll MC. The complement system in regulation of adaptive immunity. Nat Immunol. 2004;5(10):981–6.
105. Ricklin D, Hajishengallis G, Yang K, Lambris JD. Complement: a key system for immune surveillance and homeostasis. Nat Immunol. 2010;11(9):785–97.
106. Edelman GM. Antibody structure and molecular immunology. Scand J Immunol. 1991;34(1):1–22.
107. Porter RR. Lecture for the Nobel Prize for physiology or medicine 1972: Structural studies of immunoglobulins. 1972. Scand J Immunol. 1991;34(4):381–9.
108. Harris LJ, Larson SB, Hasel KW, Day J, Greenwood A, McPherson A. The three-dimensional structure of an intact monoclonal antibody for canine lymphoma. Nature. 1992;360(6402):369–72.
109. Davies DR, Cohen GH. Interactions of protein antigens with antibodies. Proc Natl Acad Sci U S A. 1996;93(1):7–12.
110. Wilson IA, Stanfield RL. Antibody-antigen interactions: new structures and new conformational changes. Curr Opin Struct Biol. 1994;4(6):857–67.
111. Alfano M, Poli G. Role of cytokines and chemokines in the regulation of innate immunity and HIV infection. Mol Immunol. 2005;42(2):161–82.
112. Kunkel EJ, Butcher EC. Chemokines and the tissue-specific migration of lymphocytes. Immunity. 2002;16(1):1–4.
113. Matsukawa A, Hogaboam CM, Lukacs NW, Kunkel SL. Chemokines and innate immunity. Rev Immunogenet. 2000;2(3):339–58.
114. Alon R, Feigelson S. From rolling to arrest on blood vessels: leukocyte tap dancing on endothelial integrin ligands and chemokines at sub-second contacts. Semin Immunol. 2002;14(2):93–104.
115. Johnston B, Butcher EC. Chemokines in rapid leukocyte adhesion triggering and migration. Semin Immunol. 2002;14(2):83–92.
116. Svanborg C, Godaly G, Hedlund M. Cytokine responses during mucosal infections: role in disease pathogenesis and host defence. Curr Opin Microbiol. 1999;2(1):99–105.
117. Ley K. Leukocyte adhesion to vascular endothelium. J Reconstr Microsurg. 1992;8(6):495–503.
118. Springer TA. Adhesion receptors of the immune system. Nature. 1990;346(6283):425–34.
119. Kumanovics A, Takada T, Lindahl KF. Genomic organization of the mammalian MHC. Annu Rev Immunol. 2003;21:629–57.
120. Gaur LK, Nepom GT. Ancestral major histocompatibility complex DRB genes beget conserved patterns of localized polymorphisms. Proc Natl Acad Sci U S A. 1996;93(11):5380–3.
121. Bouvier M. Accessory proteins and the assembly of human class I MHC molecules: a molecular and structural perspective. Mol Immunol. 2003;39(12):697–706.
122. Bouvier M, Wiley DC. Importance of peptide amino and carboxyl termini to the stability of MHC class I molecules. Science. 1994;265(5170):398–402.
123. Fremont DH, Hendrickson WA, Marrack P, Kappler J. Structures of an MHC class II molecule with covalently bound single peptides. Science. 1996;272(5264):1001–4.
124. Rudensky A, Preston-Hurlburt P, Hong SC, Barlow A, Janeway Jr CA. Sequence analysis of peptides bound to MHC class II molecules. Nature. 1991;353(6345):622–7.
125. Kawai T, Akira S. Toll-like receptors and their crosstalk with other innate receptors in infection and immunity. Immunity. 2011; 34(5):637–50.
126. Janeway Jr CA. Approaching the asymptote? Evolution and revolution in immunology. Cold Spring Harb Symp Quant Biol. 1989;54(Pt 1):1–13.
127. Blasius AL, Beutler B. Intracellular toll-like receptors. Immunity. 2010;32(3):305–15.
128. Pifer R, Benson A, Sturge CR, Yarovinsky F. UNC93B1 is essential for TLR11 activation and IL-12-dependent host resistance to Toxoplasma gondii. J Biol Chem. 2011;286(5):3307–14.
129. Akira S, Uematsu S, Takeuchi O. Pathogen recognition and innate immunity. Cell. 2006;124(4):783–801.
130. Kawai T, Akira S. The role of pattern-recognition receptors in innate immunity: update on Toll-like receptors. Nat Immunol. 2010;11(5):373–84.
131. Barton GM, Kagan JC. A cell biological view of Toll-like receptor function: regulation through compartmentalization. Nat Rev Immunol. 2009;9(8):535–42.
132. Ting JPY, Lovering RC, Alnemri ES, Bertin J, Boss JM, Davis BK, et al. The NLR gene family: a standard nomenclature. Immunity. 2008;28(3):285–7.

133. Elinav E, Strowig T, Henao-Mejia J, Flavell RA. Regulation of the antimicrobial response by NLR proteins. Immunity. 2011;34(5): 665–79.
134. Lechtenberg BC, Mace PD, Riedl SJ. Structural mechanisms in NLR inflammasome signaling. Curr Opin Struct Biol. 2014;29C: 17–25.
135. Coulombe F, Divangahi M, Veyrier F, de Leseleuc L, Gleason JL, Yang Y, et al. Increased NOD2-mediated recognition of N-glycolyl muramyl dipeptide. J Exp Med. 2009;206(8):1709–16.
136. Sabbah A, Chang TH, Harnack R, Frohlich V, Tominaga K, Dube PH, et al. Activation of innate immune antiviral responses by Nod2. Nat Immunol. 2009;10(10):1073–80.
137. Fritz JH, Girardin SE, Fitting C, Werts C, Mengin-Lecreulx D, Caroff M, et al. Synergistic stimulation of human monocytes and dendritic cells by Toll-like receptor 4 and NOD1- and NOD2-activating agonists. Eur J Immunol. 2005;35(8):2459–70.
138. Kanneganti TD, Body-Malapel M, Amer A, Park JH, Whitfield J, Franchi L, et al. Critical role for Cryopyrin/Nalp3 in activation of caspase-1 in response to viral infection and double-stranded RNA. J Biol Chem. 2006;281(48):36560–8.
139. Fritz JH, Ferrero RL, Philpott DJ, Girardin SE. Nod-like proteins in immunity, inflammation and disease. Nat Immunol. 2006;7(12): 1250–7.
140. Strowig T, Henao-Mejia J, Elinav E, Flavell R. Inflammasomes in health and disease. Nature. 2012;481(7381):278–86.
141. Davis BK, Wen H, Ting JP. The inflammasome NLRs in immunity, inflammation, and associated diseases. Annu Rev Immunol. 2011;29:707–35.
142. Agostini L, Martinon F, Burns K, McDermott MF, Hawkins PN, Tschopp J. NALP3 forms an IL-1beta-processing inflammasome with increased activity in Muckle-Wells autoinflammatory disorder. Immunity. 2004;20(3):319–25.
143. Martinon F, Burns K, Tschopp J. The inflammasome: a molecular platform triggering activation of inflammatory caspases and processing of proIL-beta. Mol Cell. 2002;10(2):417–26.
144. Schroder K, Tschopp J. The inflammasomes. Cell. 2010;140(6): 821–32.
145. Bauernfeind FG, Horvath G, Stutz A, Alnemri ES, MacDonald K, Speert D, et al. Cutting edge: NF-kappaB activating pattern recognition and cytokine receptors license NLRP3 inflammasome activation by regulating NLRP3 expression. J Immunol. 2009; 183(2):787–91.
146. Yoneyama M, Kikuchi M, Natsukawa T, Shinobu N, Imaizumi T, Miyagishi M, et al. The RNA helicase RIG-I has an essential function in double-stranded RNA-induced innate antiviral responses. Nat Immunol. 2004;5(7):730–7.
147. Yoneyama M, Kikuchi M, Matsumoto K, Imaizumi T, Miyagishi M, Taira K, et al. Shared and unique functions of the DExD/H-box helicases RIG-I, MDA5, and LGP2 in antiviral innate immunity. J Immunol. 2005;175(5):2851–8.
148. Saito T, Hirai R, Loo YM, Owen D, Johnson CL, Sinha SC, et al. Regulation of innate antiviral defenses through a shared repressor domain in RIG-I and LGP2. Proc Natl Acad Sci U S A. 2007;104(2):582–7.
149. Loo YM, Gale Jr M. Immune signaling by RIG-I-like receptors. Immunity. 2011;34(5):680–92.
150. Saito T, Owen DM, Jiang F, Marcotrigiano J, Gale Jr M. Innate immunity induced by composition-dependent RIG-I recognition of hepatitis C virus RNA. Nature. 2008;454(7203):523–7.
151. Uzri D, Gehrke L. Nucleotide sequences and modifications that determine RIG-I/RNA binding and signaling activities. J Virol. 2009;83(9):4174–84.
152. Weis WI, Drickamer K. Structural basis of lectin-carbohydrate recognition. Annu Rev Biochem. 1996;65:441–73.
153. Zelensky AN, Gready JE. The C-type lectin-like domain superfamily. FEBS J. 2005;272(24):6179–217.
154. Osorio F, Reis e Sousa C. Myeloid C-type lectin receptors in pathogen recognition and host defense. Immunity. 2011;34(5):651–64.
155. Robinson MJ, Sancho D, Slack EC, LeibundGut-Landmann S, Reis e Sousa C. Myeloid C-type lectins in innate immunity. Nat Immunol. 2006;7(12):1258–65.
156. Rogers NC, Slack EC, Edwards AD, Nolte MA, Schulz O, Schweighoffer E, et al. Syk-dependent cytokine induction by Dectin-1 reveals a novel pattern recognition pathway for C type lectins. Immunity. 2005;22(4):507–17.
157. Mocsai A, Ruland J, Tybulewicz VL. The SYK tyrosine kinase: a crucial player in diverse biological functions. Nat Rev Immunol. 2010;10(6):387–402.
158. Choudhuri K, Dustin ML. Signaling microdomains in T cells. FEBS Lett. 2010;584(24):4823–31.

The Innate Immunity

2

Haoyu Sun, Cheng Sun, and Zhigang Tian

Contents

Innate immunity refers to the naturally formed innate immune defensive functions through evolution, which makes up the first line of defense against microbial pathogens. Innate immune system is the natural immune system formed by an organism during a long period of time through evolution, and is mainly composed of the epithelial barrier, the innate immune cells, and the innate immune molecules. It mainly discriminates self from nonself by the pattern recognition mechanism of innate immune system, resulting in the initiation of innate immune responses. The major effector functions of the innate immune response include defense against infectious agents, induction of inflammatory responses, and contribution to the activation, effector functions, and regulation of the adaptive immune responses.

2.1 Epithelial Barrier: The First Line of Defense

Skin and mucosal epithelia comprise the first defensive barrier against foreign pathogens, which prevent pathogens from crossing the epithelia and colonizing tissues through physical, chemical, and microbiological barriers.

2.1.1 Physical Barrier

Epithelial cells are joined together by tight junctions, forming a physical barrier between the external world that contains pathogens and the internal environment of the body. Epithelia comprise of the skin and mucosal epithelia; the latter lines the gastrointestinal, respiratory, and urogenital tracts. The epithelial surfaces serve as the first line of defense to guard our bodies, and repair rapidly if wounded. Infection occurs when pathogens pass through this barrier; the most apparent way is through wounds and burns where the skin is broken, and pathogens pass through this physical barrier and enter the body; however, it is rather a challenge to cross this barrier in the absence of wounding. Pathogens enter the body

H. Sun • C. Sun • Z. Tian (✉)
Institute of Immunology, School of Life Sciences and Medical Center, University of Science and Technology of China, Hefei, China
e-mail: tzg@ustc.edu.cn

X.-H. Gao, H.-D. Chen (eds.), *Practical Immunodermatology*, DOI 10.1007/978-94-024-0902-4_2

most often through the internal mucosal epithelia. In the absence of epithelial disruption, pathogens may cross the epithelial barrier by binding to molecules on the epithelial surfaces or adhering to these surfaces. The mucosal epithelia secrete mucus that may prevent pathogens from adhering to the epithelia, and pathogens coated in mucus can be expelled in the flow of mucus driven by the waving of epithelial cilia in the lining of respiratory tract [1–4].

2.1.2 Chemical Barrier

Secretions of the skin and mucosal epithelia include a variety of chemical substances that can either inhibit microbial growth or kill the microorganisms. For example, lysozyme and phospholipase A are antibacterial enzymes that are being secreted in tears and saliva; the hydrochloric acids in gastric juice, the digestive enzymes, and the fatty acids of sebaceous glands all contribute to a chemical barrier against infection; α-defensins, the antibacterial and antifungal peptides made by Paneth cells, provide chemical barrier for the small intestine, while β-defensins are mainly present in the respiratory and urogenital tracts, skin, and tongue; antimicrobial proteins are also secreted into the fluids and coat the surface of pathogens to make them more easily phagocytosed by macrophages in the lung and gut.

2.1.3 Microbiological Barrier

The healthy epithelial surfaces also contain a large population of normally nonpathogenic bacteria, known as commensal bacteria. The commensal bacteria compete with pathogens for nutrients and attachment sites on epithelial cells. Commensal bacteria stimulate the epithelial cells to produce antimicrobial peptides that help to strengthen the barrier function of epithelia.

2.2 Pattern Recognition in Innate Immunity

2.2.1 PRRs and PAMPs

Recognition of microbial pathogens, infected cells, senescent cells, and tumor cells by immune cells is mediated by pattern-recognition receptors (PRRs) that recognize molecular structures that are broadly shared by pathogens, known as pathogen-associated molecular patterns (PAMPs), inducing nonspecific host-defensive responses necessary for killing infectious microbes [5, 6]. PRRs may present on the surface of phagocytes and dendritic cells, intracellular compartment, or even in the serum; they directly recognize the repeating patterns of molecular structures present on the surface of microorganisms known as PAMPs or repeating patterns of molecular structures present on the surface of dead cells and senescent cells known as damage-associated molecular patterns (DAMPs). PRRs are germline-encoded receptors that mediate swift biological responses. Upon PRR-PAMP recognition, pathogens are being ingested and killed by these phagocytes without the aid of adaptive immunity. There are four major classes of PRRs: (1) the soluble (free) receptors that are present in the serum (MBL, LBP); (2) the membrane-bound phagocytic receptors that are present on the phagocytes and recognize pathogen surfaces directly to mediate capturing, uptake, and presentation of antigens (mannose receptor (MR), scavenger receptor (SR), etc.); (3) the membrane-bound signaling receptors that are present on phagocytes and signal the presence of pathogens to induce the activation of proinflammatory pathways (toll-like receptor); and (4) the cytoplasmic signaling receptors that are present in the cytoplasm and signal the presence of pathogens to induce the activation of proinflammatory pathways (NLR, RLR) [6–8] (Table 2.1).

Table 2.1 Classification of PRRs in the innate immune system

Classification	Distribution	Major members
Soluble receptors	Humoral fluid, blood	MBL, CRP, LBP
Phagocytic receptors	Cell membrane	CLR, MR, SR, CR, FcR, fMLP
Signaling receptors	Cell membrane	TLR1, TLR2, TLR4, TLR5, TLR6, TLR10
	Endosome, lysosome	TLR3, TLR7, TLR8, TLR9, TLR11
	Cytoplasm	NLR, RLR

MBL mannose-binding lectin, *CRP* C-reactive protein, *LBP* LPS-binding protein, *CLR* C-type lectin receptor, *MR* mannose receptor, *SR* scavenger receptor, *CR* complement receptor, *FcR* Fc receptor, *fMLP* formyl-methionine-leucyl-phenylalanine, fMet-Lei-Phe, *TLR* Toll-like receptor, *NLR* nucleotide-binding, oligomerization domain (NOD)-like receptor, *RLR* retinoic acid-inducible gene (RIG)-I-like receptor

2.2.2 Pattern Recognition

Innate immunity can distinguish self from nonself by discriminating between the surface molecules displayed on the pathogens and those of the host; however, it lacks antigen-specific recognition of the adaptive immunity. Binding between the receptor and pathogen components is the main way to activate a very rapid innate immune response. For example, mannose-binding lectin (MBL), a free protein present in the blood plasma, can discriminate between self and nonself due to its special recognition system. It recognizes a fixed orientation of mannose or fucose residues, as well as their spacing, that is found only on microorganisms and not on host cells, and serves as coating in the process of opsonization. Macrophage mannose receptor can bind certain sugars on the surface of many bacteria and viruses and functions as a phagocytic receptor to stimulate the ingestion of pathogens [1–4, 9]. An important TLR that recognizes common bacteria and works in the innate immunity is TLR-4. They usually express on macrophages, and together with the help of CD14 and MD-2, recognize lipopolysaccharides (LPS). Initially, LPS in the body fluids is bound by LPS-binding protein (LBP), which transfers LPS to CD14 on the surface of phagocytes as a complex, and this CD14:LPS complex interacts with the TLR-4:MD-2 complex, resulting in the activation of transcription factor NFkB in the cell nucleus. In addition, chemotactic receptors may guide cells to the site of infection. As part of the innate system, they also induce the production of effector molecules that contribute to induced innate immune responses, and proteins that influence the initiation of subsequent adaptive immune responses [6, 10, 11].

2.3 Innate Immune Responses to Infection

2.3.1 Three Phases of an Immune Response

The immune response against an initial infection occurs in three phases: the innate phase, the early induced innate response, and the adaptive immune response. The first two phases rely on the recognition of pathogens by PRRs of the innate immune system, whereas the adaptive immune response involves variable antigen-specific receptors of the adaptive immune system. Pathogens are recognized by innate immune cells, and this recognition leads to various effector mechanisms that are all regulated by PRRs.

2.3.2 Induction of Innate Immune Responses

Innate immune responses are mainly induced by proinflammatory cytokines and chemokines secreted by phagocytes in response to pathogen recognition; the release of these proinflammatory cytokines and chemokines is controlled by the ability of phagocytes to discriminate between self and nonself. Cytokines and chemokines are responsible for local inflammation, the recruitment of effector cells, the containment of local infection, and the initiation of an adaptive immune response. They act together in the early phase to recruit more phagocytic cells to the site of infection, among which neutrophils are usually the first ones being recruited, leading to the recognition and killing of the pathogens. While, on the other hand, monocytes and immature dendritic cells arrive later.

Tissue macrophages secrete a range of cytokines after activation, resulting in a variety of local and systemic effects on the immune system. The major cytokines produced by macrophages in response to pathogen recognition include IL-1β, TNF-α, IL-6, CXCL18, and IL-12, which all contribute to fever and the production of acute phase response proteins, including mannose-binding lectin, C-reactive protein, fibrinogen, and pulmonary surfactant protein. Among the cytokines being secreted, IL-1β activates vascular endothelium and lymphocytes, causes local tissue destruction, and increases access of effector cells; TNF-α activates vascular endothelium and increases vascular permeability, leading to increased entry of IgG, complement, and cells to tissues and increased fluid drainage to lymph nodes; IL-6 activates lymphocytes and increases antibody production; CXCL18 recruits neutrophils, basophils, and T cells to the site of infection; and IL-12 activates NK cells and induces the differentiation of $CD4^+$ T cells into Th1 cells.

Viral infection leads to the production of type I interferon that serves to inhibit viral replication, increases MHC class I expression and antigen presentation, and activates dendritic cells, macrophages, and NK cells. Activated NK cells secrete IFN-γ that influences the response of CD4 T cells, leading to their differentiation into inflammatory Th1 cells that in turn activate macrophages. Cells infected by intracellular pathogens also show altered expression of MHC class I molecules, leading to their destruction as they are labeled "nonself" by NK cells. The ligands for activating receptor NKG2D are also upregulated on cells infected with intracellular bacteria or viruses, leading to the activation of NK cells and the destruction of infected cells.

Recognition of different pathogens by phagocytes and dendritic cells involves signaling through different receptors, resulting in a variety of cytokines produced and immune cells activated. They can either clear the infection or retain it until an adaptive response takes place. Cytokines, chemokines, cell adhesion molecules, and immune cells of the innate immune system all contribute to the development of an induced innate response [1–4].

References

1. Paul WE. Fundamental immunology. 7th ed. Philadelphia: Wolters Kluwer Health: Lippincot Williams & Wilkins; 2012.
2. Murphy K. Janeway's immunology. 8th ed. New York: Garland Science; 2011.
3. Abbas AK, Lichtman AH, Pillai S. Cellular and molecular immunology. 6th ed. Philadelphia: Saunders; 2010.
4. Parslow TG, Stites DP, Terry AI, Imboden JB. Medical immunology. 10th ed. New York: McGraw-Hill/Appleton & Lange; 2001.
5. Janeway Jr CA. Approaching the asymptote? Evolution and revolution in immunology. Cold Spring Harb Symp Quant Biol. 1989;54(Pt 1):1–13.

6. Kawai T, Akira S. Toll-like receptors and their crosstalk with other innate receptors in infection and immunity. Immunity. 2011; 34(5):637–50.
7. Elinav E, Strowig T, Henao-Mejia J, Flavell RA. Regulation of the antimicrobial response by NLR proteins. Immunity. 2011;34(5): 665–79.
8. Loo YM, Gale Jr M. Immune signaling by RIG-I-like receptors. Immunity. 2011;34(5):680–92.
9. Osorio F, Reis e Sousa C. Myeloid C-type lectin receptors in pathogen recognition and host defense. Immunity. 2011;34(5): 651–64.
10. Akira S. Pathogen recognition by innate immunity and its signaling. Proc Jpn Acad Ser B Phys Biol Sci. 2009;85(4):143–56.
11. Barton GM, Kagan JC. A cell biological view of Toll-like receptor function: regulation through compartmentalization. Nat Rev Immunol. 2009;9(8):535–42.

The Adaptive Immunity

3

Haoyu Sun, Cheng Sun, and Zhigang Tian

Contents

Adaptive immunity develops during the lifetime of an organism as an adaptation to infection with certain pathogens, also referring to as the acquired immunity. Adaptive immune response is highly antigen specific, although it is relatively slow, it is highly efficient at antigen clearance, and therefore it is also termed as specific immunity. Immune cells participating in the adaptive immunity include T and B cells. T and B cells are activated after antigen recognition, followed by proliferation and differentiation that lead to the production of effector cells and molecules, which eventually clear foreign substances from the system.

An adaptive immune response is characterized by: (1) specificity: lymphocytes may discriminate between different antigens and develop specific immune response against each epitope; (2) diversity: lymphocyte clones with varied antigen-specific receptors may recognize a variety of antigens in the environment, each of which leads to a distinct antigen-specific immune response; (3) memory: the immune response being produced upon initial contact with an antigen is called the primary immune response; while a faster and stronger immune response being produced upon second challenge with the same antigen is called the secondary immune response; the occurrence of such immunological memory is mainly caused by the swift activation, proliferation, and production of effector cells and molecules induced by re-exposure of memory lymphocytes to the same antigen; (4) homeostasis: the immune response induced by the immune system against foreign antigens gradually attenuates as time goes by and antigens are being cleared, restoring to the resting state; homeostasis is sustained mainly because of the inefficiency in activating lymphocytes as antigens are being cleared and the activation of regulatory mechanisms by antigens or immune responses; (5) self-tolerance: one of the most typical characters of the immune system is its ability to distinguish and clear nonself-antigens without inducing an immune response against self-antigens, and this unresponsiveness to self-antigens is generally referred to as self-tolerance.

Based on the immune cells that are involved and the products of an adaptive immune response, it may be classified

H. Sun • C. Sun • Z. Tian (✉)
Institute of Immunology, School of Life Sciences and Medical Center, University of Science and Technology of China, Hefei, China
e-mail: tzg@ustc.edu.cn

X.-H. Gao, H.-D. Chen (eds.), *Practical Immunodermatology*, DOI 10.1007/978-94-024-0902-4_3

into cell-mediated adaptive immunity and humoral adaptive immunity. During an adaptive immune response, T and B cells recognize antigens through their unique antigen receptors. B-cell receptors (BCRs) recognize antigens directly, while T-cell receptors (TCRs) only recognize antigens that are bound to MHC molecules on the surface of other cells. This typical feature of TCRs acquires through antigen presenting cells (APCs) that capture, process, and present antigens in recognition [1–4].

3.1 Antigen Processing and Presentation

Antigen processing and presentation are the basis for initiating an adaptive immune response. Antigen processing involves the generation of peptides from an intact antigen that are then combined with MHC molecules to form peptide:MHC class I/II complexes. Antigen presentation involves the displaying of these peptides at the cell surface by MHC molecules for T cells to recognize [5–7].

3.1.1 Antigen Presenting Cells

Antigen presenting cells are capable of capturing and processing antigens, followed by presenting these processed antigens in the form of antigenic peptide:MHC molecule complexes for immune cells to recognize. A variety of cells may function as APCs. APCs are divided into "professional" and "nonprofessional" APCs according to their ability to express MHC class II molecules and costimulatory molecules.

3.1.1.1 Professional APCs

Three types of cells are classified as professional APCs, including dendritic cells, macrophages, and B cells. They constitutively express MHC class II molecules and costimulatory molecules; however, each of them distributes differently, processes and presents different antigen epitopes, and performs different effector functions in activating T cells. Dendritic cells are the strongest APCs that may induce naïve T cell activation, and their main effector function is to initiate an adaptive immune response. Macrophages mainly present antigens to activated T cells and memory T cells, while exerting minimum effector function in the activation of naïve T cells. B cells efficiently internalize specific antigens and present T cell epitopes as antigenic peptide:MHC class II complexes to specific Th2 cells. While B cells are presenting these antigens to Th cells, they are also being activated with the help of Th cells, inducing immune responses against TD-Ag.

3.1.1.2 Nonprofessional APCs

Several other cell types can be induced to express MHC class II molecules or costimulatory molecules, including epithelial cells, endothelial cells, fibroblasts, etc.

3.1.1.3 Target Cells

MHC class I molecules are expressed on most nucleated cells. These cells present antigens to $CD8^+$T cells (mainly cytotoxic T cells) and serve as the targets of a cytotoxic response. Therefore these cells are referred to as target cells, including intracellular pathogen-infected cells, virus-infected cells, tumor cells, etc. [1–4].

3.1.2 Antigen Processing and Presentation

There are four distinct antigen processing and presentation pathways based on the antigen source and property:MHC class I pathway (endogenous antigen); MHC class II pathway (exogenous antigen); nonclassic antigen presenting pathway/cross-presentation pathway; and CD1-related lipid antigen presenting pathway (lipid antigen). MHC class I and MHC class II pathways are the main pathways of antigen processing and presentation.

3.1.2.1 Endogenous and Exogenous Antigens

Antigens that are being processed and presented by APCs are classified into endogenous and exogenous antigens based on their distinct sources. Endogenous antigens are usually generated inside of target cells (all somatic cells) such as the viral proteins generated in virus-infected cells, tumor antigens generated in tumor cells, etc. Exogenous antigens are cellular, bacterial, and protein antigens being captured by APCs [1–4].

3.1.2.2 Stages of Antigen Processing

Four stages are involved in the processing of endogenous and exogenous antigens: (1) antigen uptake ensures the access of antigens and pathogens to intracellular pathways of degradation; (2) degradation involves limited proteolysis of antigens to peptides; (3) peptide:MHC complex formation involves the loading of peptides onto MHC molecules; (4) antigen presentation involves the transportation and expression of peptide:MHC complexes on the surface of APCs for recognition by T cells.

3.1.2.3 MHC Class I Pathway

MHC class I molecules are expressed on all somatic cells (professional APCs, nonprofessional APCs, and target cells); therefore, these cells present their endogenous antigens to $CD8^+$ T cells mainly through MHC class I pathway. Endogenous antigen peptides are generated from proteins degraded in the cytosol by proteasome. These peptides are actively transported from the cytosol to the endoplasmic reticulum by ATP-binding protein TAP and are then available for binding by partly folded MHC class I molecules that are held tethered to TAP. Such binding between peptides and MHC class I molecules is necessary for MHC class I molecules to complete their folding and leave the endoplasmic reticulum to the cell surface. The peptide:MHC class I complexes are recognized by CD8+ T cells, allowing for the detection and elimination of cytosolic pathogens such as viruses (Table 3.1) (Fig. 3.1) [8–11].

3.1.2.4 MHC Class II Pathway

MHC class II molecules are expressed on all professional APCs; therefore, these cells present their captured exogenous antigens to CD4+ T cells mainly through MHC class II pathway. Extracellular antigens are taken up by APCs from extracellular space into membranous endosomal vesicles known as endosomes in the cell. The pH of the endosomes decreases progressively after engulfing pathogens, which activates proteases in acidified vesicles to degrade engulfed material into peptides. However, MHC class II molecules do not bind these peptides because they are targeted by a trimeric polypeptide, called the invariant chain (Ii). Ii binds to MHC class II molecule and blocks the binding of peptides and unfolded proteins in the endoplasmic reticulum. After transport into an acidified vesicle, Ii is cleaved in the presence of active proteases, leaving a short peptide fragment called the CLIP (class II-associated invariant-chain peptide) still bound to MHC class II molecule. The class II-like molecule HLA-DM binds to MHC class II:CLIP complex, catalyzing the release of CLIP and the binding of antigenic peptide. Newly synthesized MHC class II molecules pass through such acidified vesicles, bind peptide fragments of the antigen, and then transport the binding peptides to the cell surface. The peptide:MHC class II complexes are recognized by CD4+ T cells, inducing various specialized effector functions (Table 3.1) (Fig. 3.1) [12, 13].

Table 3.1 Features of MHC class I and MHC class II pathways of antigen processing and presentation

	MHC class I pathway	MHC class II pathway
Source of antigens	Intracellular Cytosolic proteins	Extracellular Endosomal/lysosomal proteins
Size of antigenic peptides	8–10 aa	13–18 aa
Degradation	Cytosol	Endocytic vesicles
Types of APCs	Nucleated cells	DCs, B cells, macrophages
Binding of peptides	MHC class I molecules	MHC class II molecules
Site of peptide loading	Endoplasmic reticulum	Specialized vesicular compartment
Molecular chaperones	TAP1, 2, Er57, tapasin, calnexin, calreticulin	Invariant chain, HLA-DM
Responsive T cells	CD8+ T cells	CD4+ T cells

3.1.2.5 Nonclassic Antigen Presenting Pathway

Nonclassic antigen presenting pathway is also called the cross-presentation pathway, referring to the process of exogenous antigens being presented to CD8+ T cells through MHC class I pathway after capturing and processing by APCs [14].

3.1.2.6 CD1-Related Lipid Antigen Presenting Pathway

Certain cells are capable of binding and presenting microbial lipid and glycolipid antigens to CD1-restricted T cells (known as NKT cells) through a small family of nonclassic MHC class I molecules called the CD1 molecules. These molecules are expressed on dendritic cells, monocytes, some thymocytes, and hematopoietic cells (Fig. 3.1) [1–4].

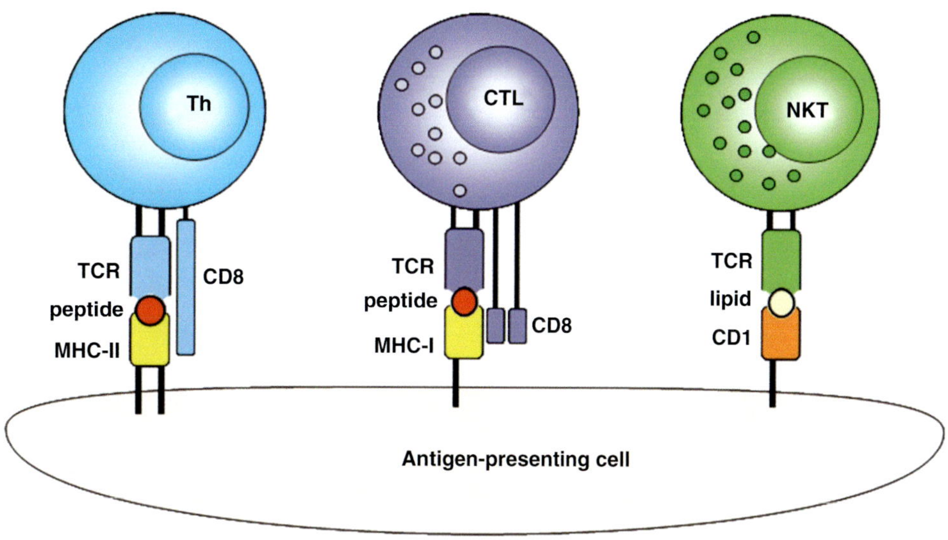

Fig. 3.1 Antigen presentation. *Th* helper T cell, *CTL* cytotoxic T lymphocytes, *NKT* NK T cell

3.2 T Cell-Mediated Immunity

Cell-mediated immunity is also known as cellular immunity, which is mediated by T cells. The immune responses mediated by T cells are divided into three phases: the first phase involves recognition of antigens and activation of naïve T cells in the peripheral lymphoid organs; the second phase involves the expansion of antigen-specific lymphocytes and their differentiation into effector and memory lymphocytes; the third phase involves the effector functions of $CD4^+$ and $CD8^+$ T cells: the effector $CD4^+$ T cells respond to antigens by producing cytokines that activate macrophages to destroy intracellular pathogens and promote the activation of specific B cells and Ig class switching; the effector $CD8^+$ T cells contribute to immune protection against virus-infected cells and tumor cells by producing cytolytic molecules and cytokines [15–18].

3.2.1 Antigen Recognition by T Cells

Antigen recognition refers to the specific binding between TCR and peptide:MHC complex presented by APC. T cells cannot recognize complete protein antigen, they can only recognize antigen in the form of a complex of a foreign peptide bound to an MHC class I/II molecule. T-cell receptor not only interacts with antigenic peptide but also with polymorphic features of the MHC molecule displaying it, and this dual specificity underlies the MHC restriction of T cell responses. T cells fall into two major classes depending on the expression of the cell surface proteins CD4 and CD8, which contribute to distinct effector functions based on their ability to recognize different classes of MHC molecules. CD8 is carried by cytotoxic T cells and recognizes MHC class I molecules, whereas CD4 is carried by helper T cells and recognizes MHC class II molecules. CD4 and CD8 are also referred to as the coreceptors (Fig. 3.2) [1].

3.2.2 T Cell Activation

APCs deliver different signals to activate naïve T cells after recognition of peptide:MHC complexes on the surface of these cells. The activation and proliferation of naïve T cells on their first encountering with specific antigens is often

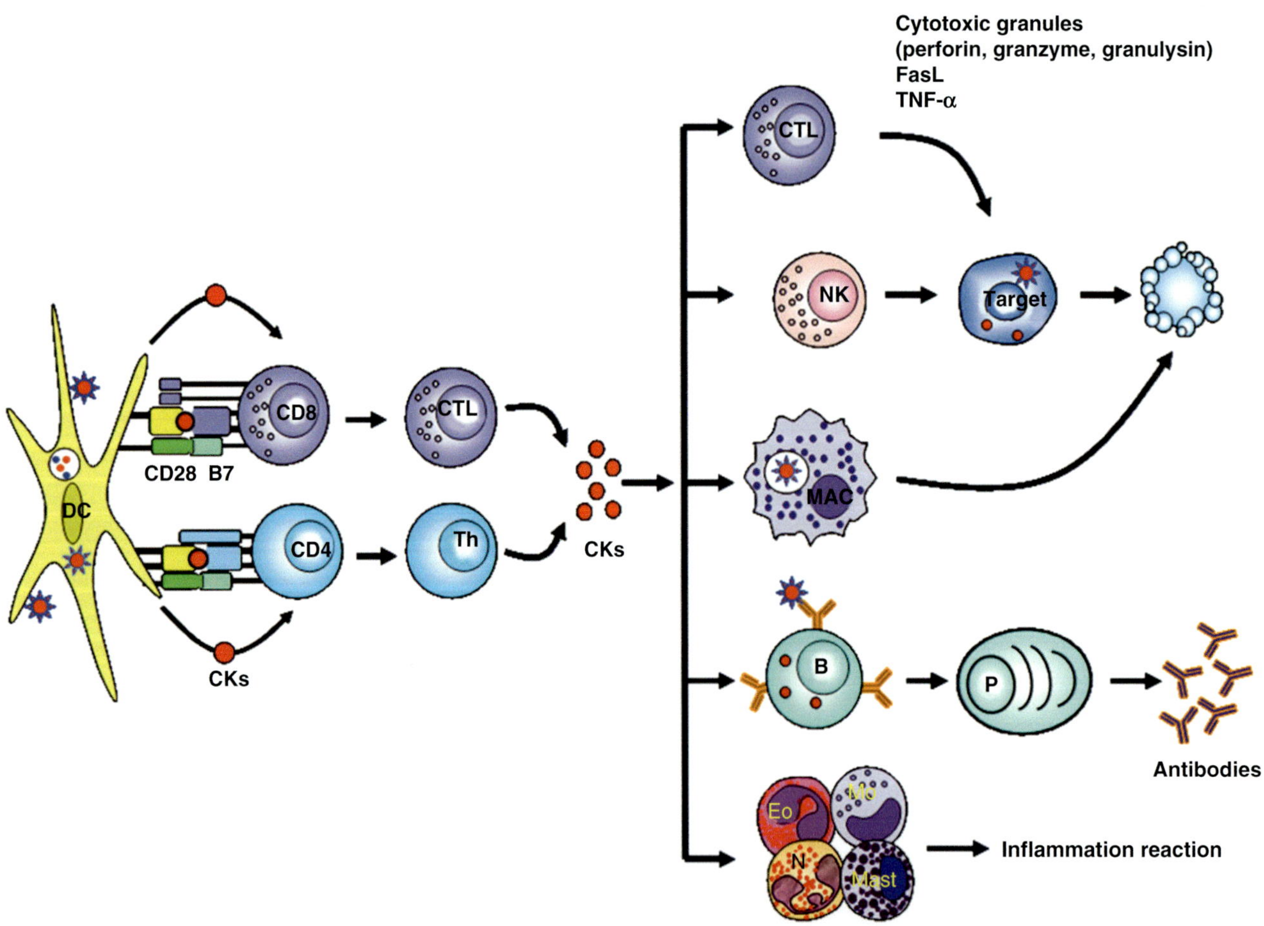

Fig. 3.2 T cell-mediated immune responses and effector functions. *CKs* cytokines, *Th* helper T cell, *CTL* cytotoxic T lymphocytes, *MAC* macrophage, *N* neutrophil, *Eo* eosinophil, *mast* mast cell, *B* B cell, *P* plasma cells, *NK* NK cell, *Mo* monocyte

referred to as priming. Two kinds of signals are involved in the activation of naïve T cells: signal 1 involves antigen-specific signals derived from the recognition of a specific peptide:MHC complex by the TCR; signal 2 involves costimulatory signals derived from the interaction between costimulatory molecules on APCs and T cells, including B7 (CD80/86) and CD28/CTLA-4; PD-L1/PD-L2 and PD-1/PD-2; ICOSL and ICOS; CD40 and CD40L, CD226 (DNAM-1)/TIGIT; and CD155 (PVR)/CD112 (PVRL2, nectin-2), etc., which may either positively or negatively regulate the activation of T cells [19, 20]. Absence of costimulation during antigen recognition leads to functional inactivation (also called anergy) of peripheral T cells. This dual-signal requires both receptor ligation and costimulation by the same APC, it helps to prevent naïve T cells from responding to self-antigens on tissue cells, which lack costimulatory activity. This is also considered one of the most important mechanisms in self-tolerance; therefore, the induction or inhibition of T cell anergy may become effective strategy in interfering pathological processes including allograft rejection, autoimmune disease, tumor, etc. The best characterized costimulatory molecules involved in signal 2 are the B7 molecules that bind to CD28 on T cells. After pairing with CD28 on activated T cells, B7 molecules induce expression of the T cell growth factor interleukin-2 (IL-2) and the high affinity IL-2 receptor that are specialized in the proliferation and differentiation of activated T cells (Fig. 3.2). On the other hand, coinhibitory molecule CTLA-4, also known as CD152, is structurally related to CD28 and can be induced on T cells to compete with CD28 for the interaction with B7 molecules [21]. The expression of CTLA-4 upregulates in activated T cells and it binds to B7 molecules with higher affinity than with CD28 (around 20- to 100-folds), thus inhibits downstream Akt pathway and prevents the costimulatory signal necessary for IL-2 production, which in turn inhibits T cell growth and proliferation [20, 22–25]. This is an important mechanism in self-regulation and protection, it benefits the induction of appropriate immune responses and effector functions and the termination of immune responses in time. CTLA-4 is also constitutively expressed on Treg cells and has a central role in the stability and function of regulatory T cells [21, 26].

3.2.3 T Cell Differentiation and Effector Functions

Activated T cells proliferate and expand under the effects of dual signals and IL-2, and they further differentiate into different effector T cells under the influence of various cytokines, including IL-1, IL-2, IL-4, IL-10, IL-12, IL-15, IFN-γ, etc., in order to perform different effector functions. These cytokines provide signal 3 for T cell activation (Fig. 3.2).

3.2.3.1 CD4$^+$ T Cells: Differentiation and Effector Functions

Naïve CD4$^+$ T cells are activated by peptide:MHC class II complexes and costimulatory molecules, they differentiate into different CD4$^+$ T cell subsets under the regulation of various cytokines in the local environment. Polarized differentiation determines the type of cells they become and the effector functions they are engaging in.

Th1 Cells When infected by intracellular pathogens (Virus, Protoza, Mycobacterium, Leishmania, etc.), innate immune responses initiate and induce the secretion of cytokines such as IL-12 and IFN-γ by activated macrophages and NK cells. IL-12 and IFN-γ bind to their receptors on Th0 cells, activate transcription factor T-bet that induces Th0 cells to differentiate into Th1 cells. Th1 subset owns dual functions. On the one hand, activated Th1 cells may secrete various cytokines that participate in the activation, proliferation, and differentiation of T, B, NK cells, and macrophages, inducing protective responses against pathogens. On the other hand, activated Th1 cells may secrete various cytokines that recruit and activate monocytes/macrophages and lymphocytes that gathered at the site of infection to mediate inflammatory reaction or delayed-type hypersensitivity, inducing pathological responses against pathogens. Th1 cells play important roles in cell-mediated immunity by activating macrophages and releasing various cytokines that clear intracellular pathogens. Lymphotoxin and TNF-α secreted by Th1 cells may activate neutrophils and enhance their ability to phagocytose and kill pathogens. IL-2, TNF-β, and IFN-γ secreted by Th1 cells may promote the proliferation of Th1 cells, Th2 cells, CTLs, and NK cells, amplifying the effector functions of cell-mediated immunity. IFN-γ also promotes class switching of activated B cells to produce opsonizing antibodies (IgG1 and IgG3), enhancing phagocytosis and killing of intracellular pathogens by macrophages through opsonization.

Th2 Cells Infections by extracellular pathogens (virus, bacteria, worm, etc.), and exposure to allergens, may activate pDCs, mast cells, eosinophils, basophils, etc., that secrete IL-4. IL-4 activates transcription factor GATA-3 that induces Th0 cells to differentiate into Th2 cells. Th2 subset plays important roles in response against parasites and in antibody production, a major part of humoral immunity. IL-4, IL-10, IL-13, IL-15, etc., secreted by Th2 cells, together with the binding of CD40L to CD40 on B cells, promote B cells to differentiate into antibody-secreting plasma cells. IL-4 and IL-15 may induce immunoglobulin class switching to IgE, which activate mast cells, eosinophils, and basophils that participate in allergic responses and antiparasitic infections. IL-4 and IL-13 may induce the secretion of TGF-β and IL-10 by macrophages, promoting the formation of collagens that are involved in tissue repairing and fibrosis.

Th17 Cells Infections by extracellular pathogens and fungi may stimulate DCs to secrete inflammatory cytokines such as TGF-β, IL-6, IL-23, etc., which in turn activate transcription factor RORγt that induces Th0 cells to differentiate into Th17 cells. Th17 cells contribute to protection against extracellular pathogens and fungal infections and are considered proinflammatory as they express high levels of proinflammatory cytokine IL-17, as well as IL-6, IL-21, IL-22, IL-26, TNF-α, and CXCL8 that recruits acute inflammatory cells to the site of infection [27]. IL-17 stimulates various types of cells to participate in host immune defense, and also participates in pathogenesis of certain diseases [28, 29].

Tfh Cells Cytokines IL-21 and IL-6 may induce the expression of transcription factor Bcl6 that drives Th0 cells to differentiate into Tfh cells. Tfh cells express CXCR5 and migrate to follicles of the peripheral lymphoid organs to help B cells to activate. Tfh cells secrete IL-21 and express high levels of IL-21R, CD40L, and ICOS. Activated B cells in the germinal center express ICOSL that binds to ICOS on Tfh cells, together with the influence of IL-21, Tfh cells can help B cells to survive, proliferate, and differentiate into antibody-secreting plasma cells in the germinal center. Tfh cells can improve antibody production, class switching, and antibody affinity maturation of B cells.

Th9 Cells Th9 is considered as a distinct subset. Cytokine IL-4 induces Th0 cells to differentiate into Th9 cells, while TGF-β induces interconversion of Th2 cells into Th9 cells [30], which may be further enhanced by IL-1 [28, 31–34]. More recently, IL-1 family members have been shown to be able to trigger an IL-4-independent Th9 differentiation [29, 33]. IL-9 secreted by Th9 cells has both physiological and pathophysiological functions. Th9 cells may play a protective role in antiextracellular parasite and antitumor [34–36] and in controlling fibrosis and mucosal wound healing [29, 37]. On the other hand, Th9 cell-derived IL-9 was shown to favor allergic asthma, especially upon induction of IL-13 and edotoxin [38]. In addition, IL-9-mediated recruitment of Th17 cells participate in the pathogenesis of autoimmune diseases (such as EAE) [34].

Th22 Cells Th22 cells arise from the stimulation of naïve T cells in the presence of IL-6 and TNF-α or the presentation of antigens in the context of pDCs, and their differentiation depends on the transcription factor AHR (aryl hydrocarbon receptor) [29, 39–41]. Th22 is an important T cell subset in the skin. These cells express CCR6 and the skin homing receptors CCR4 and CCR10, allowing infiltration into the skin [39, 42]. Th22 cells are not only observed in normal skin but are also enriched in inflamed skin [26, 43], especially in the epidermal compartment as compared to dermis in patients with inflammatory skin diseases [26, 44]. These observations suggest Th22 cell-derived IL-22 contributes not only to skin homeostasis but also the pathogenesis of skin diseases [45].

Treg Cells Natural regulatory T (nTreg) cells are a subset of T cells formed in the thymus; alternatively, induced regulatory T (iTreg) cells are induced in the periphery from $CD4^+$ T cells in the presence of TGF-β [46, 47]. Treg cells are most commonly characterized by the expression of transcription factor Foxp3. They are primarily responsible for controlling immune responses and are critical to the development and maintenance of self-tolerance, elimination of autoreactive cells, prevention of autoimmune diseases, and maintenance of immune homeostasis [48, 49]. Treg cells suppress the activation and expansion of $CD4^+$ Th cells, differentiation of cytotoxic $CD8^+$ T cells, and activation of B cells [49–53]. In the context of transplantation, Treg cells are vital to the induction and maintenance of allograft tolerance [47].

3.2.3.2 $CD8^+$ T Cells: Differentiation and Effector Functions

Naïve $CD8^+$ T cells recognize antigenic peptides, which are loaded in the cytosolic compartment in the context of MHC class I molecules [1, 18]. The differentiation of naïve $CD8^+$ T cells not only requires the specific recognition between TCR and peptide:MHC class I complex, but also the costimulatory signals and/or the help of Th cells.

$CD8^+$ T Cell Activation

$CD8^+$ T cells may be activated in two ways depending on their demand for Th cells. One way is the activation of naïve $CD8^+$ T cells by mature DCs with high intrinsic costimulatory activity without the help of Th cells. These naïve $CD8^+$ T cells require stronger costimulatory signals to be activated than do naïve $CD4^+$ T cells. In certain viral infections, DCs are fully activated and directly induce $CD8^+$ T cells to produce IL-2 required for their proliferation and differentiation without the help of Th cells. This property of DCs has been exploited to generate cytotoxic T cell responses against tumors. The other way is the activation of naïve $CD8^+$ T cells requiring the help of Th cells. In most viral infections, $CD8^+$ T cells recognize antigenic peptides on virus-infected APCs expressing weak costimulatory molecules, these $CD8^+$ T cells become activated only in the presence of Th cells recognizing related antigens on the same APCs. APCs are then activated by Th cells, inducing higher expression of costimulatory signals that compensate for inadequate costimulation of naïve $CD8^+$ T cells, Th cells may also produce abundant IL-2 to promote the proliferation and differentiation of $CD8^+$ T cells.

T Cell-Mediated Cytotoxicity

$CD8^+$ cytotoxic T cells (CTLs) are specialized in defense against intracellular pathogens (especially viruses) and mutated cells, by direct killing of infected cells and tumor cells through the induction of apoptosis or cell lysis. They store preformed cytotoxins in specialized cytotoxic granules and the release of cytotoxins is tightly focused at the site of contact with the target cells, thus killing them without harming any uninfected cells nearby. CTLs may kill any pathogen-infected cells by recognizing foreign peptides presented by MHC class I molecules on the surface of target cells and four principle mechanisms are involved in T cell-mediated cytotoxicity (Fig. 3.2): (1) The calcium-dependent release of specialized cytotoxic granules containing three types of cytotoxic effector proteins: perforin, granzyme, and granulysin. These proteins are stored in the cytotoxic granules in an active form but are not functioning until after their release. Perforin acts in the delivery of granzyme into target cell; granzyme induces apoptosis in almost any type of target cell; and granulysin, which only expresses in humans, exhibits antimicrobial activity, and induces apoptosis in target cell at high concentrations. These proteins allow cytotoxic T cells to attack and destroy virtually any cell infected with cytosolic pathogens. (2) Another way to induce apoptosis on some target cells is through Fas-Fas ligand interaction. The membrane bound Fas ligands, expressed by $CD8^+$ T cells, bind to their Fas on target cells and kill the designated cells. (3) CTLs may also induce apoptosis of target cells by interacting with TNFR1 expressed on target cells through TNF-α. (4) Cytotoxic T cells produce IFN-γ that inhibits viral replication and is an important inducer of MHC class I molecule expression and macrophage activation. Cytotoxic T cells kill infected target cells without harming normal cells, which is crucial in terms of minimizing tissue damage while allowing complete clearance of infected cells. Once $CD8^+$ T cells have differentiated into CTLs, they can respond to their target cells without costimulation.

3.3 The Humoral Immune Response

The humoral immune response is mediated by antibodies and protects the extracellular space. Upon the entrance of extracellular pathogens, BCRs recognize and bind to antigens, with the help of T cells and their cytokines, antigen-specific B cells activate, proliferate, and differentiate into antibody-secreting plasma cells and memory B cells. Plasma cells can produce antigen-specific antibodies into the extracellular space, leading to the destruction of extracellular pathogens and the prevention of spreading intracellular infections. The humoral immune response can be broadly classified into two major categories based on different types of antigens: the immune response against thymus-dependent antigens (TD-Ag) that requires help of T cells, and the immune response against thymus-independent antigens (TI-Ag) that does not require help of T cells [1–4].

3.3.1 B Cell-Mediated Immune Response to TD-Ag

TD-Ag is unable to induce a humoral immune response in animals or humans lacking T cells; therefore, help of T cells is necessary for the induction of an immune response to TD-Ag.

3.3.1.1 TD-Ag Recognition and Presentation by B Cells

The B-cell receptors (BCRs) may directly recognize and bind to a vast variety of specific antigenic epitopes. Antigen recognition of BCR is different from that of TCR in three ways: first, BCR can recognize many chemical structures other than proteins; second, BCR can recognize the natural conformation of a full antigen, or the special conformation of exposed epitopes after antigen degradation; third, B cell recognition does not rely on the processing and presentation by APCs and is not MHC restricted. TD-Ag bound by BCR on the B cell internalizes and returns to the cell surface as peptide:MHC class II complex, helper T cell recognizes this complex and then delivers activating signals to B cell, leading to the proliferation and differentiation of the B cell. The B cell can only be activated by helper T cell that recognizes the same antigen, known as linked recognition (Fig. 3.3).

3.3.1.2 B Cell Activation

Two signals are required for B cell activation: the first signal (signal 1) in B cell activation, also known as the antigen stimulation signal, is delivered by specific recognition between TD-Ag and the BCR (including BCR-Igα and Igβ complexes and B-cell coreceptors CD19, CD21, CD81). The binding between BCR and its specific TD-Ag initiates signal 1, which is delivered by Igα and Igβ and transferred into B cell. The second signal (signal 2) in B cell activation, also known as the costimulatory signal, is delivered by costimulatory molecules that can fully activate B cell. B cell responsiveness to an antigen is greatly enhanced by signaling through the B-cell coreceptor complex.

One particularly important set of costimulatory molecules involved in signal 2 are the TNF family member CD40 expressing on B cells and CD40L expressing on activated Th cells. B cells present peptide:MHC complexes to Th cells, and the interaction between antigen-binding B cells and Th cells leads to the expression of B-cell stimulatory molecule CD40L on Th cells. Binding of CD40 by CD40L helps to drive resting B cells into the cell cycle and respond to TD antigens (Fig. 3.3). B cells that have bound antigens become selectively trapped in the right location to maximize their chance of encountering Th cells that can activate them. Antigen-stimulated B cells that fail to interact with Th cells recognizing the same antigens die within 24 h. In addition, CD30 and CD30L (CD153), 4-IBB, and 4-IBBL, etc., are

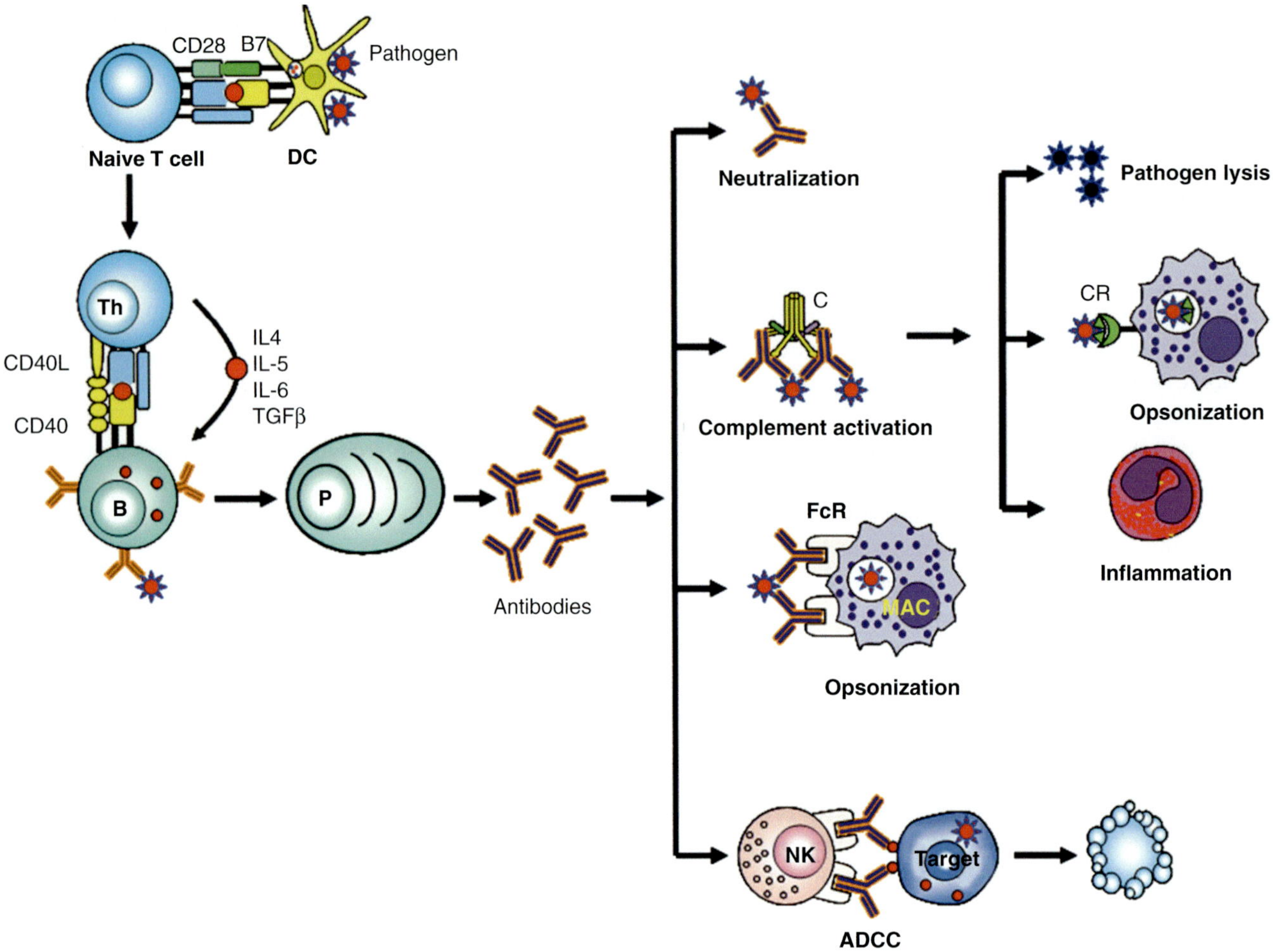

Fig. 3.3 The humoral immune response to TD-Ag and the effector functions of antibodies. *Th* helper T cell, *B* B cell, *P* plasma cells, *NK* NK cell, *MAC* macrophage, *FcR* Fc receptor, *C* complement, *CR* complement receptor, *ADCC* antibody-dependent cell-mediated cytotoxicity

also sets of costimulatory molecules that may participate in the interaction between B cells and Th cells.

A variety of cytokine receptors are expressed on activated B cells, which respond to cytokines secreted by activated Th cells. B cell stimulatory cytokines IL-4, IL-5, IL-6, and TGF-β secreted by activated Th cells induce B cell proliferation and are essential in the formation of germinal center and further differentiation of B cells into antibody-secreting plasma cells (Fig. 3.3). Alternatively, activated B cells can also become memory B cells. Therefore, cytokines are also known as the third signal in B cell activation.

3.3.1.3 B Cell Differentiation and Maturation

Circulating B cells migrate into primary lymphoid follicle of the peripheral lymphoid tissues, where follicular helper T (Tfh) cells help B cells to further activate and proliferate to ultimately form a germinal center (GC). GC is usually formed 3–4 weeks after initial TD-Ag exposure, and serves as an important place for humoral immune responses. Rapid proliferating B cells, also called the centroblasts, are characterized by rapid cell division and proliferation (divide every 6–8 h), downregulated expression of surface Ig, stable expression of CXCR4 and CXCR5, and somatic hypermutation of their Ig genes. The centroblasts divide and proliferate to produce daughter cells known as the centrocytes, characterized by upregulated expression of surface Ig and sustained expression of CXCR5, they stop dividing and receive costimulatory signals from T cells and follicular DCs (FDCs). Massive proliferating centroblasts aggregate and form the dark zone of GC, while slower proliferating centrocytes, Tfh cells, and FDCs form the light zone of GC. Resting B cells are being pushed to the periphery of the follicle, forming the mantle zone.

Activated B cells enter the light zone after somatic hypermutation. In the light zone, centrocytes continue to differentiate with the synergic help of FDCs and Tfh cells and complete their affinity maturation through positive selection. Only those minority clones with enhanced BCR affinity and expression of antiapoptotic proteins may survive. Selective cells with higher affinity surface Ig expression differentiate into antibody-secreting plasma cells or memory B cells through class switching, while others undergo apoptosis. Class switching is antigen induced, and is directly regulated by cytokines secreted by Th cells. For instance, Th2 cell-derived IL-4 favors class switching to IgG1 and IgE, TGF-β favors class switching to IgG2b and IgA; Th1 cell-derived IFN-γ favors class switching to IgG2a and IgG2. Class switching is the basis for the production of various antibodies with different effector functions. Somatic hypermutation and class switching play important roles in the diversity of antibodies.

Plasma cells can secrete abundant antibodies against specific antigens. They lack the expression of BCR and MHC class II molecule; therefore, they do not interact with either antigens or Th cells (Fig. 3.3). Some of the plasma cells are short lived and remain in the lymphoid organs, while the majority of the plasma cells are long lived and migrate to the bone marrow to continue their antibody production. Some of the B cells differentiate into memory B cells, which are long-lived descendants of cells that were once stimulated by antigens and had proliferated in the GC. Memory B cells leave the GC, enter the bloodstream, and recirculate in the system, where they can be activated very fast upon second challenge with the same antigen, leading to abundant production of antigen-specific antibodies.

3.3.2 B Cell-Mediated Immune Response to TI-Ag

Many microbial constituents, such as bacterial polysaccharides, polymeric proteins, and lipopolysaccharides (LPS), can activate naïve B cells and induce antibody production in the absence of Th cells. These microbial antigens are known as thymus-independent or TI antigens because they can induce humoral immune responses without the help of T cells. B cells responding to TI-Ag do not undergo affinity maturation, they cannot develop into memory B cells and they only produce IgM. TI antigens can be classified into TI-1 and TI-2 antigens based on the mechanisms of activation.

3.3.2.1 B Cell-Mediated Immune Response to TI-1 Ag

TI-1 antigens such as LPS and bacterial DNA can directly induce division of most B cells without antigen specificity, this is commonly known as polyclonal activation. TI-1 antigens are often referred to as B cell mitogens because they bind to mitogen receptors on B cells and induce the proliferation and differentiation of B cells without helper T cells. They can activate both immature and mature B cells leading to low affinity IgM production. They may induce polyclonal B cell responses at high concentration and induce antigen-specific antibody responses to those TI-1 antigen specific B cells at low concentration.

3.3.2.2 B Cell-Mediated Immune Response to TI-2 Ag

TI-2 antigens are highly repetitive structures on the bacterial cells including bacterial cell wall and capsular polysaccharides. TI-2 antigens are mainly recognized by B1 cells and they can only activate mature B1 cells. Multiple cross-linking of the BCR by TI-2 antigens can lead to IgM production. A cytokine released by activated DCs, known as BAFF, can augment antibody production against TI-2 antigens and induce class switching to IgG.

3.3.3 Effector Functions of the Humoral Immune Response

The extracellular space is protected by the humoral immune response. Antibodies produced by plasma cells cause the destruction of extracellular pathogens and prevent the spreading of intracellular infections. Antibodies fulfill their effector functions through neutralization, complement activation, opsonization, destruction of antibody-coated pathogens via Fc receptors, etc.

First, antibodies can inhibit toxicity of toxic molecules or infectivity of pathogens by binding to them, a process termed neutralization. For example, high-affinity IgG and IgA antibodies can neutralize bacterial toxins and inhibit infectivity of viruses. Antibodies can block adherence of bacteria to host cells and prevent pathogenic intrusion. Neutralization by antibodies is important in preventing pathogens and bacterial toxins from entering cells. Second, antibodies can coat the surfaces of pathogens to make them more easily ingested by phagocytes, a process termed opsonization. Third, antibodies of appropriate isotype can activate the classical pathway of complement by binding to pathogens. Complement proteins bound to the pathogen surface opsonize the pathogen by binding complement receptors on phagocyte; these antibodies can strongly enhance opsonization of pathogens. Other complement components recruit phagocytic cells to the site of infection, and the terminal components of complement can directly kill certain bacterial cells. Complement receptors are important in the removal of immune complexes from the circulation. The last but also the most important effector function of antibodies is the destruction of antibody-coated pathogens via Fc receptors. Fc receptors on phagocytes are activated by antibodies bound to the surface of pathogens, enabling ingestion and destruction of pathogens through phagocytosis, granule release, or both. Fc receptors comprise a family of proteins, each of which recognizes immunoglobulins of a particular isotype. Pathogens coated with IgG or IgA antibodies are recognized and destroyed by macrophages and neutrophils because their Fc receptors bind the constant regions of IgG or IgA. Whereas mast cells, basophils, and activated eosinophils bind IgE antibodies via the high-affinity Fcε receptors. IgE-mediated activation of accessory cells has an important role in antiparasitic infection and allergy. Binding to the Fc receptor also induces the production of microbicidal agents in the intracellular vesicles of the phagocytes. NK cells can recognize and destroy antibody-coated target cells in a process termed antibody-dependent cell-mediated cytotoxicity (ADCC). Most ADCC are mediated by NK cells expressing Fc receptor FcγRIII (CD16) on their surface and play an important role in defense against viral infections (Fig. 3.3).

References

1. Paul WE. Fundamental immunology. 7th ed. Philadelphia: Wolters Kluwer Health/Lippincot Williams & Wilkins; 2012.
2. Murphy K. Janeway's immunology. 8th ed. New York: Garland Science; 2011.
3. Abbas AK, Lichtman AH, Pillai S. Cellular and molecular immunology. 6th ed. Philadelphia: Saunders; 2010.
4. Parslow TG, Stites DP, Terry AI, Imboden JB. Medical immunology. 10th ed. New York: McGraw-Hill/Appleton & Lange; 2001.
5. Sercarz EE, Maverakis E. Mhc-guided processing: binding of large antigen fragments. Nat Rev Immunol. 2003;3(8):621–9.
6. Wang JH, Reinherz EL. Structural basis of T cell recognition of peptides bound to MHC molecules. Mol Immunol. 2002;38(14):1039–49.
7. Zamoyska R. CD4 and CD8: modulators of T-cell receptor recognition of antigen and of immune responses? Curr Opin Immunol. 1998;10(1):82–7.
8. Gromme M, Neefjes J. Antigen degradation or presentation by MHC class I molecules via classical and non-classical pathways. Mol Immunol. 2002;39(3–4):181–202.
9. Williams A, Peh CA, Elliott T. The cell biology of MHC class I antigen presentation. Tissue Antigens. 2002;59(1):3–17.
10. Schubert U, Anton LC, Gibbs J, Norbury CC, Yewdell JW, Bennink JR. Rapid degradation of a large fraction of newly synthesized proteins by proteasomes. Nature. 2000;404(6779):770–4.
11. Rock KL, York IA, Saric T, Goldberg AL. Protein degradation and the generation of MHC class I-presented peptides. Adv Immunol. 2002;80:1–70.
12. Villadangos JA. Presentation of antigens by MHC class II molecules: getting the most out of them. Mol Immunol. 2001;38(5): 329–46.
13. Lennon-Dumenil AM, Bakker AH, Wolf-Bryant P, Ploegh HL, Lagaudriere-Gesbert C. A closer look at proteolysis and MHC-class-II-restricted antigen presentation. Curr Opin Immunol. 2002;14(1):15–21.
14. Ackerman AL, Cresswell P. Cellular mechanisms governing cross-presentation of exogenous antigens. Nat Immunol. 2004;5(7): 678–84.
15. Cooper AM. Cell-mediated immune responses in tuberculosis. Annu Rev Immunol. 2009;27:393–422.
16. Kaufmann SH. Tuberculosis vaccines: time to think about the next generation. Semin Immunol. 2013;25(2):172–81.
17. Stenger S, Hanson DA, Teitelbaum R, Dewan P, Niazi KR, Froelich CJ, et al. An antimicrobial activity of cytolytic T cells mediated by granulysin. Science. 1998;282(5386):121–5.
18. Prezzemolo T, Guggino G, La Manna MP, Di Liberto D, Dieli F, Caccamo N. Functional signatures of human CD4 and CD8 T cell responses to mycobacterium tuberculosis. Front Immunol. 2014;5:180.
19. Bottino C, Castriconi R, Pende D, Rivera P, Nanni M, Carnemolla B, et al. Identification of PVR (CD155) and Nectin-2 (CD112) as cell surface ligands for the human DNAM-1 (CD226) activating molecule. J Exp Med. 2003;198(4):557–67.
20. Joller N, Peters A, Anderson AC, Kuchroo VK. Immune checkpoints in central nervous system autoimmunity. Immunol Rev. 2012;248(1):122–39.
21. Bour-Jordan H, Esensten JH, Martinez-Llordella M, Penaranda C, Stumpf M, Bluestone JA. Intrinsic and extrinsic control of peripheral T-cell tolerance by costimulatory molecules of the CD28/B7 family. Immunol Rev. 2011;241(1):180–205.
22. Alegre ML, Noel PJ, Eisfelder BJ, Chuang E, Clark MR, Reiner SL, et al. Regulation of surface and intracellular expression of CTLA4 on mouse T cells. J Immunol. 1996;157(11):4762–70.
23. Paterson AM, Vanguri VK, Sharpe AH. SnapShot: B7/CD28 costimulation. Cell. 2009;137(5):974–4.e1.
24. Walunas TL, Bakker CY, Bluestone JA. CTLA-4 ligation blocks CD28-dependent T cell activation. J Exp Med. 1996;183(6):2541–50.
25. Linsley PS, Brady W, Urnes M, Grosmaire LS, Damle NK, Ledbetter JA. CTLA-4 is a second receptor for the B cell activation antigen B7. J Exp Med. 1991;174(3):561–9.
26. Eyerich S, Eyerich K, Pennino D, Carbone T, Nasorri F, Pallotta S, et al. Th22 cells represent a distinct human T cell subset involved in epidermal immunity and remodeling. J Clin Invest. 2009;119(12): 3573–85.
27. Wuthrich M, Deepe Jr GS, Klein B. Adaptive immunity to fungi. Annu Rev Immunol. 2012;30:115–48.
28. Sie C, Korn T, Mitsdoerffer M. Th17 cells in central nervous system autoimmunity. Exp Neurol. 2014; 262(A):18-27.
29. Bouchery T, Kyle R, Ronchese F, Le Gros G. The differentiation of CD4(+) T-helper cell subsets in the context of Helminth parasite infection. Front Immunol. 2014;5:487.
30. Veldhoen M, Uyttenhove C, van Snick J, Helmby H, Westendorf A, Buer J, et al. Transforming growth factor-beta 'reprograms' the differentiation of T helper 2 cells and promotes an interleukin 9-producing subset. Nat Immunol. 2008;9(12):1341–6.
31. Schmitt E, Beuscher HU, Huels C, Monteyne P, van Brandwijk R, van Snick J, et al. IL-1 serves as a secondary signal for IL-9 expression. J Immunol. 1991;147(11):3848–54.
32. Schmitt E, Germann T, Goedert S, Hoehn P, Huels C, Koelsch S, et al. IL-9 production of naive CD4+ T cells depends on IL-2, is synergistically enhanced by a combination of TGF-beta and IL-4, and is inhibited by IFN-gamma. J Immunol. 1994;153(9):3989–96.
33. Uyttenhove C, Brombacher F, Van Snick J. TGF-beta interactions with IL-1 family members trigger IL-4-independent IL-9 production by mouse CD4(+) T cells. Eur J Immunol. 2010;40(8):2230–5.
34. Schmitt E, Klein M, Bopp T. Th9 cells, new players in adaptive immunity. Trends Immunol. 2014;35(2):61–8.
35. Purwar R, Schlapbach C, Xiao S, Kang HS, Elyaman W, Jiang X, et al. Robust tumor immunity to melanoma mediated by interleukin-9-producing T cells. Nat Med. 2012;18(8):1248–53.
36. Lu Y, Hong S, Li H, Park J, Hong B, Wang L, et al. Th9 cells promote antitumor immune responses in vivo. J Clin Invest. 2012;122(11):4160–71.
37. Lo Re S, Lison D, Huaux F. CD4+ T lymphocytes in lung fibrosis: diverse subsets, diverse functions. J Leukoc Biol. 2013;93(4):499–510.
38. Kerzerho J, Maazi H, Speak AO, Szely N, Lombardi V, Khoo B, et al. Programmed cell death ligand 2 regulates TH9 differentiation and induction of chronic airway hyperreactivity. J Allergy Clin Immunol. 2013;131(4):1048–57, 57 e1–2.
39. Duhen T, Geiger R, Jarrossay D, Lanzavecchia A, Sallusto F. Production of interleukin 22 but not interleukin 17 by a subset of human skin-homing memory T cells. Nat Immunol. 2009;10(8): 857–63.

40. Ramirez JM, Brembilla NC, Sorg O, Chicheportiche R, Matthes T, Dayer JM, et al. Activation of the aryl hydrocarbon receptor reveals distinct requirements for IL-22 and IL-17 production by human T helper cells. Eur J Immunol. 2010;40(9):2450–9.
41. Veldhoen M, Hirota K, Christensen J, O'Garra A, Stockinger B. Natural agonists for aryl hydrocarbon receptor in culture medium are essential for optimal differentiation of Th17 T cells. J Exp Med. 2009;206(1):43–9.
42. Trifari S, Kaplan CD, Tran EH, Crellin NK, Spits H. Identification of a human helper T cell population that has abundant production of interleukin 22 and is distinct from T(H)-17, T(H)1 and T(H)2 cells. Nat Immunol. 2009;10(8):864–71.
43. Nograles KE, Zaba LC, Guttman-Yassky E, Fuentes-Duculan J, Suarez-Farinas M, Cardinale I, et al. Th17 cytokines interleukin (IL)-17 and IL-22 modulate distinct inflammatory and keratinocyte-response pathways. Br J Dermatol. 2008;159(5):1092–102.
44. Res PC, Piskin G, de Boer OJ, van der Loos CM, Teeling P, Bos JD, et al. Overrepresentation of IL-17A and IL-22 producing CD8 T cells in lesional skin suggests their involvement in the pathogenesis of psoriasis. PLoS One. 2010;5(11):e14108.
45. Fujita H. The role of IL-22 and Th22 cells in human skin diseases. J Dermatol Sci. 2013;72(1):3–8.
46. Chen W, Jin W, Hardegen N, Lei KJ, Li L, Marinos N, et al. Conversion of peripheral CD4+CD25- naive T cells to CD4+CD25+ regulatory T cells by TGF-beta induction of transcription factor Foxp3. J Exp Med. 2003;198(12):1875–86.
47. Abdoli R, Najafian N. T helper cells fate mapping by co-stimulatory molecules and its functions in allograft rejection and tolerance. Int J Organ Transplant Med. 2014;5(3):97–110.
48. Campbell DJ, Koch MA. Phenotypical and functional specialization of FOXP3+ regulatory T cells. Nat Rev Immunol. 2011; 11(2):119–30.
49. Ohl K, Tenbrock K. Regulatory T cells in systemic lupus erythematosus. Eur J Immunol. 2014;45:344–55.
50. Takahashi T, Tagami T, Yamazaki S, Uede T, Shimizu J, Sakaguchi N, et al. Immunologic self-tolerance maintained by CD25(+)CD4(+) regulatory T cells constitutively expressing cytotoxic T lymphocyte-associated antigen 4. J Exp Med. 2000;192(2):303–10.
51. Thornton AM, Shevach EM. CD4+CD25+ immunoregulatory T cells suppress polyclonal T cell activation in vitro by inhibiting interleukin 2 production. J Exp Med. 1998;188(2):287–96.
52. McNally A, Hill GR, Sparwasser T, Thomas R, Steptoe RJ. CD4+CD25+ regulatory T cells control CD8+ T-cell effector differentiation by modulating IL-`omeostasis. Proc Natl Acad Sci U S A. 2011;108(18):7529–34.
53. Lim HW, Hillsamer P, Banham AH, Kim CH. Cutting edge: direct suppression of B cells by CD4+ CD25+ regulatory T cells. J Immunol. 2005;175(7):4180–3.

Immunotolerance and Immunoregulation

4

Haoyu Sun, Cheng Sun, and Zhigang Tian

Contents

H. Sun • C. Sun
Institute of Immunology, School of Life Sciences and Medical Center, University of Science and Technology of China, Hefei, China

Z. Tian (✉)
Institute of Immunology, School of Life Sciences and Medical Center, University of Science and Technology of China, Hefei, China
e-mail: tzg@ustc.edu.cn

4.1 Immunotolerance

The immune system clears pathogens and microorganisms by responding to antigen stimulation under normal circumstances; this is often referred to as the positive immune response. In contrast, the immune system may develop "unresponsiveness" specific to certain antigens after antigen stimulation, which is often referred to as immunological tolerance (immunotolerance), or negative immune response. Antigens that can induce immunotolerance are generally known as tolerogens [1–4]. Immunotolerance can also be defined by the complete absence or partial inhibition of a potentially harmful adaptive immune response. It operates continuously in order to protect mammals not only from the deleterious attack of self-tissues, but also from the rejection of semiallogeneic offspring and uncontrolled immune responses against foreign antigens [5–9]. Immunotolerance can be classified into either natural immunotolerance or acquired immunotolerance based on the characteristics of its formation or it can be classified into either central tolerance or peripheral tolerance based on the stage and location of its formation.

4.1.1 Natural Immunotolerance

Natural immunotolerance is formed during embryonic stage or shortly after birth. During embryonic development, immature T and B cells are stimulated by either self-antigens or foreign antigens, despite the source of stimulation, they all contribute to immunotolerance to specific antigens. Reexposure to these antigens after birth results in "unresponsiveness" of the immune system. Natural immunotolerance may persist for a very long period of time and is very hard to be broken [1–4].

4.1.2 Acquired Immunotolerance

Acquired immunotolerance develops when T and B cells that are originally responsive to antigens lose their responsiveness

X.-H. Gao, H.-D. Chen (eds.), *Practical Immunodermatology*, DOI 10.1007/978-94-024-0902-4_4

under the influence of a variety of factors, producing abnormally low or even no response to these antigens. This type of immunotolerance often fades away as the influential factors weakened, restores appropriate immune responses to these antigens. Acquired immunotolerance can be artificially induced after repeated injection of specific antigens, or the tolerogens. Two main factors contributing to the development of acquired immunotolerance are the antigen and the host system [1–4].

4.1.2.1 Antigens

Antigens are the primary source to induce acquired immunotolerance, which usually depends on the dosage, type, persistency, epitope property, and the way of administration of antigens.

Dosages of Antigen Administration Different dosages of antigen administration surely affect the formation of immunotolerance, this was initially reported by Mitchison in 1964, he discovered that only appropriate dosage of BSA can result in the production of specific antibodies when injecting mice with different dosages. Immunotolerance can be induced by very low dosage or very high dosage of antigen administration, which are often referred to as the low-zone tolerance or high-zone tolerance. The low-zone tolerance is formed due to insufficient dosage of antigens in activating T and B cells. The high-zone tolerance is formed due to overactivation of lymphocytes and induction of apoptosis or the activation of inhibitory T cells that inhibit the immune responses. Low dosage of TD antigens may induce T cell tolerance – the low-zone tolerance, while high dosage of TD antigens may induce both T- and B-cell tolerance – the high-zone tolerance. T cell tolerance usually requires about 100–10,000 times lower antigen dosage than that of B cells, and it happens very fast and persists for months to years; B cells, on the other hand, require a much higher dosage to form tolerance and it happens very slow and only persists for weeks.

Types and Epitopes of the Antigen Type of antigens also affects the formation of immunotolerance. For example, the naturally soluble proteins are composed of monomers and aggregates, antibody production can only be induced when injecting mice with full BSA, but not with BSA monomers alone; this is because protein monomers alone are difficult to be caught and presented to T cells, and B cells cannot produce specific antibodies without the help of T cells. In addition, different antigen epitopes also contribute to the formation of immunotolerance. For example, HEL epitope composed of N terminus amino acids induces activation of Treg cells, while epitope composed of C terminus amino acids induces activation of Th cells. Deleting three amino acids at the N terminus of HEL may eliminate the epitope that activates Treg cells, which in turn activates Th cells that further help B cells to produce specific antibodies. The epitope that induces the activation of Treg cells is also called tolerogenic epitope.

Ways of Antigen Administration Organism shows different levels of susceptibility to different ways of administration: intravenous injection of antigens is the easiest way to induce tolerance, followed by intraperitoneal injection, intramuscular injection, and finally subcutaneous injection that is considered the hardest way to induce tolerance. Oral administration induces systemic tolerance.

Persistent Presence of the Antigen Persistent presentation of autoantigens to T cells without costimulatory signals from APCs results in overactivation of T cells and induction of apoptosis, inducing specific tolerance of T cells to these autoantigens.

4.1.2.2 Host Factors

Besides antigen factors, host factors such as age, developmental stages, physiological status, and genetic background all contribute to the formation of immunotolerance [1–4].

4.1.3 Central Tolerance

Recognition of self-antigens by immature lymphocytes in the thymus and bone marrow during embryonic stage or shortly after birth leads to negative signals causing death or inactivation of the lymphocytes, resulting in self-tolerance to self-antigens known as the central tolerance. Central tolerance is an important mechanism underlying the induction of self-tolerance in lymphocytes developing in the thymus and bone marrow. Self-reactive thymocytes are deleted from the repertoire during T cell development in the thymus, and autoreactive B cells undergone a similar process in the bone marrow, a process known as negative selection.

4.1.3.1 Central T-Cell Tolerance

During the development in the thymus, immature T cells pass positive selection and undergo clonal deletion after recognizing self-antigens, forming central T cell tolerance.

4.1.3.2 Central B-Cell Tolerance

Immature B cells expressing IgM alone bind to self-antigens during negative selection in the bone marrow, resulting in cell death or inactivation that leads to the formation of central B-cell tolerance. There are four possible mechanisms underlying central B-cell tolerance depending on the nature of self-antigens being recognized: cell death by apoptosis or clonal deletion; production of a new receptor by receptor editing; induction of a permanent state of unresponsiveness, or anergy to an antigen; and a state of immunological ignorance. Immature B cells recognizing multivalent self-antigens undergo programmed cell death or apoptosis (clonal deletion), these cells may also undergo receptor editing to get rid of self-reactive receptor specificity. Immature B cells binding to self-antigens capable of cross-linking BCRs are rendered unresponsiveness to the antigens (anergic) and bear little surface IgM. They migrate to the periphery where they express IgD but remain anergic and they are rapidly lost in case of a competition with other B cells. Immature B cells whose antigens are inaccessible or recognizing monovalent/soluble self-antigens with low affinity do not receive any signal and mature normally. Such cells are potentially self-reactive; however, they are said to be clonally ignorant because they cannot be activated although their ligands are present [1–4].

4.1.4 Peripheral Tolerance

Peripheral tolerance refers to the "unresponsiveness" of mature T and B cells upon encountering either endogenous or exogenous antigens. Although central tolerance may eliminate the majority of autoreactive lymphocytes, it is not perfect. Undeleted autoreactive lymphocytes from central tolerance are restrained by the peripheral tolerance once they have entered peripheral lymphoid organs. Several mechanisms contribute to the peripheral tolerance, including clonal deletion, clonal anergy, clonal ignorance, antigen segregation, regulation by immune cells and cytokines, etc. Clonal deletion and clonal anergy also happen in the periphery, but from a very different perspective.

4.1.4.1 Clonal Deletion

Clonal deletion occurs when either the concentration of self-antigens or the affinity of lymphocytes toward self-antigens is very high. Autoreactive T cells binding to their self-antigen peptide:MHC complexes or autoreactive B cells binding to their self-antigens with high affinity induces extensive cross-linking between TCRs or BCRs, leading to the programmed cell death of these autoreactive lymphocytes through clonal deletion.

4.1.4.2 Clonal Anergy

Autoreactive T cells binding to their self-antigens provide the first signal for T cell activation; however, without sufficient second signal from APCs, these T cells transit into the state of anergy. Similarly, autoreactive B cells may undergo anergy in the absence of the help signal from Th cells during activation.

4.1.4.3 Clonal Ignorance

Low concentration of self-antigens, low affinity of lymphocytes toward self-antigens, ineffective presentation of self-antigens, or isolation of autoreactive lymphocytes from self-antigens by biological barrier may contribute to the unresponsiveness of autoreactive lymphocytes and the coexistence of both in the system without inducing any autoimmunity, referring to as clonal ignorance.

4.1.4.4 Antigen Segregation

From an immunological perspective, certain parts of the system are special in that they develop their own tolerance to prevent reject reaction of allograft tissues after transplantation and these tissues may survive for a very long term. These sites are often referred to as the immunologically privileged sites, and the occurrence of such sites is usually due to: (1) isolation of tissue cells from entering circulation and immune cells from entering isolated sites by biological barrier; (2) induction of Th2 type responses that suppress Th1 type responses by local microenvironment; (3) apoptosis of Fas-expressing lymphocytes by binding to Fas ligands; and (4) inhibition of T cell responses by producing inhibitory cytokines or expressing PD-1 ligands [1–4].

4.1.4.5 Role of Immune Cells

Regulatory T cells play an important role in immunotolerance. Specialized autoreactive nTreg cells developed in the thymus may carry out their regulatory functions by direct cell-to-cell contact. iTreg cells induced from naïve self-reactive T cells in the peripheral mainly fulfill their regulatory function by secreting IL-10 and TGF-β. In addition, various immune cells such as dendritic cells, macrophages, and NK cells all participate in the formation and maintenance of immunotolerance. They contribute to the homeostasis of the microenvironment either directly or indirectly (see Sect. 4.2) [9–13].

4.1.4.6 Role of Immune Molecules

A variety of immune molecules participate in the formation of immunotolerance, including inhibitory receptors, coinhibitory receptors, cytokines, etc., they play an important role in the maintenance of immunotolerance and homeostasis of the microenvironment (see Sect. 4.2) [14].

The induction or breaking of immunotolerance is usually associated with a variety of diseases, the balance between immune tolerance and immune response is critical in terms of pathology. Patients with autoimmune diseases are likely to be cured by restoring immunotolerance against self-antigens, while patients with chronic infections and tumors are likely to be cured by breaking pathologic tolerance to restore normal immune responses. Induction of immunotolerance is often accomplished by administration of antigens, use of soluble antigens or antagonist peptides, inhibition of costimulatory signals, induction of Th2 type responses etc. Breaking of immunotolerance is often accomplished by blocking inhibitory molecules, stimulating costimulatory signals, reducing Treg cells or inhibiting Treg cell functions, strengthening DC functions, and the proper usage of cytokines and antibodies.

4.2 Immunoregulation

Immunoregulation refers to the interactions between immune cells, immune cells, and immune molecules, immune system and other systems that constitute a mutually coordinating and restricting interactive network. An effective immune response is the outcome of the interplay between positive and negative regulators. In this chapter, we focus on the negative regulation of the immune response, termed as immunoregulation. Immunoregulation coordinates the entire process of immune response, involving various immune molecules (antibody, complement, cell surface receptor, cytokine, etc.), immune cells (T cells, B cells, NK cells, DC, and macrophage), and the immune-endocrine-nervous systems.

4.2.1 Immunoregulation by Antibodies and Complements

4.2.1.1 Antibodies

Antibodies have been shown to exert feedback control on the immune response. Antibodies produced in response to specific antigen stimulations may inhibit humoral immune responses, referring to as the antibody negative feedback effect. IgG antibodies can suppress the immune responses via direct antibody blocking or antibody feedback. IgG complexed with an antigen and a surface Fc receptor (FcγRII) on B cell leads to the cross-linking of FcγRII with BCR, which may suppress the signaling of the BCR [1–4].

4.2.1.2 Complements

Complement system has evolved to aid in the host defense by directly damaging invading pathogens and by inducing tissue inflammation. The regulatory control of the system is critical in preventing complement-mediated destruction of the host tissues. The feedback effect involves certain regulatory proteins of the complement system that strictly control the activation of the system, preventing unnecessary damages to the tissues [1–4].

4.2.2 Immunoregulation by Inhibitory and Coinhibitory Receptors

Membrane surface receptors can be broadly classified into activating receptors and inhibitory receptors. Activating receptors are often accompanied by ITAM that contributes to the recruitment of protein tyrosine kinase (PTK), which in turn initiates activating signal transduction. In contrast, inhibitory receptors bearing ITIM that recruits protein tyrosine phosphatase (PTP) results in the blocking of the activating signal transduction. ITIM often works as a feedback control to ensure proper amount of immune responses by negative regulation while permitting limited activation signals for effective immune functions. Besides inhibitory receptors, coinhibitory receptors are also important in terms of negative regulation and they have recently been recognized as promising therapeutic targets in cancer, as blocking their signaling pathways may enhance antitumor immune responses [15, 16].

4.2.2.1 CTLA-4

CTLA-4 (cytotoxic T lymphocyte-associated protein 4) is a coinhibitory receptor expressed on the surface of CD4 and CD8 T cells as well as on $CD25^+Foxp3^+$ Treg cells [17]. CTLA-4 is a member of the CD28 immunoglobulin superfamily and competes with CD28 for the binding of its ligands B7-1 (CD80) and B7-2 (CD86) [18]. CD28 delivers a positive costimulatory signal that is essential for optimal T cell proliferation and effector functions as well as the prevention of programmed cell death [19–21]. In contrast, CTLA-4 delivers a coinhibitory signal by binding to the same set of ligands (CD80 and CD86) as CD28 with a much higher affinity [22]. CTLA-4 does not express on naïve or resting T cells, but its expression upregulates on the cell surface after T cell activation for at least 24 h and induces a negative signal in T cells [22–25]. Engagement of CTLA-4 inhibits T cell proliferation and activation and induces T cell unresponsiveness, anergy, and tolerance [26]. In addition to direct regulation of T cell responses, CTLA-4 can indirectly regulate T cell responses by modulating the function of Treg cells, which also contribute to the limitation of T cell activation and induction of self-tolerance [15]. Absence of CTLA-4 induces early lethality and multiorgan autoimmunity, suggesting that its role as a key molecule for the regulation of autoimmune diseases [22, 26, 27].

4.2.2.2 PD-1

PD-1 (programmed death-1) is a member of the Ig superfamily and expressed on T cells, B cells, NKT cells, monocytes, DCs upon activation, and immature thymocytes during thymic development [28]. PD-1 binds to two ligands, namely PD-L1 and PD-L2. PD-L1 is expressed on a wide range of hematopoietic as well as nonhematopoietic cells, while the expression of PD-L2 can be induced on DCs, macrophages, bone marrow-derived mast cells, and B1 cells [29, 30]. PD-1 binds to PD-L1 and PD-L2, which suppresses downstream phosphoinositide 3-kinase (PI3K) and Akt signaling via ITIM that in turn inhibits T cell proliferation and activation [18]. PD-1 is induced by TCR signaling and its expression is maintained by persistent antigenic stimulation such as chronic viral infection, cancer, or autoimmunity [31]. PD-1 is the first coinhibitory receptor to be linked with an exhausted T cell phenotype and blockade of PD-1 pathway partially reverses the dysfunctional state and restores T cell effector functions [32].

4.2.2.3 TIGIT

TIGIT (T cell immunoreceptor with Ig and ITIM domains) is also known as Vsig9, Vstm3, or WUCAM, it is a member of the CD28 family that mainly expresses on T cells (particularly on memory T cells, Tfh cells, and Treg cells) and NK cells with an immunoglobulin variable (IgV) domain, a transmembrane domain, and an ITIM that binds to poliovirus receptor (PVR; CD155), nectin-2 (CD112), and possibly nectin-3 (CD-113) [14, 33–39]. CD155 and CD112 mainly express on APCs with CD155 also expressing on a variety of nonhematopoietic cells and was found to be upregulated on a number of tumors [12, 40, 41]. Both ligands of TIGIT are shared with CD226, a costimulatory receptor expressing on T cells [42]. CD226/TIGIT and their ligands CD155/CD112 therefore form a network, with CD226 delivering a positive signal while TIGIT delivering a negative signal. TIGIT can also directly inhibit T cell proliferation in the absence of APCs through its intrinsic effects and promotes T cell maintenance and survival by driving expression of cytokine receptors and anti-apoptotic molecules [35, 38, 43]. TIGIT might therefore play an important role in regulating the threshold of T cell activation and maintaining peripheral tolerance. TIGIT also directly inhibits cytotoxicity of NK cells in both human and mouse, and negatively regulates NK cell activation in vivo by interacting with CD155 expressed on the surface of Kupffer cells [16, 27, 34, 44–46].

4.2.2.4 Tim-3

Tim-3 (T cell Ig and mucin domain 3) is specifically expressed on Th1 cells with a lower expression on Th17 cells but not on Th2 cells [47–50]. Tim-3 binds to its ligand Galectin-9, a β-galactose binding protein that when bound induces calcium influx, cell aggregation, and cell death in vitro [51]. Administration of galectin-9 in vivo causes selective loss of IFN-γ-producing T cells [27, 51]. Blocking of Tim-3 signaling by Tim-3-Ig fusion protein results in hyperproliferation of Th1 cells and increased release of Th1 cytokines IFN-γ and IL-2 [52]. Therefore, Tim-3 serves as an inhibitory molecule that controls proinflammatory Th1 and possibly Th17 responses and prevents uncontrolled inflammation and immunopathology. Tim-3 has recently gained its attention in chronic viral infections and cancer [53–59]. In these settings, Tim-3 marks exhausted T cells that are characterized by failure to proliferate and exert effector functions upon antigen encountering. Furthermore, coexpression of Tim-3 and PD-1 is associated with more severe T cell exhaustion, whereas PD-1^{+}Tim-3^{-} T cells still retain some effector functions [55, 56, 60–62]. In such scenario, blockade of PD-1 only partially restores T cell function, while combined blockade of Tim-3 and PD-1 synergistically improves T cell responses [27, 55, 56].

4.2.2.5 FcγRII

BCR is the activating receptor that mediates antigen recognition and positive signal transduction for B cells. While FcγRII bearing ITIM is the inhibitory receptor that negatively regulates specific humoral immune responses through cross-linking with the BCR and antigen-antibody (antigen-specific) complex. The antigen-antibody complex simultaneously interacts with the BCR (through antigen) and FcγRII (through antibody), which in turn induces inhibitory signals.

4.2.2.6 NK Cell Inhibitory Receptors

NK cells express multiple inhibitory receptors on their surfaces, including KIR, CD94/NKG2A, ILT family, etc. Inhibitory receptors distinguish normal from diseased cells by self: MHC class I molecules, which named the “missing-self” model. Inhibitory receptors provide an educational signal that generates functional NK cells. Different regulatory NK cell subsets are found and enriched in the immunotolerant organs, and recent findings on different regulatory NK cell subsets have indicated the unique role of NK cells in the maintenance of homeostasis [10, 11].

4.2.3 Immunoregulation by Immune Cells

Immune cells regulate immune responses either directly or indirectly through cell-cell contact or cytokine secretion in order to maintain normal immune functions and homeostasis of the microenvironment.

4.2.3.1 Treg Cells

One of the most important regulatory immune cells is the regulatory T cell that may downregulate immune responses, maintain self immunotolerance, and inhibit the progression of autoimmune diseases. Treg cells can inhibit the proliferation of T cells via direct cell-cell contact, for example, they can mediate lysis of T cells and APCs through granzyme B and perforin-dependent method; in addition, they can also negatively regulate APCs by reducing costimulatory signals and inhibiting antigen presentation; furthermore, they can inhibit the expression of IL-2 and other cytokines by secreting inhibitory cytokines such as IL-10 and TGF-β.

4.2.3.2 Th1, Th2, and Th17 Cells

IFN-γ secreted by Th1 cells activates transcription of Th1-specific transcription factor T-bet, which in turn promotes the production of IFN-γ while inhibits the production of IL-4. In contrast, IL-4 secreted by Th2 cells activates the transcription of Th2-specific transcription factor GATA-3, which in turn promotes the production of IL-4 while inhibits the production of IFN-γ. Therefore, Th1 and Th2 cells may negatively regulate each other to main homeostasis of the system. Cytokines secreted by Th17 cells also participate in the regulation of immune cells and play an important role in the progression of inflammation and autoimmune diseases.

4.2.3.3 Breg Cells

Breg cells is another source of inhibitory cytokines IL-10 and TGF-β and thus are also considered an important part in immunoregulation [63]. Breg cells are activated by binding to TLR and inhibit both T cells and DCs in mice [64]. In humans, Breg cells are activated via CD40 molecules and binding to TLR also impairs the differentiation of monocytes into immature DCs, the maturation of immature DCs into mature DCs, and the ability of mature DCs to stimulate T cells [65]. Human Breg cells reduce the proliferation of CD4 T cells and enhance the expression of Foxp3 and CTLA-4 in Treg cells by cell-to-cell contact [63, 66]. Furthermore, they can block the switch of IgM to IgG by inhibiting the effects of Th cells, and those Breg cells expressing CD1d can stimulate NKT cells to exert regulatory effects [67–69].

4.2.3.4 Dendritic Cells

DCs are critical in balancing tolerance and immunity by integrating environmental signals [9, 70–72]. DC-mediated regulation and tolerance can be segregated into four layers: central tolerance, $Foxp3^+$ Treg cells, anergy/deletion, and feedback regulation. They influence each other and can be differentially regulated, which maintain normal immune functions and homeostasis between immune responses against pathogens and restraining autoimmunity [9]. Regulatory mechanisms underlying DC regulation can be preformed via the induction of Treg cells and the production of IL-10, TGF-β, retinoic acid (RA), etc. For example, a subpopulation of DCs is recently identified and characterized by the expression of CD11b and CD103. These $CD11b^+CD103^+$ DCs are present in the lamina propria (LP) of the small and large intestines and migrate to the draining lymph nodes to induce Treg cells through the release of RA and TGF-β and the expression of indoleamine 2,3-dioxygenase [73–76].

4.2.3.5 Macrophages

M2 macrophages are generally accompanied by high levels of scavenger, mannose, and galactose type receptors. They are the key players in the maintenance of tissue homeostasis by clearing apoptotic or senescent cells, remodeling and repairing tissues, and secreting inhibitory cytokines such as IL-10 and TGF-β in case of immunoregulation. A subpopulation of macrophages characterized by $CD11c^+CX3CR1^+F4/80^+$ phenotype is monocyte-derived and anti-inflammatory in nature [77]. They express high levels of IL-10 that is required for re-stimulation of Treg cells *in situ* and inhibit T cell proliferation via a contact-dependent mechanism [76, 78, 79]. $CX3CR1^+$ macrophages are very efficient at antigen capturing and they transfer antigens to $CD103^+$ DCs followed by $CD103^+$ DCs' migration to the draining lymph nodes where they can induce Treg cells. Inhibition of the transfer would result in the failure of Treg cell differentiation and oral tolerance establishment [76].

4.2.3.6 NK Cells

The regulatory effects of NK cells are critical in maintaining immune homeostasis and mediating pathogenesis of autoimmunity. NK cells may prime, influence, and regulate the activities of an adaptive immune response via cytokines secretion or cell-to-cell contact [80–82]. NK cells may mediate immunoregulation through several mechanisms: (1) silence of antigen-specific responses by lysis of DCs and T cells or induced apoptosis of activated T cells; (2) inhibition of autoreactive T cell functions by secretion of type II cytokines such as IL-5 and IL-13 (NK2 subset); (3) suppression of T cell responses via producing immunosuppressive cytokines (such as TGF-β and IL-10); (4) inhibition of T cell proliferation by up-regulating the cell cycle inhibitor p21, resulting in a G0/G1 stage cell arrest; (5) elaboration of inhibitory effects through regulatory cell populations such as NKT cells or Treg cells [10, 80, 81, 83–88].

4.2.4 Immunoregulation by AICD

Generally, immune responses and effector functions against specific antigens are not long-lived, once the antigen is cleared, the immune system has to restore its balance. Therefore, effector cells also need to be inhibited or eliminated. Activated T cells may undergo activation-induced cell death (AICD), a spontaneously apoptosis induced after activated T cells have fulfilled their effector functions. It is a highly specific negative regulation process involving the interaction between Fas and FasL that only works on activated and proliferated immune cells with a purpose to restrain massive proliferation of antigen-specific lymphocytes. Apoptotic cells are then cleared by macrophages [1–4].

4.2.5 Immunoregulation by the Immune-Endocrine-Nervous Systems

Other ways of immunoregulation include interactions between immune-endocrine-nervous systems to main a stable microenvironment. Cytokines such as IL-1, IL-2, IL-6, TNF-α, TGF-α, IFN-α, IFN-β, and IFN-γ secreted by neurons and endocrines cells affect immune cells directly; these cells may also regulate immune cells by secreting neurotransmitters and endocrine hormones. On the other side, cytokines such as IL-1, IL-6, TNF-α, etc., secreted by immune cells affect neurons and endocrine cells, and they may also regulate nervous and endocrine systems by secreting hormones and neuropeptides [1–4].

References

1. Paul WE. Fundamental immunology. 7th ed. Philadelphia: Wolters Kluwer Health/Lippincot Williams & Wilkins; 2012.
2. Murphy K. Janeway's immunology. 8th ed. New York: Garland Science; 2011.
3. Abbas AK, Lichtman AH, Pillai S. Cellular and molecular immunology. 6th ed. Philadelphia: Saunders; 2010.
4. Parslow TG, Stites DP, Terry AI, Imboden JB. Medical immunology. 10th ed. New York: McGraw-Hill/Appleton & Lange; 2001.
5. Goodnow CC, Sprent J, Fazekas de St Groth B, Vinuesa CG. Cellular and genetic mechanisms of self tolerance and autoimmunity. Nature. 2005;435(7042):590–7.
6. Trowsdale J, Betz AG. Mother's little helpers: mechanisms of maternal-fetal tolerance. Nat Immunol. 2006;7(3):241–6.
7. Erlebacher A. Immune surveillance of the maternal/fetal interface: controversies and implications. Trends Endocrinol Metab TEM. 2010;21(7):428–34.
8. Berod L, Puttur F, Huehn J, Sparwasser T. Tregs in infection and vaccinology: heroes or traitors? J Microbial Biotechnol. 2012; 5(2):260–9.
9. Mayer CT, Berod L, Sparwasser T. Layers of dendritic cell-mediated T cell tolerance, their regulation and the prevention of autoimmunity. Front Immunol. 2012;3:183.
10. Tian Z, Gershwin ME, Zhang C. Regulatory NK cells in autoimmune disease. J Autoimmun. 2012;39(3):206–15.
11. Sun H, Sun C, Tian Z, Xiao W. NK cells in immunotolerant organs. Cell Mol Immunol. 2013;10(3):202–12.
12. Sun C, Sun H, Zhang C, Tian Z. NK cell receptor imbalance and NK cell dysfunction in HBV infection and hepatocellular carcinoma. Cell Mol Immunol. 2014;12:292–302.
13. Italiani P, Boraschi D. From monocytes to M1/M2 macrophages: phenotypical vs functional differentiation. Front Immunol. 2014;5:514.
14. Sun H, Sun C, Xiao W. Expression regulation of co-inhibitory molecules on human natural killer cells in response to cytokine stimulations. Cytokine. 2014;65(1):33–41.
15. Wing K, Onishi Y, Prieto-Martin P, Yamaguchi T, Miyara M, Fehervari Z, et al. CTLA-4 control over Foxp3+ regulatory T cell function. Science. 2008;322(5899):271–5.
16. Bi J, Zhang Q, Liang D, Xiong L, Wei H, Sun R, et al. T-cell Ig and ITIM domain regulates natural killer cell activation in murine acute viral hepatitis. Hepatology. 2014;59(5):1715–25.
17. Avogadri F, Yuan J, Yang A, Schaer D, Wolchok JD. Modulation of CTLA-4 and GITR for cancer immunotherapy. Curr Top Microbiol Immunol. 2011;344:211–44.
18. Naidoo J, Page DB, Wolchok JD. Immune modulation for cancer therapy. Br J Cancer. 2014;111:2214–9.
19. Cerdan C, Martin Y, Courcoul M, Brailly H, Mawas C, Birg F, et al. Prolonged IL-2 receptor alpha/CD25 expression after T cell activation via the adhesion molecules CD2 and CD28. Demonstration of combined transcriptional and post-transcriptional regulation. J Immunol. 1992;149(7):2255–61.
20. de Boer M, Kasran A, Kwekkeboom J, Walter H, Vandenberghe P, Ceuppens JL. Ligation of B7 with CD28/CTLA-4 on T cells results in CD40 ligand expression, interleukin-4 secretion and efficient help for antibody production by B cells. Eur J Immunol. 1993; 23(12):3120–5.
21. Boise LH, Minn AJ, Noel PJ, June CH, Accavitti MA, Lindsten T, et al. CD28 costimulation can promote T cell survival by enhancing the expression of Bcl-XL. Immunity. 1995;3(1):87–98.
22. Linsley PS, Brady W, Urnes M, Grosmaire LS, Damle NK, Ledbetter JA. CTLA-4 is a second receptor for the B cell activation antigen B7. J Exp Med. 1991;174(3):561–9.
23. Waterhouse P, Penninger JM, Timms E, Wakeham A, Shahinian A, Lee KP, et al. Lymphoproliferative disorders with early lethality in mice deficient in Ctla-4. Science. 1995;270(5238):985–8.
24. Freeman GJ, Borriello F, Hodes RJ, Reiser H, Hathcock KS, Laszlo G, et al. Uncovering of functional alternative CTLA-4 counter-receptor in B7-deficient mice. Science. 1993;262(5135):907–9.
25. Alegre ML, Noel PJ, Eisfelder BJ, Chuang E, Clark MR, Reiner SL, et al. Regulation of surface and intracellular expression of CTLA4 on mouse T cells. J Immunol. 1996;157(11):4762–70.
26. Perez VL, Van Parijs L, Biuckians A, Zheng XX, Strom TB, Abbas AK. Induction of peripheral T cell tolerance in vivo requires CTLA-4 engagement. Immunity. 1997;6(4):411–7.
27. Joller N, Peters A, Anderson AC, Kuchroo VK. Immune checkpoints in central nervous system autoimmunity. Immunol Rev. 2012;248(1):122–39.
28. Nishimura H, Agata Y, Kawasaki A, Sato M, Imamura S, Minato N, et al. Developmentally regulated expression of the PD-1 protein on the surface of double-negative (CD4-CD8-) thymocytes. Int Immunol. 1996;8(5):773–80.
29. Chen C, Qu QX, Huang JA, Zhu YB, Ge Y, Wang Q, et al. Expression of programmed-death receptor ligands 1 and 2 may contribute to the poor stimulatory potential of murine immature dendritic cells. Immunobiology. 2007;212(3):159–65.
30. Zhong X, Tumang JR, Gao W, Bai C, Rothstein TL. PD-L2 expression extends beyond dendritic cells/macrophages to B1 cells enriched for V(H)11/V(H)12 and phosphatidylcholine binding. Eur J Immunol. 2007;37(9):2405–10.
31. Agata Y, Kawasaki A, Nishimura H, Ishida Y, Tsubata T, Yagita H, et al. Expression of the PD-1 antigen on the surface of stimulated mouse T and B lymphocytes. Int Immunol. 1996;8(5):765–72.
32. Barber DL, Wherry EJ, Masopust D, Zhu B, Allison JP, Sharpe AH, et al. Restoring function in exhausted CD8 T cells during chronic viral infection. Nature. 2006;439(7077):682–7.
33. Yu X, Harden K, Gonzalez LC, Francesco M, Chiang E, Irving B, et al. The surface protein TIGIT suppresses T cell activation by promoting the generation of mature immunoregulatory dendritic cells. Nat Immunol. 2009;10(1).48–57.
34. Stanietsky N, Simic H, Arapovic J, Toporik A, Levy O, Novik A, et al. The interaction of TIGIT with PVR and PVRL2 inhibits human NK cell cytotoxicity. Proc Natl Acad Sci U S A. 2009;106(42):17858–63.
35. Levin SD, Taft DW, Brandt CS, Bucher C, Howard ED, Chadwick EM, et al. Vstm3 is a member of the CD28 family and an important modulator of T-cell function. Eur J Immunol. 2011;41(4):902–15.
36. Boles KS, Vermi W, Facchetti F, Fuchs A, Wilson TJ, Diacovo TG, et al. A novel molecular interaction for the adhesion of follicular CD4 T cells to follicular DC. Eur J Immunol. 2009;39(3): 695–703.
37. Stengel KF, Harden-Bowles K, Yu X, Rouge L, Yin J, Comps-Agrar L, et al. Structure of TIGIT immunoreceptor bound to poliovirus receptor reveals a cell-cell adhesion and signaling mechanism that requires cis-trans receptor clustering. Proc Natl Acad Sci U S A. 2012;109(14):5399–404.
38. Joller N, Hafler JP, Brynedal B, Kassam N, Spoerl S, Levin SD, et al. Cutting edge: TIGIT has T cell-intrinsic inhibitory functions. J Immunol. 2011;186(3):1338–42.
39. Stanietsky N, Mandelboim O. Paired NK cell receptors controlling NK cytotoxicity. FEBS Lett. 2010;584(24):4895–900.
40. Mendelsohn CL, Wimmer E, Racaniello VR. Cellular receptor for poliovirus: molecular cloning, nucleotide sequence, and expression

of a new member of the immunoglobulin superfamily. Cell. 1989;56(5):855–65.
41. Casado JG, Pawelec G, Morgado S, Sanchez-Correa B, Delgado E, Gayoso I, et al. Expression of adhesion molecules and ligands for activating and costimulatory receptors involved in cell-mediated cytotoxicity in a large panel of human melanoma cell lines. Cancer Immunol Immunother CII. 2009;58(9):1517–26.
42. Bottino C, Castriconi R, Pende D, Rivera P, Nanni M, Carnemolla B, et al. Identification of PVR (CD155) and Nectin-2 (CD112) as cell surface ligands for the human DNAM-1 (CD226) activating molecule. J Exp Med. 2003;198(4):557–67.
43. Lozano E, Dominguez-Villar M, Kuchroo V, Hafler DA. The TIGIT/CD226 axis regulates human T cell function. J Immunol. 2012;188(8):3869–75.
44. Liu S, Zhang H, Li M, Hu D, Li C, Ge B, et al. Recruitment of Grb2 and SHIP1 by the ITT-like motif of TIGIT suppresses granule polarization and cytotoxicity of NK cells. Cell Death Differ. 2013;20(3):456–64.
45. Stanietsky N, Rovis TL, Glasner A, Seidel E, Tsukerman P, Yamin R, et al. Mouse TIGIT inhibits NK-cell cytotoxicity upon interaction with PVR. Eur J Immunol. 2013;43(8):2138–50.
46. Bi J, Zheng X, Chen Y, Wei H, Sun R, Tian Z. TIGIT safeguards liver regeneration through regulating natural killer cell-hepatocyte crosstalk. Hepatology. 2014;60(4):1389–98.
47. Monney L, Sabatos CA, Gaglia JL, Ryu A, Waldner H, Chernova T, et al. Th1-specific cell surface protein Tim-3 regulates macrophage activation and severity of an autoimmune disease. Nature. 2002;415(6871):536–41.
48. Chen Y, Langrish CL, McKenzie B, Joyce-Shaikh B, Stumhofer JS, McClanahan T, et al. Anti-IL-23 therapy inhibits multiple inflammatory pathways and ameliorates autoimmune encephalomyelitis. J Clin Invest. 2006;116(5):1317–26.
49. Hastings WD, Anderson DE, Kassam N, Koguchi K, Greenfield EA, Kent SC, et al. TIM-3 is expressed on activated human CD4+ T cells and regulates Th1 and Th17 cytokines. Eur J Immunol. 2009;39(9):2492–501.
50. Nakae S, Iwakura Y, Suto H, Galli SJ. Phenotypic differences between Th1 and Th17 cells and negative regulation of Th1 cell differentiation by IL-17. J Leukoc Biol. 2007;81(5):1258–68.
51. Zhu C, Anderson AC, Schubart A, Xiong H, Imitola J, Khoury SJ, et al. The Tim-3 ligand galectin-9 negatively regulates T helper type 1 immunity. Nat Immunol. 2005;6(12):1245–52.
52. Sabatos CA, Chakravarti S, Cha E, Schubart A, Sanchez-Fueyo A, Zheng XX, et al. Interaction of Tim-3 and Tim-3 ligand regulates T helper type 1 responses and induction of peripheral tolerance. Nat Immunol. 2003;4(11):1102–10.
53. Golden-Mason L, Palmer BE, Kassam N, Townshend-Bulson L, Livingston S, McMahon BJ, et al. Negative immune regulator Tim-3 is overexpressed on T cells in hepatitis C virus infection and its blockade rescues dysfunctional CD4+ and CD8+ T cells. J Virol. 2009;83(18):9122–30.
54. Jones RB, Ndhlovu LC, Barbour JD, Sheth PM, Jha AR, Long BR, et al. Tim-3 expression defines a novel population of dysfunctional T cells with highly elevated frequencies in progressive HIV-1 infection. J Exp Med. 2008;205(12):2763–79.
55. Jin HT, Anderson AC, Tan WG, West EE, Ha SJ, Araki K, et al. Cooperation of Tim-3 and PD-1 in CD8 T-cell exhaustion during chronic viral infection. Proc Natl Acad Sci U S A. 2010;107(33): 14733–8.
56. Sakuishi K, Apetoh L, Sullivan JM, Blazar BR, Kuchroo VK, Anderson AC. Targeting Tim-3 and PD-1 pathways to reverse T cell exhaustion and restore anti-tumor immunity. J Exp Med. 2010;207(10):2187–94.
57. Fourcade J, Sun Z, Benallaoua M, Guillaume P, Luescher IF, Sander C, et al. Upregulation of Tim-3 and PD-1 expression is associated with tumor antigen-specific CD8+ T cell dysfunction in melanoma patients. J Exp Med. 2010;207(10):2175–86.
58. Zhou Q, Munger ME, Veenstra RG, Weigel BJ, Hirashima M, Munn DH, et al. Coexpression of Tim-3 and PD-1 identifies a CD8+ T-cell exhaustion phenotype in mice with disseminated acute myelogenous leukemia. Blood. 2011;117(17):4501–10.
59. Ngiow SF, von Scheidt B, Akiba H, Yagita H, Teng MW, Smyth MJ. Anti-TIM3 antibody promotes T cell IFN-gamma-mediated antitumor immunity and suppresses established tumors. Cancer Res. 2011;71(10):3540–51.
60. Wherry EJ. T cell exhaustion. Nat Immunol. 2011;12(6):492–9.
61. Crespo J, Sun H, Welling TH, Tian Z, Zou W. T cell anergy, exhaustion, senescence, and stemness in the tumor microenvironment. Curr Opin Immunol. 2013;25(2):214–21.
62. Takamura S, Tsuji-Kawahara S, Yagita H, Akiba H, Sakamoto M, Chikaishi T, et al. Premature terminal exhaustion of Friend virus-specific effector CD8+ T cells by rapid induction of multiple inhibitory receptors. J Immunol. 2010;184(9):4696–707.
63. Kessel A, Haj T, Peri R, Snir A, Melamed D, Sabo E, et al. Human CD19(+)CD25(high) B regulatory cells suppress proliferation of CD4(+) T cells and enhance Foxp3 and CTLA-4 expression in T-regulatory cells. Autoimmun Rev. 2012;11(9):670–7.
64. Lo-Man R. Regulatory B, cells control dendritic cell functions. Immunotherapy. 2011;3(4 Suppl):19–20.
65. Morva A, Lemoine S, Achour A, Pers JO, Youinou P, Jamin C. Maturation and function of human dendritic cells are regulated by B lymphocytes. Blood. 2012;119(1):106–14.
66. Yang M, Rui K, Wang S, Lu L. Regulatory B cells in autoimmune diseases. Cell Mol Immunol. 2013;10(2):122–32.
67. Klinker MW, Lundy SK. Multiple mechanisms of immune suppression by B lymphocytes. Mol Med. 2012;18:123–37.
68. Poe JC, Smith SH, Haas KM, Yanaba K, Tsubata T, Matsushita T, et al. Amplified B lymphocyte CD40 signaling drives regulatory B10 cell expansion in mice. PLoS One. 2011;6(7):e22464.
69. Berthelot JM, Jamin C, Amrouche K, Le Goff B, Maugars Y, Youinou P. Regulatory B cells play a key role in immune system balance. Joint Bone Spine Rev Rhum. 2013;80(1):18–22.
70. Banchereau J, Steinman RM. Dendritic cells and the control of immunity. Nature. 1998;392(6673):245–52.
71. Hawiger D, Inaba K, Dorsett Y, Guo M, Mahnke K, Rivera M, et al. Dendritic cells induce peripheral T cell unresponsiveness under steady state conditions in vivo. J Exp Med. 2001;194(6):769–79.
72. Probst HC, McCoy K, Okazaki T, Honjo T, van den Broek M. Resting dendritic cells induce peripheral CD8+ T cell tolerance through PD-1 and CTLA-4. Nat Immunol. 2005;6(3):280–6.
73. Sun CM, Hall JA, Blank RB, Bouladoux N, Oukka M, Mora JR, et al. Small intestine lamina propria dendritic cells promote de novo generation of Foxp3 T reg cells via retinoic acid. J Exp Med. 2007;204(8):1775–85.
74. Coombes JL, Siddiqui KR, Arancibia-Carcamo CV, Hall J, Sun CM, Belkaid Y, et al. A functionally specialized population of mucosal CD103+ DCs induces Foxp3+ regulatory T cells via a TGF-beta and retinoic acid-dependent mechanism. J Exp Med. 2007;204(8):1757–64.
75. Matteoli G, Mazzini E, Iliev ID, Mileti E, Fallarino F, Puccetti P, et al. Gut CD103+ dendritic cells express indoleamine 2,3-dioxygenase which influences T regulatory/T effector cell balance and oral tolerance induction. Gut. 2010;59(5):595–604.
76. Mazzini E, Massimiliano L, Penna G, Rescigno M. Oral tolerance can be established via gap junction transfer of fed antigens from CX3CR1(+) macrophages to CD103(+) dendritic cells. Immunity. 2014;40(2):248–61.
77. Rivollier A, He J, Kole A, Valatas V, Kelsall BL. Inflammation switches the differentiation program of Ly6Chi monocytes from antiinflammatory macrophages to inflammatory dendritic cells in the colon. J Exp Med. 2012;209(1):139–55.
78. Hadis U, Wahl B, Schulz O, Hardtke-Wolenski M, Schippers A, Wagner N, et al. Intestinal tolerance requires gut homing and

expansion of FoxP3+ regulatory T cells in the lamina propria. Immunity. 2011;34(2):237–46.
79. Kayama H, Ueda Y, Sawa Y, Jeon SG, Ma JS, Okumura R, et al. Intestinal CX3C chemokine receptor 1(high) (CX3CR1(high)) myeloid cells prevent T-cell-dependent colitis. Proc Natl Acad Sci U S A. 2012;109(13):5010–5.
80. Moretta A, Marcenaro E, Parolini S, Ferlazzo G, Moretta L. NK cells at the interface between innate and adaptive immunity. Cell Death Differ. 2008;15(2):226–33.
81. Zhang C, Zhang J, Tian Z. The regulatory effect of natural killer cells: do "NK-reg cells" exist? Cell Mol Immunol. 2006;3(4):241–54.
82. Lanier LL. NK cell recognition. Annu Rev Immunol. 2005;23:225–74.
83. Andoniou CE, Coudert JD, Degli-Esposti MA. Killers and beyond: NK-cell-mediated control of immune responses. Eur J Immunol. 2008;38(11):2938–42.
84. Johansson S, Berg L, Hall H, Hoglund P. NK cells: elusive players in autoimmunity. Trends Immunol. 2005;26(11):613–8.
85. Flodstrom-Tullberg M, Bryceson YT, Shi FD, Hoglund P, Ljunggren HG. Natural killer cells in human autoimmunity. Curr Opin Immunol. 2009;21(6):634–40.
86. Perricone R, Perricone C, De Carolis C, Shoenfeld Y. NK cells in autoimmunity: a two-edg'd weapon of the immune system. Autoimmun Rev. 2008;7(5):384–90.
87. Lunemann A, Lunemann JD, Munz C. Regulatory NK-cell functions in inflammation and autoimmunity. Mol Med. 2009;15(9–10):352–8.
88. Sun C, Fu B, Gao Y, Liao X, Sun R, Tian Z, et al. TGF-beta1 down-regulation of NKG2D/DAP10 and 2B4/SAP expression on human NK cells contributes to HBV persistence. PLoS Pathog. 2012;8(3):e1002594.

Immnopathology

5

Cheng Sun, Haoyu Sun, and Zhigang Tian

Contents

The original version of this chapter was revised.
An erratum to this chapter can be found at
DOI 10.1007/978-94-024-0902-4_16

C. Sun • H. Sun
Institute of Immunology, School of Life Sciences and Medical Center, University of Science and Technology of China, Hefei, China

Z. Tian (✉)
Institute of Immunology, School of Life Sciences and Medical Center, University of Science and Technology of China, Hefei, China
e-mail: tzg@ustc.edu.cn

5.1 Immunodeficiency Diseases

Immunodeficiency disease refers to the condition when one or more components of the immune system are defective either due to inheritance or other acquired reasons. Immunodeficiency diseases are usually classified into two groups: the primary immunodeficiency disease (PIDD), also known as the inherited immunodeficiency disease, and the secondary immunodeficiency disease, also known as the acquired immunodeficiency disease (AIDD). Primary immunodeficiencies are caused by mutations in genes controlling the immune response, and thus are inherited and passed on through bloodline. While on the other hand, secondary immunodeficiencies are caused by the consequences of other diseases, environmental factors, or even adverse medical interventions. Both primary and secondary immunodeficiencies induce malfunctions of the immune system, causing partial or completely lack of defense against pathogenic infections. There are few common features of all immunodeficiency diseases: first, they are usually accompanied by recurrent, chronic, and uncontrolled infections; second, they are usually accompanied by autoimmunity, hypersensitivity, and inflammatory diseases; third, people with IDDs are usually more susceptible to tumors; and fourth, IDDs tend to be inherited [1–4].

5.1.1 Primary Immunodeficiency Diseases

Primary immunodeficiency diseases are caused by either the inherited mutations in genes of the immune system or the developmental defects in the immune system, and are usually seen in infants. Most of the gene defects causing primary immunodeficiencies are recessive, and many are caused by mutations in the gene on the X chromosome.

5.1.1.1 Severe Combined Immunodeficiency Disease (SCID)

Severe combined immunodeficiency disease (SCID) is a rare autosomal recessive or X-linked inherited disease featuring

X.-H. Gao, H.-D. Chen (eds.), *Practical Immunodermatology*, DOI 10.1007/978-94-024-0902-4_5

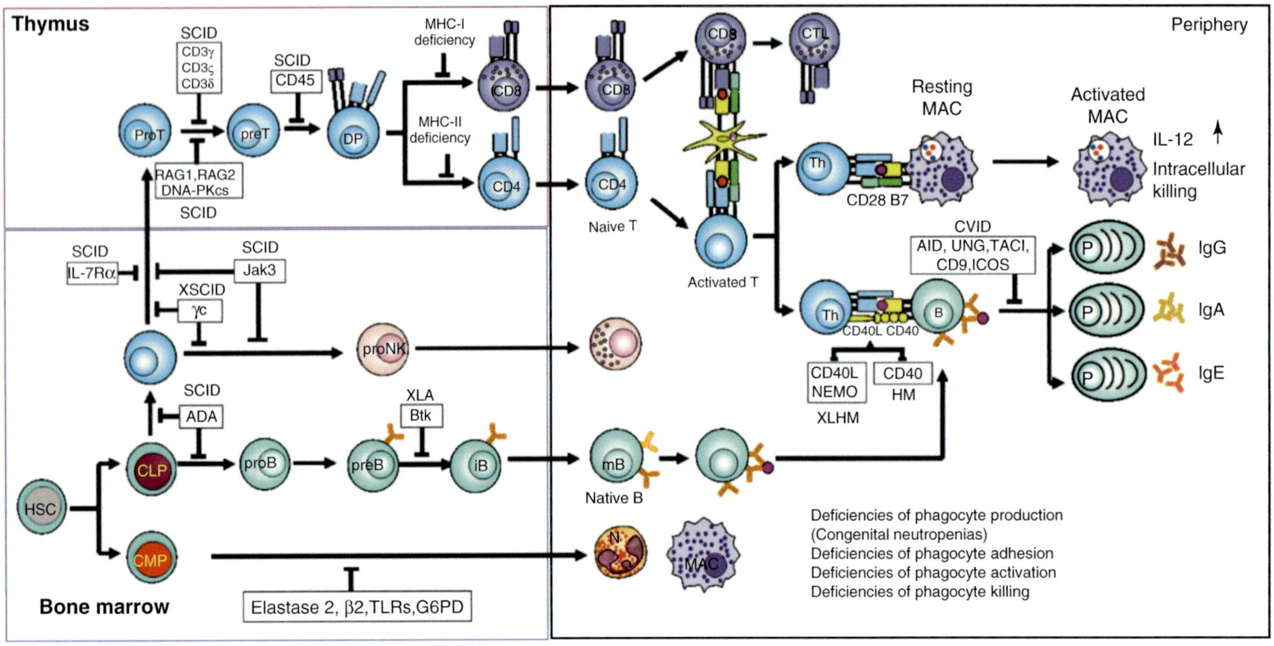

Fig. 5.1 Immunodeficiencies in T cell, B cell, and phagocyte. Mutations in genes encoding indicated proteins (indicated in the boxes) are known to cause human immunodeficiency diseases. *HSC* hematopoietic stem cell, *CLP* common lymphoid progenitor, *CMP* common myeloid progenitor, *Pro T* progenitor T cell, *Pre T* precursor T cell, *DP T cell* double-positive T cell, *Pro B* progenitor B cell, *Pre B* precursor B cell, *iB* immature B cell, *mB* mature B cell, *P* plasma cell, *MAC* macrophage, *N* neutrophil, *SCID* severe combined immunodeficiency, *XSCID* X-linked SCID, *CVID* common variable immunodeficiency, *XLA* X-linked agammaglobulinemia, *HM* Hyper IgM syndrome, *XLHM* X-linked hyper IgM syndrome

mainly by the combined deficiencies in both T and B cells. It is usually caused by defects in T- and B-cell development or the lack of cell-cell interactions. Patients with SCID lack both specific T-cell-dependent antibody responses and cell-mediated immune responses, and thus are unable to develop immunological memory [5, 6]. SCID may be further grouped into three categories: X-linked SCID (XSCID), recombinant activating gene (RAG) deficiency, and adenosine deaminase (ADA) deficiency (Fig. 5.1).

XSCID XSCID is the most common form of SCID. Patients with XSCID possess a genetic defect in interleukin-2 receptor (IL-2R) common gamma chain (γc), which is shared by many cytokine receptors, including those for IL-2, IL-4, IL-7, IL-9, IL-15, and IL-21. These cytokine receptors are involved in different signaling pathways that regulate differentiation, development, and maturation of T and B cells. Genetic defect causes failure of T and NK cell development, and due to the lack of help from T cells, B cells cannot secrete antibodies although their cell number is normal. Autosomal recessive defect in kinase Jak3 results in the development of abnormal T and NK cells but normal development of B cells, while defect in IL-17 receptor α chain (IL-17Rα) results in impaired development of T cells but normal development of B and NK cells (Fig. 5.1).

RAG Deficiency Defects in either the *RAG-1* or *RAG-2* gene result in the failure of antigen receptor gene rearrangement that induces an arrest of lymphocyte development [7]. Therefore, genetically engineered mice with defects in the *RAG* genes and patients who lack functional RAG proteins suffer a complete lack of T and B cells. Genetically engineered *scid* mice possess defects in the enzyme DNA-dependent protein kinase (DNA-PKcs) that is also involved in antigen receptor gene rearrangement. A mutation in the protein Artemis in some people acts in the same pathway as DNA-PKcs (Fig. 5.1).

ADA and PNP Deficiency Adenosine deaminase (ADA) deficiency and purine nucleotide phosphorylase (PNP) deficiency are autosomally inherited SCID, defects in these enzymes result in the accumulation of nucleotide metabolites that are toxic to developing T and B cells (Fig. 5.1).

5.1.1.2 Defects in T Cell Development and TCR Signaling

Genetic defects in either TCR signaling or thymic function blocking T cell development may result in severe immunodeficiencies.

DiGeorge Syndrome A disorder in which the thymic epithelium is developed abnormally that leads to SCID. Patients with this syndrome lack proper inductive thymic environment so that their T cells cannot mature properly. Although they possess normal levels of serum immunoglobulin, both cell-mediated immunity and T-cell-dependent antibody production are impaired.

MHC Class II Deficiency Individuals who lack the expression of MHC class II molecules are considered MHC class II deficiency. These patients suffer from severe immunodeficiency due to the lacking of MHC class II molecules in the thymus, which in turn prohibits positive selection and development of $CD4^+$ T cells. APCs in these patients also lack the expression of MHC class II molecules and therefore the few $CD4^+$ T cells that developed normally in the thymus cannot be stimulated by antigens. However, the expression of MHC class I molecules and the development of $CD8^+$ T cells are normal.

MHC Class I Deficiency Individuals who lack the expression of MHC class I molecules on the cell surfaces are considered MHC class I deficiency. The absence of MHC class I molecules on the surface of thymic epithelial cells results in a lack of $CD8^+$ T cells expressing α:β TCR. However, the expression of MHC class II molecules and the development of $CD4^+$ T cells are normal.

Defects in TCR Signaling Mutations in the tyrosine phosphatase CD45 may cause defects in lymphocyte signaling that in turn result in severe immunodeficiency. Humans and mice with CD45 deficiency exhibit reduced peripheral T cell number and abnormal B cell maturation. Defects in the signaling of TCR complex (CD3γ, CD3δ, CD3ε, and CD3ζ) that block the activation of T cells in the early thymic development can cause severe immunodeficiency (Fig. 5.1). Patients with mutations in the CD3δ, CD3ε, or CD3ζ chain of the CD3 complex possess defective pre-TCR signaling and fail to progress to the double-positive stage of the thymic development.

5.1.1.3 Antibody Deficiencies

Antibody deficiencies are often associated with impaired generation of antibodies and defective antibody functions. They are usually characterized by low levels or complete lack of immunoglobulin in the patient serum. Abnormal antibody production and defective antibody functions are caused by defects in either B- or T-cell activation and function. Antibody deficiencies lead to severe and consistent infections due to inability to opsonize the bacteria, therefore, deficiencies in antibody production and function severely affect the defense against bacteria requiring opsonization for clearance. Antibody deficiencies also affect the neutralization of viruses that enter the system (Fig. 5.1).

XLA X-linked agammaglobulinemia (XLA) is the most common type of PIDD that involves antibody deficiency, the defective gene in XLA encodes a B cell signaling transduction molecule Bruton tyrosine kinase (Btk) that plays key role in the early differentiation of normal B cells and the activation of mature B cells. XLA is characterized by low levels of Ig in the serum and significant decrease or absence of B cells in the periphery often seen in male infants, in female patients of a mutant *btk* gene, all B cells have the normal X chromosome as the active X due to natural selection (Fig. 5.1).

HM Hyper IgM syndrome (HM) is characterized by normal B- and T-cell development, high serum levels of IgM, and very limited antibody responses to pathogens requiring helper T cells. The most common form of HM is X-linked hyper IgM syndrome (XLHM), which is caused by mutations in the gene encoding CD40 ligand or NEMO (also known as IKKγ) that result in either CD40 ligand deficiency or NEMO deficiency. Studies have shown that mutations at different points in the CD40-CD40L signaling pathway may lead to a similar combined immunodeficiency syndrome (Fig. 5.1).

CVID Common variable immunodeficiency (CVID) is the most frequent symptomatic PIDD in adults, in which the functions of both B and T cells are impaired. It is often characterized by low levels of immunoglobulins including IgM, IgG, and IgA, and is caused by dysfunction of T cells in providing effective help for B cells to generate immunoglobulins and perform class switching (Fig. 5.1). Patients with CVID are susceptible to recurrent infections, and they have abnormal antibody responses and decreased serum immunoglobulin. Autoimmune diseases and gastrointestinal diseases also occur in some patients with CVID [8, 9]. The condition in patients with CVID is not as severe as some of the other immunodeficiencies, and most of them are not generally diagnosed until adulthood [10, 11].

5.1.1.4 Phagocyte Deficiencies

Defects in the adherence and phagocytosis of phagocytes lead to their functional deficiencies that allow the wide spreading of bacterial infections. There are three types of phagocyte immunodeficiencies, each caused by genes that encode proteins controlling the production, interaction, and killing, respectively.

Defects in Neutrophil Production The deficiencies in neutrophil production include severe congenital neutropenias and cyclic neutropenias. The neutrophil number is consistently low in patients with congenital neutropenia, while the neutrophil number fluctuates between normal and very low or none during an approximate cycle time of 21 days in patients with cyclic neutropenia. Mutations in human neutrophil elastase (ELA2) lead to production of dysfunctional elastases, which induce the production of a toxic intracellular protein that blocks neutrophil maturation, it is the cause for cyclic neutropenia and most severe congenital neutropenia (Fig. 5.1).

Defects in Phagocyte Migration The migration of phagocytes requires four stages and deficiencies in the proteins involved in each of these stages can inhibit the migration of phagocytes to extravascular sites of infection. For example, deficiency in the integrin common β2 subunit CD18 abolishes the adherence ability of leukocytes to endothelium, which in turn prevents the migration of leukocytes to sites of infection; deficiency in the Rac2 protein that regulates neutrophil activation and cytoskeletal function also prevents neutrophil migration. Another type of immunodeficiency involves the genes that affect the ability of killing intracellular bacteria or ingesting extracellular bacteria (Fig. 5.1).

CGD Chronic granulomatous disease (CGD) is a commonly seen phagocyte immunodeficiency disease that is caused by the defects in respiratory burst. Most of them are X-linked inherited and dominate the male population, while few of them are autosomal recessive and distribute equally among males and females. Genetic defects affecting NADPH oxidase expressed in neutrophils and monocytes can cause CGD, the killing process is inhibited and bacteria ingested by phagocytes can remain alive and reproduce continuously in the cell, they may also spread throughout the body along with phagocytes. Patients with CGD have recurrent, severe bacterial infections that may lead to the formation of granuloma.

5.1.1.5 Complement Deficiencies

Complement deficiencies are often autosomal recessive and such genetic defects affecting components involved in the complement activation, regulatory proteins, or complement receptors may lead to defective humoral immune functions [12, 13]. For example, defects in the complement regulatory protein C1-inhibitor (C1INH) may cause a syndrome known as hereditary angioneurotic edema; and defects in decay-accelerating factor (DAF) and CD59 lead to paroxysmal nocturnal hemoglobinuria.

5.1.2 Secondary Immunodeficiency Diseases

Comparing to primary immunodeficiency, secondary immunodeficiency is more common and is the major cause of infection and death. Secondary immunodeficiency is not inherited; it is usually induced by starvation, tumors related to the immune system, long term or large dosage of antibiotics, and few specific infections [14]. The most typical case of secondary immunodeficiency is acquired immune deficiency syndrome (AIDS).

5.1.2.1 HIV and AIDS

Acquired immune deficiency syndrome (AIDS) is caused by the infection of human immunodeficiency virus (HIV) that leads to gradual loss of immune competence [15]. The disease is characterized by higher susceptibility to infection with opportunistic pathogens, development of malignant tumors, and neurological defects, accompanied by a significant decrease in $CD4^+$ T cell number. HIV is a retrovirus with two types identified: HIV-1 and HIV-2. Around 95 % of AIDS worldwide is caused by the M (main) group of HIV-1, the other two groups are named O (outlier) and N (non-M, non-O). The HIV genome is composed of nine genes flanked by long terminal repeat (LTR) sequences. The three major genes are *gag*, *pol*, and *env*. The *gag* gene encodes the structural proteins of the viral core and *pol* encodes the enzymes involved in viral replication. The *gag* and *pol* together give rise to polyproteins that are then cleaved into functional proteins. The *env* gene encodes the viral envelope glycoproteins and gives rise to gp160 that is then cleaved into gp120 and gp41, which are then assembled into the viral envelope. HIV shows marked genetic variability and causes AIDS progressively over time. HIV infection is usually transmitted by sexual intercourse, blood, and mother-to-baby at birth or through breast milk [1–4].

5.1.2.2 Pathogenesis of HIV Infection

HIV infection affects predominantly the immune system and the brain. The dominant immunologic feature of HIV infection is the progressive depletion of $CD4^+$ T cells, thereby reversing the normal CD4:CD28 ratio and inexorably cause immunodeficiency.

Entrance of HIV Particle HIV mainly evades host cells expressing surface marker CD4, including $CD4^+$ T cells, monocytes/macrophages, and dendritic cells. Here, CD4 acts as a surface receptor for the virus, HIV enters the cell by binding to the CD4 molecule on the host cell through its viral glycoprotein gp120. CD4 then alters gp120 so that it also binds to a chemokine such as CXCR4 expressed on T cell, or CCR5 expressed on macrophage and dendritic cell, that serves as coreceptor for HIV entry, forming a CD4-gp120-CCR5/CXCR4 complex, which induces a conformational change in gp120 that then exposes another viral glycoprotein gp41 [16–18]. The hydrophobic sequences at the N-terminus of gp41 then insert into the plasma membrane and draw the virus envelop and plasma membrane closer for the fusion of the viral envelope and the cell's plasma membrane, allowing the entrance of the viral core into the cytoplasm [17].

Replication of HIV Particle Replication of HIV occurs only in activated T cells. HIV particle contains two complete RNA genomes and numerous copies of essential enzymes. Once the viral core has entered cell, it releases the RNA genome, which is reverse-transcribed into a complementary DNA (cDNA) by the viral reverse transcriptase and then integrates into the host-cell chromosome by the viral integrase. The integrated cDNA copy is known as the provirus. The transcription of the provirus is initiated when transcription factors NF-κB and NFAT induced by the activation of $CD4^+$ T cells bind to the proviral LTR, producing spliced mRNAs encoding various regulatory proteins, including Rev and Tat. Tat and Rev both bind to RNA transcript in which Tat stabilizes them in a form that can be translated while Rev transports them to the cytosol. These singly spliced or unspliced transcripts are translated to the structural proteins of the virus. These unspliced transcripts are packaged with these proteins to form various new particles. These newly formed viral particles then bud from the cellular membrane, each enclosed in a membrane envelope.

Depletion of $CD4^+$ T Cells The main consequence of HIV infection is the destruction of $CD4^+$ T cells. The number of $CD4^+$ T cells decreases significantly in patients with HIV, along with alterations in their functions such as reduced secretion of IL-2, lower expression of IL-2 receptors, lower responses to antigen stimulation, etc. There are at least three dominant ways to induce $CD4^+$ T cell depletion: first, direct cytopathic effects of HIV; second, indirect killing by $CD8^+$ CTLs, ADCC effect, etc.; and third, HIV-induced apoptosis of infected cells. HIV may induce apoptosis of infected cells through the following mechanisms: first, infected cells become more sensitive to Fas signaling that induces apoptosis; second, HIV induces the expression of gp120 that promotes the infusion of infected cells and $CD4^+$ T cells which in turn accelerates cell death; third, HIV-infected cells are recognized and killed by CTLs; and fourth, ADCC effect by gp120-specific antibodies or the complement activation. The body gradually becomes more susceptible to opportunistic infections as the number of $CD4^+$ T cells decreases.

Immune Escape of HIV HIV is very hard to conquer because it can survive and replicate chronically in the body by evading immune recognition and responses through different mechanisms. First, HIV mutates rapidly while replicating, producing different variants that spread in the lymphoid tissues where infected $CD4^+$ T cells, macrophages, and dendritic cells are found. Second, DC-specific intracellular adhesion molecule grabbing nonintegrin (DC-SIGN) acts as a receptor for HIV that can both increase the infectivity and sustain the infectivity of HIV. Third, HIV may either replicate or lie latently in the infected cells without expressing HIV protein on the cell surface.

5.1.2.3 Immune Responses to HIV

Both humoral and cell-mediated immune responses specific to HIV occur in HIV-infected individuals. However, these immune responses fail to eradicate all viruses and the infection eventually overwhelms the immune system in most people. During the acute phase of HIV infection, an immune response is generated against the virus. It is characterized by the activation of specific $CD8^+$ CTLs that kill HIV-infected cells followed by antibody responses to various HIV antigens, however, there is little evidence suggesting the benefits of antibodies in controlling the infection [17, 19, 20]. Eventually, the levels of antibody and HIV-specific CTLs decline, with progressively increased HIV in the peripheral blood.

5.1.2.4 Disease Progression of HIV Infection

Most individuals infected with HIV progress over time to AIDS. The acute phase of an infection is clinically characterized by an influenza-like illness in most cases, with a marked decrease in the number of circulating $CD4^+$ T cells and the occurrence of viremia, that is, an abundance of virus detected in the peripheral blood, followed by adaptive immune responses that control the acute illness and largely restore the levels of $CD4^+$ T cells but do not eradicate the virus. By 3–4 months after infection, patients with HIV passed the acute phase and moves to the asymptomatic phage (phase of clinical latency), in which the virus continues to replicate without any appearance of the disease, it results in a gradual decline in the number and function of $CD4^+$ T cells [18]. Opportunistic infections and other symptoms become more frequent when the number of $CD4^+$ T cells falls to about 500 cells μl^{-1}. The infection then enters the symptomatic phase. When the number of $CD4^+$ T cells falls below 200 cells μl^{-1}, the patient is considered AIDS and results in death eventually.

5.1.2.5 Control of AIDS

Cure of AIDS is very difficult because HIV can rapidly develop resistance to antiviral drugs due to its high variability. Once a drug is delivered, variants conferring resistance to the drug emerge and expand until the earlier levels of virus are regained [21, 22]. Vaccination against HIV is an attractive solution, however, there poses many difficulties. The main problem is the genomic diversity of HIV strain that proliferates extremely rapidly even in the existence of strong cytotoxic T cells and antibody responses. HIV directly impairs $CD4^+$ T cells and also pushes these effector T cells to become exhausted. On the other hand, lacking of a good animal model and potential HIV neutralizing antibody impedes the research progress. Therefore, the prevention of HIV transmission through public education is the only way right now to prevent the spread of HIV so that AIDS can be controlled.

5.2 Allergy and Allergic Diseases

Hypersensitivity reactions are inflammatory reactions induced by adaptive immune responses that cause tissue damage and functional disorder in response to harmless environmental antigens such as food, pollen, and drug [23]. Harmful immunologically mediated hypersensitivity reactions are generally known as allergic reactions. They may be classified into type I, II, III, and IV. Type I hypersensitivity reaction is caused by IgE-mediated immediate reaction, mainly characterized by rapid activation of mast cells; type II and type III hypersensitivity reactions are mediated by IgG; type IV hypersensitivity reaction is mediated by T lymphocytes, which also refers to as delayed-type hypersensitivity (DTH) (Fig. 5.2) [1–4, 24].

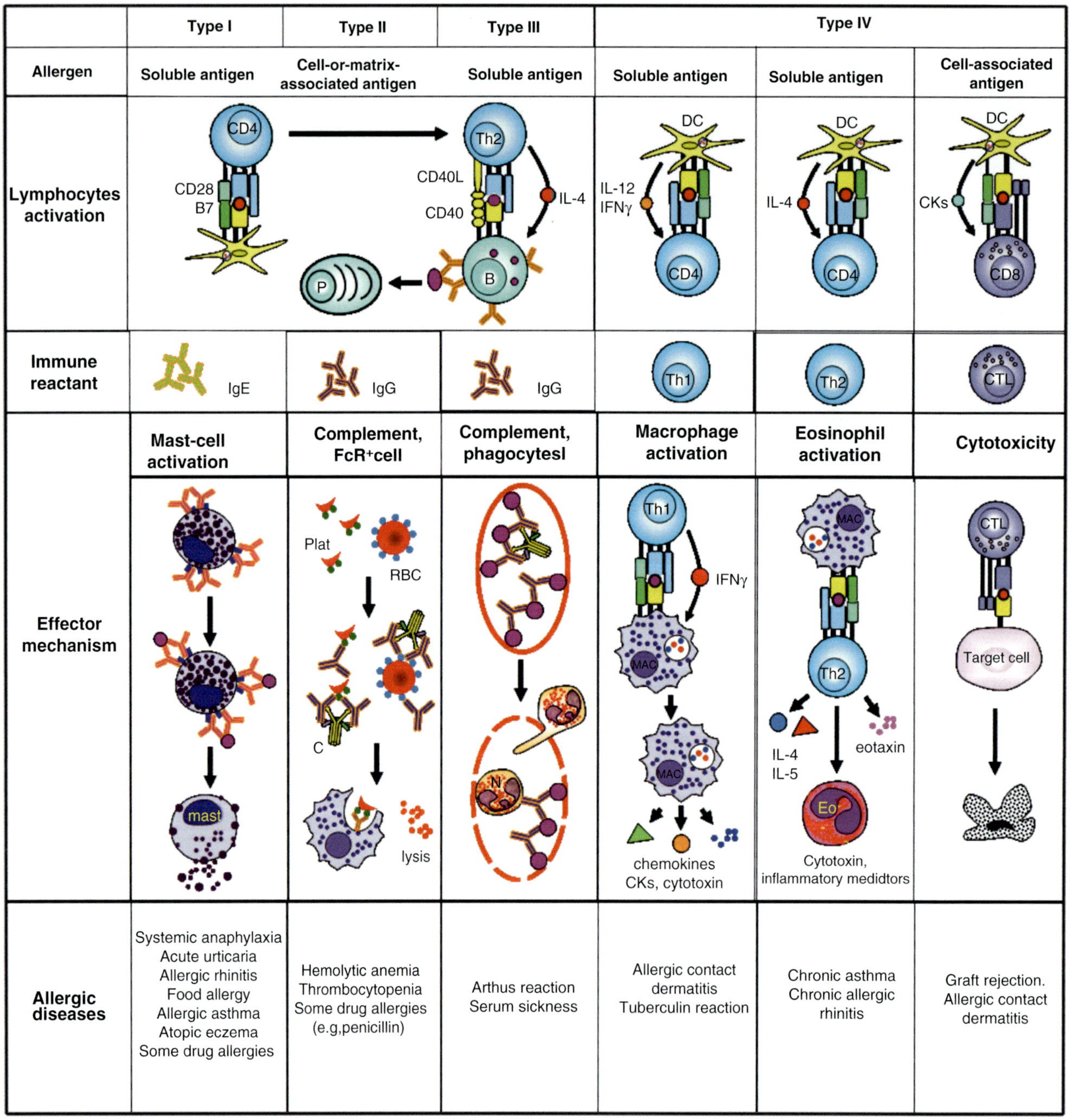

Fig. 5.2 Four types of hypersensitivity disease are mediated by immune reactions causing tissue damage. *Plat* platelets, *RBC* red blood cell, *N* neutrophil, *Eo* eosinophil, *mast* mast cell, *B* B cell, *P* plasma cell, *MAC* macrophage, *C* complement, *CKs* cytokine

5.2.1 Allergen

The innocuous antigens such as those of food, pollen, and house dust are also known as allergens, they normally enter the body at very low doses by diffusion across the mucosal surface. They can be classified into four types based on their sources: pharmaceutical and chemical allergens, inhaled allergens, alimental allergens, and few enzymes that may also act as allergens in type I sensitivity reactions. Some of the allergens are full antigens such as pollen proteins, while others are haptens such as penicillin. Although allergens act in a similar way as the other antigens, they are more likely to induce a Th2 type response and the production of IgE.

5.2.2 Type I Hypersensitivity Reactions

Type I hypersensitivity reaction is also known as allergy, the commonest type of hypersensitivity, which is immediate reaction induced by IgE-mediated bioactive agent production of mast cells and basophils. It often results in disturbing physiological functions without any damages to the cells or the tissues. It is highly inherited and exhibits significant individual differences among the whole population. There are two stages in type I hypersensitivity reaction: sensitization and allergic reaction [24, 25].

5.2.2.1 Sensitization

Sensitization refers to the sensitized state of target cells induced by the binding between IgE and FcεRI. Upon the first contact of an individual with an allergen, the person becomes sensitized to the allergen by producing IgE antibodies. The binding between IgE and the high-affinity FcεRI on either mast cells or basophils makes the body sensitized to this specific allergen. IgE-bound cells are known as sensitized cells, these cells stay sensitized for the whole period of sensitization, which may persist for several months or longer. Once IgE is produced in response to an allergen, re-exposure to the allergen triggers an allergic response.

5.2.2.2 Allergic Reaction

Allergic reaction refers to the degranulation of target cells and release of bioactive mediators induced by allergen cross-linking their EcεRI-bound IgE. Upon the second contact of an individual with the same allergen, it binds to IgE directly on the sensitized cells, leading to the degranulation of sensitized cells. Activated sensitized cells release bioactive mediators, which are either inside of the granules (histamine and kininogenase) or newly formed after cell activation (PGD2, LTs, PAF, and cytokines), that in turn induce a type I hypersensitivity reaction.

5.2.2.3 Stages of an Allergic Reaction

Allergic reactions can be divided into immediate reaction, late-phase reaction, and chronic allergic reaction.

Acute Allergic Reaction Acute allergic reaction is also known as the immediate reaction, it happens within few minutes after encountering an allergen, which activates sensitized mast cells in the local tissues, inducing their degranulation, leading to the expansion of the vascular smooth muscles and increased secretion of mucous glands.

Delayed Allergic Reaction Delayed allergic reaction is also known as the late-phase reaction, which happens few hours after acute allergic reaction. During delayed allergic reaction, activated mast cells synthesize new inflammatory mediators such as PGD2 and LT and release them into tissues, causing the infiltration of inflammatory cells.

Chronic Allergic Reaction Chronic allergic reaction is the result of repeated stimulations by the same allergen. Inflammatory mediators released by mast cells and basophils recruit other leukocytes, mainly Th2 type cells and eosinophils, to the site of allergic inflammation, which may result in a Th2-type hypersensitivity reaction (Fig. 5.2).

5.2.2.4 IgE-Mediated Allergic Diseases

Systemic Anaphylactic Shock The commonly seen type I hypersensitivity reaction disease is the anaphylactic shock. Anaphylactic shock is a serious acute systemic hypersensitivity reaction induced after encountering allergen that results in a number of symptoms including low blood pressure, choking, short of breath, and without proper treatment in time may even cause shock that leads to death. Anaphylactic shock can be either caused by drug such as penicillin or serum such as diphtheria antitoxin.

Atopy Atopy is the general name for a group of diseases that are often local hypersensitivity reactions, including asthma, allergic rhinitis, food allergy, atopic dermatitis, and eczema, etc. Patients with such diseases possess abnormally high levels of circulating IgE, secreted form of FcεII and eosinophils, accompanied by increased levels of FcεII expression on the lymphocytes and mast cells. The occurrence of such diseases is highly related to genetic inheritance and environmental factors [24, 25].

5.2.2.5 Prevention and Therapeutic Applications

The simplest way to prevent allergy is to find the allergens and avoid the contact. For patients already suffering with type I hypersensitivity reaction, desensitization treatment helps to eliminate or alleviate allergy by either transferring serum containing antibodies against allergens to patients or using different dosages of allergens to actively immune patients to induce production of antibodies against these allergens. Other therapeutic applications include inhibition of the synthesis and release of bioactive mediators, antagonism of bioactive mediators, and improvement of the reactivity of effector organs [26].

5.2.3 Type II Hypersensitivity Reactions

Type II hypersensitivity reactions are usually caused in susceptible individuals by innocuous antigens that bind to the surface of circulating blood cells or platelets. Antibodies specific to these innocuous antigens can mediate cell destruction by activating the complement system or through ADCC. This type of reaction is best exemplified by blood-transfusion reactions, in which host antibodies react with foreign antigens on the incompatible transfused blood cells and mediate destruction of these cells. Type II hypersensitivity reactions are mainly associated with allergic diseases including transfusion reaction, hemolytic disease of the new born, drug-induced hemolytic anemia, and thrombocytopenia. *Hemolytic anemia* refers to antibody-mediated destruction of red blood cells while *thrombocytopenia* refers to antibody-mediated destruction of platelets. They can be caused by certain drugs, including the antibiotics penicillin and cephalosporin, in which the drug binds to the cell surface and serves as a target for anti-drug IgG antibodies that leads to an allergic reaction (Fig. 5.2).

5.2.4 Type III Hypersensitivity Reactions

Type III hypersensitivity reactions are caused by the deposition of antigen:antibody complexes, or immune complexes (ICs), that generally facilitate the clearance of antigens by phagocytic cells. In some cases, however, larger ICs are cleared from the circulation leaving small ICs deposited in the blood vessel walls (Fig. 5.2). The immune complexes ligate Fc receptors on leukocytes to activate these cells. They also activate complement system to produce complement fragments that interact with complement receptors on leukocytes to activate and attract these cells to the site of inflammation. IC-mediated diseases are often systemic, with limited or none specificity toward any particular tissue or organ. Type III hypersensitivity reactions are mainly associated with allergic diseases including Arthus reaction, serum sickness, and drug reactions (penicillin and sulfonamide).

Arthus Reaction Arthus reaction is a local type III hypersensitivity reaction triggered in the skin of sensitized individuals who possess IgG antibodies against the sensitizing antigen. Circulating IgG antibodies diffuse into the skin and form immune complexes upon intradermal or subcutaneous antigen injection into the skin. The ICs may mediate an acute Arthus reaction within 4–8 h. During the development of the reaction, localized tissue and vascular damages result in an accumulation of fluid (edema) and red blood cells at the site. The severity of the reaction can vary from mild swelling and redness to tissue necrosis.

Serum Sickness Serum sickness is a systemic type III hypersensitivity reaction that results from the injection of large quantities of foreign protein that leads to a humoral response.

It is frequently followed by the administration of therapeutic horse antiserum and is clinically characterized by chills, fever, rash, arthritis, and sometimes glomerulonephritis. All these effects are transient and resolve when the foreign protein is cleared.

5.2.5 Type IV Hypersensitivity Reactions

Type IV hypersensitivity reactions are also known as delayed-type hypersensitivity (DTH) reactions, which are mediated by antigen-specific T cells. TDH reactions are elicited by Th1 cells and $CD8^+$ T cells, which secrete cytokines (IFN-γ, TNF-α, chemokines, etc.) that activate macrophages and induce inflammation. In $CD8^+$ T cell-mediated TDH reactions, $CD8^+$ TCLs directly kill target cells bearing MHC class I:peptide complex. T cell-mediated tissue damage may also accompany strong protective immune response against persistent pathogenic infections, especially against intracellular microbes that resist eradication by phagocytes and antibodies. Type IV hypersensitivity reactions can be grouped into three syndromes based on the route of antigen entrance: the antigen is injected into the skin in delayed-type hypersensitivity; the antigen is absorbed into the skin in contact hypersensitivity; and the antigen is absorbed by the gut in gluten-sensitive enteropathy (celiac disease) (Fig. 5.2). In addition to TDH reactions, type I hypersensitivity-mediated chronic allergic reaction may lead to Th2-type IV hypersensitivity in which Th2 type cells release cytokines and eosinophils release effector molecules that all result in persistent edema.

Delayed-Type Hypersensitivity The tuberculin test is a prototypic delayed-type hypersensitivity reaction. It is a Th1-type IV hypersensitivity reaction that is used to determine whether an individual has previously been infected with *Mycobacterium tuberculosis*. Intradermal injection of small amounts of tuberculin may lead to a hypersensitivity reaction that lasts over 24–72 h in people who have been exposed to the bacterium *M. tuberculosis*, either by infection or by immunization with the BCG vaccine. This response is mediated by chemokines and cytokines released by antigen-stimulated Th1 cells (Fig. 5.2).

Contact Hypersensitivity Contact hypersensitivity is an immune-mediated local inflammatory reaction in the skin caused by direct skin contact with certain antigens (allergic contact dermatitis) or through oral uptake of the antigens (systemic allergic contact dermatitis). Allergic contact dermatitis can be mediated by either $CD4^+$ or $CD8^+$ T cells, depending on the pathway by which antigen is processed. Typical antigens are highly reactive haptens, such as small molecular chemicals (poison ivy, DNFB) and small metal ions (nickel, chromate), that can easily penetrate intact skin to bind with self proteins, creating hapten:protein complexes that can be processed to hapten:peptide complexes for T cells to recognize. There are two stages in a cutaneous hypersensitivity response: sensitization and elicitation. During the sensitization phase, cutaneous Langerhans cells (DCs) take up and process antigens, followed by their migration to the regional lymph nodes, where they activate T cells with the consequent production of memory T cells in the dermis. During the elicitation phase, a following exposure to the sensitizing haptens leads to antigen presentation to memory T cells and the release of T cell cytokines (IFN-γ, IL-17, etc.). These cytokines further stimulate keratinocytes of the epidermis to release cytokines (IL-1, IL-6, TNF-α, etc.) and chemokines (CXCL8, etc.) that may enhance the inflammatory response by attracting more monocytes and T cells and inducing the maturation of monocytes into macrophages (Fig. 5.2). Contact with poison ivy produces a $CD8^+$ T-cell response to a chemical in the poison ivy leaf called pentadecacatechol. The chemical crosses the cell membrane and attaches to the intracellular protein to form a complete antigen. It is then processed and delivered to the cell surface as MHC:peptide to be readily recognized by $CD8^+$ T cells that cause damage either by killing the eliciting cells or by secreting cytokines such as IFN γ (Fig. 5.2).

Gluten-Sensitive Enteropathy (Celiac Disease) Celiac disease refers to a chronic condition of the upper small intestine caused by an immune response directed at α-gliadin, a protein that presents in the wheat, oats, and barley. Celiac disease possesses features of both Th1-type IV hypersensitivity reaction and autoimmunity. It is strongly genetic predisposed, with more than 95% of patients expressing HLA-DQ2 allele. The unusual structure of the peptide binding groove of HLA-DQ2 molecule allows the strong binding of peptides containing negatively charged residues at certain positions, however, α-gliadin converts selected glutamine residues to negatively charged glutamic acids by deamidation of the peptides through the enzyme tissue transglutaminase (tTG) and the formation of peptide:HLA-DQ2 complex, which then activate antigen-specific IFN-γ producing $CD4^+$ T cells that lead to intestinal inflammation.

5.3 Autoimmune Diseases

The normal immune system has the ability to distinguish "self" from "non-self", induces immune responses against nonself antigens and minimum or no responses against self-antigens, this is generally referred to as the immunological tolerance. During the state of immunological tolerance, certain amount of autoreactive T lymphocytes and autoantibodies are still present in the peripheral lymphoid system. They are important in maintaining immunological homeostasis, such remaining responses to self are called autoimmunity [1–4]. Autoimmunity diseases (AID) occur when immunological tolerance breaks down under the influence of some internal and external factors, leading to the generation of effector cells and molecules that destroy self-tissues. Autoimmune disease usually develops into chronic disease because of the difficulty to clear autoantigens from the body completely [27].

5.3.1 Classification

Autoimmunity diseases can be broadly classified into organ-specific autoimmune diseases and systemic autoimmune diseases (Table 5.1). Organ-specific autoimmune diseases are restricted to particular organ mainly due to specific interactions with organ-specific autoantigens, while on the other hand, systemic autoimmune diseases affect multiple tissues and organs by interacting with non-specific autoantigens.

Table 5.1 Systemic and organ-specific autoimmune diseases

Systemic autoimmune diseases	Organ-specific autoimmune diseases
Rheumatoid arthritis (RA)	Insulin dependent diabetes mellitus I (IDDM)
Systemic lupus erythematosus (SLE)	Multiple sclerosis (MS)
Scleroderma	Myasthenia gravis (MG)
Ankylosing sponaylitis	Graves' disease
Primary Sjögren's syndrome	Hashimoto thyroditis
Mixed essential cryoglobulinemia	Autoimmune pernicious anemia
Polymyositis	Autoimmune hemolytic anemia (AIHA)
	Autoimmune thrombocytopenic purpura
	Autoimmune Addison's disease
	Goodpasture's syndrome
	Vitiligo
	Pemphigus vulgaris
	Crohn's disease
	Psoriasis

5.3.2 Characteristics

Autoimmune diseases are usually characterized as follows: the most important immunologic abnormality is the presence of high levels of autoantibodies and/or autoreactive T lymphocytes at the pathologic site of tissues. Autoimmune diseases can be passively transferred through serum or lymphocyte transfusion [1–4, 28]. These diseases affect predominantly females and are usually triggered in genetically susceptible individuals by environmental factors such as infections. The diseases are chronic and progressive and are often observed in the form of autoimmune-overlap syndromes. The causes of most diseases are still unknown.

5.3.3 Mechanisms Underlying the Development of Autoimmune Diseases

There are many mechanisms in preventing autoimmunity diseases, each is effective in preventing anti-self response, while all of them together provide efficient protection against autoimmunity without over-inhibiting the response against pathogens. However, failure in anyone of these mechanisms may induce breakdown of the immune tolerance. First, defects in the clearance of autoreactive lymphocyte clones induce reactions with autoantigens. Second, breakdown of immunological ignorance induces immune responses against autoantigens that are usually low-affinity and low-expression. Third, polyclonal activation of lymphocytes by certain microorganisms or superantigens leads to autoimmune responses (polyclonal activation of autoreactive B lymphocytes induces production of autoantibodies). Fourth, inhibition of activation induced cell death (AICD) leads to the failure of apoptosis that in turn induces persistency of the effector lymphocytes. Fifth, defects in regulatory T lymphocytes lead to abnormal immune responses. Sixth, non-APCs with abnormal expression of MHC class II molecules may present autoantigens to autoreactive T lymphocytes. Each one of these conditions or several combined may induce immune responses against "self", which further develop into autoimmune diseases [29].

5.3.4 Factors Affecting the Development of Autoimmune Diseases

Although the mechanisms that induce autoimmune diseases are still unclear, they are thought to result from a variety of causes including genetic susceptibility and environmental triggers that lead to the breakdown of the natural tolerance, which in turn leads to the activation of autoreactive lymphocytes, production of autoantibodies, and/or autoreactive T lymphocytes that attack tissues, and the development of autoimmune diseases [30, 31].

5.3.4.1 Antigen-Related Factors

Antigen-related factors may induce the development of autoimmune diseases.

Exposure of Sequestered Antigens Lymphocytes specific to secluded antigens or sequestered antigens, that is, isolated autoantigens in the immunologically privileged sites, are not induced with immune tolerance during the development of immune system and are present in the peripheral lymphoid organs. During surgery, injury, or infection, sequestered antigens may be released into the blood and lymph fluids to induce the activation of autoreactive T lymphocytes.

Changes in Autoantigens Biological, physical, and chemical factors induce changes in autoantigens, leading to the production of autoantibodies and autoreactive T lymphocytes specific to these autoantigens.

Molecular Mimicry Certain microorganisms may possess same or similar antigen epitopes as human cells, immune responses against these microorganisms may also attack human cells with the same or similar antigen epitopes during an infection, a process known as molecular mimicry.

Epitope Spreading A single antigen possesses several epitopes, including dominant epitope and cryptic epitope. Dominant epitope is the first one to induce an immune response, followed by cryptic epitope. Epitope spreading refers to the induction of an immune response against cryptic epitope in case of a failure of antigen clearance by dominant epitope, and epitope spreading induces continuous immune responses against hidden autoantigens that further severe the disease.

5.3.4.2 Genetic Factors

The susceptibility of autoimmune diseases is strongly associated with genetic factors. Genes affecting autoantigen availability and clearance, apoptosis, signaling threshold, cytokine expression, and costimulatory molecule expression may all involve in the process.

MHC Molecules Among all the genetic loci that could contribute to autoimmune diseases, MHC molecule is the most consistently associating factor [32]. For example, certain peptide binding groove of HLA molecules cannot interact with antigenic self-peptide, inducing failure in the apoptosis of autoreactive T cells during the negative selection, which results in extremely activated autoreactive T cells.

Non-MHC Genes Certain non-MHC genes also play an important role in various autoimmune diseases. For example, deficiencies in complement component C1q and/or C4 lead to reduced ability in clearing immune complexes, which results in an increased risk of SLE. Genetic defects in signal transduction, cytokine expression, coinhibitory molecule, etc., may all result in autoimmune diseases.

5.3.4.3 Other Factors

The susceptibility of autoimmune diseases is also linked to sexuality. Certain diseases show a significant difference between males and females, for example, the sex ratio of patients with SLE (female:male) is 10 ~ 20:1, suggesting a specific role of sex hormones in the pathogenesis. Besides sexuality, age also takes part in which elder people tend to develop autoimmune diseases much more often than young people [29]. Environmental factors such as toxins, drugs, viral, or bacterial infections may all contribute to the initiation of autoimmune syndromes [33, 34]. Random event is required to trigger autoimmunity; however, genetic predisposition represents, in part, an increased chance of occurrence of this random event.

5.3.5 Mechanisms Underlying the Pathogenesis of Autoimmune Diseases

Autoreactive lymphocytes and autoantibodies play an important role in the pathogenesis of autoimmune diseases. The mechanisms of tissue damage are similar to type II, III, and IV hypersensitive reactions. Both B and T cells are involved in most autoimmune diseases although a particular type of response may predominate in causing tissue damage.

5.3.5.1 Autoantibody-Mediated Tissue Damage

Tissue damages in autoantibody-mediated autoimmune diseases are primarily due to type II hypersensitivity reactions involving antibodies against cellular/matrix antigens or cell-surface receptors, inducing damages specific to cells or tissues where these antigens are present. These autoantibodies bind to self cells and cause damages either alone or through complement activation. Type II hypersensitivity-associated autoimmune diseases mainly include autoimmune hemolytic anemia, autoimmune thrombocytopenic purpura, Graves' disease, myasthenia gravis, Goodpasture's syndrome, pemphigus vulgaris, acute rheumatic fever, etc.

5.3.5.2 Autoantigen:Autoantibody Complex-Mediated Tissue Damage

Tissue damages in autoantigen:autoantibody complex-mediated autoimmune diseases are primarily due to type III hypersensitivity reactions involving the deposition of circulating immune complexes that results in complement activation and the release of mediators from receptor-bearing cells. The immune complexes are composed of soluble autoantigens and their cognate autoantibodies. These autoimmune diseases are systemic and are characterized by autoimmune vasculitis-inflammation of the blood vessels. Type III hypersensitivity-associated autoimmune diseases mainly include mixed essential cryoglobulinemia, systemic lupus erythematosus (SLE), rheumatoid arthritis (RA), etc., in which SLE is associated with both type II and type III mechanisms, while RA is associated with both type III and type IV mechanisms.

5.3.5.3 Autoreactive T Lymphocyte-Mediated Tissue Damage

Several organ-specific autoimmune diseases are caused by type IV hypersensitivity reactions in which Th1 cells and/or cytotoxic T cells are directly involved in the tissue damage. Type IV hypersensitivity-associated autoimmune diseases mainly include insulin-dependent diabetes mellitus I (IDDM), rheumatoid arthritis, multiple sclerosis, Crohn's disease, and psoriasis, etc.

5.3.6 Therapeutic Applications

Autoimmune diseases are the outcome of abnormality of the immune tolerance; therefore, the basic therapeutic applications to fight autoimmune diseases include elimination of factors inducing abnormality of the immune tolerance, inhibition of immune responses against self-antigens, and rebuilding of immune tolerance specific to self-antigens [35].

References

1. Paul WE. Fundamental immunology. 7th ed. Philadelphia: Wolters Kluwer Health/Lippincot Williams & Wilkins; 2012.
2. Murphy K. Janeway's immunology. 8th ed. New York: Garland Science; 2011.
3. Abbas AK, Lichtman AH, Pillai S. Cellular and molecular immunology. 6th ed. Philadelphia: Saunders; 2010.
4. Parslow TG, Stites DP, Terry AI, Imboden JB. Medical immunology. 10th ed. New York: McGraw-Hill/Appleton & Lange; 2001.
5. Rucci F, Poliani PL, Caraffi S, Paganini T, Fontana E, Giliani S, et al. Abnormalities of thymic stroma may contribute to immune dysregulation in murine models of leaky severe combined immunodeficiency. Front Immunol. 2011;2(15):1–13.
6. Casanova JL, Abel L. Primary immunodeficiencies: a field in its infancy. Science. 2007;317(5838):617–9.
7. Niehues T, Perez-Becker R, Schuetz C. More than just SCID – the phenotypic range of combined immunodeficiencies associated with mutations in the recombinase activating genes (RAG) 1 and 2. Clin Immunol. 2010;135(2):183–92.
8. Losi CG, Silini A, Fiorini C, Soresina A, Meini A, Ferrari S, et al. Mutational analysis of human BAFF receptor TNFRSF13C

(BAFF-R) in patients with common variable immunodeficiency. J Clin Immunol. 2005;25(5):496–502.
9. Yu GP, Chiang D, Song SJ, Hoyte EG, Huang J, Vanishsarn C, et al. Regulatory T cell dysfunction in subjects with common variable immunodeficiency complicated by autoimmune disease. Clin Immunol. 2009;131(2):240–53.
10. Bacchelli C, Buckridge S, Thrasher AJ, Gaspar HB. Translational mini-review series on immunodeficiency: molecular defects in common variable immunodeficiency. Clin Exp Immunol. 2007;149(3):401–9.
11. Castigli E, Wilson SA, Garibyan L, Rachid R, Bonilla F, Schneider L, et al. TACI is mutant in common variable immunodeficiency and IgA deficiency. Nat Genet. 2005;37(8):829–34.
12. Unsworth DJ. Complement deficiency and disease. J Clin Pathol. 2008;61(9):1013–7.
13. Knight AK, Cunningham-Rundles C. Inflammatory and autoimmune complications of common variable immune deficiency. Autoimmun Rev. 2006;5(2):156–9.
14. Notarangelo LD. Primary immunodeficiencies. J Allergy Clin Immunol. 2010;125(2 Suppl 2):S182–94.
15. Chinen J, Shearer WT. Secondary immunodeficiencies, including HIV infection. J Allergy Clin Immunol. 2010;125(2 Suppl 2): S195–203.
16. Espert L, Denizot M, Grimaldi M, Robert-Hebmann V, Gay B, Varbanov M, et al. Autophagy is involved in T cell death after binding of HIV-1 envelope proteins to CXCR4. J Clin Invest. 2006;116(8):2161–72.
17. Shen L, Siliciano RF. Viral reservoirs, residual viremia, and the potential of highly active antiretroviral therapy to eradicate HIV infection. J Allergy Clin Immunol. 2008;122(1):22–8.
18. Brenchley JM, Schacker TW, Ruff LE, Price DA, Taylor JH, Beilman GJ, et al. CD4+ T cell depletion during all stages of HIV disease occurs predominantly in the gastrointestinal tract. J Exp Med. 2004;200(6):749–59.
19. Thompson MA, Aberg JA, Cahn P, Montaner JS, Rizzardini G, Telenti A, et al. Antiretroviral treatment of adult HIV infection: 2010 recommendations of the International AIDS Society-USA panel. JAMA. 2010;304(3):321–33.
20. Paul ME, Mao C, Charurat M, Serchuck L, Foca M, Hayani K, et al. Predictors of immunologic long-term nonprogression in HIV-infected children: implications for initiating therapy. J Allergy Clin Immunol. 2005;115(4):848–55.
21. Baker BM, Block BL, Rothchild AC, Walker BD. Elite control of HIV infection: implications for vaccine design. Expert Opin Biol Ther. 2009;9(1):55–69.
22. Kitahata MM, Gange SJ, Abraham AG, Merriman B, Saag MS, Justice AC, et al. Effect of early versus deferred antiretroviral therapy for HIV on survival. N Engl J Med. 2009;360(18):1815–26.
23. Kay AB. 100 years of 'Allergy': can von Pirquet's word be rescued? Clin Exp Allergy. 2006;36(5):555–9.
24. Jamieson M. Imagining 'reactivity': allergy within the history of immunology. Stud Hist Philos Biol Biomed Sci. 2010;41(4): 356–66.
25. von Mutius E, Vercelli D. Farm living: effects on childhood asthma and allergy. Nat Rev Immunol. 2010;10(12):861–8.
26. Ponsonby AL, Kemp A. Investigation of the hygiene hypothesis: current issues and future directions. Allergy. 2008;63(5):506–8.
27. Cooper GS, Bynum ML, Somers EC. Recent insights in the epidemiology of autoimmune diseases: improved prevalence estimates and understanding of clustering of diseases. J Autoimmun. 2009;33(3–4):197–207.
28. Davidson A, Diamond B. Autoimmune diseases. N Engl J Med. 2001;345(5):340–50.
29. Sinha AA, Lopez MT, McDevitt HO. Autoimmune diseases: the failure of self tolerance. Science. 1990;248(4961):1380–8.
30. Noseworthy JH, Lucchinetti C, Rodriguez M, Weinshenker BG. Multiple sclerosis. N Engl J Med. 2000;343(13):938–52.
31. Zhao ZS, Granucci F, Yeh L, Schaffer PA, Cantor H. Molecular mimicry by herpes simplex virus-type 1: autoimmune disease after viral infection. Science. 1998;279(5355):1344–7.
32. Javierre BM, Hernando H, Ballestar E. Environmental triggers and epigenetic deregulation in autoimmune disease. Discov Med. 2011;12(67):535–45.
33. Richard-Miceli C, Criswell LA. Emerging patterns of genetic overlap across autoimmune disorders. Genome Med. 2012;4(1):6.
34. Cho JH, Gregersen PK. Genomics and the multifactorial nature of human autoimmune disease. N Engl J Med. 2011;365(17):1612–23.
35. Hayter SM, Cook MC. Updated assessment of the prevalence, spectrum and case definition of autoimmune disease. Autoimmun Rev. 2012;11(10):754–65.

Part II

Skin Immune System

1.1 Overview

The skin is destined to serve as the defense organ against harmful stimuli from either the outside or inside of the body. Its resistance to the stimuli is accomplished by its resident components with inherent physio-chemical-biological properties, as well as through the coordinated actions with recruited or recirculating cells or molecules from other sites of the body, especially from the immune system. Every cellular components of the skin has its unique ontogeny and featured roles in the skin, for example, keratinocytes are mainly involved in barrier function, melanocytes in pigment production, Langerhans cells are classic antigen presenting cells in the epidermis, to name a few. Here, the authors reiterated the basic functions of the individual cellular components in the skin, and particularly described their roles as immunocompetent cells in the context of skin immune system. Consequently, a number of immune-related molecules, either from the skin or from circulation, are detailed in this part of the book.

1.2 The Concept of Skin Immune System

The concept of skin immune system (SIS) was first proposed by Bos, et al. in 1986. By definition, SIS is the denomination of the complexity of immune response-associated cells present in normal human skin. These cells are either resident, recruited or recirculating cells in the skin. In addition, humoral factors, a wide variety of inflammatory and immune mediators, either constitutively produced in the skin or reaches the skin by circulation, are also part of the SIS. Cellular and humoral factors in SIS are able to act in both innate and adaptive immune responses.

Cells in the Skin

6

Xiaoqin Wang, Xing-Hua Gao, Xilin Zhang, Li Zhou, Qing-Sheng Mi, Yuxiao Hong, Bing Song, Naomi McGovern*, Shawn Lim*, Mark B.Y. Tang, Florent Ginhoux, Jinyan Wang, Changlong Lu, Song Zheng, Jianjun Qiao, Hong Fang, George Man, and Mao-Qiang Man

Contents

*Both authors are contributed equally.

X. Wang (✉)
Department of Dermatology, Shengjing Hospital of China Medical University, Shenyang, Liaoning, China
e-mail: wangxq55@hotmail.com

X.-H. Gao, MD, PhD • Y. Hong (✉) • B. Song • S. Zheng (✉)
Department of Dermatology, No.1 Hospital of China Medical University, Shenyang, Liaoning, China
e-mail: yuxiao228@hotmail.com; nyaadzs@163.com

X. Zhang
Henry Ford Immunology Program, Henry Ford Health System, Detroit, MI 48202, USA

Department of Dermatology, Henry Ford Health System, Detroit, MI 48202, USA

Department of Dermatology, Second Military Medical University Changhai Hospital, 168 Changhai Rd, Shanghai 200433, China

L. Zhou • Q.-S. Mi (✉)
Henry Ford Immunology Program, Henry Ford Health System, Detroit, MI 48202, USA

Department of Dermatology, Henry Ford Health System, Detroit, MI 48202, USA

Department of Internal Medicine, Henry Ford Health System, Detroit, MI 48202, USA
e-mail: qmi1@hfhs.org

X.-H. Gao, H.-D. Chen (eds.), *Practical Immunodermatology*, DOI 10.1007/978-94-024-0902-4_6

N. McGovern • F. Ginhoux (✉)
Singapore Immunology Network (SIgN), Agency for Science, Technology and Research (A*STAR), National Skin Centre, 1 Mandalay Road, Singapore, 308205, Singapore
e-mail: Florent_ginhoux@immunol.a-star.edu.sg

S. Lim
Singapore Immunology Network (SIgN), Agency for Science, Technology and Research (A*STAR), Singapore, Singapore

L'Oreal Research and Innovation, Singapore, Singapore

M.B.Y. Tang
National Skin Centre, 8A Biomedical Grove Biopolis,Singapore, Singapore, 138648

J. Wang, PhD • C. Lu, MD, PhD (✉)
Department of Immunology, China Medical University, Shenyang, Liaoning, China
e-mail: changlonglyu@hotmail.com

J. Qiao • H. Fang (✉)
Department of Dermatology, The First Affiliated Hospital, School of Medicine, Zhejiang University, Hangzhou 310003, China
e-mail: fanghongzy@sina.com

G. Man
Dermatology Service, Veterans Affairs Medical Center San Francisco, San Francisco, CA, USA

M.-Q. Man (✉)
Dermatology Service, Veterans Affairs Medical Center San Francisco, San Francisco, CA, USA

University of California San Francisco, School of Medicine|, San Francisco, CA, USA
e-mail: maoqiangman@hotmail.com

6.1 Keratinocytes in Skin Immune System

Xiaoqin Wang and Xing-Hua Gao, MD, PhD

6.1.1 Introduction

The normal epidermis is a terminally differentiated, stratified squamous epithelium. The major cell, making up about 95 % of all, is the keratinocyte (KC), which moves progressively from basal layer toward the skin surface, forming several well-defined layers during its transit [1]. The epidermis can be divided into four distinct layers: stratum basale, stratum spinosum, stratum granulosum, and stratum corneum. A pale clear to pink layer above the granular called stratum lucidum exists in the palms and soles.

The stratum basale is a single layer of columnar cells, resting on a basement membrane. In normal skin, about 30 % of basal cells are preparing for division.

The stratum spinosum has the specialized function of producing keratin, a complex filamentous protein that not only forms the surface coat of epidermis but also is the structural protein of hair and nails. Many lamellar granules appear in the superficial keratinocytes of this layer.

The stratum granulosum normally consists of two or three layers of cells that are flatter than those in the spinous layer, and has more tonofibrils. In addition to the keratin filament system, keratinocytes of the granular zone contain keratohyaline granules, composed of amorphous particulate material of high sulfur protein content.

The stratum corneum, which is made of flattened corneocytes, provides an effective barrier to invasion by infectious agents and toxic chemicals and to water loss.

6.1.2 Immunological Roles of Keratinocytes in Skin

As a dynamic interface between our body and its environment, the skin provides many distinct functions. One of the key functions of epidermis is to form a barrier against the external environment. The cornified envelope formed from terminal differentiation of keratinocytes is rendered highly insoluble by the formation of glutamyl-lysyl isodipeptide bonds between envelope proteins, catalyzed by transglutaminases [2]. As a protective barrier, the cornified envelope can protect internal tissues against exposure to trauma, bacteria, ultraviolet (UV) radiation, temperature extremes, and toxins.

Under the stimulus of external antigens, KCs secrete proinflammatory cytokines and chemokines to attract leukocytes from the circulation to the inflammatory site. Moreover, in order to regulate the proliferation and differentiation of epidermal cells and to support the recruiting and function of Langerhans cells (LCs), KCs help to maintain the homeostasis of skin [3].

In addition to inducing dendritic cells (DCs) migration, keratinocytes can modulate the T cell response by modulating skin-resident DCs. The modulating effect of keratinocyte-derived thymic stromal lymphopoietin (TSLP) on DCs is the best example [4]. TSLP expressed by keratinocytes may be a key contributor to atopic dermatitis [5]. In response to inflammation, the receptor activator of –NF-kB ligand (RANKL) is expressed by keratinocytes, which increases the number of regulatory T (T_{Reg}) cells most likely through effects on LCs that express RANK [6]. Keratinocytes participate in not only promoting but also suppressing T_{Reg} cell responses. Cathelicidin secreted by keratinocytes can inhibit hyaluronan-induced cytokine release [7].

6.1.3 Immunity-Associated Markers and Molecules on Keratinocytes

Resting epidermal keratinocytes do not express the co-stimulatory molecule B7-1. High levels of MHC class I and II but low levels of B7-1 are expressed on activated keratinocytes. Transgenic overexpression of B7-1 on keratinocytes leads to exaggerated contact hypersensitivity, which indicates that altered regulation of B7-1 gene expression by epidermal cells may account for skin "hyper responsiveness" encountered in some chronic dermatologic disorders [8, 9]. Keratinocytes can secrete IL-10, an immunosuppressive cytokine that inhibits contact hypersensitivity [10].

Keratinocytes have been shown to express most functional TLRs. Expression of TLR4 and TLR9 reported in human keratinocytes has been controversial in the past [11–13]. Except TLR7 and TLR8, keratinocytes have been shown to express TLRs1–6 and 9 [14], and this allows them to respond to TLR4-triggering haptens, such as DNFB and nickel [15].

KCs express several kinds of receptors: Fc receptors such as FcgRI, FcgRII, and FcgRIII, complement receptors [16, 17], mannose receptor [18], and other molecules that potentially aid internalization, for example, $\alpha5\beta1$ fibronectin-binding integrin [19].

In many inflammatory dermatoses, KCs are known to express human leukocyte antigen-DR (HLA-DR) and intercellular adhesion molecule-1 (ICAM-1), which is in close association by the infiltration of T cells, a phenomenon demonstrating that KCs play an important role in skin immune system and actively mediate various kinds of biological responses [20].

6.1.4 Keratinocytes and Innate Immune Responses

Epidermis, a safeguard on the surface of the skin, is composed of keratinocytes that are regarded as a structural part of the innate immune system. Keratinocytes can protect us against environmental damage such as pathogens, UV radiation, heat and water loss, and so on. Keratinocyte stem cells (KSCs) play a key role in maintaining the normal structure and function of both the epidermis and hair follicles. They are important players in many inherited and acquired skin disorders [21].

In the course of differentiation, keratinocytes constantly divide and gradually transform themselves into corneal cells forming horny layer, which consists of protein-filled corneal envelopes (keratin, filaggrin, etc.) and a lipid-rich extracellular matrix. Filaggrin have an important role in gathering cytoskeletal proteins that form the cornified cell envelope. If it is absent, the barrier function is defective, which is determined by increased loss of water through the epidermis. The corneal layer constitutes a physical barrier that protects the body against environmental irritation.

Lamellar granules are secreted from the keratinocytes. They are vesicles filled with phospholipid components that constitute the skin's water barrier. The dark keratohyalin granules forming a hard encasing due to aggregation are made of insoluble proteins. They have anti-proteases, which defend the body against proteases released by bacteria trying to invade the skin. In the stratum spinosum, the keratinocytes produce massive amounts of desmosomes, which provide secure cell–cell cohesion and construct a barrier against friction and abrasion. Keratinized epithelium provides a better barrier against infection than nonkeratinized epithelium [22].

As is well-known, skin plays a passive role as a mechanical barrier in innate immunity. Studies on keratinocytes offered increasing evidences that epidermal cells have an active role in initiating host defense [23]. Recent research probes into the mechanisms related to keratinocytes' functions in innate immune. The protective function of keratinocytes is largely due to its production of antimicrobial peptides (AMPs). Two well-studied families of AMPs are human b-defensins (hBDs) and human cathelicidin (hCAP18/LL-37). The expression of AMPs on keratinocytes is either constitutively (hBD-1) or during inflammation (LL-37 and hBD-2, −3) [24–29]

Keratinocytes are the first active participants in the skin immune response. They express many pattern recognition receptors (PRRs) that recognize microbes through recognition of conserved molecular entities such as lipoproteins, nucleic acids, cell wall components, and flagella. At steady state, keratinocytes express a number of antimicrobial peptides, cytokines, and chemokines. Activating PRRs can rapidly increase the expression of these molecules, leading to direct antimicrobial effects as well as recruitment and education of additional immune cells [30].

6.1.5 Keratinocytes and Adaptive Immunity

Keratinocytes not only participate early in inflammation by providing first-line innate mechanisms, but also contribute to adaptive immune responses that may be associated with skin disorders. They may serve as antigen-presenting cells, produce downregulating factors such as interleukin-1 receptor antagonist (IL-Ra), and α-MSH (α-melanocyte stimulating hormone) [31]. They can promote type 1 T-helper cell responses in the skin by producing IL-23 [32]. They may induce a type 2 T cell response by production of the cytokine thymic stromal lymphopoietin (TSLP) [5].

Keratinocytes produce various kinds of cytokines, such as interleukins, growth factors, colony-stimulating factors, and chemokines. Under normal conditions, most of the cytokines are not synthesized or remain in the cytoplasm. External stimuli, such as trauma, bacterial infections, chemical substances, or ultraviolet irradiation can promote the production and release of these cytokines from keratinocyte. Cytokines secreted from keratinocytes regulate the immune and inflammatory responses through their receptors on KC, Langerhans cells, dermal fibroblasts and endothelial cells, and infiltrating T cells [3].

Keratinocytes produce cytokines either constitutively or upon induction. The cytokines secreted from keratinocytes include interleukins such as IL-1, −6, −7, −8, −10, −12, −15, −18, and −20, tumor necrosis factor-a (TNF), TGFb1, and interferon (IFN)a, b, and c. According to their function, the cytokines can be classified as pro-inflammatory, T cell trophic, or immunomodulatory, or as ligands for the cytokine receptors [33, 34].

In summary, keratinocytes have abundant cytokines and chemokines that can participate in the innate and adaptive immune responses. Keratinocytes can interact with immune cells directly and affect there functions indirectly through influence on cutaneous dendritic cells.

6.2 Langerhans Cells and Other Dendritic Cells in Skin

Xilin Zhang, Li Zhou, and Qing-Sheng Mi

6.2.1 Introduction

Dendritic cells (DCs) are professional antigen-presenting cells (APCs) involved in initiating T cell response and peripheral tolerance. Skin DCs represent a heterogeneous cell population residing at the interphase with the external environment and constitute 1–3% of the total cells in skin [35]. Canonically, immature skin DCs capture and process antigens, and then migrate to the nearby draining lymph nodes where they undergo maturation and present antigens to naïve T cells, inducing T cell priming. Skin DCs predominantly regulate skin immunity together with lymphocytes and keratinocytes, and regulate different skin disease pathogenesis [36].

As the sole DC subset in the epidermis, LCs constitutively express the characteristic lectin receptor langerin (encoded by Cd207 gene), which is associated with Birbeck granules. They also express the adhesion molecules E-cadherin and epithelial-cell adhesion molecule (EpCAM) for anchoring to neighboring keratinocytes [37] as well as the mouse lectin CD205 or major histocompatibility complex (MHC) I-like molecule CD1a in humans for antigen capture and processing [38, 39]. The dDCs are a mixed group of distinct subpopulations with specialized functions, and their classification is quite complicated due to the expression of different cell markers. The mouse dDCs can be simply divided into two subpopulations, langerin$^+$ DCs and langerin$^-$ DCs based on the expression of langerin [40–42] (Fig. 6.1), while human dDCs are subcategorized into CD1c$^+$CD14$^-$ dDCs, CD1c$^+$CD14$^+$ dDCs, and CD141$^+$ dDCs [43, 44]. Plasmacytoid DCs (pDCs) are atypical DCs that are essentially absent in the normal skin but recruited from peripheral circulation under inflammatory conditions [45]. They are characterized by their potency to produce large amounts of type I interferons (IFN), especially in response to viral infection [46]. Distinct phenotypic markers of skin DC subsets are listed in Table 6.1 [47–50].

6.2.2 Ontogeny and Homeostasis of LCs

LCs were first discovered by Paul Langerhans in 1868 and initially postulated as neurons. In 1961, ultrastructural studies identified cytoplasmic Birbeck granules as a specific feature of LCs and suggested that LCs were "effete" melanocytes instead of neurons. In 1967, Wolff and Winkelmann [51] detected ATPase activity on the surface of LCs, firstly demonstrating the leukocyte nature of LCs. Later on, Stingl, Rowden, and Klareskog [52–54] found that LCs expressed Fc and complement receptors together with MHC-II molecules, whereas Katz and Frelinger groups [55, 56] proposed a bone marrow (BM) origin of LCs by chimera studies. However, LCs were not recognized as a member of the DC system until 1985 by Gerold Schuler and Ralph Steinman [57], which was 12 years after DCs were originally discovered in the spleens of mice [58].

Ever since, whether LCs stem from BM-derived hematopoietic stem cells (HSCs) or extra-embryonic yolk sac (YS) macrophages has been a topic of considerable debate [59]. Latest lineage-tracing studies uncovered that adult mouse LCs are mainly derived from embryonic fetal liver monocytes with a minor contribution of YS-derived macrophages [60]. Likewise, the heterogeneous human LC progenitors appear at 7 weeks estimated gestational age, when hematopoiesis is active in the yolk sac, fetal liver, and aorta-gonad-mesonephros region while still inactive in the BM [61, 62]. In mice, ATPase$^+$ CD45$^+$CD115$^+$CD11b$^+$ LC

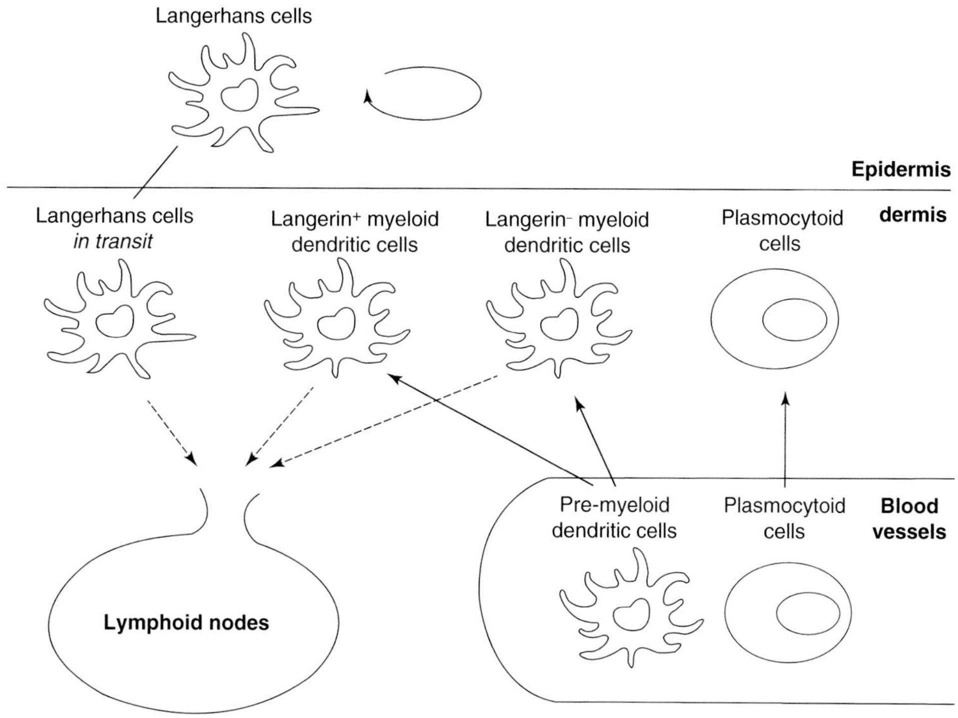

Fig. 6.1 Mouse skin dendritic cells. Under steady state, skin dendritic cells including Langerhans cells and Langerin$^{+/-}$ myeloid dendritic cells persistently migrate to skin-draining lymph nodes via afferent lymphatics. While epidermal Langerhans cells self-renew at a slow speed, Langerin$^{+/-}$ myeloid dendritic cells are supplemented by circulating precursor pre-myeloid dendritic cells. Plasmocytoid dendritic cells are essentially absent in the normal skin but recruited from peripheral blood under inflammatiory conditions

Table 6.1 Phenotypic markers of skin DC subsets

	Localization	Cell type	Phenotypic markers
Mouse	Epidermis	Langerhans cells	CD45$^+$, CD11b$^+$, CD11c$^+$, MHC-II$^+$, CD205$^+$, langerin$^+$, E-cadherin$^+$, EpCAM$^+$, CD103$^-$
	Dermis	Langerin$^-$ myeloid DCs	CD45$^+$, CD11b$^{+/-}$, CD11c$^+$, MHC-II$^+$, CD205$^+$, langerin$^-$, E-cadherin$^-$, EpCAM$^-$, CD103$^-$
		Langerin$^+$ myeloid DCs	CD45$^+$, CD11b^{low}, CD11c$^+$, MHC-II$^+$, CD205$^+$, langerin$^+$, E-cadherin$^-$, EpCAM$^-$, CD103$^+$, DC-SIGN$^+$
		Plasmacytoid DCs[a]	CD45$^+$, CD11b-, CD11c^{int}, B220$^+$
Human	Epidermis	Langerhans cells	CD45$^+$, CD11b$^+$, CD11c$^+$, MHC-II$^+$, CD1a$^+$, langerin$^+$, E-cadherin$^+$, EpCAM$^+$
	Dermis	CD1c$^+$CD14$^-$ myeloid DCs	CD45$^+$, CD11b$^+$, CD11c$^+$, MHC-II$^+$, CD1a$^{+/-}$, langerin$^-$, CD1c$^+$, CD14$^-$
		CD1c$^+$CD14$^+$ myeloid DCs	CD45$^+$, CD11b$^+$, CD11c$^+$, MHC-II$^+$, langerin$^-$, CD1c$^+$, CD14$^+$, DC-SIGN$^+$
		CD141$^+$ myeloid DCs	CD45$^+$, CD11c$^{low\ to\ int}$, MHC-II$^+$, langerin$^-$, CD1c^{low}, CD14$^-$, CD141^{high}
		Plasmacytoid DCs[a]	CD45$^+$, CD11b-, CD11c$^-$,CD123$^+$, CD303$^+$, CD304$^+$

DC Dendritic cell, *DC-SIGN* DC-specific ICAM3-grabbing non-integrin, *EPCAM* Epithelial cell adhesion molecule
[a]Plasmacytoid DCs are recruited to the dermis under inflammation conditions

precursors appear between the embryonic day (E) 16.5 and E18.5 [63, 64]. They acquire MHC class II and CD11c expression at postnatal day (P) 0 and langerin expression around P4. Subsequently, the newly differentiated LCs multiply more than tenfold, reaching a plateau at P10. In humans, ATPase$^+$ HLA-DR$^+$ leukocytes are first discovered in the skin

Table 6.2 Transcription factors in LC development and maintenance

Transcription factor	Transcription factor family	Function	Ref
ID2	Inhibitor of DNA-binding family protein containing HLH domains	ID2 null mice lack LCs and Langerin$^+$ DCs; its role during inflammatory-state remains variant	[42, 75]
RUNX3	RUNT domain family of transcription factors	In RUNX3 null mice, epidermal LCs are absent and the remaining DCs display accelerated maturation with increased efficacy in T cell priming	[76]
IRF8 (ICSBP)	Interferon-regulatory factor; interferon consensus sequence-binding protein	IRF8 null mice present decreased LC ratio, slowed down DC migration, and impaired CHS response. Controversial results	[77]
IRF2	Interferon-regulatory factor; interferon consensus sequence-binding protein	IRF2 null mice exhibit a selective cell autonomous deficiency in epidermal CD4$^+$ LCs and splenic CD4$^+$CD11b$^+$ DCs	[78]
PU.1 (SFPI1, SPI1)	ETS-domain transcription factor; binds to PU box sequences	PU.1 deficiency not only affects steady-state LCs, which BM also fails to repopulate the skin under inflammatory conditions	[79]
STAT5	Signal transducer and activator of transcription	TGF-β1-induced inhibition of STAT5 activity is required for initial LC commitment, although terminal differentiation of already committed pre-LC calls for a higher level of STAT5	[80]
C/EBP	CCAAT/enhancer binding protein (C/EBP)	Dominant-negative C/EBP switched myeloid cell fate from granulocytes/macrophages to LCs. Co-expressed C/EBP would abrogate PU.1-induced LC differentiation from human CD34$^+$ HPCs	[81]

of 6–7 week embryos. These precursor cells sequentially express MHC class II and CD1c at 9 weeks, followed by CD1a and langerin around 12–13 weeks [65]. Meanwhile, they continue to proliferate until birth.

After the initial proliferation phase, LC replenishment is differentially referred as "steady state" and "inflamed state." Under normal circumstances, an extremely slow LC regeneration is conducted by scattered in situ proliferative units [66]. After skin injuries, "short-term" LCs, which develop from peripheral blood Gr-1^{hi} monocytes, and BM-derived "long-term" LCs would transiently or stably reconstitute the LC compartment, respectively [67]. However, either monocytes [68] or BM-derived precursors [40] could still supplement transgene-induced LC shortage during steady state. In inflamed state, LC repopulation can also occur without external input or it displays mixed origins from both local and circulating precursors [64]. The detailed mechanism of exogenous LC input remains elusive.

Transforming growth factor-β1 (TGF-β1) is a crucial factor in LC development and maintenance. It is required for in vitro LC differentiation from various sources, including BM, blood monocytes, and human cord blood CD34$^+$ hematopoietic progenitor cells. Both the TGF-β1 and TGFβRII null mice exhibited a profound LC loss [69, 70]. In CD11cCre-TGF-βRI^{del} mice, LCs disappeared within the first week after birth with increased expression of co-stimulatory and pro-motility molecules, suggesting that TGF-β1 helps to maintain the immature status of epidermal LCs [71]. Colony-stimulating factor-1 receptor (CSF-1R) affects both steady-state and inflamed-state LC homeostasis [72]. Intriguingly, whereas inflammation-induced LC repopulation is dependent on its ligand Csf-1, another high-affinity ligand interleukin-34 (IL-34) specially determines normal LC development. Unlike CSF-1R, the deletion of TGF-β1 exerted no impairment on the BM's potential to generate LCs in vivo [73].

Despite the detailed understanding of LC homeostasis, the underlying transcription regulation remains elusive. We found that the canonical TGF-β1/Smad pathways are probably not required for LC differentiation [74]. Published transcription factors involved in LC development and maintenance are listed in Table 6.2.

6.2.3 Ontogeny and Homeostasis of Other Skin DCs

Unlike LCs, both skin dDCs and pDCs are short-lived and radiosensitive, and the cells from BM-derived HSC pool constantly repopulate these subsets [82]. Fms-related tyrosine kinase 3 (FLT3) is first induced in a subset of HSCs, which polarize into lymphoid-primed multipotent progenitors (LMPPs) [83]. LMPPs further differentiate into common lymphoid-restricted progenitors (CLPs) or common myeloid-restricted progenitors (CMPs). Skin dDCs and pDCs primarily derive from CMPs, while a minority of DCs (~10 %) in lymphoid organs can develop from CLPs [84]. The first precursor downstream of the CMPs that still retains DC potential is termed as macrophage dendritic cell precursors (MDPs), which can generate dDCs and pDCs as well as monocytes and macrophages [85]. The MDP is the direct progenitor of a purely DC-restricted precursor called common dendritic cell progenitor (CDP) [86]. CDP highly expresses CSF-1R and Flt3 resembling MDP but with a lower expression of the stem-cell factor receptor c-Kit [87]. CDPs further differentiate into immature pre-mDCs and pre-pDCs. Pre-mDCs then leave BM and seed in lymphoid and non-lymphoid tissues such as skin, where they proceed to become mature counterparts. To the contrary, pre-pDCs mature in the BM, and then travel to the periphery via blood circulation. However, immature pDCs can somehow be redirected to become mDCs [88]. Differentiation into distinct dDC subsets in skin is considered as a final step, which helps to maintain the stability or plasticity of the DC pool in skin. The complex network of transcription factors involved in different developmental stages has been intensively reviewed in previous excellent reviews [48, 89].

6.2.4 Skin LCs and Langerin$^+$ dDCs: Immunogenic or Tolerogenic?

DCs were traditionally considered as solely immunogenic. Similar to other tissue DCs, LCs were first thought to only mediate protective immunity, predominantly responsible for contact hypersensitivity (CHS) [90, 91]. Granulocyte/macrophage colony-stimulating factor (GM-CSF) and interleukin (IL)-1 were found to have potent impact on the viability, maturation, and function of cultured murine LCs, indicating that external stimuli facilitate the immunogenic capacity of LCs [92, 93]. This consensus was recently challenged by research results from LC-ablation mouse models. Langerin-diphtheria toxin receptor (DTR) mice (using mouse langerin promoter), which lacked LCs, langerin$^+$ dDCs, and lymphoid-resident CD8α^+langerin$^+$ DCs, showed similar or diminished ear swelling responses compared to wild-type mice [94, 95], while Langerin-diphtheria toxin subunit A (DTA) mice (using human Langerin promoter), which only deplete skin LCs, exhibited more severe ear inflammation [96]. Likewise, Langerin-DTR mice sensitized 7 or 13 days after DT injection, with only LCs absent, developed normal contact dermatitis [97]. Therefore, it appears that efficient CHS responses essentially require langerin$^+$ dDCs instead of LCs. In spite of this, recent studies demonstrated that LCs could induce CHS response by themselves if hapten did not reach langerin$^+$ dDCs or langerin$^+$ dDCs were absent [98, 99], suggesting functional redundancy of LCs and langerin$^+$ dDCs in mediating CHS.

Accumulated evidence suggests that LCs may primarily act as tolerogenic immunocytes. CD4$^+$ T cells responding to antigen presentation by activated LCs initially proliferated but then were deleted, even in the presence of potent adjuvants [100]. LCs can also promote the activation of regulatory T (Treg) cells under inflammatory situations [101, 102]. Consistently, systemically applied glucosteroids enhanced LC secretion of TGF-β1, which resulted in the expansion of Treg cells [103]. Furthermore, incompetence of LCs to defend viral infection is also noted.

In contrast to its tolerogenic function, LCs are capable of eliciting priming immunity to infectious yeast or bacteria. Using a *Candida albicans* skin infection model, LCs were sufficient for the generation of antigen-specific T-helper-17 (Th17) cells while, to the contrary, Langerin$^+$ dDCs favored the generation of cytotoxic lymphocytes and Th1 cells [104]. In the fungi infection setting, MyD88-dependent signals are required for the full activation and function of LCs [105]. In humans, LCs stimulated both Treg cells and effector T cells in response to *C. albicans* infection [106]. LCs could also induce humoral immunity toward *Staphylococcus aureus* by sampling extending dendrites through tight junctions between keratinocytes and sampling pathogenic exfoliative toxins [107]. Furthermore, the mice lacking only langerin$^+$ dDCs were still protected from infection. Together, LCs not only exert important immuno-tolerogenic functions, but can also selectively promote immune defense.

In contrast, Langerin$^+$ dDCs are prone to mediate immune protection, with a major role to cross-present antigen to CD8$^+$ T cells and initiate CTL responses. The most widely used system to assess cross-presentation included the protein ovalbumin (OVA) and ova-specific OT-I (CD8) transgenic T cells. Utilizing Langerin-DTR mice, which were adoptively transferred with OT-I cells, application of OVA onto the shaved flank skin at 1 day after DT administration led to compromised OT-I proliferation, while application of OVA at 7 day, when part of Langerin$^+$ dDCs restored to the dermis, resulted in comparable proliferation [108]. Another study found that Langerin$^+$ dDCs are able to cross-present keratinocyte-derived antigens without the assistance of LCs [50].

6.2.5 Other Skin DC Functions

In humans, CD1a$^+$CD14$^-$ dDCs display a mature phenotype capable of inducing allogeneic naïve CD4$^+$ and CD8$^+$ T cell proliferation [43, 109], while CD1a$^+$CD14$^+$ dDCs are less mature than their CD1a$^+$ counterparts with reduced ability to prime T cell immunity yet enhanced capacity to uptake antigens [110]. Human CD141$^+$ dDCs are superior at cross-presenting antigens to CD8$^+$ T cells, indicating a functional homology to mouse langerin$^+$ dDCs [44]. Unlike other CD1a$^+$ dDCs, CD141$^+$ dDCs can also mediate CD4$^+$ T cells to produce type 2 cytokines through OX40 ligand [111]. Although pDCs have limited antigen-presentation function [112], they are potent immunomodulating cells in multiple skin diseases. pDCs are able to recognize single-stranded RNA and DNA derived from invaded pathogens through toll-like receptor (TLR) 7 and TLR9 [113], and subsequently secrete large amounts of type I IFN [114]. The antimicrobial peptide LL37-self-DNA complexes were strong triggers of type I IFN production by pDCs, which may drive autoimmunity in psoriasis [115]. pDCs can also produce type I IFN and IL-6 in response to the autoantibody–nucleic acid complexes in systemic lupus erythematous (SLE), promoting autoreactive B cell responses [116].

6.2.6 Conclusion

Skin DCs are comprised of multiple heterogeneous subpopulations, which cooperate to regulate immune responses. Insight into their development and function might provide practical solutions to the diverse spectrum of skin diseases, including infection and cancer as well as allergic and autoimmune disease.

6.3 Melanocytes in Skin Immune System

Yuxiao Hong, Bing Song, and Xing-Hua Gao, MD, PhD

6.3.1 Introduction

The epidermis in skin is composed of three major resident cell types: melanocytes, keratinocytes, and Langerhans cells [117]. Melanocytes are melanin-producing cells that are derived from the neural crest and migrate during embryological development to become localized in the epidermis, including hair follicles where they release pigment for skin and hair [118].

In human epidermis, melanocytes reside in the basal layer of epidermis, and each melanocyte is surrounded by a group of about 35 neighboring keratinocytes, forming the so-called epidermal melanin unit [117, 119, 120]. Microscopically, mature melanocytes are oval or fusiform, dendritic cells, smaller than keratinocytes. The cytoplasm of melanocytes contains specialized membrane-bound organelles called melanosomes, which produce melanin [121]. The melanosomes produced by melanocytes are disseminated via elongated melanocytic dendrites to the neighboring keratinocytes of the epidermal melanin unit [122]. Within keratinocytes, melanosomes are positioned preferentially above the nuclear DNA in such a way that they form a protective screen against ultraviolet (UV) radiation [122].

Melanocytes and their production of melanin pigment (a process termed melanogenesis) have important roles in cutaneous physiology [123]. The most obvious and most studied function of melanocytes is to synthesize melanin, which confers color on skin and hair and protects epidermal cells from UV radiation-induced changes in DNA structure [119]. However, recent evidence has shown that melanocytes are also active players in the skin immune system, that they participate in immune responses, and that they have immunomodulatory properties.

6.3.2 Immunological Roles for Melanocytes in Skin

Histologically, melanocytes, along with keratinocyte and Langerhans cells, are positioned strategically within the epidermis, the outermost layer of skin. These three cells of the epidermis, sometimes called the "cutaneous troika," form a physical barrier that protects the skin from pathogens and and from other types of injury. The strategic positioning of melanocytes in the epidermis offers opportunities to encounter potentially harmful stimuli from outside, and it raises the possibility that melanocytes respond to potentially hostile environment insults, in addition to UV radiation. The dendritic nature and large surface area of melanocytes, coupled with their strategic location in the superficial layers of skin, raise the possibility that they are immunologically important cells in the skin immune system [119, 124]. Clinically, it is noteworthy that fungal infections are more common in individuals with fair skin than in those with dark skin [125]. This leads us to hypothesize that melanocytes and melanization, during which melanin is produced in melanocyte, have immunological impact on the skin immune system.

6.3.3 Immunity-Associated Markers and Molecules on Melanocytes

Toll-like receptors (TLRs) are a class of conserved receptors that recognize pathogen-associated molecular patterns (PAMPs) present in microbes, and they are known to play important roles in host defense [126, 127]. Normal human melanocytes express functional TLRs such as TLRs 2–5, 7, 9, and 10 [128–130]. Upon ligation of TLRs with LPS, for example, melanocytes may trigger NF-kB and/or MAPK (mitogen-activated protein kinase) signaling pathways [130, 131], thereby producing several pro-inflammatory cytokines and chemokines [128, 130]. These cytokines and chemokines (Table 6.3) from stimulated melanocytes may modulate the recruitment and activation of different immune cells in the skin. The expression of functional TLRs on melanocytes suggests that they may act as early sensors in immune responsiveness.

Some melanocytes cell lines also express major histocompatibility complex class II molecules [133]. Intercellular adhesion molecules such as intercellular adhesion molecules (ICAM-1) and CD40 have also been shown to be expressed

Table 6.3 Cytokines and chemokines expressed by stimulated melanocytes when challenged by stimulants.

Cells	Stimulants	Cytokines and chemokines expressed by melanocytes after stimulation	References
Primary human epidermal melanocytes	LPS	IL-1β,TNF-α	[132]
Primary human epidermal melanocytes	IL-1β	IL-6, TNF-α	[132]

by melanocytes [124, 134]. ICAM-1 is the ligand for leukocyte function associated antigen (LFA-1), which mediates non-antigen-specific cell contact. This contact is essential for helper T cell function, interactions between APC and lymphocytes, cell-mediated cytotoxicity, and antibody-dependent cellular cytotoxicity [124]. CD40 antigen plays a key role in T-cell-dependent activation, proliferation, and differentiation of B cells. Upon CD40 ligation, melanocytes upregulate expression of their co-stimulating and adhesion molecules, indicating that they are likely to be immunocompetent [124].

6.3.4 Melanocytes and Innate Immune Responses

There is a link between immunity and melanization. Melanization, the production of melanin, involves stepwise oxidation of the amino acid tyrosine and downstream aromatic compounds [135]. Melanization plays important protective roles in many species since many toxic intermediates may be produced, including semiquinones, dopaquinone, indolequinones, as well as many reactive oxygen species [136]. These intermediate compounds are believed to exert strong antimicrobial activities, and melanin, the end-product of melanization, may have the capacity to trap, inhibit, and even kill invading bacteria and other microorganisms [125, 137, 138]. Melanin may also play an immunoregulatory role. It has been found to have immunomodulatory activities through inhibition of pro-inflammatory cytokine production by T-lymphocytes and monocytes, as well as by fibroblasts and endothelial cells [139, 140].

The transfer of acidified organelles corresponding to melanosomes from melanocytes to neighboring keratinocytes in outer portions of the epidermis may have a role in acidifying the stratum corneum in darkly pigmented skin. Acidity in the stratum corneum could enhance skin barrier function and the integrity/cohesion of the stratum corneum; it might also exert antimicrobial function [141].

In response to various stimuli, melanocytes secrete a wide range of immunological molecules, including inducible nitric oxide synthase [142, 143], inflammatory cytokines, and chemokines [128, 132, 144]. These cytokines and chemokines from stimulated melanocytes may affect keratinocytes, lymphocytes, fibroblasts, mast cells, and endothelial cells in the skin. Melanocytes could also regulate skin immune response by producing and releasing several immunosuppressive molecules such as α-MSH [132]. a-MSH has a wide array of effects including anti-inflammatory as well as immunomodulatory activities [145, 146].

6.3.5 Melanocytes and Adaptive Immunity

It has been demonstrated that melanocytes are capable of phagocytosis [147]. Moreover, melanosomes have functional and structural similarities to lysosomes, and have been considered as indeed specialized melanosomes [130, 148, 149]. It is commonly believed that phagocytosis is an important step for antigen processing and presentation. Phagocytosis by melanocytes may be the first step in antigen presentation. Furthermore, it has been demonstrated that cultured normal human skin melanocytes are capable of processing and presenting the mycobacterial protein HSP65 and whole cell sonicate of *Mycobacterium leprae* to $CD4^+$ T cells in an Ag-specific and MHC class II-restricted manner, indicating that melanocytes could function as nonprofessional antigen-presenting cells in vivo [150].

Taken together, accumulating evidence supports the concept that melanocytes are not only professional melanin-producing cells but are also active players in the skin immune system. The immunological potential of melanocytes in the skin immunity is far from being fully explored. Additional work will be required to develop a comprehensive understanding of the underappreciated role played by melanocytes in the skin immune system.

6.4 Dermal Monocyte-Derived Cells and Macrophages: Organization, Immune Function, and Relation to the Dendritic Cell Compartment

Naomi McGovern, Shawn Lim, Mark B.Y. Tang, and Florent Ginhoux

6.4.1 Introduction

The skin is one of the largest organs of the body in contact with the external environment and is constantly exposed to a diverse array of microorganisms as well as potentially harmful environmental agents, such as chemicals and toxins. Consequently, the two major layers of the skin, the epidermis and the dermis, are specially adapted to fulfill their respective roles: while the epidermis is considered primarily for its physically protective properties, the underlying dermis is an important immune interface and is populated with specialized resident immune cell subsets. The dermal immune compartment is tasked with ensuring tissue integrity upon infection and inflammation, as well as shaping adaptive cutaneous immune responses to commensals and pathogens. Understanding how immune cells dynamically sense and respond to these threats to the human body, while maintaining tolerance to commensals and itself, is meaningful both from an immunological and therapeutic perspective.

Pathogen sensing and presentation, as well as initiation and regulation of the ensuing immune response, are the specialized functions of antigen-presenting cells (APCs), which belong to the mononuclear phagocyte system (MPS). The APC network comprises a heterogeneous population of mononuclear phagocytes, including monocytes, macrophages, and dendritic cells (DCs). Together, APCs play a crucial role in tissue homeostasis and local immunity; they act as a bridge between innate and adaptive arms of the immune system and are considered the primary regulators of any immune response to self and foreign proteins, pathogens, vaccines, and tumors. APCs are distributed throughout the body but are especially abundant beneath barrier tissues, including the skin and mucosae. As separate-but-related parts of the MPS, some functions and phenotypic features of the APC subpopulations are shared by more than one cell type, a fact that has historically made them difficult to distinguish. However, among the APCs, DCs are unique in their ability to initiate adaptive immunity following detection of a pathogenic threat; they are equipped with a panel of uptake and pathogen-sensing receptors that enables them to take up pathogen-derived proteins and convert them to peptides for cell surface display to T cells, while simultaneously processing pathogen-type-specific information that is used to optimally polarize the type of T cell response. Meanwhile, tissue-resident macrophages are primarily recognized for their role as phagocytic scavengers, clearing erythrocytes and cellular debris, but are also involved in an array of other processes that contribute to development, homeostasis, and tissue repair [151]. Moreover, macrophages are important components of both the innate and adaptive immune response, particularly through presentation of antigen to T cells. Alongside tissue-resident macrophages in the MPS sit the monocyte-derived cells, termed CD14$^+$ cells. CD14$^+$ cells share many functional properties with tissue-resident macrophages as will be discussed below, but unlike self-renewing tissue-resident macrophages, CD14$^+$ cells are derived from blood-precursors [152].

Alongside these general properties of the mononuclear phagocytes, the specific populations of APCs that reside within the tissues exhibit a degree of specialization that enables them to fulfill the demands of their microenvironmental/biological niche. Within the skin, the broadest division is made between APCs resident in the epidermis and the dermis. Langerhans cells were the first cutaneous APC type to be recognized, and have been extensively characterized [153], while in contrast it is only relatively recently that we have begun to understand the complexity and importance of the dermal APC compartment. The dermis of human skin in the steady state contains a dense network of diverse mononuclear phagocytes, which we now know is comprised of a population of nonmigratory tissue-resident macrophages, two migratory DC subsets (CD141$^+$ DCs and CD1c$^+$ DCs), and the CD14$^+$ tissue-resident monocyte-derived cells (termed CD14$^+$ cells herein). The latter were long considered a third DC subpopulation, but new data have confirmed their distinction from the DC populations and the nonmigratory tissue-resident macrophages in terms of both ontogeny and function [152] (Fig. 6.2). In addition, under inflammatory conditions the resident populations are supplemented by an influx of inflammatory cells with features of both DCs and macrophages, which exhibit notable plasticity and versatility in their functions (Fig. 6.2).

Understanding APCs' interrelations, functions, and regulation is central to understanding how immune responses are generated and regulated both in health and disease. This is particularly pertinent in the case of the skin given its crucial barrier and immune-modulatory roles; moreover there is growing evidence that some common skin pathologies have an immune component, spotlighting APCs as potential targets for therapeutic intervention. Here we will discuss recent advances that have led to an important redefinition of the dermal MPS and have dramatically changed our comprehension of how immunity is regulated in the skin. In particular, we will highlight the pivotal studies that have challenged our understanding of dermal monocyte-derived cells and the distinct contributions of macrophages, DCs, and CD14$^+$ cells to skin integrity and immunity. Finally, we will discuss how the APC network is modified in inflammation and the role of monocyte-derived cells and tissue-resident macrophages in cutaneous inflammatory diseases.

6.4.1.1 Defining Characteristics of Dermal Macrophages, Dendritic Cells, and Monocyte-Derived Cells

While collectively the tissue-resident macrophages, DCs, and monocyte-derived cells form the dermal compartment of the MPS, each discrete subpopulation differs in aspects of

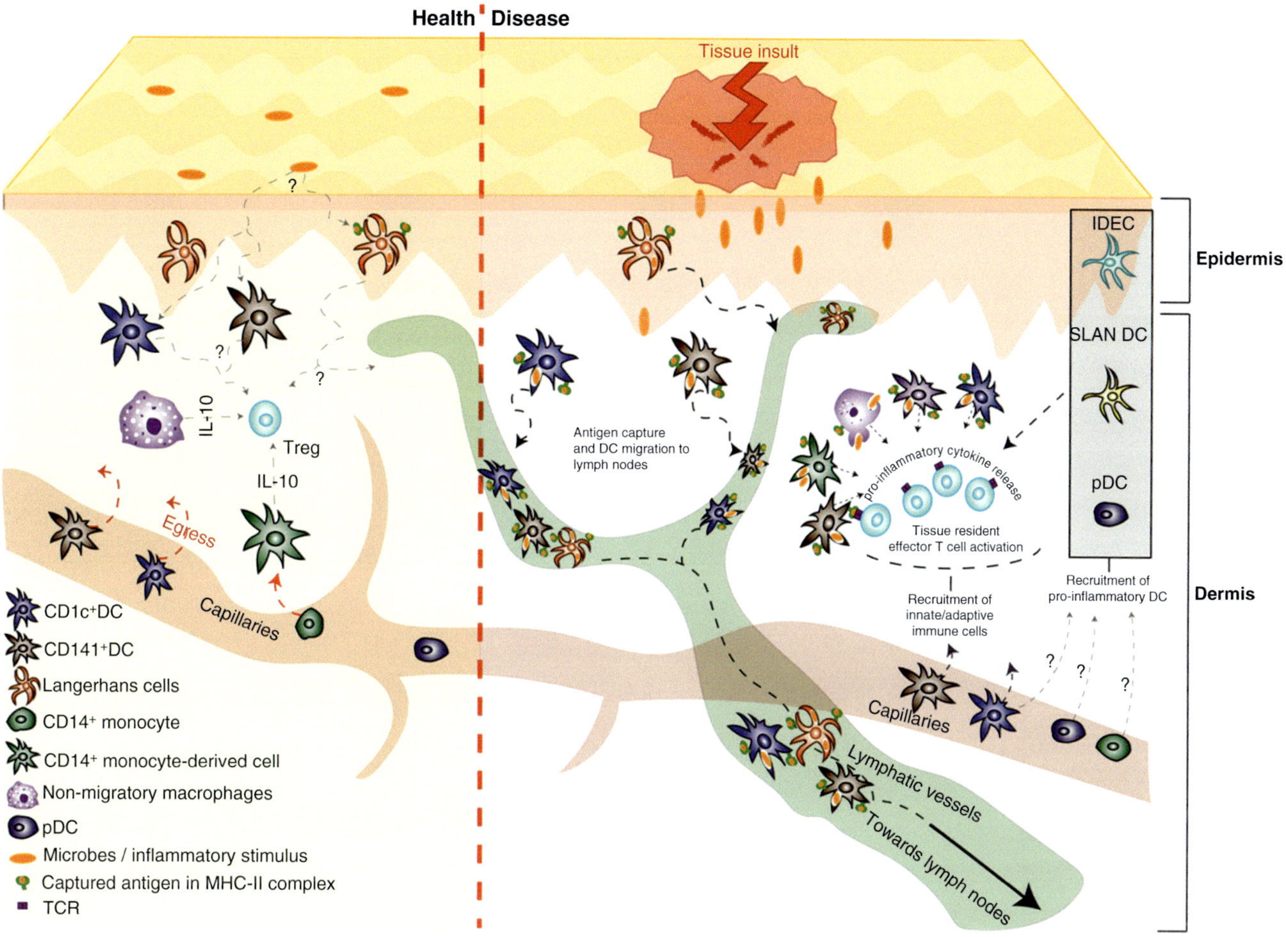

Fig. 6.2 The antigen-presenting cell compartment of human skin in the steady state and inflammation. In steady state, patrolling DCs and monocytes egress from the capillaries to replenish the dermal population. Dermal DC subsets, monocyte-derived cells, and tissue-resident macrophages continuously probe the local microenvironment, releasing cytokines and factors to help maintain tissue homeostasis. Langerhans cells (LCs) in the epidermis orchestrate the appropriate response to commensals and other antigen sources that penetrate the skin surface at a low intensity. Upon inflammation, increased numbers of DCs and monocytes are recruited, egressing from the capillaries into the tissue and promoting inflammation. Upon activation and antigen capture, DCs migrate via the lymphatic vessels to the lymph nodes. Depending on the nature of the inflammatory stimulus, additional APC subsets are present in the skin, including IDECs, inflammatory DCs and plasmacytoid DCs. The origin of these cells remains unclear. Dendritic cells (*DCs*), Langerhans cells (*LCs*), antigen-presenting cells (*APCs*), inflammatory dendritic epidermal cells (*IDECs*). Dashed grey lines indicate relationships that require confirmation

ontogeny, phenotype, function, and localization. Traditionally, human dermal APCs were studied by immuno-histochemical analysis of skin sections [154, 155]. Wang et al. have recently provided invaluable information on their anatomical localization *in situ* [156]. Alongside, flow cytometry analysis of dermal APCs collected from skin samples has revealed intricate subset-specific surface molecule expression profiles (Table 6.4). This technique has significant advantages over traditional immuno-histochemical staining methods, including the ability to precisely interrogate the expression of multiple markers simultaneously from a single specimen and to exclude false positive or negative signals from nonviable cells. Thus, while earlier studies on cutaneous APCs lacked the resolution to delineate the different cellular subsets, significant progress has recently been made in this regard.

Using flow cytometry, dermal APCs are identifiable as $CD45^+$, HLA-DR^+ leukocytes, lacking expression of T cell (CD3) and B cell (CD19 and CD20) markers [157, 158] (Table 6.4). Due to their high melanin content and large vacuoles (*see cytospin in* Table 6.4), which confer high autofluorescence and side-scatter area (SSC-A) in flow cytometry, tissue-resident macrophages (also known as melanophages) can be identified within the HLA-DR^+ fraction [159]. In addition, dermal macrophages abundantly express factor XIIIa (FXIIIa), CD163 (a scavenger receptor for the hemoglobin–haptoglobin complex) [154, 159, 160], the hyaluronan receptor LYVE-1 [156], CD26 (Dipeptidyl peptidase-4 (DPP4)) [152] and CD14 [159], while lacking CD11c, CD1a, and CD1c [159]. Meanwhile, both of the dermal DC populations (named $CD141^+$ DC and $CD1c^+$ DC) as well as $CD14^+$

Table 6.4 Surface marker expression profile of human dermal antigen-presenting cell subsets. Surface markers used to identify human dermal APC subsets are indicated in the table. Dermal APCs do not express the lineage markers CD3, CD19, or CD20. The highlighted boxes (blue, red, grey, and brown) display the combination of markers that are commonly used to identify the specific subset of interest

Dermal antigen-presenting cell characterization

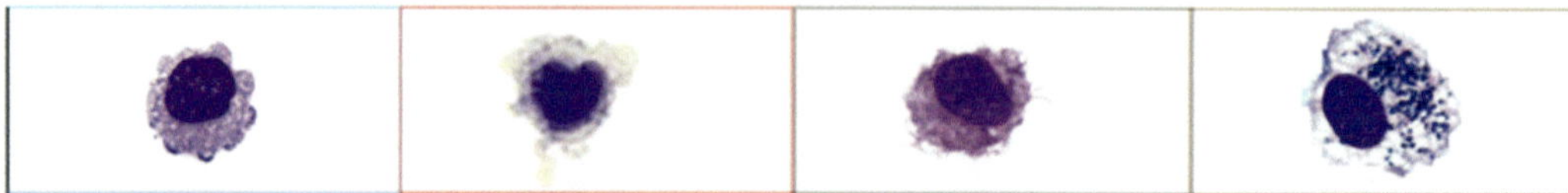

	CD1c⁺ DC	CD141⁺ DC	CD14⁺ cells	Macrophages
CD45	+	+	+	+
HLA-DR	+	+	+	+
Autofluorescence	lo	lo	lo	hi
Side-scatter area	lo	lo	lo	hi
CD14	-	-	+	+
CD1a	+	lo/-	lo/-	-
CD1c	+	-/+	lo/-	-
CD141	+/-	++	+/lo	+/lo
CD11c	+	lo/-	+	lo/-
CD26	-	+	-	lo/+
SIRPα	+	-	+	+
CD163	-	-	+	+
FXIIIa	-	-	lo/-	+
Lyve-1	-	-	-	+
CD11b	+	-	+	+
CD64	+	-	+	+
CD68	lo/+	ND	+	+
CD206	lo/+	ND	+	+
CD209	-	-	+	+
CD169	lo/-	-	+	+
Melanin	-	-	lo/-	hi

cells exhibit low auto-fluorescence and low SSC-A [152, 159, 161]. Although CD141⁺ DCs, as their name would imply, are most commonly identified by their high CD141 (thrombomodulin, BDCA-3) expression, it should be noted that other cells, including CD1c⁺ DCs and CD14⁺ cells, also express variable levels of CD141 [161] (Table 6.4). While CD14 expression allows straightforward separation of CD141⁺ DCs from CD14⁺ cells, CD141⁺ DCs can express low levels of CD1c (BDCA-1) and CD11c (Integrin αX) resulting in some phenotypic overlap with the CD1c⁺ DC subset. However, more in-depth analysis can successfully separate the two dermal DC subsets: surface markers that are expressed by CD141⁺ DCs but not CD1c⁺ DCs include CD26 (Dipeptidyl peptidase-4 (DPP4)) [162], cell-adhesion molecule 1 (CADM1, nectin-like 2 Necl-2) [163, 164], the C-type lectin Clec9a (DNGR1) [165, 166], and the chemokine receptor XCR1 [167, 168]. Of these four, CD26 is the most reliably expressed on the surface of CD141⁺ DCs following their extraction from the skin by collagenase digestion (*N. McGovern and F. Ginhoux own observations*). In addition to high CD11c and CD1c expression, dermal CD1c⁺ DCs also abundantly express SIRPα (CD172α) and CD11b (Mac-1) [152, 159, 169]. Migratory Langerhans cells within the dermal layer can be most readily distinguished from dermal DCs by their low to negative labeling for CD11c and high CD1a and langerin expression [161]. When trying to distinguish CD1c+ DCs from Langerhans cells, it should be noted that CD1c+ DCs can also upregulate CD1a and langerin to a certain degree, hence extra caution is required for distinguishing these subsets [170, 171]. Phenotypically, CD14+ cells possess a phenotype intermediate between monocytes and dermal macrophages: similar to these cell types, CD14+ cells express CD163, and in common with dermal macrophages they express CD209 (DC-SIGN), low levels of FXIIIa [152, 159], and lack surface expression of LYVE-1 [156] and CD26 [152] (Table 6.4).

6.4.1.2 The Distinction Between Dermal CD14+ Cells and Bona Fide Dendritic Cells

By definition, DCs are bone-marrow-derived [159] and are equipped with the molecular sensors and antigen-processing machinery required for their specialized immune-stimulatory and modulatory roles. Another defining property of tissue-resident DCs is their ability to migrate to the lymph node and present peptide antigens bound to HLA-DR to lymphocytes. Upon maturation and activation, tissue-resident DCs migrate to the lymph node, present these antigens to lymphocytes and release specific cytokines, thereby initiating and directing the immunological response. Hence, through their migration to lymph nodes and programming of adaptive immunity, CD141+ and CD1c+ DCs are central to the initiation and regulation of immune responses in the skin.

Since dermal CD14+ cells share expression of HLA-DR and several other markers with DCs and are similarly able to migrate spontaneously from dermal explants *ex vivo*, they were long considered a type of DC [155, 160, 172]. However, additional study of their functional properties led to the conclusion that they are not in fact DCs. Surface expression of CCR7 is crucial for DC migration to the lymph nodes; however, CD14+ cells do not express CCR7, even upon restimulation [152, 161, 173]. Pivotally, CD14+ cells have yet to be convincingly identified in the migratory DC fraction of lymph nodes [174, 175], in afferent lymph [176], or within lymphatic vessels of cultured skin explants [152]. Finally, microarray transcription profiling of cutaneous APCs has revealed that skin CD14+ cells transcriptionally align more closely with human monocytes and macrophages than DCs [152]. These data collectively suggest that dermal CD14+ cells, unlike *bona fide* DCs, do not migrate to the lymph node but instead act locally, moderating immune responses within the tissue. This is an important clarification for the field as the fact that CD14+ cells were long considered true DCs immediately implied a prototypic functional specialization in line with such an identity, and therefore drove research predominantly in that direction. Now that we know CD14+ cells are in fact monocyte-derived and more closely related to macrophages, new hypotheses can be generated and tested to elucidate their immune functions and role in disease, as will be discussed below.

6.4.1.3 Functional Properties of Dermal Monocyte-Derived CD14+ Cells and Macrophages

The immunological properties of CD14+ cells have been determined from a number of studies utilizing either primary cells from *ex vivo* cultures or cells generated in vitro from CD34+ hematopoietic stem cells (HSCs) [152, 159, 177–182]. Several investigators have shown that, in agreement with their non-DC status, both dermal macrophages and dermal CD14+ cells are far less able to induce allogeneic T cell proliferation than are dermal DCs [177, 179, 183]. Consistent with this observation, dermal CD14+ cells exhibit a broadly tolerogenic phenotype, expressing high levels of the immunoregulatory receptor immunoglobulin-like transcript 3 (ILT-3), as well as releasing biologically relevant amounts of the immune-regulatory cytokine IL-10 [177, 184, 185] (Fig. 6.2). Indeed, it seems that IL-10 produced by dermal CD14+ cells directly relates to their impaired ability to induce allogeneic T cell proliferation relative to the CD1c+ DC subset [184], confirming data from Banchereau et al. [186]. Dermal CD14+ cells can also induce the differentiation of regulatory T cells (Treg) with immunosuppressive capacity both when generated in vitro and when transferred into mice, in vivo [184]. However, upon stimulation with *Candida albicans*, dermal CD14+ cells, macrophages, and DCs all induce memory T cell proliferation and cytokine (IL-17, IL-22 IFN-γ, IL-4) production to a similar extent [152], highlighting the exquisite sensitivity and responsiveness of these cells. Taken together, these data suggest a model of dermal CD14+ cell function whereby monocytes entering the tissue from local blood vessels during the steady state differentiate into dermal CD14+ cells that act locally to help maintain tissue homeostasis by secreting IL-10 and promoting Treg induction. Upon detection of an immunological threat however, as shown with *C. albicans*, CD14+ cells can trigger local pro-inflammatory responses to help restrain the infection [152].

Similar to CD14+ cells, tissue-resident macrophages also play an important role in maintaining healthy tissue homeostasis. Although the gene expression profile of macrophages overlaps with that of CD14+ cells to a certain degree, they possess a distinct morphology (see cytospin profile in Table 6.4), phenotype (as discussed above), functional profile, and ontogeny. In the steady state, the primary role of dermal macrophages is to scavenge for degradation products in order to maintain tissue function and homeostasis as well as to contribute to immune tolerance by secreting the immune-regulatory cytokine IL-10 (Fig. 6.2). However, following immune challenge and inflammation they become activated, markedly increasing their phagocytic capacity, antimicrobial activity [187], and release of pro-inflammatory cytokines and chemokines that recruit and activate other immune cells [187–189]. In the skin specifically, macrophages play a central role in the response to diverse stimuli, including allergens, microbes, and UV irradiation as we will discuss below. Upon tissue injury and healing, macrophages are important for tissue repair through their scavenger activity and cytokine production [190]. Thus, dysregulation of the dermal macrophage response is a major contributor to the pathogenesis of inflammatory skin diseases such as psoriasis and atopic dermatitis [191].

6.4.1.4 Ontogeny of Macrophages and Dermal CD14⁺ Cells

Defining the ontogenic pathways of APC populations enables us to make sense of their interrelationships, commonalities, and distinguishing features both individually and within the broader context of tissue homeostasis and immune regulation. Fundamental to our understanding of the origins and development of human macrophages, DC and monocyte have been quantified in immune-deficient patients and those that have undergone hematopoietic stem cell transplantation (HSCT). Studies from patients lacking circulating DCs and monocytes as a result of genetic mutations in GATA2 or IRF8 are also depleted in their tissue DCs and $CD14^+$ cells [192, 193]. Additionally, the cytotoxic therapy used to suppress the bone marrow of HSCT patients prior to transplant results in absolute monocytopenia, accompanied by the loss of $CD14^+$ cells and DCs from the skin, while macrophage populations are reduced only by approximately 50% [152]. These data indicate that monocyte and DC precursors are both derived from the bone marrow, and that blood-circulating cells seed the tissues with their monocyte and DC populations. Interestingly, upon bone marrow transplant into these patients, the kinetics of $CD14^+$ cell reconstitution within the skin are different from those of DCs: while $CD14^+$ cells are rapidly reconstituted within skin in the early recovery phase post-HSCT, the kinetics of DC recovery are much slower [152]. These findings further highlight the distinct precursor–progeny relationships of dermal DCs and $CD14^+$ cells and provide direct evidence of the monocytic origin of dermal $CD14^+$ (Fig. 6.2).

Gene array data and transcript profiling of all blood and skin macrophage, DC, and monocyte subsets has also proven invaluable in delineating their origins and developmental pathways. Dermal $CD14^+$ cells express a gene set that overlaps significantly with that of dermal macrophages and $CD14^+$ blood monocytes, but is notably distinct from that of blood and skin DCs [152, 161]. Moreover, upon culture with primary endothelial cells, $CD14^+$ monocytes upregulate expression of certain surface molecules and adopt morphological changes characteristic of dermal $CD14^+$ cells [152]. These data are consistent with the conclusions drawn from transplant recipients and in vitro functional analyses, namely, $CD14^+$ cells derive from blood monocytes that differentiate into macrophage-like cells following extravasation into the skin (Fig. 6.2), and are not classical DCs as thought before.

In contrast to dermal DCs and $CD14^+$ cell populations, the tissue-resident macrophages are self-renewing [159], and, as in the mouse, are thought to be largely derived from fetal progenitors that seed the tissue prior to birth [194]. Macrophage-like cells can be detected from 3 weeks estimated gestational age (EGA) in the human fetal yolk sac [195, 196] and in fetal skin by 9 weeks EGA [197, 198], before hematopoiesis becomes fully established in the bone marrow at 10 weeks EGA. In this regard, Langerhans cells (LCs) also represent an interesting cell population: studies in HLA-mismatched patients after either BM or limb transplant showed that LCs in the human adult self-renew, maintaining their population independently of blood-derived precursors [199, 200], similar to tissue macrophages. Arising from fetal progenitors, most likely in the yolk sac [198, 201], LCs have been detected in fetal skin from just 6–7 weeks EGA [202]. Moreover, considering again the experiments in bone marrow transplant recipients, macrophage populations in the skin are reduced by only 50% while DCs and $CD14^+$ cell populations are decimated, further suggesting some independence of the adult macrophage population from bone marrow precursors and a degree of self-renewal capacity [152]. While several lines of evidence support this conclusion, whether skin-resident macrophages arise predominantly from self-renewing fetal cells or from recruited monocytes remains to be defined.

6.4.1.5 Aligning Mouse and Human Monocyte and Macrophage Subsets

For understanding the human relevance of findings from experiments in animal models, it is important that we can align cell subsets across species, especially between human and mouse [203]. Studies have shown that human $CD141^+$ DCs are homologous to murine $CD103^+/CD8^+$ DCs [161, 165, 167, 168, 204] and are highly efficient at cross-presenting antigen to $CD8^+$ T cells [161, 165, 167, 168, 204, 205]. Meanwhile, $CD1c^+$ DCs are homologous to murine $CD11c^+CD4^+$ DCs in the spleen and $CD11b^+CD24^+CD64^-$ DCs in non-lymphoid tissues [206], and are highly efficient at stimulating $CD4^+$ T cells [169, 206].

However, until recently it had not been possible to identify a mouse equivalent of human dermal $CD14^+$ cells. This was largely because mouse dermal monocyte-derived cells were indistinguishable from other cellular subsets, until Tamatounour et al. developed a high resolution method allowing the distinction of macrophage, DCs and monocyte-derived cells within the mouse [207]. Using this model they directly demonstrated that murine dermal monocyte-derived cells are continuously generated by extravasated Ly-$6C^{hi}$ monocytes, further supporting the notion that human dermal $CD14^+$ cells are of monocytic origin. Comparative transcriptomic analysis using microarray data generated in mice and humans has now shown that human $CD14^+$ cells have the highest enrichment score with the mouse dermal DC and macrophage fraction, of which approximately 90 % and 80–90 %, respectively, are monocyte-derived cells. Collectively, these studies provide substantial evidence that the murine homologs of human CD14$^+$ cells are dermal monocyte-derived cells. Further development of this work will now aid in elucidating the immunological role of monocyte-derived cells within the dermal layer of human skin, both in health and disease.

6.4.1.6 Monocyte-Derived Cells and Macrophages in Cutaneous Inflammation

Cutaneous APCs have a range of potent biological capabilities, including eliciting inflammation, antigen presentation, phagocytosis, and tissue homeostasis and repair. Thus, they, and/or their dysregulation, have long been implicated in the pathogenesis of dermatological diseases [208–210]. In particular, there has been much interest in the potential role of dermal APCs in the heterogeneous set of pathologies that are characterized by aberrant T cell infiltration, activation, and inflammation, which includes several inflammatory, autoimmune and lymphoproliferative skin diseases. As well as DCs and tissue-resident macrophages, in recent years the focus of dermal disease research has expanded to monocyte-derived cells recruited during inflammation as awareness has grown of the important role that recruited monocyte-derived cells play in such settings [174].

6.4.1.7 Dermal APCs in Atopic Dermatitis

Atopic dermatitis (AD) is one of the most common skin inflammatory disorders, with a prevalence of 2–5 % in adults and approximately 10 % in children [211, 212]. Characteristic signs and symptoms of AD include chronic relapsing itchy, red, inflamed skin lesions accompanied by dysfunction in the skin barrier, which renders patients susceptible to recurrent microbial infections [213]. The etiology of AD is multifactorial, but two hypotheses exist as to the driving biological process underlying this condition: skin barrier dysfunction and dysfunctional immune regulation. There is evidence to support important roles for both, and perhaps also for their interaction. Filaggrin is an epidermal protein whose normal function is required for the maintenance of the epidermal barrier, and loss of function mutations in the filaggrin gene are the strongest known genetic risk factor for AD susceptibility [214, 215]. Defects in barrier integrity such as those caused by filaggrin mutation render the epidermis permissive to allergens, irritants, and opportunistic agents, which in turn can activate cutaneous APCs, thereby triggering a robust inflammatory response [214].

The inflammation that characterizes AD consists of a massive infiltration of immune cells, including CD4$^+$ memory T cells, eosinophils, DCs, and macrophages. Markedly more DCs, monocytes, and macrophages are present in lesional skin of AD patients compared to unaffected or normal skin [216, 217] (Fig. 6.2). Importantly, distinct profiles of APC subsets can be found in healthy compared to diseased skin [208–210]. Unique inflammatory dendritic epidermal cells (IDECs), with abundant expression of the high-affinity receptor for IgE (FCεR1), have been described in AD [218], and their precise phenotyping has allowed the differentiation between extrinsic and intrinsic forms of the condition [219]. Indeed, IDECs have been shown to play a critical role in perpetuating the chronic inflammatory response characteristic of AD (Fig. 6.2). However, whether IDECs arise from monocytes or represent an independent population of inflammatory DCs remains to be investigated. Elevated expression of IgE and FCεR1 expression is also observed on APCs in the AD dermal infiltrate [220], consistent with the established knowledge that IgE-mediated sensitization is the basis of the food and environmental allergen response frequently observed in AD.

Dermal macrophages are also implicated in the pathogenesis of AD. Kiekens et al. used CD68 and RFD7 to identify macrophages in AD lesional and non-lesional skin, and found that this cell type was significantly more abundant in AD skin compared with healthy skin, as well as in acute lesional skin compared with non-lesional skin from the same donor [217]. Furthermore, CD68$^+$ macrophages in lesional skin exhibited elevated expression of the mannose receptor (MR/CD206) and the scavenger receptor CD36, a phenotype consistent with a heightened macrophage activation state in AD. More recently, Sugaya et al. showed that the number of macrophages expressing CD163 was higher in AD lesional skin compared to normal skin [221]. This is particularly intriguing as CD163, alongside CD206, is considered a marker of "alternatively activated" macrophages, a subset normally associated with resolution of inflammation and wound healing. Th2 cytokines such as IL-4 and IL-13 are known to trigger the differentiation of these alternatively activated macrophages, and indeed a dysregulated Th2-type response is one of the hallmarks of AD. Thymic stromal lymphopoietin (TSLP), an IL-17-related cytokine, is highly elevated in the lesional skin of AD patients as compared to non-lesional or normal skin, and was found to drive activation of CD11c$^+$ DCs to trigger production of Th2 cytokines by T helper cells, thereby contributing to AD pathology [222]. Although keratinocytes were thought to be the main source of TSLP in AD skin, dermal injection of allergen into normal skin of atopic individuals triggered TSLP expression by CD68$^+$ macrophages [223]. Finally, Han and colleagues demonstrated, in a mouse model of allergic airway inflammation, that TSLP acts directly on quiescent macrophages to promote differentiation to the alternatively activated phenotype in an IL-13-dependent manner [224]. While it is clear that macrophages are intimately engaged in the processes of

AD, their relative contribution toward pathological inflammation versus resolution of the AD inflammatory response remains unknown.

Rather than considering AD as a manifestation of either epidermal barrier dysfunction or immune dysfunction, there is increasing appreciation that the interaction of these two factors is likely to be a significant contributing factor. The compromised epidermal barrier of AD skin renders sufferers susceptible to recurrent opportunistic infections, and indeed there is a strong correlation between AD severity and infection of lesional skin by *Staphylococcus aureus* [225–227]. A dysregulated response to microbial infection might also be involved. Macrophage recognition of gram-positive bacteria such as *S. aureus* occurs via membrane-bound TLR-2, and macrophages (and monocytes) from AD patients appear to be impaired in TLR-2 expression, and had reduced production of the pro-inflammatory cytokines IL6 and IL-1β following stimulation with bacterial components [228, 229]. Hence, treating both inflammation and infection is critical in the management of AD, especially during disease flares. In addition, genetic polymorphisms in TLR-2 are present in a significant fraction of AD patients, typically correlating with a more severe disease phenotype [230]. Interestingly, monocytes from AD patients carrying the TLR-2 R753Q polymorphism produced significantly more IL-6 and IL-12 in response to TLR-2 stimulation compared to their wild-type counterparts. In contrast, IL-6 production in monocytes of patients with the homozygous TLR-2 A-16934 T mutation was reduced [231]. Collectively, the data suggest that an imbalance in TLR-2 signaling is implicated in the increased susceptibility to bacterial skin infections observed in AD patients, but the exact mechanism remains to be elucidated.

6.4.1.8 Psoriasis

Psoriasis is a common chronic skin inflammatory condition characterized by the presence of well-demarcated scaly red plaques that result from epidermal hyper-proliferation, secondary to a prolific inflammatory cell infiltration of the skin. In contrast to AD, where the Th2 response is thought to play a key role, the conventional understanding of the pathogenesis of psoriasis is that excessive production of Th1 cytokines by T cells leads to dysregulated keratinocyte proliferation and differentiation. This theory was initially supported by the observation that bone marrow transplantation from a psoriatic individual into a previously unaffected individual was sufficient to elicit disease symptoms; conversely psoriatic patients who received bone marrow transplants from an unaffected donor experienced resolution of their lesions [232, 233]. However, more recent evidence has challenged this traditional T-cell-centric view, demonstrating the importance of other immune cell types, cytokines and keratinocyte signal transduction, as will be discussed in the following section.

Psoriatic skin is in fact a highly atypical immune environment in several respects. Inflammatory immune cells including $CD1c^+$ DCs, $CD3^+$ T cells, and $CD163^+$ macrophages are between two and four times more abundant in psoriasis plaques compared to non-lesional skin [154]. In addition, plasmacytoid DCs, which are not present in healthy skin and are normally associated with the clearance of viral infections, have been found in inflammatory psoriatic lesions [234, 235] (Fig. 6.2). Moreover, a specific inflammatory APC subset has been characterized in psoriasis, so-called SLAN (6-sulfo LacNAc) DCs, which accumulate in psoriatic skin and can drive strong Th17/Th1 T cell responses, promoting the disease [236, 237] (Fig. 6.2). The term "SLAN DC" relates to the presence of the Sulpho LacNAc (SLAN) carbohydrate modification of the P selectin glycoprotein ligand 1 (PSGL-1) on the cell surface. Blood $SLAN^+$ DCs produce Th17-polarizing inflammatory cytokines, including IL-1β, IL-23, and IL-6, while the presence of $SLAN^+$ DCs in inflamed tissues may be linked to several immunopathological conditions including psoriasis [236], lupus erythematosus [237], and multiple sclerosis [238]. In psoriatic skin lesions, $SLAN^+$ DCs produce the inflammatory cytokines TNF-α and iNOS [236] upon stimulation and can drive Th17 polarization of allogeneic T cells [235, 236], which could have a functional role in exacerbating the disease.

The finding that SLAN expression is otherwise restricted to a subfraction of the minor $CD14^{low}CD16^+$ blood monocyte population [239, 240] has since led to questions as to the true nature of $SLAN^+$ DCs. While $SLAN^+$ DCs are known to be highly pro-inflammatory and to possess some DC-like features [236, 241], preliminary gene array analysis indicates that they are most likely monocyte-derived [240], and their relative inefficiency at antigen presentation similarly argues against them being true DCs [240, 242]. Hence, they might more accurately be considered as a type of patrolling tissue monocyte that is recruited into inflamed tissues and has significant pro-inflammatory properties [243]. Whether $SLAN^+$ DCs truly arise from monocytes or represent an independent population of inflammatory DCs remains to be unequivocally confirmed.

There is some evidence that macrophages in psoriasis and in AD share common phenotypic features, which could be important in understanding their roles in such conditions. $CD163^+$ macrophages in psoriasis also express CD206, FXIIIa, and RFD7 [189]. However, immunofluorescence imaging showed that psoriasis macrophages express the products of IFN-γ responsive genes including STAT-1, CXCL9 and high levels of HLA-DR, suggesting a possible contribution to pathogenic inflammation in this condition. In addition, $CD68^+$ monocytes/macrophages isolated from psoriasis lesions were found to express IL-23, which is essential for induction of the Th17 response [243]. Interestingly, the selective elimination of epidermal macrophages in an induced mouse model of psoriasis resulted in attenuation of disease symptoms, but this appeared to be independent of IFN-γ-driven macrophage activation [244]. Thus, macrophages were clearly involved in disease pathogenesis, but their precise role remained undefined. Using a different mouse model, Wang and his colleagues found evidence to suggest that $CD4^{+}$ T cells activated in the dermis drive the activation of dermal macrophages, which then produce high levels of TNF-α responsible for the physiological changes in psoriatic skin [245]. In support of this hypothesis, TNF-α signaling blockade returned inflammatory cell numbers to levels comparable with non-lesional skin and reduced epidermal hyperplasia [246]. The association of macrophages specifically with production of TNF-α in psoriasis was suggested through immunohistochemical examination of psoriatic lesions, which revealed that macrophages express TNF-α at a high level, in contrast to other myeloid cells within the dermis [247]. TNF-α was shown to induce keratinocyte production of TGF-α [248], which acts in an autocrine manner to stimulate keratinocyte proliferation through binding of the epidermal growth factor receptor [249].

The production of TNF-α by psoriatic macrophages may also serve a second indirect but important function in the condition. TGF-α induces expression of the gene encoding the potent pro-angiogenic factor VEGF in keratinocytes in vitro, which is elevated in the epidermis of psoriatic skin [250]. High VEGF expression is consistent with the characteristic dilation and increase in dermal vasculature that is a prominent feature of psoriasis lesions. Furthermore, activated macrophages secrete a variety of cytokines such as FGF-2, GM-CSF, PDGF, and TGF-α that support various phases of angiogenesis, including proliferation of endothelial cells and facilitation of capillary differentiation [251]. Thus, macrophages can be considered to both drive and maintain several of the pathological processes controlling the manifestation of psoriasis, both directly through their pro-inflammatory actions and indirectly, by driving keratinocyte proliferation and the expansion of the local blood vasculature.

6.4.1.9 Graft-Versus-Host Disease

Graft-versus-host disease (GVHD) is a clinically significant potential complication of allogeneic HSCT, which often has a component of dermatologic manifestation. In the acute phase, GVHD can manifest as diffuse erythematous macules and blisters, and in the chronic phase, a lichenoid eruption. The severity of GVHD correlates with a stronger infiltration of macrophages in the skin lesions [252], and studies on skin biopsies from patients undergoing HSCT show that these macrophages originate from the recipient rather than from the donor. As APCs, macrophages may potentiate GVHD through presentation of host-specific tissue antigens. Additionally, dermal macrophages potently activate and stimulate proliferation of $CD8^{+}$ T cells; these two mechanisms are thought to be the main contributors to the severity of GVHD [159]. In a murine model of chronic GVHD, $F4/80^{+}CSF\text{-}1R^{+}CD206^{+}iNOS^{+}$ cells with a phenotype indicative of monocyte-derivation infiltrated the skin, and their depletion using an anti-CSF-1R (colony-stimulating factor 1, M-CSFR, C115) monoclonal antibody markedly reduced cutaneous GVHD [253]. In summary, not only are macrophages clearly instrumental to the development of cutaneous GVHD, but targeting their depletion through CSF-1 signaling after transplantation may be a promising strategy for the prevention and treatment of this debilitating disease.

6.4.1.10 Wound Healing

Wound healing in healthy skin is a multistage process that is intricately intertwined with, and reliant upon, a functional immune system. In the acute phase immediately after skin injury, immune cells quickly infiltrate the wound site and respond by inducing a highly pro-inflammatory milieu to combat pathogens and remove tissue debris and necrotic cells. This is followed-up by an anti-inflammatory phase that promotes the formation of granulation tissue and initiates the process of re-epithelialization and restoration of the skin barrier. Finally, the cytokine-rich environment of the wound space promotes abundant deposition of extracellular matrix by fibroblasts, to regenerate the dermis and return tensile strength to the tissue [254]. Chronic wounds such as diabetic or venous leg ulcers arise from the failure or dysregulation in the delicate balance of this coordinated cellular response [255–257].

The significance of macrophage response in all phases of wound healing was demonstrated by conditionally deleting macrophages at different time points prior to or following experimental wounding of mice. Macrophage depletion before wounding resulted in impairments in cytokine production, in granulation tissue formation, in re-epithelialization, and delayed wound closure [256, 258, 259]. This is unsurprising as innate immune cells such as neutrophils and macrophages are the first to infiltrate the injury site, producing pro-inflammatory cytokines including TNF-α, IL-1β, and IL-6, as well as nitric oxide to support the acute antimicrobial and cytotoxic host defense. Although highly relevant in the acute phase, overstimulation or persistence of this pro-inflammatory response has been linked to delayed or impaired wound healing. Sindrilaru and colleagues established an iron-overload macrophage mouse model that mimics macrophages found in human chronic venous leg ulcers, and demonstrated that such macrophages persist in an unrestrained pro-inflammatory state. This resulted in elevated TNF-α and oxidative stress that induced premature senescence in dermal fibroblasts, eventually leading to impaired wound healing [260]. Understanding the regulation of prolonged inflammatory activation of macrophages will be the first step toward using this knowledge for clinical benefit.

Aside from their role in the acute inflammatory phase, depletion of macrophages during the formation of granulation tissue results in delayed wound closure associated with a defect in vascularization and maturation of the granulation tissue [261]. During this phase, differentiation of anti-inflammatory macrophages is induced in response to phagocytic clearance of apoptotic neutrophils with subsequent release of TGF-β1 [262, 263]. This phagocytic interaction between neutrophils and macrophages is dependent on β_2 integrin-mediated adhesion, and patients with syndromes associated with lack of functional β_2 integrin spontaneously develop skin ulcerations that are slow to heal [264, 265]. Macrophage-derived TGF-β_1 is a chemotactic agent that recruits and promotes fibroblast proliferation as well as induces the deposition of collagen, which is linked to formation of fibrotic tissue. On the other hand, IL-10 and VEGF produced by these same anti-inflammatory macrophages are responsible for dampening of the inflammatory response as well as promoting endothelial cell recruitment and differentiation into new vasculature [256, 262, 265]. It thus appears that macrophage phenotype must evolve dynamically to meet the spatial and temporal requirements of the wound microenvironment if optimal healing is to occur [254].

6.4.1.11 Conclusion

Cutaneous APCs play a significant role in the priming and driving of immune responses in many common, high-burden, inflammatory skin diseases. Dermal monocyte-derived $CD14^+$ cells and tissue-resident nonmigratory macrophages are particularly important in the regulation of local immune responses and the maintenance of tissue homeostasis. A better understanding and awareness of their differential roles in an inflammatory setting may aid in the identification of new therapeutic targets to improve our ability to resolve pathological inflammation and improve patient treatment outcomes.

6.5 Endothelial Cells

Jinyan Wang, PhD and Changlong Lu, MD, PhD

Endothelial cells (ECs) are a heterogeneous populations that form a single layer called endothelium, which lines the vasculature and lymphatic systems forming a semipermeable barrier between blood or lymph within vessels and the surrounding tissues. Endothelium is a highly specialized, dynamic, disseminated organ that serves as a physical barrier [266].

The involvement of endothelial cells into a variety of physiological functional processes to maintain vascular tone, blood pressure, and blood flow rate at the steady state of the body has been clearly described [267]. These physical function of endothelial cells is mediated by several kinds of mediators, such as nitric oxide, prostacyclin, and endothelin. The production of these mediators are tightly regulated to maintain the balance of either vasodilation or vasoconstriction [268]. Endothelial cells also play key role in the regulation of coagulation cascade. Under normal physiological conditions, ECs inhibit the activation of pro-coagulation by expression of a variety of inhibitory molecules, such as factor X, thrombin, and fibrin; alternatively, once the endothelium is injured, the endothelial cells quickly transforms to a pro-coagulant state by inducing tissue factors that initiate the extrinsic coagulation cascade [269].

As constituents of physical barrier, endothelial cells have an essential role in modulating vascular permeability that controls the cells to move into and out of the circulatory system by the endothelium permeability through the interactions among different epithelial cells by paracellular and transcellular ways. The structure of blood vascular endothelium varies in different locations; for example, the resting cutaneous blood vessels composed of a continuous monolayer of endothelial cells, which are covered with pericytes, form tight and adherents junctions [270]. Under normal physical conditions, endothelium basal permeability only allows for the easy diffusion of solutes such as glucose, ions, and other metabolites to underlying cells. In contrast, endothelial permeability increases, allowing for excess trafficking of immune cells to migrate into the tissues, which may contribute to the initiation of tissue inflammation [271]. Inflammatory responses include a series of process that are characterized by redness, swelling, heat, and pain at the site of inflammation. In this condition, endothelial cells are activated to express distinct extent of cell-adhesion molecules that promote the binding of circulating leukocytes extravagate into the tissues; considerable amounts of plasma proteins enter from circulation into the tissue, leading to tissue edema and pain. The alterations of epithelial cells are initiated by the pro-inflammatory cytokines and chemokine produced by activated macrophages, such as tumor necrosis factor-α(TNF-α),IL-1ß, IL-6, IL-8, and others [272]. Binding of these cytokines to receptors on endothelial cells upregulate the expression of adhesion molecules such as E-selectin, intercellular adhesive molecule-1 (ICAM-1), and vascular cell-adhesion molecule-1 (VCAM-1), allowing rolling and attachment of leukocytes to the epithelium [273].

Recent studies have extensively demonstrated that endothelial cells function as immune cells that play an important role in initiation of inflammation and mediating immune responses [274]. Immune responses are complex processes in which immune cells recognize and respond to antigen stimulation leading to elimination of antigen. By mechanism of actions, immune responses can be classified into two categories, innate immune response that relies on a limited number of receptors expressed on innate immune cells such as pattern recognition receptors (PRRs), including TLRs and NLRs, as well as secreted proteins such as cytokines, complements that are encoded in the germ line that recognize features common to many pathogens, which initiate rapid immune responses against pathogens. In contrast, adaptive immune response is mediated by T lymphocytes and/or B lymphocytes, cells expressing clonally distributed antigen receptors that are capable of fine distinctions between different antigens. Innate immune responses provide initial defenses and also contribute to the induction of adaptive immune responses [275].

Endothelial cells are considered as sentinels of the innate immune system, which form the first line in the circulation of the host to interact with microbial components. Endothelial cells express diverse PRRs such as TLRs and NLRs on their surface, which recognize the component of pathogen-associated molecular patterns (PAMPs), leading to activation of endothelial cells [276]. Activated endothelial cells show enhanced expression of pattern recognition receptors (PRRs), sequentially increasing the expression of diverse adhesive molecules, which results in increased capacity to interact with circulating leukocytes for transendothelial migration (TEM). Transendothelial migration not only promotes the migration of circulating leukocyte into the inflammatory tissue, but also enhances the expression of co-stimulatory molecules associated with antigen presentation and activation of monocytes [277]. Activated endothelial cells are able to produce inflammatory cytokines such as IL-1, IL-8, and monocyte chemotactic protein-1 (MCP-1) in response to lipopolysaccharide (LPS) stimulation [278]. TLR4 and CD14 expressed on the surface of endothelial cells are required for LPS binding. Endothelial cells can express TLR2, TLR3, TLR7, TLR8, and TLR9 to contribute recognition of pathogen-associated molecular pattern of pathogen, including lipopolysaccharides and viral and bacterial RNA and DNA [279]. Thus, activated endothelial cells play an essential role in the initiating of innate immune response.

Endothelial cells also play roles in initiating adaptive immunity. It has been well documented that endothelial cells play a clear role in antigen presentation [280, 281]. Endothelial cells have been considered as conditional antigen-presenting cells (APCs). Antigen presentation of endothelial cells requires MHC molecules, which structurally possess antigen-binding groove, to present antigen peptides to T cells. MHC class I molecules, constitutively expressed by all nucleated cells, present endogenous antigen to $CD8^{+}T$ cells, and MHC class II molecules that expressed on professional APCs, such as dendritic cells, macrophage and B cells, and induced expression on conditional APCs which present exogenous antigen to $CD4^{+}T$ cells. It is clear that endothelial cells express MHC class II molecules in response to stimulation by inflammatory mediators, such as IFN-γ [282]. Antigens in the context of MHC molecules provide the first signal for T cell activation. The second signal for T cells' activation is provided by co-stimulatory molecules on endothelial cells, such as CD80 and CD86 molecules. Lozanoska-Ochser B et al. demonstrated that freshly isolated human islet endothelial cells constitutively expressed CD86 and ICOS ligand, but not CD80 or CD40 co-stimulatory molecules; co-culture of human islet endothelial cells with $CD4^{+}T$ cells facilitate the proliferation of CD4 + T cells in the presence of CD3 molecules. These proliferation of $CD4^{+}T$ cells was completely abrogated by anti-CD86 mAbs, indicating that CD86 molecules on endothelial cells play key role in the activation of activated $CD4^{+}T$ cells [283]. The importance of endothelial cells function as APCs is highlighted in studies of allo-transplantation in which endothelium MHC and co-stimulator molecule expressions trigger allogeneic memory T cells' activation, leading to allograft rejection [284]. In addition to expression of MHC molecules and CD80/CD86 molecules, endothelial cells also express other co-stimulatory molecules, such as CD40, PD-1 ligand PD-L1. A recent study indicated that lymphatic endothelial cells (LECs) actively scavenge and cross-present foreign exogenous Ags to cognate $CD8^{+}T$ cells under homeostatic conditions. Upregulation of MHC class I molecules and PD-L1on LECs upon antigen recognition leads to $CD8^{+}T$ cell proliferation and activation. However, activated $CD8^{+}T$ cells exhibit early-stage apoptosis and dysfunctional activated phenotype, causing dysfunctional activation of $CD8^{+}T$ cells under homeostatic conditions, suggesting LECs main tain tolerance to draining peripheral antigens through cross-presentation of such antigens [285]. These studies indicated that endothelial cells act as conditional antigen-presenting cells to stimulate T cells' activation, and thus serve as link to bridge innate immunity and adaptive immunity.

Endothelial cells produce diverse kinds of cytokines in response to different stimulators. Cytokines are small-molecular-weight proteins produced by cells with bioactivity on target cells that bind to its receptor with high affinity. Binding of cytokine to its receptor on the endothelial cells changes the endothelial cell behavior and properties through autocrine, paracine, and endocrine manner. Activated endothelial cell has been showed to produce distinct sets of either pro-inflammatory or inflammatory inhibitory cytokines, including inflammatory cytokines, IL-1, IL-3, IL-5, IL-6, IL-8, and G-CSF and inhibitory cytokines, IL-10, TGF-ß [286, 287]. These cytokines play important roles in the regulation of the strength and type of immune responses and participate in the initiation of inflammation.

In addition to cytokine production in response to distinct stimuli, activated endothelial cells release microparticles (MP) [288]. Microparticles are small vesicles from plasma membrane, diameter usually 0.1–1.5 μm, which could be produced by different cell types during cell activation or apoptosis. Endothelial MP (EMP), found in high levels in plasma in activated endothelial cells, are responsible for numerous immune inflammatory cutaneous diseases, such as atopic dermatitis, sepsis, and multiple sclerosis. It has been clearly demonstrated that EMP can enhance T cell activation and potentiate antigen presentation, proposing a novel role for endothelial cells for the pathogenesis of inflammatory diseases and its possible complications of infectious diseases [289]. EMP expressed a variety of molecules necessary for antigen presentation and T cell activation, such as MHC class II, CD40, ICOSL, and β2-microglobulin; however, activation of T cells by EMPs is dependent on adhesive molecules VCAM-1 and ICAM-1.

The function of endothelial cells are tightly regulated; dysregulated activation or partial regulation of endothelial cells lead to impaired vascular relaxation, increased leukocyte adhesion, enhanced endothelial permeability, generation of thrombotic state, and overactivation of T cells. Thus, dysfunction of endothelial cells has been closely linked to the pathogenesis of inflammatory cutaneous diseases, including psoriasis and dermatitis.

The involvement of dysfunctional endothelial cells contributing to the development of psoriasis has been recently described. Circulating endothelial cells and microparticles, as a sign of endothelial dysfunction, was significantly increased in psoriasis patients as compared with normal controls [290]. CARD14 is a scaffolding protein that regulates NF-kB activation; mutations in CARD14 gene lead to enhanced NF-kB activation in psoriasis patients [291]. A recent study demonstrated [292] that CARD14 molecules were highly expressed on dermal endothelial cells and also expressed on non-dermal endothelial cells such as aortic endothelial cells in psoriasis. CARD14 molecules are responsible for the phosphorylation of NF-kB. Furthermore, heightened expression of CXCL10, IL-8 and CCL2 in psoriasis-associated CARD14-mutant epithelial cells suggested high NK-kB signaling associated with CARD14 mutation. These results suggested that NK-kB signaling pathway plays key role in contributing to the development of psoriasis. Inhibition of endothelial cell activation or induction of apoptosis of activated endothelial cell alleviates psoriasis-like skin inflammation [293].

Allergic dermatitis represents cutaneous diseases that characterize with antigen-specific IgE and tissue eosinophilia [294]. Cheng LE et al. demonstrated that activated basophils–endothelial interaction induced enhanced expression of VCAM-1 that facilitated accumulation of eosinophils, suggesting that interaction of endothelial cells with basophils contributes to the accumulation of eosinophils, allowing the progress of allergic dermatitis [295].

In summary, recent studies of endothelial cell phenotype and function on human and murine models have recently demonstrated that endothelial cells are enabled to function as innate immune cells and regulate the type of adaptive immune response through a variety of adhesive molecules expression, cytokine secretion that are required for controlling the trafficking of T cells, and promoting T cell either activation or tolerance. Future development of immunotherapies on cutaneous diseases that target endothelial cells should consider the key role of endothelial cells in regulation of local or systemic innate and adaptive immunity.

6.6 Mast Cells as Versatile Immune Cells in the Skin

Song Zheng and Xing-Hua Gao

Mast cells are widely recognized as critical effector cells in allergic disorders and other IgE-associated acquired immune responses. Recently, the diverse roles that these cells play in immunology have been discovered. It is now clear that mast cells are also capable of playing critical roles in both innate immunity and adaptive immunity independent of IgE, extending far beyond as key effector cells in allergy. Mast cells can be activated by a variety of stimuli and secrete rapidly both preformed and newly synthesized products with the potential to modulate the development and regulate the magnitude and the kinetics of adaptive immune responses. Thus, a picture of mast cells as both effector cells and immunomodulatory cells in immunology is established. Elucidating the mechanisms how mast cells are actively involved in a specific setting of immunity will provide pharmacological target for treating such disease, especially immune-related skin disorders.

6.6.1 Introduction

Mast cells arise from bone-marrow-derived precursors that circulate in the blood and become differentiated after entering tissues where they ultimately reside. Mature mast cells are found in most tissue of the body and they are typically most abundant at sites that are close to host–environment interfaces, such as the skin and various mucosal tissues. Due to this anatomical location, mast cells are ideally situated to act during the first line of defense against external pathogens and other environmental insults. They are long-lived cells, able to survive for months or years and, despite being terminally differentiated, they can proliferate in response to appropriate signals. Despite having a common lineage, mast cells are highly heterogeneous and phenotypically malleable cells, the intricacies of which have only begun to be defined. In mice, mast cells fall into two broad categories: mucosal and connective tissue mast cell types. Connective tissue mast cells are predominantly found in the skin and peritoneal cavity. In contrast, mucosal mast cells are found mainly in the mucosal layer of the gut and lungs. In humans, two analogous subsets of mast cells have been described [296]. These subsets of mast cells differ in their granule contents and, therefore, function; however, it is thought that the above phenotypes are plastic and interchangeable and there is still much to learn about the in vivo significance of mast cell heterogeneity. Almost all mast cells in the human skin possess granules containing both tryptase and chymase [297]. Here, we introduce facets of mast cell activation, how to study their immune functions in vivo, and general considerations of the roles that mast cells play in immunology, and then we focus on their relevant roles in skin immunology, specifically, in skin infection, skin inflammation, and skin cancers.

6.6.2 Mast Cell Activation

Upon being activated, mast cells are capable of producing a plethora of mediators – both preformed and newly synthesized. Within seconds of stimulation, mast cells can undergo degranulation, rapidly releasing preformed mediators. Shortly (within minutes) after the initiation of degranulation, mast cells can produce lipid-derived products, mainly leukotrienes and prostaglandins. Finally, over the course of hours, the transcriptional upregulation of cytokines and chemokines can be induced. Of note, mast cell activation does not necessarily lead to degranulation. Mast cell degranulation can occur in response to various external stimuli, most notably, IgE receptor cross-linking, but they also degranulate in response to complement activation, neuropeptides, and certain toxins. Mast cell degranulation can occur in two modes. In the classical anaphylactic degranulation mode, the entire contents of each granule are released by exocytosis, immediately upon mast cell activation. Alternatively, in piecemeal degranulation, partial degranulation occurs and granule contents are released in a slow, progressive manner. In addition, mast cells can replenish their granules and thus can undergo multiple rounds of degranulation, which could greatly impact the severity and perpetuation of mast-cell-mediated responses.

6.6.3 Multiple Ways of Mast Cell Activation

Mast cells respond to a wide range of "danger" signals in a rapid manner. For this purpose, these cells are armed with a large repertoire of receptors enabling them to interact both directly and indirectly with pathogens and environmental toxins.

6.6.3.1 Toll-Like-Receptor-Mediated Activation

Toll-like receptors (TLRs) are at the center of direct pathogen recognition by innate immune cells and are a critical link between innate and adaptive immunity [298]. Mast cells express a range of TLRs, including TLR2, TLR3, TLR4, TLR6, TLR7, and TLR9. Lipopolysaccharide (LPS) stimulation of rodent mast cells through TLR4 promoted cytokine production in the absence of degranulation, whereas stimulation through TLR2 by peptidoglycan (PGN) induced both degranulation and cytokine production [299]. PGN from *Staphylococcus aureus* stimulated mast cells in a TLR2-dependent manner to produce TNF-α, IL-4, IL-5, IL-6, and IL-13, but not IL-1β and intradermal injection of PGN led to increased vasodilatation and inflammation through TLR2-dependent activation of mast cells in the skin [299]. Mast cell TLR3 activation in response to poly(I:C), a double-stranded RNA analog, or double-stranded RNA virus have been demonstrated to produce chemokines to recruit NK cells via CXCL-8 [300]. In addition, mast cells are shown to produce pro-inflammatory cytokines (TNF-α and IL-6) and chemokines (RANTES, MIP-1, and MIP-2) in response to poly(I:C), R-848, and CpG oligodeoxynucleotide, which are TLR3, TLR7, and TLR9 activators, respectively [301]. Thus, mast cells are able to respond quickly to invading pathogens by elaborating chemokines and cytokines, which might be critical to recruitment and activation of innate immune cells to restrain early infection favoring the host prior to the development of adaptive immune response. Indeed, mast-cell-derived TNF-α were shown critical for survival in mouse models of bacterial infection by promotion of neutrophil influx [302, 303].

6.6.3.2 Fc-Receptor-Mediated Activation

Mast cells express receptors for the Fc portions of both IgE and IgG antibodies. IgE-mediated activation of mast cells via cross-linking by FcεRI is one of the best-known modes of mast cell activation and has been extensively studied in the context of allergic reactions. Interestingly, accumulating data indicate that monomeric IgE molecules without binding to cognate antigens can promote mast cell survival and activation [304, 305]. Human Fc receptors for IgG (FcγRs) differ in function, affinity for the Fc fragment of antibody, and in cellular distribution. There are five activating FcγRs: the high-affinity receptor FcγRI, which can bind monomeric IgG, and four low-affinity receptors (FcγRIIA, FcγRIIC, FcγRIIIA, and FcγRIIIB), which bind only to immune-complexed IgG [306]. FcγRIIB is the only inhibitory FcγR [306]. Mouse mast cells were found to express FcγRIIIA and FcγRIIB, whereas human mast cells express FcγRII (CD32) and in some cases FcγRI (CD64) but not FcγRIII (CD16) [307]. Mast cells derived in culture from human skin were reported to express FcγRIIA but not FcγRIIB and released histamine, lipid-derived mediators, and cytokines in response to stimulation by anti-FcγRIIA antibody fragments [308]. FcγRI were reported to be inducible by interferon γ (IFN-γ) in cultured human mast cells [309, 310]. FcγRs displayed on mast cells can contribute to mast cell activation in an antigen-dependent manner and such activation generally leads to degranulation, the production of lipid mediators, and the generation of various cytokines and chemokines [311].

6.6.3.3 Complement-Receptor-Mediated Activation

Mast cells have long been recognized to interact with the complement system through complement receptor 3 (CR3; also known as CD11b–CD18), CR4 (also known as CD11c–CD18), and the receptors for complement product 3a (C3aR) and C5a (C5aR, also known as CD88), and activation of mast cells through C5aR can result in degranulation [312]. In addition to their function as mast-cell-activating agents, C3a and C5a have been shown to be chemotactic for mast cells [312]. In a mouse model of acute septic peritonitis, both C3- and C4-deficient mice are more susceptible to bacterial insults [313]. C3-deficient mice also exhibited reductions in peritoneal mast cell degranulation, production of TNF-alpha, neutrophil infiltration, and clearance of bacteria, which could be recovered by treating the C3-deficient mice with purified C3 protein confirming that the defects were complement-dependent [313]. Additionally, the integrin $\alpha2\beta1$ expressed on mast cells was found to function as a receptor for the complement protein C1q. This receptor was demonstrated to be critical for mast-cell-mediated host defense to peritonitis [314].

6.6.3.4 Activation by Other Factors

Mast cells can also undergo degranulation in response to some exogenous stimuli that accompany pathogen injection into the skin or breaching of the skin barrier, such as components of snake and honeybee venoms or mosquito saliva [315]. Interestingly, after degranulation, mast cells can secrete carboxypeptidase A (CPA), which proteolytically degrades sarafotoxins, thus inactivating them, to protect the host from these insults [316]. Several host endogenous peptides, including neurotensin and endothelin-1 can also activate mast cells [315]. Of note, in mouse models of acute septic peritonitis, upon activation by these endogenous toxins, mast-cell-derived chymase and neurolysin can, in turn, degrade endothelin 1 and neurotensin, respectively, to promote host survival from sepsis [317, 318].

6.6.4 Study of Mast Cell Functions In Vivo: Mast-Cell Knock-in Mice

Kit-mutant mice, which are deficient in mast cells, can be used to analyze the in vivo functions of mast cells. The most commonly used animals for such studies are the $Kit^{W/W-v}$ mice and the more recently characterized C57BL/6-$Kit^{W-sh/W-sh}$ mice. Kit^{W} contains a point mutation that encodes a truncated KIT protein, which lacks the transmembrane domain and is therefore not expressed on the cell surface; Kit^{W-v} encodes a (Thr660Met) mutation in the KIT tyrosine kinase domain that markedly decreases the kinase activity of the receptor; and Kit^{W-sh} contains an inversion mutation of the transcriptional regulatory elements upstream of the Kit transcription start site on mouse chromosome 5. Adult $Kit^{W/W-v}$ and C57BL/6-$Kit^{W-sh/W-sh}$ mice are profoundly deficient in mast cells and melanocytes. $Kit^{W/W-v}$ mice have several other phenotypical abnormalities, such as macrocytic anemia, a decrease in the number of bone-marrow and blood neutrophils, sterility, and a marked decrease in the number of interstitial cells of Cajal, which are found in the gastrointestinal tract. By contrast, C57BL/6-$Kit^{W-sh/W-sh}$ mice are neither anemic nor sterile, and they seem to have normal numbers of bone-marrow and blood neutrophils. Because the Kit-related phenotypical abnormalities that affect lineages other than mast cells are generally milder in C57BL/6-$Kit^{W-sh/W-sh}$ mice than in $Kit^{W/W-v\ mice}$, and because C57BL/6-$Kit^{W-sh/W-sh}$ mice are fertile and are on the well-studied C57BL/6 background, they are becoming increasingly popular for studies to elucidate the roles of mast cells in vivo. Differences in the biological responses of Kit-mutant mice compared with wild-type mice might be due to any one of the abnormalities that result from the Kit mutations in these animals and they might not be specifically due to the loss of mast cells. However, the lack of mast cells in *Kit*-mutant mice can be selectively repaired by the adoptive transfer of genetically compatible, in-vitro-derived, wild-type mast cells. Such in-vitro-derived mast cells, for example, bone-marrow-derived cultured mast cells (BMMCs), can be administered intravenously or intradermally to create so-called mast cell "knock-in" mice. These mast cell knock-in mice can then be used to assess the extent to which differences in the biological responses of Kit-mutant mice compared with wild-type mice are due to the lack of mast cells in the *Kit*-mutant mice. If a mediator is selectively expressed by mast cells, and if its deletion does not significantly influence the expression of other mast cell products, then it is possible to draw conclusions about the role of that mast cell mediator in vivo by reconstitution of mast-cell-mediator-deficient BMMCs into *Kit*-mutant mice. More recently, additional mouse models have emerged in which mast cell deficiency is independent of alterations in KIT signaling [319]. Owing to the development of this new generation of mast-cell-deficient mice, some of the proposed functions of mast cells have been questioned, whereas others have been confirmed [319, 320].

6.6.5 Mast Cells in Skin Infection

At the initiation of infection, the first responsibility of mast cells is to recognize that pathogen invasion has occurred. As previously described, PGN from *S. aureus* stimulated skin mast cells in a TLR2-dependent manner to induce degranulation and produce cytokines [299]. In another mouse model of skin infection, *Pseudomonas aeruginosa* injections resulted in strikingly (>twofold) larger skin lesions in Kit^{W}/Kit^{W-v} mice than in wild-type mice, which exhibited pronounced MC degranulation at infection sites [321]. In addition, neutrophil recruitment following *P. aeruginosa* injections and bacterial clearance from sites of infection was significantly impaired in Kit^{W}/Kit^{W-v} mice compared with wild-type mice. Notably, the adoptive transfer of mast cells to the skin of Kit^{W}/Kit^{W-v} mice before *P. aeruginosa* infection resulted in normal neutrophil accumulation as well as skin lesions comparable with those in wild-type mice in both bacterial burden and size. According to these authors, these findings demonstrate that activated mast cells are crucial for the induction of protective innate immune responses to bacterial skin infections [321]. These findings are consistent with results from early studies among which mast cells as innate immune sentinel cells were shown critical for host survival in mouse models of bacterial infections [302, 303]. Furthermore, products of mast cell activation by bacterial components may also potentially promote adaptive immune response. For example, mast cell production of tumor necrosis factor (TNF) can substantially enhance T cell recruitment to local lymph nodes and the accompanying lymph node enlargement during experimental skin infection induced by dermal (footpad) injection of *Escherichia coli* [322]. Moreover, during footpad infection with *E. coli* in mast-cell-deficient mice, as compared to their mast-cell-sufficient counterparts, the serum antibody response is significantly diminished and less protective following passive immunization in a urinary tract infection model [323]. In this study, mast cells were found to recruit large numbers of dendritic cells into the infected tissue site, which eventually migrated into draining lymph nodes (DLNs). This pattern of trafficking was facilitated by MC-generated TNF, which increased the expression of E-selectin on local blood vessels because antibody blockade of E-selectin inhibited dendritic cell recruitment into the site of infection and DLNs and consequently impaired the primary humoral immune response. Pushed by these findings, the same group explored potential use of mast cell activators as adjuvants in vaccines [324, 325]. They demonstrate that subcutaneous or nasal administration of C48/80, a small-molecule MC activator, with vaccine antigens evoke large increases in antigen-specific serum immunoglobulin G (IgG) responses [324]. These responses were MC-dependent and correlated with increased dendritic cell and lymphocyte recruitment to draining lymph nodes. Nasal instillation of these formulations provided protection against vaccinia virus infection in vivo. Thus, they highlighted mast cell activators as a new class of vaccine adjuvants. Importantly, in comparison with two well-known adjuvants, CpG oligodeoxynucleotides and cholera toxin, C48/80 is a safe and effective adjuvant, when used by the intradermal route. In sum, mast cells are clearly essential for initiating both innate and adaptive immune responses to many bacterial pathogens and products. The role of mast cells in the immunity against other skin-tropic pathogens, such as virus, fungi, and protozoa, is largely unknown and awaits investigations, although few studies have touched this topic [326–328].

6.6.6 Mast Cells in Skin Inflammation

6.6.6.1 Atopic Dermatitis

Atopic dermatitis (AD) often has high serum levels of IgE and eosinophilia and patients have a high incidence of allergic rhinitis, asthma, and food allergies. Mast cells are well known as effector cells in allergies and it is expectable that mast cells are also involved in the pathogenesis of AD. Recently, an elegant study [329] found that culture supernatants of *Staphylococcus aureus* contain potent mast cell degranulation activity and δ-toxin was identified as the mast cell-degranulation-inducing factor produced by *S. aureus*. Importantly, *S. aureus* isolates recovered from patients with atopic dermatitis produced large amounts of δ-toxin. Skin colonization with *S. aureus*, but not a mutant deficient in δ-toxin, promoted IgE and IL-4 production, as well as inflammatory skin disease. Furthermore, enhancement of IgE production and dermatitis by δ-toxin was abrogated in $Kit^{W-sh/W-sh}$ mast-cell-deficient mice and restored by mast cell reconstitution. This study sheds new light on our understanding the role of mast cells contributing to the pathogenesis of AD and suggests a mechanistic link between *S. aureus*, mast cells, and AD. This study also has important clinical implications since more than 90 % of patients with AD are colonized with *S. aureus* in the lesional skin, whereas most healthy individuals do not harbor the pathogen [330].

Pruritus is one of the most prominent clinical features of AD and several lines of evidence suggest that mast cell is one of the main culprits. Clinically, the major pruritogenic mediator from mast cells, that is, histamine, turned out to be disappointing as a target of anti-itch therapeutics, while sedative antihistamines worked well both in human AD and mouse AD models [331], implicating mediators other than histamine, such as neurogenic components, get involved in itch sensation. The proximity of dermal mast cells to afferent C fiber terminals in the skin suggests a functional relation between these two cell types. Activation of the mast cell releases tryptase, which in turn activates proteinase activated receptor-2 (PAR-2) localized on C fiber terminals [332]. The activated C fibers will transmit this information to the central nervous system, where it can cause the sensation of itch [333]. Additionally, activation will lead to a local release of neuropeptides including substance P, which can specifically activate NK1 receptors on mast cells, leading to sensitization of these cells and increased production of TNF-α [333]. TNF-α in turn can sensitize nociceptive nerve endings – further evidence of the extensive cross talk between nerve and mast cells [333]. In a study, the endogenous PAR-2 agonist tryptase was increased up to fourfold in AD patients and PAR-2 was markedly enhanced on primary afferent nerve fibers in skin biopsies of AD patients [334]. Taken together, activated mast cells can substantially contribute to pruritus in AD patients via cross talk with C fibers at least by tryptase-PAR-2-substance P-TNF-α pathway.

6.6.6.2 Bullous Pemphigoid

Mast cells have a demonstrated role in bullous pemphigoid (BP), a chronic subepidermal blistering skin disease characterized by the presence of IgG autoantibodies to hemidesmosomal antigens BP230 or BP180. Passive transfer of BP230- or BP180-specific IgG leads to disease in neonatal BALB/c mice and reproduces the key clinical features of human BP, including complement deposition at the junction of the dermoepidermis, dermal inflammation, and subepidermal blistering [335]. Mast cell degranulation occurs within 60 min of antibody transfer and elicits neutrophilic infiltration and subsequent blistering of the skin in this mouse model [336]. Mast-cell-deficient or wild-type mice treated with an inhibitor of mast cell degranulation fail to develop disease, but local engraftment of $Kit^{W/Wv}$ mice with BMMCs restores the BP phenotype. In BP, mast cells triggered by complement activation appear to be a crucial source of the potent neutrophil chemoattractant CXCL8 [336, 337]. UV-B irradiation has also been shown to selectively and specifically increase CXCL8 release from mast cells in vitro [338], and this may partly explain the clinical observation that BP lesions are often precipitated by exposure to UV light. Human BP is associated with elevated serum levels of IgE autoantibodies and the presence of eosinophils in blisters. In addition, passive transfer of IgE from BP patients into athymic mice elicits the development of erythematous plaques similar to those observed in BP [339]. These data suggest a role for IgE that may act through mast cells in human BP, validated by the clinical observation that patients with BP and high serum levels of IgE responded to systemic omalizumab, a humanized mAb that inhibits IgE binding to its high-affinity receptor (FcεRI) [340, 341].

6.6.6.3 Contact Hypersensitivity

Contact hypersensitivity (CHS) to chemical haptens are highly dependent on the local density and migratory properties of epidermal Langerhans cells (LCs). In these responses, immune sensitization in the skin is enhanced by antigen-independent effects of IgE [304]. In this study, contact sensitivity was markedly impaired in $IgE^{-/-}$ mice but was restored by administration of hapten-irrelevant IgE before sensitization. Moreover, $IgE^{-/-}$ mice exhibited impairment in the reduction of dendritic cell numbers in the epidermis after hapten exposure. Diminished contact sensitivity in mice lacking FcεRI or mast cells was also observed, suggesting that levels of IgE normally present in mice favor immune sensitization via antigen-independent but FcεRI-dependent effects on mast cells. Following sensitization and challenge with the hapten FITC, both $Kit^{W/Wv}$ and $TNF^{-/-}$ mice exhibit deficits in the CHS response and show significant delays in the migration of dendritic cells (DCs) into draining lymph nodes [342]. Engraftment of mast-cell-deficient mice with wild-type but not $TNF^{-/-}$ BMMCs repairs the DC migration defect. Thus, mast cells and mast-cell-derived TNF are required for optimal expression of CHS to FITC. Taken together, these studies clearly demonstrate that mast cells may provide substantial help to skin DCs (LCs) to initiate mouse models of CHS response; however, several lines of evidence suggest that mast cells are also able to dampen CHS response. In another study, mast cells and mast-cell-derived IL-10 markedly limited the magnitude and promoted the resolution of CHS induced in response to hapten 2,4-dinitro-1-fluorobenzene (DNFB) or to urushiol, which is the hapten-containing sap of poison ivy or poison oak [343]. Mast-cell-derived IL-10 was shown to limit many aspects of these responses, including the numbers of granulocytes, macrophages, and T cells at the reaction sites, as well as local tissue swelling, epidermal hyperplasia, and, importantly, full-thickness epidermal necrosis and ulceration. These diverse roles of mast cells in CHS have been explained by the notion that mast cells might first promote the sensitization and/or elicitation phases of an immune response, and then help to limit or resolve the local tissue changes induced by antigen challenge [344].

6.6.6.4 Mast Cells and Photoimmunity

Early study showed that the ability of ultraviolet B (UVB) irradiation of the skin to induce systemic immunosuppression of CHS was markedly decreased in mast-cell-deficient mice but was restored following mast cell knock-in [345], and this result was confirmed in another study [346]. In addition, mast cells have a critical role in suppressing secondary immune reactions by UVA (320–400 nm) radiation [347]. The skin absorbs UVB, yet UV exposure induces system-wide immune suppression. How the immunosuppressive signal is transmitted from the skin to the lymph nodes is not entirely clear, but migrating mast cells have a role [348]. In an elegant study [349] using mast-cell-tracing experiments by green fluorescent protein (GFP), when mouse skin was grafted onto mast-cell-deficient mice, upon UV exposure, GFP(+) mast cells preferentially migrated into the lymph nodes draining the skin and these mast cells migrated primarily to the B cell areas of the draining nodes. Mast cells express CXCR4 and UV exposure upregulated the expression of its ligand CXCL12 by lymph node B cells. Treating UV-irradiated mice with a CXCR4 antagonist blocked mast cell migration and abrogated UV-induced immune suppression. This study indicates that UV-induced mast cell migration to draining lymph nodes, mediated by CXCR4 interacting with CXCL12, represents a key early step in UV-induced immune suppression. Mast cells also link UV radiation and inhibition of antibody formation in vivo, because UV irradiation blocks germinal center formation, antibody secretion, and follicular helper T cell function and this effect is mast-cell-dependent [350]. Again, mast-cell-derived IL-10 is indispensible for this effect, and this result is in agreement with the result of the previous study [343] led by Tsai M and Galli SJ, who reported that mast-cell-derived IL-10 limits skin pathology in contact dermatitis and chronic irradiation with ultraviolet B. Taken together, these studies suggest that mast cells may be important immune regulatory cells bridging UV radiation and immunosuppression and this effect may be also highly relevant in the pathogenesis of skin cancers, including skin squamous cell carcinomas, basal cell carcinomas, and melanomas, occurring on sun-exposed areas [351].

6.6.7 Conclusion and Perspective

The role of mast cells as critical effector cells in allergies is well established. However, recent research suggests mast cells play diverse roles in immunology. Given their multiple ways of activation and capability of production of a wide range of mediators, mast cells may be indeed versatile immune cells. However, much of what we know about mast cells' immune function comes from mast cell knock-in mouse models. Caution should be exercised when translating these results into clinical settings, since substantial difference exists between mice and the human immune system. The results of limited studies suggest that mast cells are actively involved in the pathogenesis of inflammatory skin disorders, such as atopic dermatitis, bullous pemphigoid, and contact dermatitis and skin infectious diseases, although skin is a rich source of mast cells. Further studies are awaited to elucidate the mechanism whereby mast cells participate in these conditions.

6.7 Granulocytes

Jinyan Wang, PhD and Changlong Lu, MD, PhD

Granulocytes are composed of heterogeneous populations of cells characterized by different expression of surface proteins and distinct cytoplasmic granules that contain cell-specific enzymes,cationic proteins, and other cell-specific molecules. These cells are generated from hematopoietic stem cells during the development of hematopoiesis in bone marrow [352]. According to the contents of cytoplasmic granules, granulocytes can be classified into neutrophils, eosinophils, and basophils [353]. Neutrophils constitute the majority of circulating leukocytes; these cells are released into the peripheral blood and circulate before entering into the tissue. Basophils are relatively rare in the circulation, but can be very potent in their biological function. On activation, basophils release the contents of their granules; these contents include preformed mediators such as vasoactivve amines and protease, and newly formed mediators such as arachidonic acid metabolites. These mediators increase blood vessel permeability and smooth muscle activity. Eosinphils are motile phagocytic cells that can migrate from the blood into the tissue. It is thought that these cells play an important role in the defense against multicellular parasitic organisms, including worms. The molecules released by the cytoplasmic granules of these granulocytes act as effector molecules that determine the various effector functions. Granulocytes are crucial effector cells in the innate immune system that participate in the immune defense against infectious microbes, immune surveillance to eradicate mutated or transformed cells of host, and immune homeostasis to clear dead cells or tissue repair [354]. Different types of granulocytes show distinct functions against microbes and foreign substances. Basophils and eosinophils are critical components to mediate allergic reaction induced by foreign substances. Activated basophils release various kinds of vasoactive amines, proteases, and arachidonic acid metabolites, leading to dilation of blood vessels and increased vascular permeability, and stimulate contraction of smooth muscles. Eosinophils are an important cause of tissue injury in these reactions through the release of proteases [355]. In addition to the role in innate immunity, recent studies suggested the antigen-presenting capacity of granulocyte to display peptide of allergic antigen in the context of MHC molecules to T cells, leading to activation of allergen-specific $CD4^{+}$T helper cells that contribute to the induction of hypersensitivities [356]. Current studies highlight the multifunctional potential of granulocytes to serve as direct immune defense against microbes and foreign substance and bridge the innate immunity and adaptive immunity to effectively eradicate these antigens.

6.7.1 Neutrophils

Neutrophils, which constitute 50–70% of the circulating white blood cells, are the most abundant white blood cells in the circulation in mammals. After being generated from hematopoietic stem cells by hematopoiesis in the bone marrow, they are released into the peripheral blood and circulate for 7–10 h before migrating into the tissues, where they have a life span of only a few days. In response to many types of infections, the bone marrow releases more than the usual number of neutrophils and these cells generally are the first to arrive at a site of infection and serve as the key player for initiating immune defenses and inflammation against infections [357].

Neutrophils are active phagocytic cells that contain two kinds of granules in the cytoplasm. The primary granules are larger and contain dense peroxidase, lysozyme, and various hydrolytic enzymes. The secondary granules are small and contain collagenase, lactoferrin, and lysozyme. Both primary and secondary granules fuse with phagosomes, whose contents are then digested and eliminated (e.g., ingested foreign pathogens), similar as in macrophages [358]. In addition, neutrophils express surface Fcγ receptor and C3b receptor, which can bind to the Fc portion of IgG isotype and complement C3b fragment. Binding of Fcγ receptor to IgG-conjugated antigen complex and C3b receptor to C3b-coated antigen cause increased phagocytosis and bactericidal activity of the neutrophils, facilitating opsonization by neutrophils [359].

Recent studies demonstrated that neutrophils play an important role in the pathogenesis of lupus [360]. The presence of low-density granulocytes (LDGs) in mononuclear cell of the patients correlates with lupus. Some of lupus patients showed significant amount of genes encoding these LDGs in granulocytes. LDGs in granulocytes of patients exhibited distinct properties compared to healthy granulocytes, including cytotoxicity to endothelial cells, perturbing the differentiation of endothelial progenitor cells to mature endothelial cells by enhanced type I interferon (IFNs) production. This study suggests that abnormal granulocytes formation leads to enhanced vascular damage and blunt vascular repair, which contributes to the development of systemic lupus erythematosus (SLE). Coit P et al. described the differences of neutrophils between lupus patient and healthy controls by comparison of the methylation sites across the entire genome [361]. They identified the hypomethylation of methylated CG sites of neutrophils in lupus patients compared to healthy controls; the results indicate that the hypomethylated DNA of neutrophils in patients leads to increased type-1 IFN production via Toll-like receptor-9 (TLR-9). The results suggest that epigenetic alterations in neutrophils of patients contributes to the pathogenesis of SLE.

Neutrophils are also involved in the process of wound repair. A recent study demonstrated that neutrophils mediated abscess formation in mouse skin model during cutaneous *Staphylococcus aureus* infection [362]. *S. aureus* infection induced wounds are mediated by three mechanisms: (1) robust neutrophils are recruited to the skin from the circulation, (2) prolonged neutrophils' survival within the abscess in the skin, and (3) homing of c-kit+progenitor cells to the abscess where they locally produce mature neutrophils. Increasing evidences have shown that the commensal microbiota has a high impact on individuals by modulating the development and homeostasis of host immune system. Accelerated wound healing was also associated with commensal microbiota. The absence of commensal microbiota resulted in decreased accumulation of neutrophils and increased infiltration of mast and macrophage into the wounds, suggesting that reduced accumulation of neutrophils participates in correcting in the wound-healing process [363]. Basically, neutrophils use two mechanisms to efficiently clear microbial infections, that is, phagocytosis, and destroying microbes through mechanisms generated by oxygen-dependent and oxygen-independent pathways in the granules of the cytoplasm. The release of Neutrophil Extracellular Traps (NETs) has been also recently described in the relationship between microbiota and tissue injury [364]. The NETs containing DNA, histones and antimicrobial peptides, function as effector molecules to damage epithelium. Regulation of NET production by neutrophils is mediated by exogenous glucose and glycosis in the cytoplasm, suggesting alterations of metabolic pathways by microbiota could change neutrophil cytotoxic function and wound epithelization. Tauzin S demonstrated that coordination of macrophages and neutrophils is necessary for neutrophil wound attraction through p22phox and Yes-related kinase pathway in zebrafish [365], suggesting the necessity of cooperative function of neutrophils with other innate immune cells serving to tissue damage.

Accumulating evidence suggests that neutrophils not only are activated and participate in the inflammatory process, but are also associated with the resolution of inflammatory responses. However, the role of neutrophils in the resolution of inflammatory-related skin pathology remains unclear. One study suggests that neutrophils might secrete some kinds of anti-inflammatory cytokines, such as TGF-β and soluble IL-1 receptor, which mediate suppressive effect and act to inhibit the IL-1 signaling cascade during the late phase of inflammation, respectively. As inflammatory response resolves, neutrophils undergo apoptosis and are cleared by local tissue macrophages, and finally disappear from the site of inflammation [366].

6.7.2 Basophils

Basophils are considered as granulocytes that contain large granules filled with basically basic dye positive staining proteins, so as referred to basophils. Basophils are circulating cells in the blood. They are relatively rare but can be potent in response to binding of circulating antibodies, resulting in releasing contents of granules [367]. These effector molecules share with mast cells including histamine, cytokines and lipid mediators such as prostaglandins and leukotrienes, which lead to enhanced blood vessel permeability and smooth muscle contraction [368]. The release of mediators from basophils or mast cells is tightly regulated by various factors. Basophils constantly express FcεRs on its surface, which bind to Fc portion of IgE with high affinity. Cross-linking of FcεRs on basophils by allergen-specific IgE leads to activation of basophils. Allergen-specific IgE occupy FcεRI exceed 10 % cause activation of basophils, leading to degranulation and cytokine production [369]. The binding affinity of allergen to IgE influences the activation of basophils. It is demonstrated that activated basophils appear to participate in the pathogenesis of allergic diseases and certain autoimmune diseases. A recent study indicated that binding of FcεRI on surface of basophils to IgE facilitates the amplification of autoimmune inflammation, such as lupus. Deficiency of IgE leads to reduced production of autoantibody and amelioration of organ pathologies, which was associated with decreased activation of basophils, suggesting that increased basophils associated with the presence of IgE contributed to the pathogenesis of SLE [370]. The accumulation of basophils in inflamed skin lesions is the hallmark of allergic diseases, as in atopic dermatitis, in which the mechanisms underlying skin lesion involves the degranulation and cytokine production by basophils, resulting in inflammation and tissue damage. However, it seems likely that basophils could interact with other innate/adaptive immune cells causing cutaneous lesion. This proposal has been evidenced that basophils promote cutaneous inflammation by enhance group2 innate lymphoid cell (ILC2s) mediated responses during cutaneous inflammation [371].

6.7.3 Eosinophils

Eosinophils are granulocytic leukocytes that originate from multiple hematopoietic stem cells in the bone marrow. Their cytoplasmic granules contain arginine-rich basic proteins, which can be stained by the acidic stain eosin [372]. Under steady state, a small population of eosinophils circulates in the blood; however, most eosinophils rapidly appear in the tissue, especially in the connective tissue, underneath respiratory, gut, and urogenital epithelium. Elevated eosinophils in blood and tissue compartments are associated with helminthic parasite infections as well as allergic inflammation [373]. Eosinophils express a variety of cell-surface receptors, including complement receptor C3b, cytokine receptors (such as IL-5), and Fc receptors (Fcγ receptor and Fcα receptors), which bind to complement fragment C3b, cytokine IL-5, and IgG/IgA conjugated immune complexes, respectively. Binding of receptors to its ligand causes activation of eosinophils. Activated eosinophils release the content of cytoplasmic granules, including some proteases to destroy microbes. In addition, activated eosinophils increase in the expression of various surface proteins, such as CD69 and CD62L molecules, and exhibit enhanced expression of MHC class II molecules and co-stimulatory molecules, such as CD80 and CD86, allowing antigen presentation potential to T cells. Activated eosinophils preferentially prime $CD4^{+}T$ cells to bias toward Th2 cells [374]. Activated eosinophils also play a key role in regulation of strength and type of immune responses through the production of a variety of cytokines, including inflammatory cytokines, IL-1β, TNF-α, IL-12, and inhibitory cytokines, such as IL-4, IL-10, TGF−β, and others such as a proliferation-inducing ligand (APRIL), CCL5/RANTES, GM-CSF [375]. For example, eosinophil-derived IL-1β promotes the activation and differentiation of Th17 cells [376], which are implicated in the pathogenesis of allergic airway inflammation. IL-13 is a cytokine usually derived from activated Th2 cells that contribute to the development of allergic airway response, including airway hyper-responsiveness, goblet cell hyperplasia, and mucus secretion. However, a study indicated that IL-13 derived from eosinophils integrating with IL-13 produced by T cells is responsible for the pathogenesis of allergic airway responses [377]. Deficiency of IL-13 in eosinophils leads to low airway hyper-responsiveness. TGF-β belongs to an inhibitory cytokine that suppresses the differentiation and activation of Th1 cells, Th2 cells, and $CD8^{+}T$ cells. TGF-β secreted by eosinophils promotes fibroblast proliferation and differentiation, thus leading to skin lesion repair and remodeling events in human atopic skin [378].

Besides diverse cytokines production, activated eosinophils are able to release highly toxic effector molecules, such as proteases and free radicals, which are responsible for tissue damage in allergic reactions. Activated eosinophils also synthesize and release many chemical mediators such as prostaglandins and leukotrienes, leading to prolonged highly vascular permeability and muscle contraction of the local tissue, and thus eosinophils play a key role in amplifying the inflammatory response against allergens. A recent study implicated that ROS produced by eosinophils might be responsible for the development of murine irritant contact dermatitis. The interaction of basophils with fibroblasts promotes the eosinophils recruitment and contributes to the development of skin inflammation. These results indicate that complex intercellular regulatory networks exist in the initiation of local inflammation during the pathogenesis of skin damage [379].

In summary, as innate immune cells, neutrophils, basophils, and eosinophils serve as effector cells to eliminate microbes and foreign substances. In addition to these effector functions, these cells play an important role in regulating immune responses and mediating local inflammatory response. Skin infiltrated with these cells are responsible for the tissue damage and associated with the development of various cutaneous diseases. Therefore, targeting therapies to regulate functional activity of these cells might throw light on the treatment of diverse cutaneous diseases, such as atopic disorders.

6.8 T Cells in the Skin

Changlong Lu, MD, PhD and Jinyan Wang, PhD

The barrier function of the skin is part of the function of the immune system, which evokes innate and adaptive immune responses. The skin immune system constitutes distinct types of cells including lymphocytes such as T cells (αβT cells and γδT cells), B cells, and NK cells, which determine the specificity and the type of immunity. T cells in skin can also show unresponsiveness to particular antigens, such as immunological tolerance [380].

6.8.1 αβT Cells in the Skin

Skin αβT cells have three characteristics: (1) memory phenotype, (2) skin tropism, and (3) localization of subsets. (1) Essentially all of the skin αβT cells are memory cells. They express CD45RO and CD44 (at a high level), whereas neither CD62L nor CCR7 is expressed. (2) Skin tropism is determined by expression of CLA (cutaneous lymphocyte antigen), CCR4, and CCR10 on these T cells. CLA, a modified version of PSGL-1 (P-selectin glycoprotein ligand-1), binds to E-selectin (CD62E) expressed on the endothelial cells (ECs) of post-capillary venules in the skin. CCR4 is a receptor for MDC (macrophage-derived chemokine or CCL22) and TARC (thymus and activation-regulated chemokine or CCL17). MDC is produced by skin macrophages and keratinocytes, while TARC is secreted by keratinocytes. CCR10, as a receptor for CTACK (cutaneous T-cell-attracting chemokine or CCL27), mediates chemotaxis toward CTACK, which is made of keratinocytes. (3) Distinct subsets of T cells have different predictable locations on the dermis and the perivascular area. Most CD4 T cells reside in the perivascular area; only a small amount of αβT cells are in the epidermis, which are essentially CD8 tissue-resident memory T (Trm) cells. These skin Trm cells protect the whole body from infection [381, 382]. αβT cells can be divided into two main subsets based on the expression of either CD4 or CD8 molecules.

6.8.2 CD4T Cells

Skin CD4T cells consist of diverse helper T (Th) cells including Th1, Th2, Th17, Th22, Th9, and Treg cells (immunosuppressive T cells).

Th1 cells Th1 cells dominate during the early phase of contact dermatitis [383]. They secrete IFN-γ and protect against intracellular pathogens such as Mycobacteria and viruses. IFN- γ secreted by Th1 cells promote the expressions of IL-12 receptor β1 and β2 subunits, IL-18 receptor, CXCR3, and CCR5 molecules. Differentiation of CD4 T cells to Th1 cells is regulated by IFN-γ in synergy with IL-12, IL-18, and type I IFN, that is, IFN-α and IFN- β. IL-12 activates signal transducer and activator of transcription (STAT) 4, a modifier of Th1-related genes such as IFN-γ, IL12R, and IL18R. IFN-γ activates STAT1 and reinforces Th1 cell differentiation. Activated STAT4 and STAT1 induce expression of T-bet, encoded by TBX21 gene (the master regulator for Th1 cells) [384].

Th2 cell Th2 cells play a central role in atopic diseases such as asthma, chronic rhinosinusitis, atopic dermatitis, and food allergy. They secrete IL-4, IL-5, IL-13, IL-24 (an antitumor cytokine of IL-10 family), IL-25 (IL-17E, an IL-17 family cytokine that amplifies allergic responses), and IL-31 (a pruritus-inducing IL-6 family cytokine). Isotype class-switching to IgE, mediated by Th2 cells, contributes to host defense against parasitic worms. Recent studies suggest that Th2 cells can be fully activated by collaboration with epithelial keratinocytes in the skin and group 2 innate lymphoid cells (ILC2s) [385]. Th2 cells regulate the acute- and late-phase allergic reactions mediated by IgE and eosinophils, respectively. IgE-production is stringently controlled by at least two steps. The first is mediated by Th2-cytokines, IL-4 and IL-13, which stimulate B cells through STAT6 to produce germline transcripts, a prerequisite for class-switch recombination. The second is conducted by CD40/CD40 ligand through cell-to-cell contact between Th2 and B cells, leading to completion of recombination of IgE locus [386]. IgE activates mast cells and basophils, both of which initiate the early-phase allergic response. The late-phase response is mediated by eosinophils, of which maturation, migration, activation, and survival are modulated by Th2-cytokines. Impairment of skin barrier irritates keratinocytes to produce IL- 25, IL-33 (an IL-1 family alarmin), and TSLP (thymic stromal lymphopoietin). These cytokines activate ILC2s that promptly produce IL-5, IL-9, and IL-13, leading to activation of Th2 cells [385]. Th2-cytokines are speculated to damage the skin barrier further; IL-4 and IL-13 reduce filaggrin expression of human keratinocytes in vitro; IL-31 induces pruritus, which triggers scratch-behavior leading to further barrier damages. Therefore, atopic skin diseases are complexed with a trinity of barrier abnormality, allergy/immunology, and pruritus. Th2 cells may also play a role in tumor immunity for IL-24 (melanoma-differentiation-associated antigen 7) induces apoptosis of tumor cells [387, 388]. Yet, the role Th2 cells in skin tumors awaits further investigation.

Th17 cells Th17 cells can be divided into nonpathogenic and pathogenic Th17 cells. Nonpathogenic Th17 cells express IL-17A, IL-17 F, IL-10, CCL20, and CXCR6, and are differentiated by combination of IL-6 and TGF-β1. Nonpathogenic Th17 cells become pathogenic after exposure to IL-23. Combination of IL-1β, IL-6, and IL-23 induces pathogenic Th17 cells, which express IL-17A, IL-17 F

IL-22, CCL9, and CXCR3. IL-23 occupies a central role in Th17-mediated pathogenicity, leading to autoimmune diseases such as psoriasis, rheumatoid arthritis, multiple sclerosis, and atopic dermatitis. Keratinocytes regulate differentiation and activation of Th17 cells. Irritated keratinocytes produce IL-1β and IL-6, which stimulate LCs and dermal DCs to produce IL-23 and to migrate to regional lymph nodes where Th17 cells are differentiated [394]. Skin-homing Th17 produces IL- 17A, IL-17 F, and TNF-α, which stimulate keratinocytes to produce cytokines such as IL-33, IL-36, CXCL1, CCL20, and antibacterial peptides [389].

Th22 cells Skin-homing Th22 cells express CCR4, CCR6, and CCR10. Function of this subset is ascribed to IL-22 (an IL-10-family cytokine), which operates in pro- and anti-inflammatory ways, and is also produced by Th1, Th17, and γδT cells in humans. IL-22 activates epithelial innate immune responses, which can be protective or detrimental. An example of pathogenic effect is epithelial hyperplasia in psoriasis. IL-22 promotes squamous cell carcinoma of immunocompromised patients. IL-22 and Th22 cells are involved in various skin diseases including psoriasis vulgaris, atopic dermatitis, contact dermatitis, and scleroderma [400–402]. Th22 cells are induced by IL-6 and TNF, both of which are produced by plasmacytoid DCs [390]. Specific transcription factor is not defined for Th22 cell differentiation, while aryl hydrocarbon receptor (AhR) and RORgt are at least important for production of IL-22 [391]. Th22 cells accumulate in lesions of psoriasis and atopic dermatitis. Lipid antigen (presented on CD1a by LCs) stimulates Th22 cells and mediates acanthosis [390].

Th9 cells Th9 cells are induced from Th2 or naive T cells by IL-4 and TGF-β [392]. In humans, Th9 cells in blood and tissues are skin-tropic or skin-resident memory cells that produce TNF-α, granzyme B, and IL-9. Th9 cells, with uncommon cytokines compared to other helper T cells, are specific for *Candida albicans*. Human Th9 cells transiently produce IL-9, which maximizes production of IFN-γ, IL-9, IL-13, and IL-17 by skin-tropic T cells. IL-9-producing cells are increased in psoriasis and atopic dermatitis [393].

Foxp3+regulatory T cells Foxp3+CD4+ regulatory T (Treg) cells are immunosuppressive subsets, which contain Treg(thymus-derived) and iTreg(peripherally induced) cells [394]. Foxp3 is expressed in about 20 % of CD4T cells in adult human skin in steady state and it can reach 60 % under inflammatory conditions [395]. Human skin Treg cells are nonmigratory, being associated with hair follicles [402–410]. Over time, they encounter skin-associated antigens, obtain effector-memory phenotype (CD45RO+ and high levels of CTLA4, CD25, ICOS, CD27, and BCL2), and accumulate gradually with age. Few TCRβ sequences are shared between skin Treg cells and conventional skin memory T cells, indicating that these two populations recognize different antigens. Skin Treg cells in psoriatic lesion are proliferative and express IL-17, suggesting that they can be functionally defective in inflammatory milieus [396]. Migrant CD4T cells from the skin contain a major population of Foxp3+ Treg cells with high-level expression of CD25, CD103, and GITR, and low level of CD62L (a cell-surface phenotype suggestive of memory/effector cells). These Treg cells are potent suppressors in vitro and in vivo [397]. The mechanism of Treg-cell-mediated suppression can be divided into three catalogues: humoral factor-mediated suppression, cell-contact-dependent suppression, and functional modification of APCs [398, 399]. Defects in Treg cells may cause various skin disorders including psoriasiform dermatitis, eczematous dermatitis, cheilitis, nail dystrophy, serum hyper-IgE, eosinophilia, alopecia areata, urticaria, and bullous pemphigoid [400].

Regulatory T cells without Foxp3 Tr1 and Th3 cells are both CD4+ T cells. Tr1 cells produce IL-10 and Th3 cells produce TGF-β. Tr1 cells can characteristically express LAG3 (lymphocyte activation gene-3) and CD49b. LAG3 attenuates CD4/MHC-II-mediated T cell-activation. Antigen stimulation together with IL-10 and vitamin D3 induces Tr1 cells. Th3 cells, maybe a subset of iTreg cells, are induced in animal models for oral tolerance [401, 402].

6.8.3 CD8T Cells

CD8T cells, also known as killer or cytotoxic T lymphocytes (CTLs), are the principal effector cells, which recognize antigens on MHC-I. In steady state, skin CD8T cells are essentially Trm cells (resident memory T cells), which reside in epidermis and do not enter circulation [381]. CD8 Trm cells not only poise themselves to resume attack but also are capable of maximizing their function by summoning circulating memory T cells to the site of virus reactivation or reentry [403]. Development of skin Trm cells is not fully understood. The skin CD103+CD8+T cells, which develop in epidermis under the influence of IL-15 and TGF-β, show a transcriptional profile shared with that of Trm cells [404]. CD8 Trm cells persist in the dermal–epidermal junction [403]. Effector CD8T cells are involved in various skin diseases, including contact dermatitis, psoriasis, graft versus host disease, drug eruption, and fixed drug eruption. IL-17- or IL-22-producing CD8T cells play roles in psoriasis. In addition to the eradication of virally infected cells, CD8T cells induce apoptosis of tumor cells, grafted allogeneic cells, or keratinocytes in the lesion of drug eruption. Epidermal CD8 Trm cells contribute to the pathogenesis of fixed drug eruption [405].

6.8.4 γδT Cells in the Skin

γδT cells represent a minor population of T cells, which express a distinct T cell receptor (TCR) composed of γδ chains instead of αβ chains. Unlike αβT cells, γδT cells display a restricted TCR repertoire and recognize non-peptide antigens. γδT cells act as a link between innate and adaptive immunity, because they lack precise major histocompatibility complex (MHC) restriction and seize the ability to recognize ligands that are generated during affliction [406]. γδTCR recognize non-peptide antigens like glycerolipids and other small molecules, polypeptides that are soluble or membrane-anchored, and cross-linked to major histocompatibility complex (MHC) molecules or MHC-like molecules in an antigen-independent manner [407]. Skin epidermal γδT cells, recognizing antigen expressed by damaged or stressed keratinocytes, play an indispensable role in tissue homeostasis and tissue repair through secretion of distinct growth factors. γδT cells produce keratinocyte growth factor (KGF), an important cytokine for wound repair and epithelial cell regeneration.

It has been demonstrated that human γδT cells' activation and expansion can be controlled by forkhead boxP3(FOXP3), programmed death-1(PD-1), and cytotoxic T lymphocyte antigen (CTLA)-4 both in vivo and in vitro [408]. Human Vγ9Vδ2 (also known as Vg2Vd2) T cells can be activated by metabolites from isoprenoid synthetic pathway. These include (E)-4-hydroxy-3-methyl-but-2-enyl pyrophosphate (HMBPP), exogenous prenyl pyrophosphate from bacteria and parasitic protozoa and isopentenyl pyrophosphate (IPP), and endogenous prenyl pyrophosphate derived from mevalonate pathway [406].

Effector γδT cells produce IFN-γ, TNF-α, and IL-17. IFN-γ and TNF-α enhance cell-mediated immune response and IL-17 plays a vital role in early neutrophil-mediated response. In addition, cytotoxic components such as perforin and granzymes secreted by these cells ultimately cause direct or indirect effect of cytotoxicity against infected cells [409]. They provide a wide range of defense mechanisms against microorganisms such as viruses, bacteria, and protozoa, and diseases like cancer and also in healing of wounds and burns. In addition, γδ T cells also play a role in autoimmune diseases such as rheumatoid arthritis (RA) and systemic lupus erythematosus (SLE) through antigen-presenting capacity, release of pro-inflammatory cytokines, immunomodulatory properties, interaction with Tregs, and promotion of antibody production [410].

γδT-cell-based immunotherapy strategies possess great prominence in the treatment of various diseases because of the property of their MHC-independent cytotoxicity, copious amount of cytokine release, and an immediate response in infections.

6.9 Cutaneous Microecology

Jianjun Qiao and Hong Fang

The skin, covering the surface of the human body, serves as an active border between the internal and the external environment. As a great ecosystem, the skin consists of several ecological compartments. Different microorganism groups also colonize in different parts of the skin. A better understanding of cutaneous structures will lead to a better understanding of cutaneous microecology [411, 412].

The skin is composed of three layers: epidermis, dermis, and subcutaneous tissue, with distribution of blood vessels, lymph vessels, nerves, muscles, and adnexa deriving from the epidermis. The epidermal adnexa include hair, sebaceous glands, and nails. The skin accounts for 16% in weight and 1.2–2.0 m^2 in surface area. The surface area of skin in a newborn is about 0.21 m^2 [411].

Skin is sterile upon birth. Soon after birth, various kinds of bacteria and fungi begin to colonize on the surface of skin. All these microorganisms, with a long-term co-adaptation on skin surface, can inhabit the skin for long periods of time. Although there is variance among different individuals or among different sites, the cutaneous microorganisms can keep relative balance with the skin [411]. These microorganisms are regarded as the normal microbial community of the skin. Commonly, this microbial community is nonpathogenic and constitutes an indispensable part of life. It plays a key role in maintaining the ecological balance of the skin, offering the outermost biological barrier, defending the invasion of external pathogens and participating in the physiological functions. The changes of internal or external environment to the human body will result in the damage of the microecological balance and the interactions among the normal microbial community. Such a condition facilitates the invasion of pathogens, and turns the normal microbial communities into pathogenic ones, thus leading to the production of toxin and the infectious disorders [411–413].

6.9.1 The Normal Microbial Community of Skin

6.9.1.1 The Resident Flora of Skin

Resident flora and transient flora constitute the normal microbial community of the skin. The resident flora refers to the microbe that can proliferate and inhabit the skin permanently. The transient flora refers to the microbe that inhabits the skin temporarily and which may disappear after a period of time [414–416].

The category of cutaneous normal microbial community only accounts for a very small part in the total varieties of external microorganisms. It is estimated to be 6–80,000/cm^2 on the skin. Generally, the normal microbial community of the skin locates on the outermost layer of the epidermis and the openings of hair follicles, with most microbes exist in a way of minute colony. There is great variance of cutaneous normal microbial community among different individuals as well as among different biological sites. The main categories of the cutaneous normal microbial community are listed in the following [414–416].

Coagulase-Negative Staphylococci (CNS)

Eighteen types of CNS have been isolated from the skin. The most common *CNS* is *Staphylococci epidermidis*. Other *CNS* include *S. haminis*, *S. capitis*, *S. auricularis*, *S. saccharolyticus*, *S. warneri*, *S. hemolyticus*, *S. saprophyticus*, *S. cohnii*, *S. xylosus*, and *S. simulans*. As the most dominant microbe on human skin, *S. epidermidis* is one of the main symbiotic bacteria of skin, and serves as one of the most important members of the cutaneous normal microbial community [414, 415].

S. epidermidis is most abundant on the superior part of trunk, where it accounts for more than 50% of resident Staphylococci. It is of great importance in maintaining the cutaneous microecological balance. With the disturbance of cutaneous microecology, however, it may lead to infection as an opportunistic pathogen [417].

Another important symbiotic Staphylococcus of the skin is *S. haminis*. It tends to inhabit sites with a prosperous secretion of glands, including axil, buttocks, pubic symphysis, perineum, inguina, and legs. *S. capitis* inhabits primarily on the sites of scalp, frontal region, eyebrows, face, neck, external acoustic meatus, and secretory opening of sebaceous glands, while on other sites of skin, it inhabits in the manner of transient flora [414, 417, 418].

Micrococci

Although it is not so common in skin as Staphylococci, eight types of Micrococci have been isolated in skin, including *M. luteus*, *M. varians*, *M. lylae*, *M. nishinomiyaensis*, *M. kristinae*, *M. sedentarius*, *M. agieis*, and *M. roseus*, with the most common type being *M. luteus*, which, together with *M. varians*, constitutes dominant symbiotic bacteria. *M. lylae* and *M. kristinae* are much more common in children's skin, while *M. lylae* is more common in cold seasons [414–416].

Corynebacterium

It is one of the gram-positive microbials with pleomorphism. The most common Corynebacterium is Diphtheroid, which accounts for the majority of cutaneous resident flora, and is divided into two groups: aerobic and anaerobic.

Aerobic Diphtheroid distributes on reductus and humid sites, including axil, inguina, buttocks internatal groove, interdigit, nose, pharynx, conjunctiva, and external acoustic meatus. It is more common in individuals with excessive sweat. It can be divided into two types: lipophilic and unlipophilic. The former is the predominant type, and can be accelerated in growth by oleic acid of cutaneous sebum. As one common type of lipophilic Corynebacterium, *C. minutissimum* can produce porphyrin, resulting in superficial erythrasma on the sites of axil and inguina. It was regarded as a single microbial; however, now it is clear that *C. minutissimum* is one kind of compound bacteria consisting of eight types of microbials. *C. tenuis* is the pathogen of trichomycosis axillaris, inhabiting on the hair cuticles of axillary hairs and pubic hairs in an intracellular or an intercellular way. Nevertheless, it does not damage the hair root or skin [414–416].

Anaerobic Diphtheroid is one of the resident floras in hair follicles and in sebaceous glands, and is one of the dominant categories of cutaneous normal microbes. It is commonly divided into three types. The most common one is *C. acnes*, which is the main member of the cutaneous microecological system. It plays an important role in maintaining the stability of the cutaneous microecological system and in the metabolism of cutaneous lipids. Disturbance to cutaneous microecology may result in the overproliferation of *C. acnes* [419, 420]. The quantity of the microbial corresponds to the production of sebaceous glands on sebum-rich sites such as scalp, frontal region, and upper breast and back. The amount of *C. acnes* reaches summit in the adolescent, and then it is stable in adults, and does not decrease until old age. *C. granulosum*, with a second amount in quantity (accounts for about 20 % in Corynebacterium), distributes everywhere sporadically, although it can be more easily isolated on sebum-rich sites. It is rather common in comedones, and considered as one of the pathogens of acne. Another category of Corynebacterium, *C. avidum*, tends to inhabit humid reductus sites such as axil, perineum, and nasal cavity [419, 420].

Bacillus brevis accounts for a certain percent in Corynebacterium. *B. brevis* may produce protease, and grows very quickly. It can be observed at interdigits in patients with tinea pedis, and is capable of producing awful smell on foot.

Mycoflora

Fungi, especially some yeast fungus, also account for a certain percent in the cutaneous normal microbial community. It is also recognized that Mycoflora is one of the predominant microbials in the cutaneous normal microbial community [416].

As one type of lipophilic yeast, Malassezia requires an environment of a high content of fat for growth, and olive oil is essential in the in vitro culture. There are two types of Malassezia according to shape: *Malassezia ovale* and *M. orbiculare*. Malassezia exists in the blastospore form among cutaneous normal microflora. In correspondence with the production of cutaneous lipids, it is most abundant on the back, and Malassezia turns to hyphal form after it enters the deep layers of the stratum corneum [423].

The isolating rate of Candida from oral mucous membrane is as high as 40%. The isolating rate of *Candida albicans* at normal skin is 15%. *C. parapsilosis* and *C. tropicalis* are non-lipophilic yeasts, with a higher isolating rate on interdigits. Broad-spectrum antibiotics, immunosuppressive agents, and glucocorticoids may result in proliferation of Candida and then lead to candidiasis [414–416, 424].

Protozoan

Protozoan (e.g., *Demodex folliculorum*) inhabits hair follicles and sebaceous glands, with a higher isolating rate on sebum-rich sites such as face and scalp [414, 415].

Virus

It is still a matter of debate whether virus should be included in the cutaneous normal microflora. *Herpes simplex virus* primarily lies in the border between skin and mucous membrane, such as oral lips and genital organs. The virus might exist in a latent state, which colonizes at basal cells. Generally, it is difficult for the virus to proliferate due to the local protective system; however, as soon as there is an opportunity, such as decreased resistance of host and local immune deficiency, the virus will lead to clinical conditions [414–416, 424].

6.9.1.2 The Transient Flora of Skin

Staphylococcus Aureus

Due to the natural resistance of human skin to the coagulase positive *Staphylococcus aureus*, it is very difficult for *S. aureus* to inhabit healthy skin. However, if qulitation is considered, then it is easier to trace *S. aureus* in the whole cutaneous ecological system. The positive rate of *S. aureus* on reductus sites is very high, for example, on perineal region it is 20 %, while it is higher on the nose. Persistent carriage rate in population is estimated to be 20–40 %. The carriage rate is even higher in hospitals, as well as in patients with diabetes mellitus, vein addicts, and dialysis. *S. aureus* can be found all through the skin of patients with psoriasis and atopic dermatitis. It is the most common bacterium that leads to pyogenic infection on skin and mucous membrane [418–422].

Streptococcus

A type of gram-positive bacteria, Streptococcus is spherical or orbicular in shape, with an alignment way of gemination or chain. It could be divided into three types according to the hemolytic character: α, β, and γ Streptococcus. It has various types and a wide range of distribution. Generally, α hemolytic Streptococcus or γ non-hemolytic Streptococcus can be found at nose and laryngea pharyngis of healthy individual, but is hard to be detected on smooth skin. Nevertheless, at the anaphase of newborn, the cutaneous isolating rate of α hemolytic Streptococcus or γ non-hemolytic Streptococcus is rather high. β hemolytic Streptococcus has a robust virulence and leads to pyogenic infection readily [415, 416].

Sarcina

It has a high isolating rate on the healthy skin of infants.

Neisseria

As one type of gram-negative bacteria, it has a special requirement for oxygen and produces oxidase and catalase. The isolating rate of *Neisseria* is high at nasopharynx in healthy individuals, but on skin it is rare. Only *Neisseria intracellularis* or *N. gonorrhoeae* is pathogenic to humans [414, 424].

Gram-Negative Rods

Gram-negative rods are not a common resident flora due to dryness of the skin. However, as one kind of cutaneous transient flora, it usually results from contamination of discharge of gastrointestinal tract. It can be detected in healthy individuals on sites of humid reductus such as perineum, axil, interdigit, and nasal mucosa. Mainly, it consists of the types listed in the following.

Acinetobacter

As an anaerobe, *Acinetobacter* can be found extensively in nature. It can be detected on the skin in more than 25 % of healthy individuals. The isolating rate in male is higher than in female. The quantity of *Acinetobacter* is especially higher in summer due to the increased secretion of sweat and a high humidity.

Esherichia

A group of dynamic gram-negative rods, Esherichia is regarded as one of the normal microflora in human intestinal tract. The most common type, *E. coli*, can be detected on the normal skin of infants and children. It is not pathogenic to humans; on the contrary, it helps to synthesize vitamin B and K in the intestinal tract and benefits the human body. Nevertheless, a certain type of *E. coli* may cause cutaneous infection under the condition of immunosuppression.

Proteus

As another kind of normal microflora in the human intestinal tract, *Proteus* can facilitate phagocytosis via its pilus and then result in a decreased virulence. It exists on human skin as a type of transient flora. Normally, it is nonpathogenic; however, under unusual conditions it may proliferate quickly, leading to an increased quantity, making *Proteus* opportunistic pathogenic bacteria.

Pseudomonas

It can be found extensively in nature and consists of many types, with the most important type being *Pseudomonas aruginosa*. Although it is another kind of resident flora in human intestinal tract, *P. aruginosa* is a type of transient flora on skin. The amount of *P. aruginosa* may increase significantly in immunocompromised patients or hospitalized patients. The virulence of *P. aruginosa* comes from the structural components, toxins and enzymes, which can result in infections of operative incision, burning wound, and severe drug eruption, or even worse, can lead to septicemia [425, 426].

Alkaligenes Faecalis

It is one kind of resident flora in human intestinal tract. Yet, it also can be isolated on skin in a small part of healthy individuals.

6.9.2 Factors Affecting Cutaneous Normal Microflora

There is a relatively balanced system of normal microflora on skin; however, the quantity as well as the construction of flora may change due to many influential factors. These influential factors include the interior factors, the environmental factors, and the interaction between different bacteria.

6.9.2.1 The Climate, Temperature, and Humidity

Usually, resident flora can be affected by environment and local ecologic circumstance. The alteration of temperature and humidity may influence the ecology. A higher temperature and increased humidity will lead to increased hydration of the stratum corneum.

Generally speaking, a humid environment promotes the proliferation of bacteria, while a dry environment inhibits it. It has been indicated that eligible temperature and humidity is essential for the proliferation of bacteria. A study reported that when inoculated on skin, the bacteria lived longer on wet skin than on dry skin. Bacteria on forearm skin increased 10,000 times when occluded for 24 h, with gram-negative rods, gram-negative Corynebacterium and Candida increased faster than coccobacteria. Besides, the increased temperature and humidity caused by occlusion may result in the microbial changing from normal flora to pathogens, such as yeasts (Candida and Pityrosporum) and Dermatophytes. Interestingly some bacteria, such as Nicrococcus, favor dry and cold [411, 414].

6.9.2.2 Age

Age is another important influential factor. The colonization rates of Micrococcus, Corynebacterium, and gram-negative bacteria in infants are much higher than those in children or adults. Before adolescence, cutaneous resident flora mainly consists of *S. epidermidis and S. sarcina. E. coli* can be isolated on inguina and perineum, while the isolating rate of *P. ovale* and *C. acnes* is low. However, the amount of the bacteria will increase in the next 10 years, and will be close to adult level at the age of 15. The amount of *C. acnes* also increases in the adolescence, due to the increase of sebaceous secretion and free fatty acid [411, 414, 415].

6.9.2.3 Anatomic Sites

The constitution of cutaneous normal microflora varies according to the difference of skin site. At the UV-exposed areas such as face, neck, and hands, the transient flora take advantage. While at lipid-rich areas such as face and upper trunk, lipophilic bacteria and Pityrosporum become the predominant types. As a special ecological region, the scalp has a high density for Staphylococci, *Propionibacterium acnes*, and Pityrosporum. Relatively closed areas, including axillary fossa, perineal region, and interdigit, have a higher temperature and humidity. In these special ecological sites, it is suitable for the cutaneous colonizing bacteria. The normal flora at axillary fossa includes Staphylococci and Corynebacterium, while at the perineal region it includes *C. minutissimum*, which is the pathogen for erythrasma. Many bacteria, with the majority being gram-negative bacteria, Dermatophytes and some conditional pathogenic bacteria have also been isolated at interdigit. The amount of bacteria at upper arms and upper legs is much less due to dryness. Nevertheless, there are some bacteria that can proliferate everywhere, such as *S. epidermidis* [411].

6.9.2.4 pH Value of Skin

The pH for the growth of cutaneous resident flora (mainly *S. epidermis*) ranges from 6.5 to 8.5, with the best range from 7.5 to 8. Although pH on normal adult skin is about 4.5–6, cutaneous normal microflora is tolerant to the pH and can grow well. The pH value on the skin of newborn and infants is higher than that of adults, which reaches 6.0–7.0, and is more suitable for the growth of resident flora than adults' skin. The low pH in adults' skin should be mainly attributed to the increased production of fatty acid in sebum layer. The total amount of flora on adults' skin is not less than that of infants, which results from the proliferation of lipophilic Pityrosporum and *C. diphtheroides* [411].

6.9.2.5 Oxygen and Carbon Dioxide

Anaerobic bacteria, specific aerobic bacteria, and facultative anaerobic bacteria are cutaneous normal flora. Therefore, the concentration of cutaneous oxygen and carbon dioxide is very important to the habitation of microbials. Although the epidermis is exposed to the air directly, the intracellular oxygen is supplied by dermal small vessels. Oxygen pressure in the epidermis is lower than that in artery, while carbon dioxide is comparable with that in artery, indicating that oxygen is essential for the metabolism of keratinocytes and microbials.

Some aerobic bacteria can proliferate on the skin. The concept of biofilm has been raised recently. Biofilm is a self-closed system resulting from the epidermal aggregation of microflora as well as their metabolic products. The nutrition and air are dispersed into the system, while PO_2 is present there in escalated levels. The balance alteration of the O_2 and

CO_2 pressure may lead to changes of the microbial category and quantity. For example, wafer may result in the decrease of O_2 pressure and the increase of CO_2 pressure. These changes lead to a remarkable increase in gram-negative rods and Corynebacterium [411, 415].

6.9.2.6 The Ultraviolet

The ultraviolet (UV) is capable of inhibiting or even killing some cutaneous normal microflora. In vitro study has revealed UVA with a dose of 50 mJ/cm^2 can kill Pityrosporum, and UVB with a dose of 250–900 mJ/cm^2 can kill Pityrosporum and *C. albicans*. However, Staphylococci are not sensitive to UV radiation. *S. epidermidis* cannot be killed until a dose of 900 mJ/cm^2 UVB radiation, while *S. aureus* can only be inhibited by the dose. This might explain why sunlight is helpful for seborrheic dermatitis. Both UV light and sunlight have beneficial effect on psoriasis; this might be attributed to the production of Vitamin D in skin induced by radiation, or to the direct or indirect effects of radiation on the cutaneous microbials. However, whether UV radiation can cause the alteration of cutaneous microbials requires further investigation. Previous studies have observed the effect of PUVA on psoriasis, and failed to find the significant difference of cutaneous normal microflora on local radiated area [427].

6.9.2.7 The Adhesive Power of Bacteria

The first step for microbial habitation is adhesion. The habitation ability of microbials is associated with their adhesive power. The surface molecule responsible for adhesion is named adhesin. Adhesins take effect via special receptors on the surface of the host molecule. These special receptors, with the main content being glycose or glycoconjugate, are regarded as adhesive receptors. Adhesin is the bridge between microbials and host molecules. The epidemic cells at different areas of skin have different adhesive receptors, which can explain why cutaneous normal microflora varies among different sites of skin.

Teichoic acid, one component of cell wall in Staphylococci and Streptococci, can combine with its corresponding adhesive receptor (fibronectin, Fn) on epidemic cells. Fn is a kind of glycoprotein receptor. It is revealed that adhesin may combine with Fn from at least two parts on epidermal cells, and dissolvable Fn can inhibit the combination between Streptococci and epidermal cells. Multiple receptors can combine with one single adhesin, while one single receptor can also be competitively combined with multiple adhesins.

For gram-negative bacteria, the most important adhesin is pilus, which is constituted of pilin. For example, the adhesin of *E. coli* includes common pilus, P pilus, and S pilus. Most *E. coli* express common pilus under appropriate condition, which enables the bacterium to adhere on almost all epithelial cells in human. Also, it has been proved that pilus of *Neisseria gonorrhoeae* can adhere to the epithelial cells at cervix or vagina. Increasing evidences indicate that fibril may promote the adhesion of *Streptococcus pyogenes* to epithelial cells, and the adhesive effect is related to the hydrophobicity.

For *C. albicans*, the adhesin is a kind of mannitol-protein compound, which can combine with glycoprotein protein on the surface of host and thus cause adhesion.

Not only microbial factors but also host factors can have influence on the adhesive power. Some patients are more sensitive to a certain kind of pathogen, which might be attributed to a higher adhesive power of their keratinocytes to that pathogen. It is observed that due to the increased adhesive receptors, keratinocytes in atopic dermatitis patients are more adhesive to *S. aureus* than healthy controls. Besides, among the susceptive individuals carrying *S. aureus* on nasal mucosa, the expression of HLA is intimately associated with bacteria colonization [428].

6.9.2.8 The Interactions Between Microflora

The normal cutaneous microflora serve as barrier against the invasion of bacteria, which, together with human body and the environment, constitutes a harmonious system. The mechanisms of microbial barrier are complex, including the interaction between microflora and host, and the interaction between microorganisms. Both antagonism and enhancement effect are of great importance to the integrity of this barrier and the balance of cutaneous normal microecology.

Reciprocal Enhancement Among Microflora

Corynebacterium acne and *Staphylococcus epidermidis* can both live in hair follicle and sebaceous gland. Due to the consumption of oxygen and the decrease of local pH value caused by *S. epidermidis*, it is a good condition for the proliferation of *C. acne*, while the decomposition of cutaneous keratin and the secretion of probiotics by Corynebacterium and Bacillus can also stimulate the growth of *S. epidermidis*. Besides, the decomposition of sebum by Corynebacterium and *S. epidermidis* can enhance the growth of Bacillus. It is confirmed that Nicrococcus is capable of synthesizing some nutritious factors, which then enhances the proliferation of fungi that can produce antibiotics [424].

Reciprocal Antagonism Among Microflora

The mechanisms of reciprocal antagonism between microflora include competitive consumption of nutrition among microflora, production of oxidoreduction electric potential to inhibit the growth of other microbials, competitive combination of adhesive receptor to interfere with the colonization of other bacteria, and production of inhibitory materials to restrain the growth of other bacteria. The inhibitory materials mainly include decomposed products of lipids, bacteria hydrolase, and antibiotics.

Corynebacterium acne is capable of decomposing triglyceride to free fatty acid. Long-chain free saturated fatty acid and oleic acid have inhibitory effect on *Streptococcus pyogenes* and gram-negative bacteria. Pityrosporum has the activity of lipoxygenase and can turn oleic acid to azelaic acid, which can inhibit Corynebacterium, Staphylococci, and some fungi. Propionic acid produced by Corynebacterium has inhibitory effect on *Trichophyton gypsum*. Short-chain fatty acid produced by resident flora can also have an inhibitory effect in a high local concentration [419, 420].

Corynebacterium acne may produce bacteria hydrolyses and inhibit the growth of Staphylococci and other Corynebacterium. Staphylococci can produce lysozyme and inhibit the colonization of other microorganisms [414, 415, 419, 420].

A lot of cutaneous normal microflora can synthesize antibiotics. Coagulase-negative Staphylococcus and a small quantity of Corynebacterium may produce round polypeptin, and inhibit or even kill the bacteria that are close in taxology (such as *S. aureus*). A certain kind of fungi is capable of producing antibiotics such as streptomycin, penicillin, and actinomycin, which leads to the detection of resistant bacteria around the border of dermatomycosis lesion. Some dermatophytes may produce peptide and inhibit the growth of *Bacillus brevis* or even virus, and therefore inhibit the awful smell of foot [415].

6.9.3 The Physiologic Function of Cutaneous Normal Microflora

6.9.3.1 Defense Function

The primary function of cutaneous normal microflora is protection and defense. *Corynebacterium acne* and *Staphylococcus epidermidis* are capable of decomposing the sebum and producing free fatty acids. The acids emulsify lipid membrane, which leads to the acidity of skin surface. These normal microflora orderly colonize on skin and form a biological barrier, functioning as a protection of naked epidermis from the colonization of external pathogens, thus preventing infection of host skin or even internal organs [417, 422].

6.9.3.2 Immune Function

Skin is an important immune organ. Cutaneous normal microflora can serve as natural nonspecific antigens that constantly stimulate the immune system. The stimulation enhances the immunity of the human body. *Staphylococcus epidermidis* may enhance the defense ability via inducing the immune response of host. There are evidences indicating that the inflammation clearance ability of host may decrease in the absence of the trigger effect of *S. epidermidis*. *S. epidermidis* can enable the cutaneous innate immunity via Toll-like receptor signal transduction system and produce effective response against pathogens in keratinocytes, thus preventing the skin or internal organs from being infected by pathogens [429–431].

Cutaneous normal microflora is capable of secreting antibacterial peptides, which can help the host to eliminate pathogens. *S. epidermidis* produces antibiotics that are toxic to other microbials such as *S. aureus* and group A Streptococcus. *Pseudomonas aeruginosa* is also protective for the human body, because it produces PsVP-10. It is another type of antibacterial peptides and possesses defense ability against Streptococci. *P. aeruginosa* can also produce chemical compounds such as pyocyanin, pyrrolnitrin, and oxyhydroxide phenazine. These substances kill or inhibit the growth of pathogenic fungi. They also prevent the transformation of Candida from yeast form to pathogenic hyphal form [429–432].

6.9.3.3 Nutrition Function

Intracellular glucose, water, and electrolytes (such as potassium, natrium, and calcium) supply nutrition for the growth of cutaneous microflora. Phospholipids, sterin, and keratin produced by cutaneous microflora can also be absorbed by cutaneous cells, which can enhance the growth of cells, prevent skin-aging progress and reduce wrinkles [411].

6.10 Co-regulation of Epidermal Permeability Barrier and Cutaneous Immunity

George Man and Mao-Qiang Man

The major function of skin is to serve as a protective barrier, including physical, chemical, and biological barrier, between the inside and outside of the environment. Presently, the regulatory role of the epidermal permeability barrier in cutaneous functions, including epidermal proliferation, differentiation, pathogenesis of certain dermatoses and immune function has been well demonstrated. In this chapter, the regulatory role of the epidermal permeability barrier in cutaneous immunity is summarized.

6.10.1 Epidermal Permeability Barrier

The epidermal permeability barrier, regulating the movement of water and other molecules in and out of the skin, resides in the stratum corneum, the outermost layer of the epidermis [433]. It is the permeability barrier that makes life possible in a terrestrial environment. Both corneocytes and extracellular lipids are determinants of the epidermal permeability barrier function. The corneocytes provide both the mechanical strength of the skin and a scaffold, consisting of differentiation proteins and small proline-rich proteins, for the extracellular lamellar membranes [434]. The differentiation proteins, such as filaggrin, loricrin, and involucrin, form a cornified envelope while lipids, including proximal equal moles of cholesterol, fatty acids, and sphingolipids, form extracellular lamellar membranes [435]. The majority of these lipids are synthesized as precursors (glucosylceramides, sphingomyelin, and phospholipids) by keratinocytes [436–438]. In the stratum granulosum, cholesterol and other lipid precursors together with lipid-processing enzymes, including beta-glucocerebrosidase, acid sphingomyelinase, and acid secretory phospholipase A2, are packaged in lamellar bodies, ovoid organelles [439]. To date, ATP-binding cassette transporter 12 (ABCA12) is the only known transmembrane transporter to transport glucosylceramide into lamellar bodies [440–442]. Evidence suggests that lamellar bodies originate from the Golgi apparatus because disruption of the Golgi apparatus interferes with the formation of lamellar bodies, and ABCA12 and glucosylceramide co-localize in the Golgi apparatus [442, 443]. The mechanisms whereby other components are incorporated into lamellar bodies remain unknown. Nevertheless, upon barrier requirement, lamellar bodies deliver lipids and their processing enzymes into extracellular spaces of the lower stratum corneum, where the lipid precursors are processed by their respective enzymes [444–447]. The optimal pH for these processing enzymes is acidic. The role of the epidermal permeability barrier in the pathogenesis of certain dermatoses, such as atopic dermatitis, psoriasis, and infection, is well known [448–452].

6.10.2 Epidermal Permeability Barrier and Skin Immunity

6.10.2.1 Co-regulation of Epidermal Permeability Barrier and Epidermal Cytokines

Keratinocytes can synthesize a number of cytokines, some of which benefit the permeability barrier. Studies have shown that treatment of fetal rat explants (skin from fetal rat at the age of 17 days of gestation) with IL-1β at a concentration of 50 ng/ml, or IL-1α or TNFα at a concentration of 100 ng/ml accelerated barrier formation, as indicated by an over 20 % reduction in transepidermal water loss, paralleled with decreased lanthanum penetration [453]. Similarly, addition of IL-6 at a concentration of 100 ng/ml also promotes permeability barrier formation [454]. The beneficial effects of TNF, IL-1, and IL-6 on permeability barrier function are likely attributed to upregulation of differentiation-related protein expression [453, 454]. In vivo studies demonstrated that IL-1 receptor KO rat displayed a delay in epidermal permeability barrier development [453]. In contrast, neither TNF nor IL-6 receptor KO alters permeability barrier formation [453, 454], suggesting that the TNF and IL-6 are not critical for barrier formation during fetal development.

In addition to influencing barrier formation in fetal skin, cytokines also improve the permeability barrier in adult skin. Delayed permeability barrier recovery has been shown in both aged humans and mice [455, 456]. Either intracutaneous injections of IL-1α or stimulation of IL-1α production by topical imiquimod accelerates permeability barrier recovery in aged skin [457]. The beneficial effects of IL-1α on barrier function in aged skin are attributed, in part, to stimulation of epidermal lipid production [457]. Jung et al. used the same protocol and found that IL-1α could overcome the abnormalities in the permeability barrier, stratum corneum integrity, as well as antimicrobial peptide expression induced by topical tacrolimus [458].

Cytokines benefit the permeability barrier, while the permeability barrier regulates cytokine expression. In normal mouse epidermis, TNFα is primarily expressed in the upper nucleated layers where it displays a diffuse cytosolic pattern. Barrier disruption can elevate epidermal TNFα expression as quickly as 10 min after disruption. Studies have shown that 2 h after acute disruption of the barrier with either acetone or tape-stripping, TNFα was extensively expressed throughout all of the nucleated epidermal cell layers [459]. Likewise, a significant increase in epidermal TNFα expression is also observed in essential fatty acid deficient mice, a mouse model of chronic defective barrier [459]. The barrier disruption-induced increase in TNFα is mainly 17KD, not 24–26KD, the precursor TNF protein [460]. Barrier disruption not only increases TNFα protein expression, but also increases its mRNA expression. Studies from our groups have demonstrated that barrier disruption with acetone induced a ninefold increase in epidermal TNFα mRNA expression at 2.5 h and returned to normal levels at 8 h [460]. In contrast, tape-stripping, another method of barrier disruption, only induced a fourfold increase in epidermal TNFα mRNA expression [460, 461] while the TNFα mRNA expression remained unchanged in the dermis [461]. The expression levels of epidermal TNFα mRNA in essential fatty acid deficient mice are about 6.5-fold of normal controls [460]. Artificial correction of permeability barrier function by occlusion can normalize the expression levels of TNFα mRNA in essential fatty acid deficient mice, but not in normal mice after acute barrier disruption [462]. Moreover, the expression levels of TNFα p55, not p75, receptor mRNA are also elevated 87 % at 2.5 h after acute barrier disruption with tape-stripping, and return to the normal levels at 7 h. Surprisingly, the expression levels of TNFα p55 receptor mRNA are increased again at 18 h after barrier disruption [461]. However, the expression levels of TNFα p55 receptor mRNA remain normal in essential fatty acid deficient mice and the dermis of tape-stripped normal mice. Additionally, occlusion does not alter the expression levels of epidermal TNFα p55 receptor mRNA after tape-stripping [461]. These evidences indicate that the influences of the permeability barrier on TNFα and its receptor expression vary with the methods of barrier disruption.

IL-1α is another cytokine expressed in the epidermis. In similar fashion as TNFα, the epidermal IL-1α expression is increased at 10 min and returns to normal levels by 8 h after barrier disruption [463]. Moreover, the expression levels of epidermal IL-1α are also increased in the dermis 10 min after barrier disruption, but return to normal levels by 24 h after barrier disruption [461, 463]. Similarly, the epidermal IL-1α expression in essential fatty acid deficient mice is also elevated, but primarily in the stratum corneum, following barrier disruption [463]. Again, following barrier disruption, artificial correction of permeability barrier function by occlusion lowers the expression levels of IL-1α protein [463], but not IL-1α mRNA in normal mice [462]. Interestingly, except for a reduction in the basal level of IL-1α expression, barrier disruption does not elevate the epidermal IL-1α protein expression when mice are pre-occluded for 48 h [463]. Consistently, occlusion of either normal or essential fatty acid deficient mice, which have a higher level of basal IL-1α mRNA expression [461], lowers the epidermal IL-1α mRNA expression [462]. A barrier disruption-induced increase in epidermal IL-1α expression is likely released from pre-formed pool because disruption of skin barrier at 4°C also increases IL-1α expression both in vivo and in vitro [463]. Finally, barrier disruption increases epidermal IL-1r antagonist (IL-1ra) mRNA expression [464], which cannot be prevented by occlusion. In contrast, occlusion of essential fatty acid deficient mice or normal mice lowers epidermal IL-1ra mRNA expression [462]. Collectively, barrier disruption differentially regulates IL-1α protein and its mRNA expression. In addition to TNFα and IL-1α, epidermal permeability barrier also regulates other cutaneous cytokine and receptor expression. For example, the expression levels of epidermal granulocyte – macrophage colony stimulating factor (GM-CSF) and IL-1β mRNA are elevated in both acute and chronic barrier disruption models [460]. It is worth to note that the increase in IL- Iα and β mRNA levels are maximal at 4 h [460] while the peak times for TNFα and GM-CSF are at 1 h after barrier disruption [460]. Thus, regulation of the permeability barrier in cytokine expression varies with the types of cytokines and the models of barrier disruption.

6.10.2.2 Epidermal Permeability Barrier and Epidermal Toll-Like Receptors

Toll-like receptors (TLR) play an important role in host innate immunity. To date, 10 TLRs have been identified in human. TLR2 recognizes a variety of microbial components, including lipoproteins/lipopeptides from various pathogens while TLR4 recognizes lipopolysaccharides (LPS) from gram-negative bacteria, and other ligands such as oligosaccharides of hyaluronic acid, heparan sulfate and fibrinogen [465–468]. TLR3 is implicated in virus-derived double-stranded RNA. TLR5 detects bacterial flagellin and TLR9 is required for response to unmethylated CpG DNA. Finally, TLR7 and TLR8 recognize small synthetic antiviral molecules [469, 470], and single-stranded RNA is reported to be their natural ligand [471]. TLR1-6 and 9 are expressed in human keratinocytes [472–478]. Our studies showed that repeated barrier disruption increased TLR2 expression in the epidermis, and TLR4 expression in both the epidermis and dermis [479]. TLR2 deficient mice display a delayed barrier repair [480]. Activation of TLR2,3 benefits the epidermal permeability barrier, possibly via upregulation of tight junction protein. In addition to the requirements of stratum corneum lipids and differentiation-related protein, the tight junction (TJ) and its adhesion molecules are also crucial for permeability barrier homeostasis [481–483]. For example, claudin-1-deficient mice display a higher transepidermal water loss [481, 482]. Conversely, activation of tight junctions enhances permeability barrier. In vitro, TRL2 and 3 activators increase the transepithelial electric resistance (TER) resulting from the upregulation of tight junction protein mRNA such as claudin-1, claudin-23, occludin, and zonulae occludens 1. Consistently, topical applications of TRL2 agonist accelerate permeability barrier repair in human atopic dermatitis skin, which exhibits a lower level of TRL1,2 [480]. The inverse correlation of TRL1,2 expression with TEWL has been demonstrated in atopic dermatitis. Yuki et al. [484] reported that activation of TLR1-4 and 9 with their respective ligand significantly increased TER, indicating the improvement of permeability barrier. The effects of TLR ligands on tight junction barrier could be blocked by either TLR adaptor MyD88 or the TLR neutralizing antibodies.

Recently, Borkowski et al. [485] demonstrated the role of TLR3 in epidermal permeability barrier homeostasis. Activation of TLR3 by double-stranded RNA (dsRNA) increases a whole panel of permeability-barrier-related markers. Treatment of keratinocytes with dsRNA stimulates the expression of several barrier-related genes, including ABCA12, glucocerebrosidase, acid sphingomyelinase, serine palmotyltranferase, glucosylceramide synthase, and transglutaminase 1, which play key roles in permeability barrier homeostasis. These changes are coupled with the accumulation of sphingolipid content and an increased number of lamellar bodies. In contrast, ligands for TLR2,7, 8, and 9 do not significantly alter expression of these barrier-related genes. Notably, activation of TLR3 does not change the expression level of other barrier-related genes, including involucrin, keratin 1, loricrin, and filaggrin. Gallo's group reported that activation of TLR3 stimulated tight-junction-related proteins, corneodesmosin, occludin, tight junction protein 1, and claudin 1 mRNA expression [486]. The role of TLR3 in permeability homeostasis is further demonstrated by TLR3 KO mice that display a delayed barrier repair following UVB irradiation [486]. Pertinent to tight junction barriers, the activation of the transient receptor potential cation channel subfamily V4 (TRPV4), not TRPV1 or TRPV3, induces ≈ 60 % increase in TER at 48 h after addition of 10 μM 4α-phorbol 12, 13-didecanoate in parallel with a 1.5-fold to twofold increase in claudin-4 and occludin expression [487]. Taken together, barrier disruption upregulates TLR expression, while TLRs regulate permeability barrier homeostasis via stimulation of tight junction proteins and lamellar body formation.

6.10.2.3 Co-regulation of Epidermal Permeability Barrier and Epidermal Antimicrobial Defense

As stated above, epidermal permeability barrier is clearly linked to innate immunity. The permeability barrier and antimicrobial barrier are key functions of the skin. Recent studies have shown that these functions are linked. Aberg et al. [488] showed that the expression levels of epidermal cathelicidin-related antimicrobial peptide (CAMP) and mouse β-defensin 3 (mBD3) were significantly increased 1 h after barrier disruption and returned to normal levels at 24 h. In addition, CAMP mRNA expression was increased at 1 h and mBD3 mRNA expression was increased at 4 h after barrier disruption. Ahrens et al. [489] showed that both protein and mRNA expression for mBD1,3 and 14 were increased following barrier disruption. Blockade of CAMP and mBD3 mRNA expression by occlusion further confirmed the regulatory role of the permeability barrier in CAMP and mBD3 expression [488, 489]. Barrier disruption induced increase in antimicrobial peptide expression, at least in mBD3, is likely mediated via TNFα [489]. Epidermal CAMP expression changes in parallel with permeability barrier status [490]. For example, psychological stress that compromises permeability barrier lowers CAMP expression [490]. Certain approaches that enhance permeability barrier increase epidermal antimicrobial peptide expression [458, 491–494]. In murine models, severe barrier perturbation with tape-stripping enhances *Staphylococcus aureus* skin colonization, accompanied by elevation of epidermal IL-1β, IL-6, and TNF-α [495]. The epidermal permeability barrier also prevents the invasion of certain Candida, such as *Candida tropicalis*, *C. paropsiiosis*, *C. krusei*, and *C. guilliermondi*, but not *C. albicans* and *C. stellatoidea* [496]. In humans, enhancing the epidermal permeability barrier with topical sunflower seed oil reduces the risk of skin infection [497]. The role of CAMP in permeability barrier homeostasis is demonstrated in CAMP KO mice, which exhibited impaired barrier in a tape-stripped model [488]. Thus, the epidermal permeability barrier and epidermal antimicrobial defense are co-regulated.

6.10.2.4 Epidermal Permeability Barrier Regulates Inflammatory Cell Infiltration

Part of the regulatory role of the epidermal permeability barrier in cutaneous inflammation is due to the regulation of inflammatory cell infiltration. The role of mast cells in host immune defense is well recognized. Mast cells can directly kill microorganisms by phagocytosis, produce antimicrobial peptides, induce cytokine and chemotactic factors' release, and enhance the maturation of immature dendritic cells [498–503]. Barrier disruption causes an over 50 % increase in mast cell density in dermis [503]. Interestingly, mast cell deficiency causes ≈ 160 % acceleration of barrier recovery at 2 h after barrier disruption [504]. Langerhans cells are antigen-presenting dendritic cells present in both the dermis and epidermis. Langerhans cells play critical roles in both skin antimicrobial immunity and contact allergic dermatitis [505]. It has been demonstrated that barrier disruption induces a 94–175 % increase in epidermal Langerhans cell density depending on the methods employed to disrupt the barrier while Langerhans cell density in the dermis remains unchanged [506]. The extent of barrier disruption is linearly correlated with the increase in epidermal Langerhans cell density. In murine allergic contact dermatitis model, barrier disruption also increases epidermal Langerhans cell density and enhances allergic reaction [507]. Moreover, barrier disruption stimulates Langerhans cell maturation [508]. Disruption of epidermal permeability barrier increases contact sensitivity to a variety of sensitizers, including 2,4-dinitrofluorobenzene, picryl chloride, and tetrachlorosalicylanilide, a photosensitizer, resulting from the increased epidermal permeability to these sensitizers [509]. Acute barrier disruption induces a onefold increase in IL-1 activity and

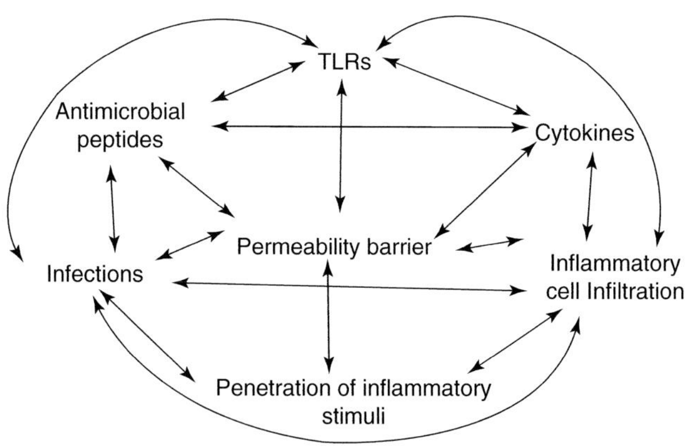

Fig. 6.3 Schematic diagram showing co-regulation of epidermal permeability barrier and cutaneous immunity

1.5-fold increase in T cell proliferation. In addition, barrier disruption upregulates the expression of major histocompatibility complex class II molecules, CD54, and CD86 in Langerhans cells. Thus, the permeability barrier regulates inflammatory cell infiltration, proliferation, and maturation.

In summary, the epidermal permeability barrier and cutaneous immunity co-regulate each other's function (Fig. 6.3). Disruption of the epidermal permeability barrier disturbs cutaneous immune homeostasis while perturbation of cutaneous immune function could compromise permeability barrier. Therefore, improvement of the epidermal permeability barrier can benefit certain immune-associated dermatoses.

References

Keratinocytes in Skin Immune System

1. Houben E, et al. A keratinocyte's course of life. Skin Pharmacol Physiol. 2007;20:122–32.
2. Candi E, et al. The cornifi ed envelope: a model of cell death in the skin. Nat Rev Mol Cell Biol. 2005;6:328–40.
3. Uchi H, et al. Cytokines and chemokines in the epidermis. J Dermatol Sci. 2000;24 Suppl 1:S29–38.
4. Liu YJ, et al. TSLP: an epithelial cell cytokine that regulates T cell differentiation by conditioning dendritic cell maturation. Annu Rev Immunol. 2007;25:193–219.
5. Soumelis V, et al. Human epithelial cells trigger dendritic cell mediated allergic inflammation by producing TSLP. Nat Immunol. 2002;3:673–80.
6. Loser K, et al. Epidermal RANKL controls regulatory T-cell numbers via activation of dendritic cells. Nat Med. 2006;12:1372–9.
7. Morioka Y, et al. Cathelicidin antimicrobial peptides inhibit hyaluronan-induced cytokine release and modulate chronic allergic dermatitis. J Immunol. 2008;181:3915–22.
8. Nasir A, et al. Exaggerated and persistent cutaneous delayed-type hypersensitivity in transgenic mice whose epidermal keratinocytes constitutively express B7-1 antigen. J Clin Invest. 1994;94:892–8.
9. Williams IR, et al. Keratinocyte expression of B7-1 in transgenic mice amplifies the primary immune response to cutaneous antigens. Proc Natl Acad Sci U S A. 1994;91:12780–4.
10. Ferguson TA, et al. Regulation of contact hypersensitivity by interleukin 10. J Exp Med. 1994;179:1597–604.
11. Kollisch G, et al. Various members of the Toll-like receptor family contribute to the innate immune response of human epidermal keratinocytes. Immunology. 2005;114:531–41.
12. Mempel M, et al. Toll-like receptor expression in human keratinocytes: nuclear factor kappaB controlled gene activation by Staphylococcus aureus is toll-like receptor 2 but not toll-like receptor 4 or platelet activating factor receptor dependent. J Invest Dermatol. 2003;121:1389–96.
13. Pivarcsi A, et al. Expression and function of Toll-like receptors 2 and 4 in human keratinocytes. Int Immunol. 2003;15:721–30.
14. Miller LS. Toll-like receptors in skin. Adv Dermatol. 2008;24:71–87.
15. Lebre MC, et al. Human keratinocytes express functional Toll-like receptor 3, 4, 5, and 9. J Invest Dermatol. 2007;127:331–41.
16. Tigalonowa M, et al. The distribution of Fc gamma RI, Fc gamma RII and Fc gamma R III on Langerhans' cells and keratinocytes in normal skin. Acta Derm Venereol. 1990;70:385–90.
17. Cauza K, et al. FcgammaRIII expression on cultured human keratinocytes and upregulation by interferon-gamma. J Invest Dermatol. 2002;119:1074–9.
18. Szolnoky G, et al. A mannose-binding receptor is expressed on human keratinocytes and mediates killing of Candida albicans. J Invest Dermatol. 2001;117:205–13.
19. Pellegrini G, et al. Expression, topography, and function of integrin receptors are severely altered in keratinocytes from involved and uninvolved psoriatic skin. J Clin Invest. 1992;89:1783–95.
20. Bos JD, et al. The skin immune system: progress in cutaneous biology. Immunol Today. 1993;14:75–8.
21. Singh A, et al. Innate immunity and the regulation and mobilization of keratinocyte stem cells: are the old players playing a new game? Exp Dermatol. 2012;21(9):660–4.
22. Abrahamsohn PA. Epithelial tissue. In: Basic histology: text and atlas. 11th ed. New York: McGraw-Hill; 2005. p. 66–89.
23. Strbo N, et al. Innate and adaptive immune responses in wound epithelialization. Adv Wound Care (New Rochelle). 2014;3(7):492–501.
24. Sorensen OE, et al. Wound healing and expression of antimicrobial peptides/polypeptides in human keratinocytes, a consequence of common growth factors. J Immunol. 2003;170:5583–9.
25. Braff MH, et al. Keratinocytes store the antimicrobial peptide cathelicidin in lamellar bodies. J Invest Dermatol. 2005;124:394–400.
26. Sayama K, et al. New mechanisms of skin innate immunity: ASK1-mediated keratinocyte differentiation regulates the expression of betadefensins, LL37, and TLR2. Eur J Immunol. 2005;35:1886–95.
27. Ali RS, et al. Expression of the peptide antibiotics human beta defensin-1 and human beta defensin-2 in normal human skin. J Invest Dermatol. 2001;117:106–11.
28. Oren A, et al. In human epidermis, beta-defensin 2 is packaged in lamellar bodies. Exp Mol Pathol. 2003;74:180–2.
29. Richard L, et al. Microbial symbiosis with the innate immune defense system of the skin. J Invest Dermatol. 2011;131(10):1974–80.
30. Gallo RL, et al. Innate barriers against infection and associated disorders. Drug Discov Today Dis Mech. 2008;5:145–52.
31. Chu AC, et al. The keratinocyte. In: Bos JD, editor. Skin immune system (SIS): cutaneous immunology and clinical immunodermatology. 3rd ed. Boca Raton: CRC Press; 2005. p. 77–99.
32. Piskin G, et al. In vitro and in vivo expression of IL-23 by keratinocytes in healthy skin and psoriasis lesions: enhanced expression in psoriatic skin. J Immunol. 2006;176:1908–15.
33. Corsini E, et al. Epidermal cytokines in experimental contact dermatitis. Toxicology. 2000;142:203–11.
34. Grone A. Keratinocytes and cytokines. Vet Immunol Immunopathol. 2002;88:1–12.

Langerhans Cells and Other Dendritic Cells in Skin

35. Banchereau J, Steinman RM. Dendritic cells and the control of immunity. Nature. 1998;392(6673):245–52.
36. Rupec RA, Boneberger S, Ruzicka T. What is really in control of skin immunity: lymphocytes, dendritic cells, or keratinocytes? facts and controversies. Clin Dermatol. 2010;28(1):62–6.
37. Tang A, et al. Adhesion of epidermal Langerhans cells to keratinocytes mediated by E-cadherin. Nature. 1993;361(6407):82–5.

38. Jiang W, et al. The receptor DEC-205 expressed by dendritic cells and thymic epithelial cells is involved in antigen processing. Nature. 1995;375(6527):151–5.
39. Hunger RE, et al. Langerhans cells utilize CD1a and langerin to efficiently present nonpeptide antigens to T cells. J Clin Invest. 2004;113(5):701–8.
40. Poulin LF, et al. The dermis contains langerin+dendritic cells that develop and function independently of epidermal Langerhans cells. J Exp Med. 2007;204(13):3119–31.
41. Shklovskaya E, Roediger B, Fazekas B, Fazekas de St Groth B. Epidermal and dermal dendritic cells display differential activation and migratory behavior while sharing the ability to stimulate CD4+ T cell proliferation in vivo. J Immunol. 2008;181(1):418–30.
42. Ginhoux F, et al. The origin and development of nonlymphoid tissue CD103+ DCs. J Exp Med. 2009;206(13):3115–30.
43. Nestle FO, et al. Characterization of dermal dendritic cells obtained from normal human skin reveals phenotypic and functionally distinctive subsets. J Immunol. 1993;151(11):6535–45.
44. Haniffa M, et al. Human tissues contain CD141hi cross-presenting dendritic cells with functional homology to mouse CD103+ nonlymphoid dendritic cells. Immunity. 2012;37(1):60–73.
45. Colonna M, Trinchieri G, Liu YJ. Plasmacytoid dendritic cells in immunity. Nat Immunol. 2004;5(12):1219–26.
46. Cella M, et al. Plasmacytoid monocytes migrate to inflamed lymph nodes and produce large amounts of type I interferon. Nat Med. 1999;5(8):919–23.
47. Helft J, et al. Origin and functional heterogeneity of non-lymphoid tissue dendritic cells in mice. Immunol Rev. 2010;234(1):55–75.
48. Belz GT, Nutt SL. Transcriptional programming of the dendritic cell network. Nat Rev Immunol. 2012;12(2):101–13.
49. Chu CC, Di Meglio P, Nestle FO. Harnessing dendritic cells in inflammatory skin diseases. Semin Immunol. 2011;23(1):28–41.
50. Henri S, et al. CD207+ CD103+ dermal dendritic cells cross-present keratinocyte-derived antigens irrespective of the presence of Langerhans cells. J Exp Med. 2010;207(1):189–206.
51. Romani N, Clausen BE, Stoitzner P. Langerhans cells and more: langerin-expressing dendritic cell subsets in the skin. Immunol Rev. 2010;234(1):120–41.
52. Klareskog L, et al. Epidermal Langerhans cells express Ia antigens. Nature. 1977;268(5617):248–50.
53. Rowden G, Lewis MG, Sullivan AK. Ia antigen expression on human epidermal Langerhans cells. Nature. 1977;268(5617):247–8.
54. Stingl G, et al. Epidermal Langerhans cells bear Fc and C3 receptors. Nature. 1977;268(5617):245–6.
55. Frelinger JG, et al. Mouse epidermal Ia molecules have a bone marrow origin. Nature. 1979;282(5736):321–3.
56. Katz SI, Tamaki K, Sachs DH. Epidermal Langerhans cells are derived from cells originating in bone marrow. Nature. 1979;282(5736):324–6.
57. Schuler G, Steinman RM. Murine epidermal Langerhans cells mature into potent immunostimulatory dendritic cells in vitro. J Exp Med. 1985;161(3):526–46.
58. Steinman RM, Cohn ZA. Identification of a novel cell type in peripheral lymphoid organs of mice. I. Morphology, quantitation, tissue distribution. J Exp Med. 1973;137(5):1142–62.
59. Chorro L, Geissmann F. Development and homeostasis of 'resident' myeloid cells: the case of the Langerhans cell. Trends Immunol. 2010;31(12):438–45.
60. Hoeffel G, et al. Adult Langerhans cells derive predominantly from embryonic fetal liver monocytes with a minor contribution of yolk sac-derived macrophages. J Exp Med. 2012;209(6):1167–81.
61. Schuster C, et al. Human embryonic epidermis contains a diverse Langerhans cell precursor pool. Development. 2014;141(4):807–15.
62. Tavian M, Peault B. Embryonic development of the human hematopoietic system. Int J Dev Biol. 2005;49(2–3):243–50.
63. Kobayashi M, et al. Development of ATPase-positive, immature Langerhans cells in the fetal mouse epidermis and their maturation during the early postnatal period. Cell Tissue Res. 1987;248(2):315–22.
64. Chorro L, et al. Langerhans cell (LC) proliferation mediates neonatal development, homeostasis, and inflammation-associated expansion of the epidermal LC network. J Exp Med. 2009;206(13):3089–100.
65. Schuster C, et al. HLA-DR+ leukocytes acquire CD1 antigens in embryonic and fetal human skin and contain functional antigen-presenting cells. J Exp Med. 2009;206(1):169–81.
66. Ghigo C, et al. Multicolor fate mapping of Langerhans cell homeostasis. J Exp Med. 2013;210(9):1657–64.
67. Sere K, et al. Two distinct types of Langerhans cells populate the skin during steady state and inflammation. Immunity. 2012;37(5):905–16.
68. Ginhoux F, et al. Langerhans cells arise from monocytes in vivo. Nat Immunol. 2006;7(3):265–73.
69. Borkowski TA, et al. A role for endogenous transforming growth factor beta 1 in Langerhans cell biology: the skin of transforming growth factor beta 1 null mice is devoid of epidermal Langerhans cells. J Exp Med. 1996;184(6):2417–22.
70. Kaplan DH, et al. Autocrine/paracrine TGFbeta1 is required for the development of epidermal Langerhans cells. J Exp Med. 2007;204(11):2545–52.
71. Kel JM, et al. TGF-beta is required to maintain the pool of immature Langerhans cells in the epidermis. J Immunol. 2010;185(6):3248–55.
72. Greter M, et al. Stroma-derived interleukin-34 controls the development and maintenance of langerhans cells and the maintenance of microglia. Immunity. 2012;37(6):1050–60.
73. Borkowski TA, et al. A role for TGFbeta1 in langerhans cell biology. Further characterization of the epidermal Langerhans cell defect in TGFbeta1 null mice. J Clin Invest. 1997;100(3):575–81.
74. Xu YP, et al. TGFbeta/Smad3 signal pathway is not required for epidermal Langerhans cell development. J Invest Dermatol. 2012;132(8):2106–9.
75. Hacker C, et al. Transcriptional profiling identifies Id2 function in dendritic cell development. Nat Immunol. 2003;4(4):380–6.
76. Fainaru O, et al. Runx3 regulates mouse TGF-beta-mediated dendritic cell function and its absence results in airway inflammation. EMBO J. 2004;23(4):969–79.
77. Schiavoni G, et al. ICSBP is critically involved in the normal development and trafficking of Langerhans cells and dermal dendritic cells. Blood. 2004;103(6):2221–8.
78. Ichikawa E, et al. Defective development of splenic and epidermal CD4+ dendritic cells in mice deficient for IFN regulatory factor-2. Proc Natl Acad Sci U S A. 2004;101(11):3909–14.
79. Chopin M, et al. Langerhans cells are generated by two distinct PU.1-dependent transcriptional networks. J Exp Med. 2013;210(13):2967–80.
80. van de Laar L, et al. Tight control of STAT5 activity determines human CD34-derived interstitial dendritic cell and langerhans cell development. J Immunol. 2011;186(12):7016–24.
81. Iwama A, et al. Reciprocal roles for CCAAT/enhancer binding protein (C/EBP) and PU.1 transcription factors in Langerhans cell commitment. J Exp Med. 2002;195(5):547–58.
82. Liu K, et al. Origin of dendritic cells in peripheral lymphoid organs of mice. Nat Immunol. 2007;8(6):578–83.
83. Adolfsson J, et al. Identification of Flt3+ lympho-myeloid stem cells lacking erythro-megakaryocytic potential a revised road map for adult blood lineage commitment. Cell. 2005;121(2):295–306.
84. Schlenner SM, et al. Fate mapping reveals separate origins of T cells and myeloid lineages in the thymus. Immunity. 2010;32(3):426–36.

85. Fogg DK, et al. A clonogenic bone marrow progenitor specific for macrophages and dendritic cells. Science. 2006;311(5757):83–7.
86. Onai N, et al. Identification of clonogenic common Flt3 + M-CSFR+ plasmacytoid and conventional dendritic cell progenitors in mouse bone marrow. Nat Immunol. 2007;8(11):1207–16.
87. Auffray C, et al. CX3CR1+ CD115+ CD135+ common macrophage/DC precursors and the role of CX3CR1 in their response to inflammation. J Exp Med. 2009;206(3):595–606.
88. Schlitzer A, et al. Identification of CCR9- murine plasmacytoid DC precursors with plasticity to differentiate into conventional DCs. Blood. 2011;117(24):6562–70.
89. Satpathy AT, et al. Re(de)fining the dendritic cell lineage. Nat Immunol. 2012;13(12):1145–54.
90. Braathen LR, Thorsby E. Studies on human epidermal Langerhans cells. I. Allo-activating and antigen-presenting capacity. Scand J Immunol. 1980;11(4):401–8.
91. Ptak W, et al. Role of antigen-presenting cells in the development and persistence of contact hypersensitivity. J Exp Med. 1980;151(2):362–75.
92. Heufler C, Koch F, Schuler G. Granulocyte/macrophage colony-stimulating factor and interleukin 1 mediate the maturation of murine epidermal Langerhans cells into potent immunostimulatory dendritic cells. J Exp Med. 1988;167(2):700–5.
93. Witmer-Pack MD, et al. Granulocyte/macrophage colony-stimulating factor is essential for the viability and function of cultured murine epidermal Langerhans cells. J Exp Med. 1987;166(5):1484–98.
94. Kissenpfennig A, et al. Dynamics and function of Langerhans cells in vivo: dermal dendritic cells colonize lymph node areas distinct from slower migrating Langerhans cells. Immunity. 2005;22(5):643–54.
95. Bennett CL, et al. Inducible ablation of mouse Langerhans cells diminishes but fails to abrogate contact hypersensitivity. J Cell Biol. 2005;169(4):569–76.
96. Kaplan DH, et al. Epidermal langerhans cell-deficient mice develop enhanced contact hypersensitivity. Immunity. 2005;23(6):611–20.
97. Bursch LS, et al. Identification of a novel population of Langerin + dendritic cells. J Exp Med. 2007;204(13):3147–56.
98. Noordegraaf M, et al. Functional redundancy of Langerhans cells and Langerin + dermal dendritic cells in contact hypersensitivity. J Invest Dermatol. 2010;130(12):2752–9.
99. Honda T, et al. Compensatory role of Langerhans cells and langerin-positive dermal dendritic cells in the sensitization phase of murine contact hypersensitivity. J Allergy Clin Immunol. 2010;125(5):1154–6. e2.
100. Shklovskaya E, et al. Langerhans cells are precommitted to immune tolerance induction. Proc Natl Acad Sci U S A. 2011;108(44):18049–54.
101. Kautz-Neu K, et al. Langerhans cells are negative regulators of the anti-Leishmania response. J Exp Med. 2011;208(5):885–91.
102. Schwarz A, et al. Langerhans cells are required for UVR-induced immunosuppression. J Invest Dermatol. 2010;130(5):1419–27.
103. Stary G, et al. Glucocorticosteroids modify Langerhans cells to produce TGF-beta and expand regulatory T cells. J Immunol. 2011;186(1):103–12.
104. Igyártó BZ, et al. Skin-resident murine dendritic cell subsets promote distinct and opposing antigen-specific T helper cell responses. Immunity. 2011;35(2):260–72.
105. Haley K, et al. Langerhans cells require MyD88-dependent signals for Candida albicans response but not for contact hypersensitivity or migration. J Immunol. 2012;188(9):4334–9.
106. Seneschal J, et al. Human epidermal Langerhans cells maintain immune homeostasis in skin by activating skin resident regulatory T cells. Immunity. 2012;36(5):873–84.
107. Ouchi T, et al. Langerhans cell antigen capture through tight junctions confers preemptive immunity in experimental staphylococcal scalded skin syndrome. J Exp Med. 2011;208(13):2607–13.
108. Wang L, et al. Langerin expressing cells promote skin immune responses under defined conditions. J Immunol. 2008;180(7):4722–7.
109. Klechevsky E, et al. Functional specializations of human epidermal Langerhans cells and CD14+ dermal dendritic cells. Immunity. 2008;29(3):497–510.
110. Angel CE, et al. CD14+ antigen-presenting cells in human dermis are less mature than their CD1a + counterparts. Int Immunol. 2007;19(11):1271–9.
111. Chun IY, et al. Human CD141 + dendritic cells induce CD4+ T cells to produce type 2 cytokines. J Immunol. 2014;193(9):4335–43.
112. Villadangos JA, Young L. Antigen-presentation properties of plasmacytoid dendritic cells. Immunity. 2008;29(3):352–61.
113. Gilliet M, Cao W, Liu Y-J. Plasmacytoid dendritic cells: sensing nucleic acids in viral infection and autoimmune diseases. Nat Rev Immunol. 2008;8(8):594–606.
114. Siegal FP, et al. The nature of the principal type 1 interferon-producing cells in human blood. Science. 1999;284(5421):1835–7.
115. Lande R, et al. Plasmacytoid dendritic cells sense self-DNA coupled with antimicrobial peptide. Nature. 2007;449(7162):564–9.
116. Banchereau J, Pascual V. Type I interferon in systemic lupus erythematosus and other autoimmune diseases. Immunity. 2006;25(3):383–92.

Melanocytes in Skin Immune System

117. Nordlund JJ. The melanocyte and the epidermal melanin unit: an expanded concept. Dermatol Clin. 2007;25(3):271–81, vii.
118. Nishimura EK. Melanocyte stem cells: a melanocyte reservoir in hair follicles for hair and skin pigmentation. Pigment Cell Melanoma Res. 2011;24(3):401–10.
119. Plonka PM, et al. What are melanocytes really doing all day long…? Exp Dermatol. 2009;18(9):799–819.
120. Tolleson WH. Human melanocyte biology, toxicology, and pathology. J Environ Sci Health C Environ Carcinog Ecotoxicol Rev. 2005;23(2):105–61.
121. Cichorek M, et al. Skin melanocytes: biology and development. Postepy Dermatol Alergol. 2013;30(1):30–41.
122. Feller L, et al. Melanin: the biophysiology of oral melanocytes and physiological oral pigmentation. Head Face Med. 2014;10(1):8.
123. Hearing VJ. Milestones in melanocytes/melanogenesis. J Invest Dermatol. 2011;131(E1):E1.
124. Lu Y, et al. Melanocytes are potential immunocompetent cells: evidence from recognition of immunological characteristics of cultured human melanocytes. Pigment Cell Res. 2002;15(6):454–60.
125. Mackintosh JA. The antimicrobial properties of melanocytes, melanosomes and melanin and the evolution of black skin. J Theor Biol. 2001;211(2):101–13.
126. Hari A, et al. Toll-like receptors: role in dermatological disease. Mediators Inflamm. 2010;2010:437246.
127. Kumar H, Kawai T, Akira S. Pathogen recognition by the innate immune system. Int Rev Immunol. 2011;30(1):16–34.
128. Yu N, et al. Cultured human melanocytes express functional toll-like receptors 2–4, 7 and 9. J Dermatol Sci. 2009;56(2):113–20.
129. Jin SH, Kang HY. Activation of Toll-like receptors 1, 2, 4, 5, and 7 on human melanocytes modulate pigmentation. Ann Dermatol. 2010;22(4):486–9.
130. Ahn JH, et al. Human melanocytes express functional Toll-like receptor 4. Exp Dermatol. 2008;17(5):412–7.
131. Ahn JH, Jin SH, Kang HY. LPS induces melanogenesis through p38 MAPK activation in human melanocytes. Arch Dermatol Res. 2008;300(6):325–9.
132. Tam I, Stepien K. Secretion of proinflammatory cytokines by normal human melanocytes in response to lipopolysaccharide. Acta Biochim Pol. 2011;58(4):507–11.

133. Smit N, et al. Expression of different immunological markers by cultured human melanocytes. Arch Dermatol Res. 1993;285(6):356–65.
134. Yohn JJ, et al. Modulation of melanocyte intercellular adhesion molecule-1 by immune cytokines. J Invest Dermatol. 1990;95(2):233–7.
135. Ebanks JP, Wickett RR, Boissy RE. Mechanisms regulating skin pigmentation: the rise and fall of complexion coloration. Int J Mol Sci. 2009;10(9):4066–87.
136. Vavricka CJ, Christensen BM, Li J. Melanization in living organisms: a perspective of species evolution. Protein Cell. 2010;1(9):830–41.
137. Fuentes M, et al. Antifungal activity of melanin in clinical isolates of Candida spp. Rev Chilena Infectol. 2014;31(1):28–33.
138. Burkhart CG, Burkhart CN. The mole theory: primary function of melanocytes and melanin may be antimicrobial defense and immunomodulation (not solar protection). Int J Dermatol. 2005;44(4):340–2.
139. Wood JM, et al. What's the use of generating melanin? Exp Dermatol. 1999;8(2):153–64.
140. Mohagheghpour N, et al. Synthetic melanin suppresses production of proinflammatory cytokines. Cell Immunol. 2000;199(1):25–36.
141. Gunathilake R, et al. pH-regulated mechanisms account for pigment-type differences in epidermal barrier function. J Invest Dermatol. 2009;129(7):1719–29.
142. Rocha IM, Guillo LA. Lipopolysaccharide and cytokines induce nitric oxide synthase and produce nitric oxide in cultured normal human melanocytes. Arch Dermatol Res. 2001;293(5):245–8.
143. Fecker LF, et al. Inducible nitric oxide synthase is expressed in normal human melanocytes but not in melanoma cells in response to tumor necrosis factor-alpha, interferon-gamma, and lipopolysaccharide. J Invest Dermatol. 2002;118(6):1019–25.
144. Miniati A, et al. Stimulated human melanocytes express and release interleukin-8, which is inhibited by luteolin: relevance to early vitiligo. Clin Exp Dermatol. 2014;39(1):54–7.
145. Luger TA, et al. New insights into the functions of alpha-MSH and related peptides in the immune system. Ann N Y Acad Sci. 2003;994:133–40.
146. Luger TA, et al. The role of alpha-MSH as a modulator of cutaneous inflammation. Ann N Y Acad Sci. 2000;917:232–8.
147. Le Poole IC, et al. Phagocytosis by normal human melanocytes in vitro. Exp Cell Res. 1993;205(2):388–95.
148. Schraermeyer U, et al. Melanin granules of retinal pigment epithelium are connected with the lysosomal degradation pathway. Exp Eye Res. 1999;68(2):237–45.
149. Orlow SJ. Melanosomes are specialized members of the lysosomal lineage of organelles. J Invest Dermatol. 1995;105(1):3–7.
150. Le Poole IC, et al. A novel, antigen-presenting function of melanocytes and its possible relationship to hypopigmentary disorders. J Immunol. 1993;151(12):7284–92.

Dermal Monocyte-Derived Cells and Macrophages: Organization, Immune Function, and Relation to the Dendritic Cell Compartment

151. Wynn TA, Chawla A, Pollard JW. Macrophage biology in development, homeostasis and disease. Nature. 2013;496:445–55.
152. McGovern N, Schlitzer A, Gunawan M, Jardine L, Shin A, Poyner E, et al. Human dermal CD14(+) cells are a transient population of monocyte-derived macrophages. Immunity. 2014;41:465–77.
153. Romani N, Brunner PM, Stingl G. Changing views of the role of Langerhans cells. J Investig Dermatol. 2012;132:872–81.
154. Zaba LC, Fuentes-Duculan J, Steinman RM, Krueger JG, Lowes MA. Normal human dermis contains distinct populations of CD11c+BDCA-1+ dendritic cells and CD163+FXIIIA+ macrophages. J Clin Invest. 2007;117:2517–25.
155. Angel CE, Lala A, Chen CJ, Edgar SG, Ostrovsky LL, Dunbar PR. CD14+ antigen-presenting cells in human dermis are less mature than their CD1a+counterparts. Int Immunol. 2007;19:1271–9.
156. Wang X-N, McGovern N, Gunawan M, Richardson C, Windebank M, Siah T-W, et al. A three-dimensional atlas of human dermal leukocytes, lymphatics, and blood vessels. J Invest Dermatol. 2013;134(4):965–74.
157. Collin M, McGovern N, Haniffa M. Human dendritic cell subsets. Immunology. 2013;140:22–30.
158. Bigley V, Spence LE, Collin M. Connecting the dots: monocyte/DC and NK subsets in human peripheral blood. Blood. 2010;116:2859–60.
159. Haniffa M, Ginhoux F, Wang XN, Bigley V, Abel M, Dimmick I, et al. Differential rates of replacement of human dermal dendritic cells and macrophages during hematopoietic stem cell transplantation. J Exp Med. 2009;206:371–85.
160. Nestle FO, Zheng XG, Thompson CB, Turka LA, Nickoloff BJ. Characterization of dermal dendritic cells obtained from normal human skin reveals phenotypic and functionally distinctive subsets. J Immunol. 1993;151:6535–45.
161. Haniffa M, Shin A, Bigley V, McGovern N, Teo P, See P, et al. Human tissues contain CD141hi cross-presenting dendritic cells with functional homology to mouse CD103+ nonlymphoid dendritic cells. Immunity Elsevier Inc. 2012;37:60–73.
162. Schutz F, Hackstein H. Identification of novel dendritic cell subset markers in human blood. Biochem Biophys Res Commun. 2014;443(2):453–7.
163. Dutertre C-A, Jourdain J-P, Rancez M, Amraoui S, Fossum E, Bogen B, et al. TLR3-responsive, XCR1+, CD141(BDCA-3)+/CD8α+−equivalent dendritic cells uncovered in healthy and simian immunodeficiency virus-infected rhesus macaques. J Immunol Am Asso Immunol. 2014;192:4697–708.
164. Galibert L, Diemer GS, Liu Z, Johnson RS, Smith JL, Walzer T, et al. Nectin-like protein 2 defines a subset of T-cell zone dendritic cells and is a ligand for class-I-restricted T-cell-associated molecule. J Biol Chem. 2005;280:21955–64.
165. Poulin LF, Salio M, Griessinger E, Anjos-Afonso F, Craciun L, Chen JL, et al. Characterization of human DNGR-1+ BDCA3+ leukocytes as putative equivalents of mouse CD8+dendritic cells. J Exp Med. 2010;207:1261–71.
166. Huysamen C, Willment JA, Dennehy KM, Brown GD. CLEC9A is a novel activation C-type lectin-like receptor expressed on BDCA3+ dendritic cells and a subset of monocytes. J Biol Chem. 2008;283:16693–701.
167. Crozat K, Guiton R, Contreras V, Feuillet V, Dutertre CA, Ventre E, et al. The XC chemokine receptor 1 is a conserved selective marker of mammalian cells homologous to mouse CD8+dendritic cells. J Exp Med. 2010;207:1283–92.
168. Bachem A, Guttler S, Hartung E, Ebstein F, Schaefer M, Tannert A, et al. Superior antigen cross-presentation and XCR1 expression define human CD11c+CD141+ cells as homologues of mouse CD8+ dendritic cells. J Exp Med. 2010;207:1273–81.
169. Watchmaker PB, Lahl K, Lee M, Baumjohann D, Morton J, Kim SJ, et al. Comparative transcriptional and functional profiling defines conserved programs of intestinal DC differentiation in humans and mice. Nat Immunol. 2014;15:98–108.
170. Bigley V, McGovern N, Milne P, Dickinson R, Pagan S, Cookson S, et al. Langerin-expressing dendritic cells in human tissues are related to CD1c+dendritic cells and distinct from Langerhans cells and CD141high XCR1+ dendritic cells. J Leukoc Biol. 2015;97:627–34.
171. Milne P, Bigley V, Gunawan M, Haniffa M, Collin M. CD1c+blood dendritic cells have Langerhans cell potential. Blood. 2015;125:470–3.

172. Lenz A, Heine M, Schuler G, Romani N. Human and murine dermis contain dendritic cells. Isolation by means of a novel method and phenotypical and functional characterization. J Clin Invest Am Soc Clin Invest. 1993;92:2587–96.
173. Angel CE, George E, Brooks AES, Ostrovsky LL, Brown TLH, Dunbar PR. Cutting edge: CD1a+antigen-presenting cells in human dermis respond rapidly to CCR7 ligands. J Immunol. 2006;176:5730–4.
174. Segura E, Valladeau-Guilemond J, Donnadieu MH, Sastre-Garau X, Soumelis V, Amigorena S. Characterization of resident and migratory dendritic cells in human lymph nodes. J Exp Med. 2012;209:653–60.
175. Angel CE, Chen CJ, Horlacher OC, Winkler S, John T, Browning J, et al. Distinctive localization of antigen-presenting cells in human lymph nodes. Blood. 2009;113:1257–67.
176. Morandi B, Bonaccorsi I, Mesiti M, Conte R, Carrega P, Costa G, et al. Characterization of human afferent lymph dendritic cells from seroma fluids. J Immunol. 2013;191:4858–66.
177. Klechevsky E, Morita R, Liu M, Cao Y, Coquery S, Thompson-Snipes L, et al. Functional specializations of human epidermal Langerhans cells and CD14+ dermal dendritic cells. Immunity. 2008;29:497–510.
178. Matthews K, Chung NP, Klasse PJ, Moore JP, Sanders RW. Potent induction of antibody-secreting B cells by human dermal-derived CD14+ dendritic cells triggered by dual TLR ligation. J Immunol. 2012;189:5729–44.
179. de Gruijl TD, Sombroek CC, Lougheed SM, Oosterhoff D, Buter J, van den Eertwegh AJ, et al. A postmigrational switch among skin-derived dendritic cells to a macrophage-like phenotype is predetermined by the intracutaneous cytokine balance. J Immunol. 2006;176:7232–42.
180. Larregina AT, Morelli AE, Spencer LA, Logar AJ, Watkins SC, Thomson AW, et al. Dermal-resident CD14+ cells differentiate into Langerhans cells. Nat Immunol. 2001;2:1151–8.
181. Caux C, Vanbervliet B, Massacrier C, Dezutter-Dambuyant C, de Saint-Vis B, Jacquet C, et al. CD34+ hematopoietic progenitors from human cord blood differentiate along two independent dendritic cell pathways in response to GM-CSF+TNF alpha. J Exp Med. 1996;184:695–706.
182. Penel-Sotirakis K, Simonazzi E, Péguet-Navarro J, Rozières A. Differential capacity of human skin dendritic cells to polarize CD4+ T cells into IL-17, IL-21 and IL-22 producing cells. PLoS One. 2012;7:e45680.
183. Morelli AE, Rubin JP, Erdos G, Tkacheva OA, Mathers AR, Zahorchak AF, et al. CD4+ T cell responses elicited by different subsets of human skin migratory dendritic cells. J Immunol. 2005;175:7905–15.
184. Chu CC, Ali N, Karagiannis P, Di Meglio P, Skowera A, Napolitano L, et al. Resident CD141 (BDCA3)+dendritic cells in human skin produce IL-10 and induce regulatory T cells that suppress skin inflammation. J Exp Med. 2012;209:935–45.
185. Klechevsky E, Flamar AL, Cao Y, Blanck JP, Liu M, O'Bar A, et al. Cross-priming CD8+ T cells by targeting antigens to human dendritic cells through DCIR. Blood. 2010;116:1685–97.
186. Banchereau J, Thompson-Snipes L, Zurawski S, Blanck JP, Cao Y, Clayton S, et al. The differential production of cytokines by human Langerhans cells and dermal CD14(+) DCs controls CTL priming. Blood. 2012;119:5742–9.
187. Mosser DM, Edwards JP. Exploring the full spectrum of macrophage activation. Nat Rev Immunol. 2008;8:958–69.
188. Mantovani A, Sica A, Sozzani S, Allavena P, Vecchi A, Locati M. The chemokine system in diverse forms of macrophage activation and polarization. Trends Immunol. 2004;25:677–86.
189. Fuentes-Duculan J, Suárez-Fariñas M, Zaba LC, Nograles KE, Pierson KC, Mitsui H, et al. A subpopulation of CD163-positive macrophages is classically activated in psoriasis. J Investig Dermatol. 2010;130:2412–22.
190. Willenborg S, Eming SA. Macrophages – sensors and effectors coordinating skin damage and repair. J Dtsch Dermatol Ges. 2014;12:214. –21–214–23.
191. Nomura I, Goleva E, Howell MD, Hamid QA, Ong PY, Hall CF, et al. Cytokine milieu of atopic dermatitis, as compared to psoriasis, skin prevents induction of innate immune response genes. J Immunol. 2003;171:3262–9.
192. Dickinson RE, Griffin H, Bigley V, Reynard LN, Hussain R, Haniffa M, et al. Exome sequencing identifies GATA-2 mutation as the cause of dendritic cell, monocyte, B and NK lymphoid deficiency. Blood. 2011;118:2656–8.
193. Hambleton S, Salem S, Bustamante J, Bigley V, Boisson-Dupuis S, Azevedo J, et al. IRF8 mutations and human dendritic-cell immunodeficiency. N Engl J Med. 2011;365:127–38.
194. Ginhoux F, Jung S. Monocytes and macrophages: developmental pathways and tissue homeostasis. Nat Rev Immunol. 2014;14:392–404.
195. Hutchins KD, Dickson DW, Rashbaum WK, Lyman WD. Localization of morphologically distinct microglial populations in the developing human fetal brain: implications for ontogeny. Brain Res Dev Brain Res. 1990;55:95–102.
196. Enzan H. Electron microscopic studies of macrophages in early human yolk sacs. Acta Pathol Jpn. 1986;36:49–64.
197. Schuster C, Vaculik C, Prior M, Fiala C, Mildner M, Eppel W, et al. Phenotypic characterization of leukocytes in prenatal human dermis. J Investig Dermatol. 2012;132:2581–92.
198. Schuster C, Vaculik C, Fiala C, Meindl S, Brandt O, Imhof M, et al. HLA-DR+ leukocytes acquire CD1 antigens in embryonic and fetal human skin and contain functional antigen-presenting cells. J Exp Med Rockefeller Univ Press. 2009;206:169–81.
199. Kanitakis J, Morelon E, Petruzzo P, Badet L, Dubernard J-M. Self-renewal capacity of human epidermal Langerhans cells: observations made on a composite tissue allograft. Exp Dermatol Blackwell Publishing Ltd. 2011;20:145–6.
200. Bigley V, Haniffa M, Doulatov S, Wang X-N, Dickinson R, McGovern N, et al. The human syndrome of dendritic cell, monocyte, B and NK lymphoid deficiency. J Exp Med. 2011;208:227–34.
201. Hoeffel G, Wang Y, Greter M, See P, Teo P, Malleret B, et al. Adult Langerhans cells derive predominantly from embryonic fetal liver monocytes with a minor contribution of yolk sac-derived macrophages. J Exper Med Rockefeller Univ Press. 2012;209:1167–81.
202. Foster CA, Holbrook KA, Farr AG. Ontogeny of Langerhans cells in human embryonic and fetal skin: expression of HLA-DR and OKT-6 determinants. J Invest Dermatol. 1986;86:240–3.
203. Dutertre C-A, Wang L-F, Ginhoux F. Aligning bona fide dendritic cell populations across species. Cell Immunol. 2014;291:3–10.
204. Jongbloed SL, Kassianos AJ, McDonald KJ, Clark GJ, Ju X, Angel CE, et al. Human CD141+ (BDCA-3)+dendritic cells (DCs) represent a unique myeloid DC subset that cross-presents necrotic cell antigens. J Exp Med. 2010;207:1247–60.
205. Cohn L, Chatterjee B, Esselborn F, Smed-Sörensen A, Nakamura N, Chalouni C, et al. Antigen delivery to early endosomes eliminates the superiority of human blood BDCA3+ dendritic cells at cross presentation. J Exp Med Rockefeller Univ Press. 2013;210:1049–63.
206. Schlitzer A, McGovern N, Teo P, Zelante T, Atarashi K, Low D, et al. IRF4 transcription factor-dependent CD11b+dendritic cells in human and mouse control mucosal IL-17 cytokine responses. Immunity. 2013;38:970–83.
207. Tamoutounour S, Guilliams M, Montanana Sanchis F, Liu H, Terhorst D, Malosse C, et al. Origins and functional specialization of macrophages and of conventional and monocyte-derived dendritic cells in mouse skin. Immunity. 2013;39:925–38.
208. Wollenberg A, Wagner M, Günther S, Towarowski A, Tuma E, Moderer M, et al. Plasmacytoid dendritic cells: a new cutaneous

dendritic cell subset with distinct role in inflammatory skin diseases. J Invest Dermatol. 2002;119:1096–102.
209. Chu C-C, Di Meglio P, Nestle FO. Harnessing dendritic cells in inflammatory skin diseases. Semin Immunol. 2011;23:28–41.
210. Schäkel K, Hänsel A. News from dendritic cells in atopic dermatitis. Curr Opin Allergy Clin Immunol. 2011;11:445–50.
211. Odhiambo JA, Williams HC, Clayton TO, Robertson CF, Asher MI, ISAAC Phase Three Study Group. Global variations in prevalence of eczema symptoms in children from ISAAC phase three. J Allergy Clin Immunol. 2009;124:1251–8.e23.
212. Niebuhr M, Werfel T. Innate immunity, allergy and atopic dermatitis. Curr Opin Allergy Clin Immunol. 2010;10:463–8.
213. Leung DYM, Boguniewicz M, Howell MD, Nomura I, Hamid QA. New insights into atopic dermatitis. J Clin Invest Am Soc Clin Invest. 2004;113:651–7.
214. Irvine AD, McLean WHI, Leung DYM. Filaggrin mutations associated with skin and allergic diseases. N Engl J Med. 2011;365:1315–27.
215. Palmer CNA, Irvine AD, Terron-Kwiatkowski A, Zhao Y, Liao H, Lee SP, et al. Common loss-of-function variants of the epidermal barrier protein filaggrin are a major predisposing factor for atopic dermatitis. Nat Genet Nature Publishing Group. 2006;38:441–6.
216. Guttman-Yassky E, Lowes MA, Fuentes-Duculan J, Whynot J, Novitskaya I, Cardinale I, et al. Major differences in inflammatory dendritic cells and their products distinguish atopic dermatitis from psoriasis. J Allergy Clin Immunol. 2007;119:1210–7.
217. Kiekens RC, Thepen T, Oosting AJ, Bihari IC, Van De Winkel JG, Bruijnzeel-Koomen CA, et al. Heterogeneity within tissue-specific macrophage and dendritic cell populations during cutaneous inflammation in atopic dermatitis. Br J Dermatol. 2001;145:957–65.
218. Wollenberg A, Kraft S, Hanau D, Bieber T. Immunomorphological and ultrastructural characterization of Langerhans cells and a novel, inflammatory dendritic epidermal cell (IDEC) population in lesional skin of atopic eczema. J Invest Dermatol. 1996;106:446–53.
219. Oppel T, Schuller E, Günther S, Moderer M, Haberstok J, Bieber T, et al. Phenotyping of epidermal dendritic cells allows the differentiation between extrinsic and intrinsic forms of atopic dermatitis. Br J Dermatol. 2000;143:1193–8.
220. Novak N, Kraft S, Bieber T. Unraveling the mission of FcepsilonRI on antigen-presenting cells. J Allergy Clin Immunol. 2003;111:38–44.
221. Sugaya M, Miyagaki T, Ohmatsu H, Suga H, Kai H, Kamata M, et al. Association of the numbers of CD163(+) cells in lesional skin and serum levels of soluble CD163 with disease progression of cutaneous T cell lymphoma. J Dermatol Sci. 2012;68:45–51.
222. Soumelis V, Reche PA, Kanzler H, Yuan W, Edward G, Homey B, et al. Human epithelial cells trigger dendritic cell mediated allergic inflammation by producing TSLP. Nat Immunol. 2002;3:673–80.
223. Corrigan CJ, Jayaratnam A, Wang Y, Liu Y, de Waal Malefyt R, Meng Q, et al. Early production of thymic stromal lymphopoietin precedes infiltration of dendritic cells expressing its receptor in allergen-induced late phase cutaneous responses in atopic subjects. Allergy Blackwell Publishing Ltd. 2009;64:1014–22.
224. Han H, Headley MB, Xu W, Comeau MR, Zhou B, Ziegler SF. Thymic stromal lymphopoietin amplifies the differentiation of alternatively activated macrophages. J Immunol. 2013;190:904–12.
225. Leyden JJ, Marples RR, Kligman AM. Staphylococcus aureus in the lesions of atopic dermatitis. Br J Dermatol. 1974;90:525–30.
226. Bunikowski R, Mielke ME, Skarabis H, Worm M, Anagnostopoulos I, Kolde G, et al. Evidence for a disease-promoting effect of Staphylococcus aureus-derived exotoxins in atopic dermatitis. J Allergy Clin Immunol. 2000;105:814–9.
227. Breuer K, HAussler S, Kapp A, Werfel T. Staphylococcus aureus: colonizing features and influence of an antibacterial treatment in adults with atopic dermatitis. Br J Dermatol. 2002;147:55–61.
228. Niebuhr M, Lutat C, Sigel S, Werfel T. Impaired TLR-2 expression and TLR-2-mediated cytokine secretion in macrophages from patients with atopic dermatitis. Allergy Blackwell Publishing Ltd. 2009;64:1580–7.
229. Hasannejad H, Takahashi R, Kimishima M, Hayakawa K, Shiohara T. Selective impairment of Toll-like receptor 2-mediated proinflammatory cytokine production by monocytes from patients with atopic dermatitis. J Allergy Clin Immunol. 2007;120:69–75.
230. Niebuhr M, Langnickel J, Draing C, Renz H, Kapp A, Werfel T. Dysregulation of toll-like receptor-2 (TLR-2)-induced effects in monocytes from patients with atopic dermatitis: impact of the TLR-2 R753Q polymorphism. Allergy. 2008;63:728–34.
231. Oh D-Y, Schumann RR, Hamann L, Neumann K, Worm M, Heine G. Association of the toll-like receptor 2 A-16934T promoter polymorphism with severe atopic dermatitis. Allergy. 2009;64:1608–15.
232. Gardembas-Pain M, Ifrah N, Foussard C, Boasson M, Saint Andre JP, Verret JL. Psoriasis after allogeneic bone marrow transplantation. Arch Dermatol. 1990;126:1523.
233. Eedy DJ, Burrows D, Bridges JM, Jones FG. Clearance of severe psoriasis after allogenic bone marrow transplantation. BMJ. 1990;300:908.
234. Nestle FO, Gilliet M, Liu Y-J. Plasmacytoid predendritic cells initiate psoriasis through interferon- production. J Exper Med [Internet]. 2005;202:135–43. Available from: http://www.ncbi.nlm.nih.gov/pubmed/15998792.
235. Zaba LC, Krueger JG, Lowes MA. Resident and "inflammatory" dendritic cells in human skin. J Investig Dermatol. 2009;129:302–8.
236. Hänsel A, Günther C, Ingwersen J, Starke J, Schmitz M, Bachmann M, et al. Human slan (6-sulfo LacNAc) dendritic cells are inflammatory dermal dendritic cells in psoriasis and drive strong TH17/TH1 T-cell responses. J Allergy Clin Immunol. 2011;127:787.–94.e1–9.
237. Hänsel A, Günther C, Baran W, Bidier M, Lorenz H-M, Schmitz M, et al. Human 6-sulfo LacNAc (slan) dendritic cells have molecular and functional features of an important pro-inflammatory cell type in lupus erythematosus. J Autoimmun. 2013;40:1–8.
238. Thomas K, Dietze K, Wehner R, Metz I, Tumani H, Schultheiß T, et al. Accumulation and therapeutic modulation of 6-sulfo LacNAc(+) dendritic cells in multiple sclerosis. Neurol Neuroimmunol Neuroinflamm Lippincott Williams Wilkins. 2014;1:e33. –3.
239. Ziegler-Heitbrock L, Hofer TPJ. Toward a refined definition of monocyte subsets. Front Immunol Frontiers. 2013;4:23.
240. Cros J, Cagnard N, Woollard K, Patey N, Zhang SY, Senechal B, et al. Human CD14dim monocytes patrol and sense nucleic acids and viruses via TLR7 and TLR8 receptors. Immunity. 2010;33:375–86.
241. Schakel K, Kannagi R, Kniep B, Goto Y, Mitsuoka C, Zwirner J, et al. 6-Sulfo LacNAc, a novel carbohydrate modification of PSGL-1, defines an inflammatory type of human dendritic cells. Immunity. 2002;17:289–301.
242. Schäkel K, von Kietzell M, Hänsel A, Ebling A, Schulze L, Haase M, et al. Human 6-sulfo LacNAc-expressing dendritic cells are principal producers of early interleukin-12 and are controlled by erythrocytes. Immunity. 2006;24:767–77.
243. Lee E, Trepicchio WL, Oestreicher JL, Pittman D, Wang F, Chamian F, et al. Increased expression of interleukin 23 p19 and p40 in lesional skin of patients with psoriasis vulgaris. J Exp Med. 2004;199:125–30.
244. Stratis A, Pasparakis M, Rupec RA, Markur D, Hartmann K, Scharffetter-Kochanek K, et al. Pathogenic role for skin macro-

phages in a mouse model of keratinocyte-induced psoriasis-like skin inflammation. J Clin Invest. 2006;116:2094–104.
245. Wang H, Peters T, Kess D, Sindrilaru A, Oreshkova T, van Rooijen N, et al. Activated macrophages are essential in a murine model for T cell-mediated chronic psoriasiform skin inflammation. J Clin Invest. 2006;116:2105–14.
246. Gottlieb AB, Chamian F, Masud S, Cardinale I, Abello MV, Lowes MA, et al. TNF inhibition rapidly down-regulates multiple proinflammatory pathways in psoriasis plaques. J Immunol. 2005;175:2721–9.
247. Nickoloff BJ, Karabin GD, Barker JN, Griffiths CE, Sarma V, Mitra RS, et al. Cellular localization of interleukin-8 and its inducer, tumor necrosis factor-alpha in psoriasis. Am J Pathol. 1991;138:129–40.
248. Valyi-Nagy I, Jensen PJ, Albelda SM, Rodeck U. Cytokine-induced expression of transforming growth factor-alpha and the epidermal growth factor receptor in neonatal skin explants. J Invest Dermatol. 1992;99:350–6.
249. Schultz GS, White M, Mitchell R, Brown G, Lynch J, Twardzik DR, et al. Epithelial wound healing enhanced by transforming growth factor-alpha and vaccinia growth factor. Science. 1987;235:350–2.
250. Detmar M, Brown LF, Claffey KP, Yeo KT, Kocher O, Jackman RW, et al. Overexpression of vascular permeability factor/vascular endothelial growth factor and its receptors in psoriasis. J Exp Med. 1994;180:1141–6.
251. Sunderkötter C, Nikolic T, Dillon MJ, van Rooijen N, Stehling M, Drevets DA, et al. Subpopulations of mouse blood monocytes differ in maturation stage and inflammatory response. J Immunol. 2004;172:4410–7.
252. Nishiwaki S, Terakura S, Ito M, Goto T, Seto A, Watanabe K, et al. Impact of macrophage infiltration of skin lesions on survival after allogeneic stem cell transplantation: a clue to refractory graft-versus-host disease. Blood. 2009;114:3113–6.
253. Alexander KA, Flynn R, Lineburg KE, Kuns RD, Teal BE, Olver SD, et al. CSF-1-dependant donor-derived macrophages mediate chronic graft-versus-host disease. J Clin Invest. 2014;124:4266–80.
254. Sindrilaru A, Scharffetter-Kochanek K. Disclosure of the culprits: macrophages-versatile regulators of wound healing. Adv Wound Care (New Rochelle). 2013;2:357–68.
255. Brancato SK, Albina JE. Wound macrophages as key regulators of repair: origin, phenotype, and function. Am J Pathol. 2011;178:19–25.
256. Mirza R, DiPietro LA, Koh TJ. Selective and specific macrophage ablation is detrimental to wound healing in mice. Am J Pathol. 2009;175:2454–62.
257. Brem H, Tomic-Canic M. Cellular and molecular basis of wound healing in diabetes. J Clin Invest. 2007;117:1219–22.
258. Leibovich SJ, Ross R. The role of the macrophage in wound repair. A study with hydrocortisone and antimacrophage serum. Am J Pathol. 1975;78:71–100.
259. Goren I, Allmann N, Yogev N, Schürmann C, Linke A, Holdener M, et al. A transgenic mouse model of inducible macrophage depletion: effects of diphtheria toxin-driven lysozyme M-specific cell lineage ablation on wound inflammatory, angiogenic, and contractive processes. Am J Pathol. 2009;175:132–47.
260. Sindrilaru A, Peters T, Wieschalka S, Baican C, Baican A, Peter H, et al. An unrestrained proinflammatory M1 macrophage population induced by iron impairs wound healing in humans and mice. J Clin Invest. 2011;121:985–97.
261. Lucas T, Waisman A, Ranjan R, Roes J, Krieg T, Müller W, et al. Differential roles of macrophages in diverse phases of skin repair. J Immunol. 2010;184:3964–77.
262. Lucas M, Stuart LM, Savill J, Lacy-Hulbert A. Apoptotic cells and innate immune stimuli combine to regulate macrophage cytokine secretion. J Immunol. 2003;171:2610–5.
263. Fadok VA, Bratton DL, Konowal A, Freed PW, Westcott JY, Henson PM. Macrophages that have ingested apoptotic cells in vitro inhibit proinflammatory cytokine production through autocrine/paracrine mechanisms involving TGF-beta, PGE2, and PAF. J Clin Invest. 1998;101:890–8.
264. Anderson DC, Schmalsteig FC, Finegold MJ, Hughes BJ, Rothlein R, Miller LJ, et al. The severe and moderate phenotypes of heritable Mac-1, LFA-1 deficiency: their quantitative definition and relation to leukocyte dysfunction and clinical features. J Infect Dis. 1985;152:668–89.
265. Peters T, Sindrilaru A, Hinz B, Hinrichs R, Menke A, Al-Azzeh EAD, et al. Wound-healing defect of CD18(−/−) mice due to a decrease in TGF-beta1 and myofibroblast differentiation. EMBO J. 2005;24:3400–10.

Endothelial Cells

266. Jaffe EA. Cell biology of endothelial cells. Hum Pathol. 1987;18(3):234–9.
267. Davidson SM. Endothelial mitochondria and heart disease. Cardiovasc Res. 2010;88(1):58–66.
268. Moncada S, Higgs EA. Nitric oxide and the vascular endothelium. Heidelberg: Springer; 2006.
269. Cines DB, Pollak ES, Buck CA, Loscalzo J, Zimmerman GA, McEver RP, Pober JS, Wick TM, Konkle BA, Schwartz BS, et al. Endothelial cells in physiology and in the pathophysiology of vascular disorders. Blood. 1998;91(10):3527–61.
270. Aird WC. Phenotypic heterogeneity of the endothelium: I. Structure, function, and mechanisms. Circ Res. 2007;100:158–73.
271. Bazzoni G, Dejana E. Endothelial cell-to-cell junctions: molecular organization and role in vascular homeostasis. Physiol Rev. 2004;84(3):869–901.
272. Lee WL, Liles WC. Endothelial activation, dysfunction and permeability during severe infections. Curr Opin Hematol. 2011;18(3):191–6.
273. Jackson JR, Seed MP, Kircher CH, et al. The codependence of angiogenesis and chronic inflammation. FASEB J. 1997;11:457–65.
274. Mai J, Virtue A, Shen J, Wang H, Yang XF. An evolving new paradigm: endothelial cells – conditional innate immune cells. J Hematol Oncol. 2013;6:61.
275. Kenneth M. Janeway's immune biology. 8th ed. Garland Science, Taylor & Francis Group, New York, LLC; 2013. p. 47.
276. Opitz B, Eitel J, Meixenberger K, Suttorp N. Role of Toll-like receptors, NOD-like receptors and RIG-I-like receptors in endothelial cells and systemic infections. Thromb Haemost. 2009;102(6):1103–9.
277. Ancuta P, Moses A, Gabuzda D. Transendothelial migration of CD16+ monocytes in response to fractalkine under constitutive and inflammatory conditions. Immunobiology. 2004;209(1–2):11–20.
278. Anand AR, Cucchiarini M, Terwilliger EF, Ganju RK. The tyrosine kinase Pyk2 mediates lipopolysaccharide-induced IL-8 expression in human endothelial cells. J Immunol. 2008;180(8):5636–44.
279. Tsou TC, Liou SH, Yeh SC, Tsai FY, Chao HR. Crucial role of Toll-like receptors in the zinc/nickel-induced inflammatory response in vascular endothelial cells. Toxicol Appl Pharmacol. 2013;273(3):492–9.
280. Geppert T, Lipsky P. Antigen presentation by interferon-gamma-treated endothelial cells and fibroblasts: differential ability to function as antigen-presenting cells despite comparable Ia expression. J Immunol. 1985;135:3750–62.
281. Rothermel AL, Wang Y, Schechner J, Mook-Kanamori B, Aird WC, Pober JS, Tellides G, Johnson DR. Endothelial cells present antigens in vivo. BMC Immunol. 2004;5:5.

282. Leeuwenberg JF, Van Damme J, Meager T, Jeunhomme TM, Buurman WA. Effects of tumor necrosis factor on the interferon-gamma-induced major histocompatibility complex class II antigen expression by human endothelial cells. Eur J Immunol. 1988;18(9):1469–72.
283. Klingenberg R, Autschbach F, Gleissner C, Giese T, Wambsganss N, Sommer N, Richter G, Katus HA, Dengler TJ. Endothelial inducible costimulator ligand expression is increased during human cardiac allograft rejection and regulates endothelial cell-dependent allo-activation of CD8+ T cells in vitro. Eur J Immunol. 2005;35(6):1712–21.
284. Lozanoska-Ochser B, Klein NJ, Huang GC, Alvarez RA, Peakman M. Expression of CD86 on human islet endothelial cells facilitates T cell adhesion and migration. J Immunol. 2008;181(9):6109–16.
285. Hirosue S, Vokali E, Raghavan VR, Rincon-Restrepo M, Lund AW, Corthésy-Henrioud P, Capotosti F, Halin Winter C, Hugues S, Swartz MA. Steady-state antigen scavenging, cross-presentation, and CD8+ T cell priming: a new role for lymphatic endothelial cells. J Immunol. 2014;192(11):5002–11.
286. Krishnaswamy G, Kelley J, Yerra L, Smith JK, Chi DS. Human endothelium as a source of multifunctional cytokines: molecular regulation and possible role in human disease. J Interferon Cytokine Res. 1999;19(2):91–104.
287. Kofler S, Nickel T, Weis M. Role of cytokines in cardiovascular diseases: a focus on endothelial responses to inflammation. Clin Sci (Lond). 2005;108(3):205–13.
288. Chironi GN, Boulanger CM, Simon A, Dignat-George F, Freyssinet JM, Tedgui A. Endothelial microparticles in diseases. Cell Tissue Res. 2009;335(1):143–51.
289. Wheway J, Latham SL, Combes V, Grau GE. Endothelial microparticles interact with and support the proliferation of T cells. J Immunol. 2014;193(7):3378–87.
290. Batycka-Baran A, Paprocka M, Krawczenko A, Duś D, Szepietowski JC. Increased number of circulating endothelial cells (CECs) in patients with psoriasis – preliminary report. J Eur Acad Dermatol Venereol. 2014;28(1):116–9.
291. Ammar M, Bouchlaka-Souissi C, Helms CA, Zaraa I, Jordan CT, Anbunathan H, Bouhaha R, Kouidhi S, Doss N, Dhaoui R, Ben Osman A, Ben Ammar El Gaied A, Marrakchi R, Mokni M, Bowcock AM. Genome-wide linkage scan for psoriasis susceptibility loci in multiplex Tunisian families. Br J Dermatol. 2013;168(3):583–7.
292. Harden JL, Lewis SM, Pierson KC, Suárez-Fariñas M, Lentini T, Ortenzio FS, Zaba LC, Goldbach-Mansky R, Bowcock AM, Lowes MA. CARD14 expression in dermal endothelial cells in psoriasis. PLoS One. 2014;9(11):e111255.
293. Forkel S, Schön M, Hildmann A, Claßen A, John SM, Danker K, Schön MP. Inositoylated platelet-activating factor (Ino-C2-PAF) modulates dynamic lymphocyte-endothelial cell interactions and alleviates psoriasis-like skin inflammation in two complementary mouse models. J Invest Dermatol. 2014;134(10):2510–20.
294. Manam S, Tsakok T, Till S, Flohr C. The association between atopic dermatitis and food allergy in adults. Curr Opin Allergy Clin Immunol. 2014;14(5):423–9.
295. Cheng LE, Sullivan BM, Retana LE, Allen CD, Liang HE, Locksley RM. IgE-activated basophils regulate eosinophil tissue entry by modulating endothelial function. J Exp Med. 2015;212(4):513–24. pii: jem.20141671. [Epub ahead of print].

Mast Cells as Versatile Immune Cells in the Skin

296. Irani AA, Schechter NM, Craig SS, DeBlois G, Schwartz LB. Two types of human mast cells that have distinct neutral protease compositions. Proc Natl Acad Sci U S A. 1986;83(12):4464–8.
297. Harvima IT, Nilsson G. Mast cells as regulators of skin inflammation and immunity. Acta Derm Venereol. 2011;91(6):644–50.
298. Trinchieri G, Sher A. Cooperation of Toll-like receptor signals in innate immune defence. Nat Rev Immunol. 2007;7(3):179–90.
299. Supajatura V, Ushio H, Nakao A, et al. Differential responses of mast cell Toll-like receptors 2 and 4 in allergy and innate immunity. J Clin Invest. 2002;109(10):1351–9.
300. Burke SM, Issekutz TB, Mohan K, Lee PW, Shmulevitz M, Marshall JS. Human mast cell activation with virus-associated stimuli leads to the selective chemotaxis of natural killer cells by a CXCL8-dependent mechanism. Blood. 2008;111(12):5467–76.
301. Matsushima H, Yamada N, Matsue H, Shimada S. TLR3-, TLR7-, and TLR9-mediated production of proinflammatory cytokines and chemokines from murine connective tissue type skin-derived mast cells but not from bone marrow-derived mast cells. J Immunol. 2004;173(1):531–41.
302. Echtenacher B, Mannel DN, Hultner L. Critical protective role of mast cells in a model of acute septic peritonitis. Nature. 1996;381(6577):75–7.
303. Malaviya R, Ikeda T, Ross E, Abraham SN. Mast cell modulation of neutrophil influx and bacterial clearance at sites of infection through TNF-alpha. Nature. 1996;381(6577):77–80.
304. Bryce PJ, Miller ML, Miyajima I, Tsai M, Galli SJ, Oettgen HC. Immune sensitization in the skin is enhanced by antigen-independent effects of IgE. Immunity. 2004;20(4):381–92.
305. Kawakami T, Kitaura J. Mast cell survival and activation by IgE in the absence of antigen: a consideration of the biologic mechanisms and relevance. J Immunol. 2005;175(7):4167–73.
306. Smith KG, Clatworthy MR. FcgammaRIIB in autoimmunity and infection: evolutionary and therapeutic implications. Nat Rev Immunol. 2010;10(5):328–43.
307. Malbec O, Daeron M. The mast cell IgG receptors and their roles in tissue inflammation. Immunol Rev. 2007;217:206–21.
308. Zhao W, Kepley CL, Morel PA, Okumoto LM, Fukuoka Y, Schwartz LB. Fc gamma RIIa, not Fc gamma RIIb, is constitutively and functionally expressed on skin-derived human mast cells. J Immunol. 2006;177(1):694–701.
309. Okayama Y, Kirshenbaum AS, Metcalfe DD. Expression of a functional high-affinity IgG receptor, Fc gamma RI, on human mast cells: Up-regulation by IFN-gamma. J Immunol. 2000;164(8):4332–9.
310. Woolhiser MR, Okayama Y, Gilfillan AM, Metcalfe DD. IgG-dependent activation of human mast cells following up-regulation of FcgammaRI by IFN-gamma. Eur J Immunol. 2001;31(11):3298–307.
311. Marshall JS. Mast-cell responses to pathogens. Nat Rev Immunol. 2004;4(10):787–99.
312. Nilsson G, Johnell M, Hammer CH, et al. C3a and C5a are chemotaxins for human mast cells and act through distinct receptors via a pertussis toxin-sensitive signal transduction pathway. J Immunol. 1996;157(4):1693–8.
313. Prodeus AP, Zhou X, Maurer M, Galli SJ, Carroll MC. Impaired mast cell-dependent natural immunity in complement C3-deficient mice. Nature. 1997;390(6656):172–5.
314. Edelson BT, Stricker TP, Li Z, et al. Novel collectin/C1q receptor mediates mast cell activation and innate immunity. Blood. 2006;107(1):143–50.
315. Abraham SN, St John AL. Mast cell-orchestrated immunity to pathogens. Nat Rev Immunol. 2010;10(6):440–52.
316. Metz M, Piliponsky AM, Chen CC, et al. Mast cells can enhance resistance to snake and honeybee venoms. Science. 2006;313(5786):526–30.
317. Maurer M, Wedemeyer J, Metz M, et al. Mast cells promote homeostasis by limiting endothelin-1-induced toxicity. Nature. 2004;432(7016):512–6.

318. Piliponsky AM, Chen CC, Nishimura T, et al. Neurotensin increases mortality and mast cells reduce neurotensin levels in a mouse model of sepsis. Nat Med. 2008;14(4):392–8.
319. Reber LL, Marichal T, Galli SJ. New models for analyzing mast cell functions in vivo. Trends Immunol. 2012;33(12):613–25.
320. Rodewald HR, Feyerabend TB. Widespread immunological functions of mast cells: fact or fiction? Immunity. 2012;37(1):13–24.
321. Siebenhaar F, Syska W, Weller K, et al. Control of Pseudomonas aeruginosa skin infections in mice is mast cell-dependent. Am J Pathol. 2007;170(6):1910–6.
322. McLachlan JB, Hart JP, Pizzo SV, et al. Mast cell-derived tumor necrosis factor induces hypertrophy of draining lymph nodes during infection. Nat Immunol. 2003;4(12):1199–205.
323. Shelburne CP, Nakano H, St John AL, et al. Mast cells augment adaptive immunity by orchestrating dendritic cell trafficking through infected tissues. Cell Host Microbe. 2009;6(4):331–42.
324. McLachlan JB, Shelburne CP, Hart JP, et al. Mast cell activators: a new class of highly effective vaccine adjuvants. Nat Med. 2008;14(5):536–41.
325. McGowen AL, Hale LP, Shelburne CP, Abraham SN, Staats HF. The mast cell activator compound 48/80 is safe and effective when used as an adjuvant for intradermal immunization with Bacillus anthracis protective antigen. Vaccine. 2009;27(27):3544–52.
326. Aoki R, Kawamura T, Goshima F, et al. Mast cells play a key role in host defense against herpes simplex virus infection through TNF-alpha and IL-6 production. J Invest Dermatol. 2013;133(9):2170–9.
327. Romo-Lozano Y, Hernandez-Hernandez F, Salinas E. Sporothrix schenckii yeasts induce ERK pathway activation and secretion of IL-6 and TNF-alpha in rat mast cells, but no degranulation. Med Mycol. 2014;52(8):862–8.
328. Maurer M, Lopez Kostka S, Siebenhaar F, et al. Skin mast cells control T cell-dependent host defense in Leishmania major infections. FASEB J. 2006;20(14):2460–7.
329. Nakamura Y, Oscherwitz J, Cease KB, et al. Staphylococcus delta-toxin induces allergic skin disease by activating mast cells. Nature. 2013;503(7476):397–401.
330. Bieber T. Atopic dermatitis. N Engl J Med. 2008;358(14):1483–94.
331. Kawakami T, Ando T, Kimura M, Wilson BS, Kawakami Y. Mast cells in atopic dermatitis. Curr Opin Immunol. 2009;21(6):666–78.
332. Steinhoff M, Vergnolle N, Young SH, et al. Agonists of proteinase-activated receptor 2 induce inflammation by a neurogenic mechanism. Nat Med. 2000;6(2):151–8.
333. Yosipovitch G, Greaves MW, Schmelz M. Itch. Lancet. 2003;361(9358):690–4.
334. Steinhoff M, Neisius U, Ikoma A, et al. Proteinase-activated receptor-2 mediates itch: a novel pathway for pruritus in human skin. J Neurosci. 2003;23(15):6176–80.
335. Leighty L, Li N, Diaz LA, Liu Z. Experimental models for the autoimmune and inflammatory blistering disease. Bullous pemphigoid. Arch Dermatol Res. 2007;299(9):417–22.
336. Chen R, Ning G, Zhao ML, et al. Mast cells play a key role in neutrophil recruitment in experimental bullous pemphigoid. J Clin Invest. 2001;108(8):1151–8.
337. Nelson KC, Zhao M, Schroeder PR, et al. Role of different pathways of the complement cascade in experimental bullous pemphigoid. J Clin Invest. 2006;116(11):2892–900.
338. Endoh I, Di Girolamo N, Hampartzoumian T, Cameron B, Geczy CL, Tedla N. Ultraviolet B irradiation selectively increases the production of interleukin-8 in human cord blood-derived mast cells. Clin Exp Immunol. 2007;148(1):161–7.
339. Fairley JA, Burnett CT, Fu CL, Larson DL, Fleming MG, Giudice GJ. A pathogenic role for IgE in autoimmunity: bullous pemphigoid IgE reproduces the early phase of lesion development in human skin grafted to nu/nu mice. J Invest Dermatol. 2007;127(11):2605–11.
340. London VA, Kim GH, Fairley JA, Woodley DT. Successful treatment of bullous pemphigoid with omalizumab. Arch Dermatol. 2012;148(11):1241–3.
341. Fairley JA, Baum CL, Brandt DS, Messingham KA. Pathogenicity of IgE in autoimmunity: successful treatment of bullous pemphigoid with omalizumab. J Allergy Clin Immunol. 2009;123(3):704–5.
342. Suto H, Nakae S, Kakurai M, Sedgwick JD, Tsai M, Galli SJ. Mast cell-associated TNF promotes dendritic cell migration. J Immunol. 2006;176(7):4102–12.
343. Grimbaldeston MA, Nakae S, Kalesnikoff J, Tsai M, Galli SJ. Mast cell-derived interleukin 10 limits skin pathology in contact dermatitis and chronic irradiation with ultraviolet B. Nat Immunol. 2007;8(10):1095–104.
344. Galli SJ, Grimbaldeston M, Tsai M. Immunomodulatory mast cells: negative, as well as positive, regulators of immunity. Nat Rev Immunol. 2008;8(6):478–86.
345. Hart PH, Grimbaldeston MA, Swift GJ, Jaksic A, Noonan FP, Finlay-Jones JJ. Dermal mast cells determine susceptibility to ultraviolet B-induced systemic suppression of contact hypersensitivity responses in mice. J Exp Med. 1998;187(12):2045–53.
346. Alard P, Kurimoto I, Niizeki H, Doherty JM, Streilein JW. Hapten-specific tolerance induced by acute, low-dose ultraviolet B radiation of skin requires mast cell degranulation. Eur J Immunol. 2001;31(6):1736–46.
347. Ullrich SE, Nghiem DX, Khaskina P. Suppression of an established immune response by UVA – a critical role for mast cells. Photochem Photobiol. 2007;83(5):1095–100.
348. Ullrich SE, Byrne SN. The immunologic revolution: photoimmunology. J Invest Dermatol. 2012;132(3 Pt 2):896–905.
349. Byrne SN, Limon-Flores AY, Ullrich SE. Mast cell migration from the skin to the draining lymph nodes upon ultraviolet irradiation represents a key step in the induction of immune suppression. J Immunol. 2008;180(7):4648–55.
350. Chacon-Salinas R, Limon-Flores AY, Chavez-Blanco AD, Gonzalez-Estrada A, Ullrich SE. Mast cell-derived IL-10 suppresses germinal center formation by affecting T follicular helper cell function. J Immunol. 2011;186(1):25–31.
351. Ch'ng S, Wallis RA, Yuan L, Davis PF, Tan ST. Mast cells and cutaneous malignancies. Mod Pathol. 2006;19(1):149–59.

Granulocytes

352. Kondo M, et al. Biology of hematopoietic stem cells and progenitors: implications for clinical application. Annu Rev Immunol. 2003;21:759–806.
353. Akashi K, Traver D, Miyamoto T, Weissman IL. A clonogenic common myeloid progenitor that gives rise to all myeloid lineages. Nature. 2000;404(6774):193–7.
354. Tam VC, Aderem A. Macrophage activation as an effector mechanism for cell-mediated immunity. J Immunol. 2014;193(7):3183–4.
355. Krishna S, Miller LS. Innate and adaptive immune responses against Staphylococcus aureus skin infections. Semin Immunopathol. 2012;34(2):261–80.
356. Wang J, Arase H. Regulation of immune responses by neutrophils. Ann N Y Acad Sci. 2014;1319:66–81.
357. Pruchniak MP, Arazna M, Demkow U. Life of neutrophil: from stem cell to neutrophil extracellular trap. Respir Physiol Neurobiol. 2013;187(1):68–73.
358. Verdrengh M, Tarkowski A. Role of neutrophils in experimental septicemia and septic arthritis induced by Staphylococcus aureus. Infect Immun. 1997;65(7):2517–21.
359. Mölne L, Verdrengh M, Tarkowski A. Role of neutrophil leukocytes in cutaneous infection caused by Staphylococcus aureus. Infect Immun. 2000;68(11):6162–7.

360. Denny MF, Yalavarthi S, Zhao W, Thacker SG, Anderson M, Sandy AR, McCune WJ, Kaplan MJ. A distinct subset of proinflammatory neutrophils isolated from patients with systemic lupus erythematosus induces vascular damage and synthesizes type I IFNs. J Immunol. 2010;184(6):3284–97.
361. Coit P, Yalavarthi S, Ognenovski M, Zhao W, Hasni S, Wren JD, Kaplan MJ, Sawalha AH. Epigenome profiling reveals significant DNA demethylation of interferon signature genes in lupus neutrophils. J Autoimmun. 2015;58:59–66. pii: S0896-8411(15)00005-0.
362. Kim MH, Granick JL, Kwok C, Walker NJ, Borjesson DL, Curry FR, Miller LS, Simon SI. Neutrophil survival and c-kit(+)-progenitor proliferation in Staphylococcus aureus-infected skin wounds promote resolution. Blood. 2011;117(12):3343–52.
363. Canesso MC, Vieira AT, Castro TB, Schirmer BG, Cisalpino D, Martins FS, Rachid MA, Nicoli JR, Teixeira MM, Barcelos LS. Skin wound healing is accelerated and scarless in the absence of commensal microbiota. J Immunol. 2014;193(10):5171–80.
364. Kruger P, Saffarzadeh M, Weber AN, Rieber N, Radsak M, von Bernuth H, Benarafa C, Roos D, Skokowa J, Hartl D. Neutrophils: between host defence, immune modulation, and tissue injury. PLoS Pathog. 2015;11(3):e1004651.
365. Tauzin S, Starnes TW, Becker FB, Lam PY, Huttenlocher A. Redox and Src family kinase signaling control leukocyte wound attraction and neutrophil reverse migration. J Cell Biol. 2014;207(5):589–98.
366. William EP. Fundamental immunology. 7th ed. Philadelphia: Wolters Kluwer health/Lippincott Williams & Wilkins; 2013.
367. Karasuyama H, Mukai K, Obata K, Tsujimura Y, Wada T. Nonredundant roles of basophils in immunity. Annu Rev Immunol. 2011;29:45–69.
368. Chirumbolo S. State-of-the-art review about basophil research in immunology and allergy: is the time right to treat these cells with the respect they deserve? Blood Transfus. 2012;10:148–64.
369. Rodríguez-Espinosa O, Rojas-Espinosa O, Moreno-Altamirano MM, López-Villegas EO, Sánchez-García FJ. Metabolic requirements for neutrophil extracellular traps (nets) formation. Immunology. 2014. doi:10.1111/imm.12437. [Epub ahead of print].
370. Dema B, Suzuki R, Rivera J. Rethinking the role of immunoglobulin E and its high-affinity receptor: new insights into allergy and beyond. Int Arch Allergy Immunol. 2014;164:271–9.
371. Kim BS, Wang K, Siracusa MC, Saenz SA, Brestoff JR, Monticelli LA, Noti M, Tait Wojno ED, Fung TC, Kubo M, Artis D. Basophils promote innate lymphoid cell responses in inflamed skin. J Immunol. 2014;193(7):3717–25.
372. Rosenberg HF, Dyer KD, Foster PS. Eosinophils: changing perspectives in health and disease. Nat Rev Immunol. 2013;13:9–22.
373. Jung Y, Rothenberg ME. Roles and regulation of gastrointestinal eosinophils in immunity and disease. J Immunol. 2014;193:999–1005.
374. Padigel UM, Lee JJ, Nolan TJ, Schad GA, Abraham D. Eosinophils can function as antigen-presenting cells to induce primary and secondary immune responses to Strongyloides stercoralis. Infect Immun. 2006;74(6):3232–8.
375. Davoine F, Lacy P. Eosinophil cytokines, chemokines, and growth factors: emerging roles in immunity. Front Immunol. 2014;5:570.
376. Esnault S, Kelly EA, Nettenstrom LM, Cook EB, Seroogy CM, Jarjour NN. Human eosinophils release IL-1ß and increase expression of IL-17A in activated CD4+ T lymphocytes. Clin Exp Allergy. 2012;42(12):1756–64.
377. Walsh ER, Thakar J, Stokes K, Huang F, Albert R, August A. Computational and experimental analysis reveals a requirement for eosinophil-derived IL-13 for the development of allergic airway responses in C57BL/6 mice. J Immunol. 2011;186(5):2936–49.
378. Phipps S, Ying S, Wangoo A, Ong YE, Levi-Schaffer F, Kay AB. The relationship between allergen-induced tissue eosinophilia and markers of repair and remodeling in human atopic skin. J Immunol. 2002;169(8):4604–12.
379. Nakashima C, Otsuka A, Kitoh A, Honda T, Egawa G, Nakajima S, Nakamizo S, Arita M, Kubo M, Miyachi Y. Basophils regulate the recruitment of eosinophils in a murine model of irritant contact dermatitis. J Allergy Clin Immunol. 2014;134(1):100–7.

T Cells in the Skin

380. Nomura T, et al. The panoply of αβT cells in the skin. J Dermatol Sci. 2014;76(1):3–9.
381. Mueller SN, et al. Memory T cell subsets, migration patterns, and tissue residence. Annu Rev Immunol. 2013;31:137–61.
382. Clark RA, et al. Skin effector memory T cells do not recirculate and provide immune protection in alemtuzumab-treated CTCL patients. Sci Transl Med. 2012;4(117):117ra7.
383. Honda T, et al. Update of immune events in the murine contact hypersensitivity model: toward the understanding of allergic contact dermatitis. J Invest Dermatol. 2013;133(2):303–15.
384. Lazarevic V, Glimcher LH. T-bet in disease. Nat Immunol. 2011;12(7):597–606.
385. Kim BS, et al. Innate lymphoid cells and allergic inflammation. Curr Opin Immunol. 2013;25(6):738–44.
386. Vercelli D. Immunoglobulin E and its regulators. Curr Opin Allergy Clin Immunol. 2001;1(1):61–5.
387. Kabashima K. New concept of the pathogenesis of atopic dermatitis: interplay among the barrier, allergy, and pruritus as a trinity. J Dermatol Sci. 2013;70(1):3–11.
388. Whitaker EL, et al. Interleukin 24: mechanisms and therapeutic potential of an anti-cancer gene. Cytokine Growth Factor Rev. 2012;23(6):323–31.
389. Kurebayashi Y, et al. Recent advances in understanding the molecular mechanisms of the development and function of Th17 cells. Genes Cells Devoted Mol Cell Mech. 2013;18(4):247–65.
390. Fujita H. The role of IL-22 and Th22 cells in human skin diseases. J Dermatol Sci. 2013;72(1):3–8.
391. Veldhoen M, et al. The aryl hydrocarbon receptor links TH17-cell-mediated autoimmunity to environmental toxins. Nature. 2008;453(7191):106–9.
392. Schmitt E, et al. Th9 cells, new players in adaptive immunity. Trends Immunol. 2014;35(2):61–8.
393. Schlapbach C, et al. Human TH9 cells are skin-tropic and have autocrine and paracrine proinflammatory capacity. Sci Transl Med. 2014;6(219):219ra218.
394. Abbas AK, et al. Regulatory T cells: recommendations to simplify the nomenclature. Nat Immunol. 2013;14(4):307–8.
395. Sather BD, et al. Altering the distribution of Foxp3(+) regulatory T cells results in tissuespecific inflammatory disease. J Exp Med. 2007;204(6):1335–47.
396. Sanchez Rodriguez R, et al. Memory regulatory T cells reside in human skin. J Clin Invest. 2014;124(3):1027–36.
397. Tomura M, et al. Activated regulatory T cells are the major T cell type emigrating from the skin during a cutaneous immune response in mice. J Clin Invest. 2010;120(3):883–93.
398. Honda T, et al. Regulatory T cells in cutaneous immune responses. J Dermatol Sci. 2011;63(2):75–82.
399. Sakaguchi S, et al. Regulatory T cells and immune tolerance. Cell. 2008;133(5):775–87.
400. Halabi-Tawil M, et al. Cutaneous manifestations of immune dysregulation, polyendocrinopathy, enteropathy, X-linked (IPEX) syndrome. Br J Dermatol. 2009;160(3):645–51.
401. Weiner HL. The mucosal milieu creates tolerogenic dendritic cells and T(R)1 and T(H)3 regulatory cells. Nat Immunol. 2001;2(8):671–2.

402. Gagliani N, et al. Coexpression of CD49b and LAG-3 identifies human and mouse T regulatory type 1 cells. Nat Med. 2013;19(6):739–46.
403. Heath WR, Carbone FR. The skin-resident and migratory immune system in steady state and memory: innate lymphocytes, dendritic cells and T cells. Nat Immunol. 2013;14(10):978–85.
404. Mackay LK, et al. The developmental pathway for CD103(+) CD8(+) tissue-resident memory T cells of skin. Nat Immunol. 2013;14(12):1294–301.
405. Shiohara T. Fixed drug eruption: pathogenesis and diagnostic tests. Curr Opin Allergy Clin Immunol. 2009;9(5):316–21.
406. Latha TS, et al. Gammadelta T cell-mediated immune responses in disease and therapy. Front Immunol. 2014;5:571.
407. Born WK, et al. Diversity of gammadelta T-cell antigens. Cell Mol Immunol. 2013;10(1):13–20.
408. Peters C, et al. Phenotype and regulation of immunosuppressive Vdelta 2-expressing gammadelta T cells. Cell Mol Life Sci. 2014;71(10):1943–60.
409. Chien YH, et al. Gammadelta T cells: first line of defense and beyond. Annu Rev Immunol. 2014;32:121–55.
410. Su D, et al. Roles of gammadelta T cells in the pathogenesis of autoimmune diseases. Clin Dev Immunol. 2013;2013:985753.

Cutaneous Microecology

411. Xiong DX: Modern microecology. Chinese science and technology, Beijing (2000).
412. Zhang X: Dermatology and venereology (8th Version). People's Health Publication, Beijing (2012).
413. You B, Chen X, Wang L. Application of cutaneous probiotic cream in facial cosmetology. 2000; Chin J Microecol,12: 45–46.
414. Grice EA, Segre JA. The skin microbiome. 2011; Nat Rev Microbiol. 9:244–253.
415. Schloss PD. Microbiology: An integrated view of the skin microbiome. Nature. 2014;514(7520):44–5.
416. Schommer NN, Gallo RL. Structure and function of the human skin microbiome. Trends Microbiol. 2013;21(12):660–8.
417. Gallo RL. S. epidermidis influence on host immunity: More than skin deep. Cell Host Microbe. 2015;17(2):143–4.
418. Zhang LJ, Guerrero-Juarez CF, Hata T, Bapat SP, Ramos R, Plikus MV, Gallo RL. Innate immunity. Dermal adipocytes protect against invasive Staphylococcus aureus skin infection. Science. 2015;347(6217):67–71.
419. Jahns AC, Lundskog B, Ganceviciene R, Palmer RH, Golovleva I, Zouboulis CC, McDowell A, Patrick S, Alexeyev OA. An increased incidence of Propionibacterium acnes biofilms in acne vulgaris: a case-control study. Br J Dermatol. 2012;167(1):50–8.
420. Kistowska M, Meier B, Proust T, Feldmeyer L, Cozzio A, Kuendig T, Contassot E, French LE. Propionibacterium acnes promotes Th17 and Th17/Th1 responses in acne patients. J Invest Dermatol. 2015;135(1):110–8.
421. Koziel J, Potempa J. Protease-armed bacteria in the skin. Cell Tissue Res. 2013;351(2):325–37.
422. Cogen AL, Nizet V, Gallo RL. (2008) Skin microbiota: a source of disease or defence? Br J Dermatol. 2008; 158: 442–455.
423. Soares RC, Zani MB, Arruda AC, Arruda LH, Paulino LC. Malassezia intra-specific diversity and potentially new species in the skin microbiota from Brazilian healthy subjects and seborrheic dermatitis patients. PLoS One. 2015;10(2):e0117921.
424. Probst AJ, Auerbach AK, Moissl-Eichinger C. Archaea on human skin. PLoS One. 2013;8(6):e65388.
425. Gorantla JN, Kumar SN, Nisha GV, Sumandu AS, Dileep C, Sudaresan A, Kumar MM, Lankalapalli RS, Kumar BS. Purification and characterization of antifungal phenazines from a fluorescent Pseudomonas strain FPO4 against medically important fungi. J Mycol Med. 2014;24(3):185–92.
426. Treat J, James WD, Nachamkin I, Seykora JT. Growth inhibition of Trichophyton species by Pseudomonas aeruginosa. Arch Dermatol. 2007;143(1):61–4.
427. Kaur A, Thatai P, Sapra B. Need of UV protection and evaluation of efficacy of sunscreens. J Cosmet Sci. 2014;65(5):315–45.
428. Sanchez DA, Nosanchuk JD, Friedman AJ. The skin microbiome: is there a role in the pathogenesis of atopic dermatitis and psoriasis. J Drugs Dermatol. 2015;14(2):127–30.
429. Zeeuwen PL, Kleerebezem M, Timmerman HM, Schalkwijk J. Microbiome and skin diseases. Curr Opin Allergy Clin Immunol. 2013;13(5):514–20.
430. Belkaid Y, Segre JA. Dialogue between skin microbiota and immunity. Science. 2014;346(6212):954–9.
431. Mathieu A, Vogel TM, Simonet P. The future of skin metagenomics. Res Microbiol. 2014;165(2):69–76.
432. Nagao K, Udey MC. Mushrooming insights into skin dendritic cell physiology. Immunity. 2015;42(2):210–3.

Co-regulation of Epidermal Permeability Barrier and Cutaneous Immunity

433. Elias PM. Stratum corneum defensive functions: an integrated view. J Invest Dermatol. 2005;125:183–200.
434. Kalinin AE, Kajava AV, Steinert PM. Epithelial barrier function: assembly and structural features of the cornified cell envelope. Bioessays. 2002;24:789–800.
435. Feingold KR. Thematic review series: skin lipids. The role of epidermal lipids in cutaneous permeability barrier homeostasis. J Lipid Res. 2007;48:2531–46.
436. Feingold KR, Man MQ, Menon GK, Cho SS, Brown BE, Elias PM. Cholesterol synthesis is required for cutaneous barrier function in mice. J Clin Invest. 1990;86:1738–45.
437. Holleran W, Feingold KR, Man MQ, Gao WN, Lee JM, Elias PM. Regulation of epidermal sphingolipid synthesis by permeability barrier function. J Lipid Res. 1991;32:1151–8.
438. Mao-Qiang M, Elias PM, Feingold KR. Fatty acids are required for permeability barrier homeostasis. J Clin Invest. 1993;92:791–8.
439. Feingold KR. The outer frontier: the importance of lipid metabolism in the skin. J Lipid Res. 2009;50:S417–22.
440. Akiyama M, Sugiyama-Nakagiri Y, Sakai K, McMillan JR, Goto M, et al. Mutations in lipid transporter ABCA12 in harlequin ichthyosis and functional recovery by corrective gene transfer. J Clin Invest. 2005;115:1777–84.
441. Mitsutake S, Suzuki C, Akiyama M, Tsuji K, Yanagi T, Shimizu H, et al. ABCA12 dysfunction causes a disorder in glucosylceramide accumulation during keratinocyte differentiation. J Dermatol Sci. 2010;60:128–9.
442. Sakai K, Akiyama M, Sugiyama-Nakagiri Y, McMillan JR, Sawamura D, Shimizu H. Localization of ABCA12 from Golgi apparatus to lamellar granules in human upper epidermal keratinocytes. Exp Dermatol. 2007;16:920–6.
443. Mao-Qiang M, Brown BE, Wu-Pong S, Feingold KR, Elias PM. Exogenous nonphysiologic vs physiologic lipids. Divergent mechanisms for correction of permeability barrier dysfunction. Arch Dermatol. 1995;131:809–16.
444. Mao-Qiang M, Feingold KR, Jain M, Elias PM. Extracelluar processing of phospholipids is required for barrier homeostasis. J Lipid Res. 1995;36:1925–35.
445. Mao-Qiang M, Jain M, Feingold KR, Elias PM. Secretory phospholipase A2 activity is required for barrier homeostasis. J Invest Dermatol. 1996;106:57–63.

446. Holleran WM, Takagi Y, Menon GK, Legler G, Feingold KR, Elias PM. Processing of epidermal glucosylceramides is required for optimal mammalian cutaneous permeability barrier function. J Clin Invest. 1993;91:1656–64.
447. Uchida Y, Hara M, Nishio H, Sidransky E, Inoue S, Otsuka F, et al. Epidermal sphingomyelins are precursors for selected stratum corneum ceramides. J Lipid Res. 2000;41:2071–82.
448. Wolf R, Orion E, Ruocco E, Ruocco V. Abnormal epidermal barrier in the pathogenesis of psoriasis. Clin Dermatol. 2012;30:323–8.
449. Wolf R, Wolf D. Abnormal epidermal barrier in the pathogenesis of atopic dermatitis. Clin Dermatol. 2012;30:329–34.
450. Ye L, Lv C, Man G, Song S, Elias PM, Man MQ. Abnormal epidermal barrier recovery in uninvolved skin supports the notion of an epidermal pathogenesis of psoriasis. J Invest Dermatol. 2014. doi:10.1038/jid.2014.205.
451. Elias PM, Williams ML, Feingold KR. Abnormal barrier function in the pathogenesis of ichthyosis: therapeutic implications for lipid metabolic disorders. Clin Dermatol. 2012;30:311–22.
452. Elias PM, Crumrine D, Paller A, Rodriguez-Martin M, Williams ML. Pathogenesis of the cutaneous phenotype in inherited disorders of cholesterol metabolism: therapeutic implications for topical treatment of these disorders. Dermatoendocrinol. 2011;3:100–6.
453. Jiang YJ, Lu B, Crumrine D, Man MQ, Elias PM, Feingold KR. IL-1alpha accelerates stratum corneum formation and improves permeability barrier homeostasis during murine fetal development. J Dermatol Sci. 2009;54:88–98.
454. Jiang YJ, Lu B, Crumrine D, Elias PM, Feingold KR. IL-6 stimulates but is not essential for stratum corneum formation and permeability barrier development during gestation. Exp Dermatol. 2010;19:e31–6.
455. Choi EH, Man MQ, Xu P, Xin S, Liu Z, Crumrine DA, et al. Stratum corneum acidification is impaired in moderately aged human and murine skin. J Invest Dermatol. 2007;127:2847–56.
456. Ghadially R, Brown BE, Sequeira-Martin SM, Feingold KR, Elias PM. The aged epidermal permeability barrier. Structural, functional, and lipid biochemical abnormalities in humans and a senescent murine model. J Clin Invest. 1995;95:2281–90.
457. Barland CO, Zettersten E, Brown BS, Ye J, Elias PM, Ghadially R. Imiquimod-induced interleukin-1 alpha stimulation improves barrier homeostasis in aged murine epidermis. J Invest Dermatol. 2004;122:330–6.
458. Jung YJ, Jung M, Kim M, Hong SP, Choi EH. IL-1α stimulation restores epidermal permeability and antimicrobial barriers compromised by topical tacrolimus. J Invest Dermatol. 2011;131:698–705.
459. Tsai JC, Feingold KR, Crumrine D, Wood LC, Grunfeld C, Elias PM. Permeability barrier disruption alters the localization and expression of TNF alpha/protein in the epidermis. Arch Dermatol Res. 1994;286:242–8.
460. Wood LC, Jackson SM, Elias PM, Grunfeld C, Feingold KR. Cutaneous barrier perturbation stimulates cytokine production in the epidermis of mice. J Clin Invest. 1992;90:482–7.
461. Wood LC, Stalder AK, Liou A, Campbell IL, Grunfeld C, Elias PM, et al. Barrier disruption increases gene expression of cytokines and the 55 kD TNF receptor in murine skin. Exp Dermatol. 1997;6:98–104.
462. Wood LC, Elias PM, Sequeira-Martin SM, Grunfeld C, Feingold KR. Occlusion lowers cytokine mRNA levels in essential fatty acid-deficient and normal mouse epidermis, but not after acute barrier disruption. J Invest Dermatol. 1994;103:834–8.
463. Wood LC, Elias PM, Calhoun C, Tsai JC, Grunfeld C, Feingold KR. Barrier disruption stimulates interleukin-1 alpha expression and release from a pre-formed pool in murine epidermis. J Invest Dermatol. 1996;106:397–403.
464. Wood LC, Feingold KR, Sequeira-Martin SM, Elias PM, Grunfeld C. Barrier function coordinately regulates epidermal IL-1 and IL-1 receptor antagonist mRNA levels. Exp Dermatol. 1994;3:56–60.
465. Takeda K, Kaisho T, Akira S. Toll-like receptors. Annu Rev Immunol. 2003;21:335–76.
466. Poltorak A, He X, Smirnova I, Liu MY, Van Huffel C, Du X, et al. Defective LPS signaling in C3H/HeJ and C57BL/10ScCr mice: mutations in Tlr4 gene. Science. 1998;282:2085–8.
467. Hoshino K, Takeuchi O, Kawai T, Sanjo H, Ogawa T, Takeda Y, et al. Cutting edge: Toll-like receptor 4 (TLR4)-deficient mice are hyporesponsive to lipopolysaccharide: evidence for TLR4 as the Lps gene product. J Immunol. 1999;162:3749–52.
468. Gao B, Tsan MF. Endotoxin contamination in recombinant human heat shock protein 70 (Hsp70) preparation is responsible for the induction of tumor necrosis factor alpha release by murine macrophages. J Biol Chem. 2003;278:174–9.
469. Jurk M, Heil F, Vollmer J, Schetter C, Krieg AM, Wagner H, et al. Human TLR7 or TLR8 independently confer responsiveness to the antiviral compound R-848. Nat Immunol. 2002;3:499.
470. Jurk M, Kritzler A, Schulte B, Tluk S, Schetter C, Krieg AM, et al. Modulating responsiveness of human TLR7 and 8 to small molecule ligands with T-rich phosphorothiate oligodeoxynucleotides. Eur J Immunol. 2006;36:1815–26.
471. Heil F, Hemmi H, Hochrein H, Ampenberger F, Kirschning C, Akira S, et al. Species-specific recognition of single-stranded RNA via toll-like receptor 7 and 8. Science. 2007;303:1526–9.
472. Kawai K, Shimura H, Minagawa M, Ito A, Tomiyama K, Ito M. Expression of functional Toll-like receptor 2 on human epidermal keratinocytes. J Dermatol Sci. 2002;30:185–94.
473. Mempel M, Voelcker V, Köllisch G, Plank C, Rad R, Gerhard M, et al. Toll-like receptor expression in human keratinocytes: nuclear factor kappaB controlled gene activation by Staphylococcus aureus is toll-like receptor 2 but not toll-like receptor 4 or platelet activating factor receptor dependent. J Invest Dermatol. 2003;121:1389–96.
474. Song PI, Park YM, Abraham T, Harten B, Zivony A, Neparidze N, et al. Human keratinocytes express functional CD14 and toll-like receptor 4. J Invest Dermatol. 2002;119:424–32.
475. Pivarcsi A, Bodai L, Réthi B, Kenderessy-Szabó A, Koreck A, Széll M, et al. Expression and function of Toll-like receptors 2 and 4 in human keratinocytes. Int Immunol. 2003;15:721–30.
476. Baker BS, Ovigne JM, Powles AV, Corcoran S, Fry L. Normal keratinocytes express Toll-like receptors (TLRs) 1, 2 and 5: modulation of TLR expression in chronic plaque psoriasis. Br J Dermatol. 2003;148:670–9.
477. Miller LS, Sørensen OE, Liu PT, Jalian HR, Eshtiaghpour D, Behmanesh BE, et al. TGF-alpha regulates TLR expression and function on epidermal keratinocytes. J Immunol. 2005;174:6137–43.
478. Köllisch G, Kalali BN, Voelcker V, Wallich R, Behrendt H, Ring J, et al. Various members of the Toll-like receptor family contribute to the innate immune response of human epidermal keratinocytes. Immunology. 2005;114:531–41.
479. Lv CZ, Man M, Zhang XJ, Feingold KR, Elias PM, Man MQ. Cutaneous expression of Toll-like receptor 2 and 4 in various dermatitis models. Chin J Dermatovenereol. 2009;23:390–2.
480. Kuo IH, Carpenter-Mendini A, Yoshida T, McGirt LY, Ivanov AI, Barnes KC, et al. Activation of epidermal toll-like receptor 2 enhances tight junction function: implications for atopic dermatitis and skin barrier repair. J Invest Dermatol. 2013;133:988–98.
481. Furuse M, Hata M, Furuse K, Yoshida Y, Haratake A, Sugitani Y, et al. Claudin-based tight junctions are crucial for the mammalian epidermal barrier: a lesson from claudin-1-deficient mice. J Cell Biol. 2002;156:1099–111.
482. Sugawara T, Iwamoto N, Akashi M, Kojima T, Hisatsune J, Sugai M, et al. Tight junction dysfunction in the stratum granulosum leads to aberrant stratum corneum barrier function in claudin-1-deficient mice. J Dermatol Sci. 2013;70:12–8.
483. Kirschner N, Rosenthal R, Furuse M, Moll I, Fromm M, Brandner JM. Contribution of tight junction proteins to ion, macromol-

ecule, and water barrier in keratinocytes. J Invest Dermatol. 2013;133:1161–9.

484. Yuki T, Yoshida H, Akazawa Y, Komiya A, Sugiyama Y, Inoue S. Activation of TLR2 enhances tight junction barrier in epidermal keratinocytes. J Immunol. 2011;187:3230–7.
485. Borkowski AW, Park K, Uchida Y, Gallo RL. Activation of TLR3 in keratinocytes increases expression of genes involved in formation of the epidermis, lipid accumulation, and epidermal organelles. J Invest Dermatol. 2013;133:2031–40.
486. Borkowski AW, Kuo IH, Bernard JJ, Yoshida T, Williams MR, Hung NJ, et al. Toll-like receptor 3 activation is required for normal skin barrier repair following UV damage. J Invest Dermatol. 2014. doi:10.1038/jid.2014.354.
487. Akazawa Y, Yuki T, Yoshida H, Sugiyama Y, Inoue S. Activation of TRPV4 strengthens the tight-junction barrier in human epidermal keratinocytes. Skin Pharmacol Physiol. 2013;26:15–21.
488. Aberg KM, Man MQ, Gallo RL, Ganz T, Crumrine D, Brown BE, et al. Co-regulation and interdependence of the mammalian epidermal permeability and antimicrobial barriers. J Invest Dermatol. 2008;128:917–25.
489. Ahrens K, Schunck M, Podda GF, Meingassner J, Stuetz A, Schröder JM, et al. Mechanical and metabolic injury to the skin barrier leads to increased expression of murine β-defensin-1, −3, and −14. J Invest Dermatol. 2011;131:443–52.
490. Rodriguez-Martin M, Martin-Ezquerra G, Man MQ, Hupe M, Youm JK, Mackenzie DS, et al. Expression of epidermal CAMP changes in parallel with permeability barrier status. J Invest Dermatol. 2011;131:2263–70.
491. Hong SP, Kim MJ, Jung MY, Jeon H, Goo J, Ahn SK, et al. Biopositive effects of low-dose UVB on epidermis: coordinate up-regulation of antimicrobial peptides and permeability barrier reinforcement. J Invest Dermatol. 2008;128:2880–7.
492. Hou M, Sun R, Hupe M, Kim PL, Park K, Crumrine D, et al. Topical apigenin improves epidermal permeability barrier homoeostasis in normal murine skin by divergent mechanisms. Exp Dermatol. 2013;22:210–5.
493. Hou M, Man M, Man W, Zhu W, Hupe M, Park K, et al. Topical hesperidin improves epidermal permeability barrier function and epidermal differentiation in normal murine skin. Exp Dermatol. 2012;21:337–40.
494. Man M, Hupe M, Mackenzie D, Kim H, Oda Y, Crumrine D, et al. A topical Chinese herbal mixture improves epidermal permeability barrier function in normal murine skin. Exp Dermatol. 2011;20:285–8.
495. Wanke I, Skabytska Y, Kraft B, Peschel A, Biedermann T, Schittek B. Staphylococcus aureus skin colonization is promoted by barrier disruption and leads to local inflammation. Exp Dermatol. 2013;22:153–5.
496. Ray TL, Wuepper KD. Experimental cutaneous candidiasis in rodents; II. Role of the stratum corneum barrier and serum complement as a mediator of a protective inflammatory response. Arch Dermatol. 1978;114:539–43.
497. Darmstadt GL, Saha SK, Ahmed AS, Chowdhury MA, Law PA, Ahmed S, et al. Effect of topical treatment with skin barrier-enhancing emollients on nosocomial infections in preterm infants in Bangladesh: a randomised controlled trial. Lancet. 2005;365:1039–45.
498. Abraham SN, St John AL. Mast cell-orchestrated immunity to pathogens. Nat Rev Immunol. 2010;10:440–52.
499. Malaviya R, Ross EA, MacGregor JI, Ikeda T, Little JR, Jakschik BA, et al. Mast cell phagocytosis of FimH-expressing enterobacteria. J Immunol. 1994;152:1907–14.
500. Di Nardo A, Vitiello A, Gallo RL. Cutting edge: mast cell antimicrobial activity is mediated by expression of cathelicidin antimicrobial peptide. J Immunol. 2003;170:2274–8.
501. von Köckritz-Blickwede M, Goldmann O, Thulin P, Heinemann K, Norrby-Teglund A, Rohde M, et al. Phagocytosis-independent antimicrobial activity of mast cells by means of extracellular trap formation. Blood. 2008;111:3070–80.
502. Mazzoni A, Young HA, Spitzer JH, Visintin A, Segal DM. Histamine regulates cytokine production in maturing dendritic cells, resulting in altered T cell polarization. J Clin Invest. 2001;108:1865–73.
503. Dudeck A, Suender CA, Kostka SL, von Stebut E, Maurer M. Mast cells promote Th1 and Th17 responses by modulating dendritic cell maturation and function. Eur J Immunol. 2011;41:1883–93.
504. Lin TK, Man MQ, Santiago JL, Park K, Roelandt T, Oda Y, et al. Topical antihistamines display potent anti-inflammatory activity linked in part to enhanced permeability barrier function. J Invest Dermatol. 2013;133:469–78.
505. Merad M, Ginhoux F, Collin M. Origin, homeostasis and function of Langerhans cells and other langerin-expressing dendritic cells. Nat Rev Immunol. 2008;8:935–47.
506. Proksch E, Brasch J, Sterry W. Integrity of the permeability barrier regulates epidermal Langerhans cell density. Br J Dermatol. 1996;134:630–8.
507. Proksch E, Brasch J. Influence of epidermal permeability barrier disruption and Langerhans' cell density on allergic contact dermatitis. Acta Derm Venereol. 1997;77:102–4.
508. Katoh N, Hirano S, Kishimoto S, Yasuno H. Acute cutaneous barrier perturbation induces maturation of Langerhans' cells in hairless mice. Acta Derm Venereol. 1997;77:365–9.
509. Nishijima T, Tokura Y, Imokawa G, Seo N, Furukawa F, Takigawa M. Altered permeability and disordered cutaneous immunoregulatory function in mice with acute barrier disruption. J Invest Dermatol. 1997;109:175–82.

Humoral Factors in the Skin

7

Umberto Cornelli, Changlong Lu, Xun Sun, Jinyan Wang, Roberto Perricone, Eleonora Ballanti, and Yun-Feng Gao

Contents

U. Cornelli (✉)
Loyola University School of Medicine-Chicago, Chicago, IL, USA
e-mail: umbertocornelli@cornelliconsulting.it

C. Lu, MD, PhD (✉) • X. Sun, MD, PhD • J. Wang
Department of Immunology, China Medical University, Shenyang, China
e-mail: changlonglyu@hotmail.com

R. Perricone (✉) • E. Ballanti
Rheumatology, Allergology and Clinical Immunology; Department of Internal Medicine, University of Rome Tor Vergata, Rome, Italy
e-mail: eleonora.ballanti@gmail.com

Y.-F. Gao
Department of Immunology of China Medical University, Shenyang, China

7.1 Oxidation and Antioxidants

Umberto Cornelli

7.1.1 Introduction

In aerobic organisms, the use of oxygen (O_2) is vital for the cellular functions that undergo a continuous alternation of oxidation and reduction processes. Oxidation consists of the removal of one or more electrons (e^-) from a given molecule, and this process can also occur without the presence of O_2. Since hydrogen (*H*) is formed by $1e^- + H^+$, by definition, the removal of one H corresponds to an oxidation, while the addition of one H corresponds to a reduction. The processes of reduction and oxidation are usually combined, one e^-(or a hydrogen atom H) passing from a donor (*oxidized element*) to an acceptor (*reduced element*), and the donor/acceptor couple is defined as a "*redox couple*".

In the context of the four fundamental elements that constitute living matter, O_2 (even 1/2 O), carbon (C), nitrogen (N), hydrogen (H), or metals, such as iron (Fe), zinc (Zn), and copper (Cu), the oxidation process is substantially reversible, since all these constituents can return to the original condition, regaining the e^- lost in the reduction process. This characteristic allows them to be used to transfer an e^- from one element to another in a process defined as "*redox exchange*".

For more complex molecules, such as amino acids, lipids, carbohydrates, or other compounds derived from their combination (i.e., proteins, lipids, DNA), the oxidation process

X.-H. Gao, H.-D. Chen (eds.), *Practical Immunodermatology*, DOI 10.1007/978-94-024-0902-4_7

Table 7.1 Some of the most common reactive species (RS) divided based on the representative element

Radical nature	Formula	Nonradical nature	Formula
Reactive oxygen species (ROS)			
Oxygen[a]	$O_2^{\bullet\bullet}$	Singlet oxygen	Δ o ΣO_2
Superoxide	$O_2^{\bullet -}$	Hydrogen peroxide	H_2O_2
Hydroxyl	$^{\bullet}OH$	Ozone	O_3
Hydroperoxyl	$HO_2^{\bullet}$	Hypochloric acid[b]	HOCl
Peroxyl	$RO_2^{\bullet}$	Hypobromous acid	HOBr
Alcoxyl	$RO^{\bullet}$	Organic hydroperoxides	ROOH
Carbonate	$CO_3^{\bullet -}$	Peroxynitrite ion	$ONOO^-$
Carbon dioxide	$CO_2^{\bullet -}$	Peroxynitrous acid[b]	ONOOH
Chloride reactive species (RClS)			
Chloride ion	$Cl^{\bullet}$	Hypochloric acid[b]	HOCl
		Nitryl chloride	NO_2Cl
		Chloramine	RNHCl
		Chloride	Cl_2
Nitrogen reactive species (RNS)			
Nitric oxide	$^{\bullet}NO$	Nitrous acid	HNO_2
Nitric dioxide	$NO_2^{\bullet}$	Peroxynitrous[b]	ONOOH
		Alkylperoxynitrite	ROONO
		Peroxynitrite ion[b]	$ONOO^-$
		Nitryl chloride	NO_2Cl

The presence of the point either to the right or the left of the formula indicates that the product is a "free radical"
[a]Represented in the form of a biradical
[b]Some reactive species appear in more than one category. The dot at the top right (sometimes left) indicates the radical nature

can lead to a structural modification, which can prelude to an *activation* (capacity to perform a specific activity) or a *deactivation* (interruption of a specific activity). In the latter case, the process could prelude to the *elimination* also.

7.1.2 Reactive Species

Reactive species (*RS*) are a large number of elements or compounds characterized by the capacity to avidly attract one e^- or H, and are described as follows:

ROS (reactive oxygen species), because the "attractor" is oxygen (O_2 or O); RNS (Reactive Nitrogen Species), if the "attractor" is nitrogen; RSS in the case of sulfur (S), RCS for carbon, RClS in the case of chloride. In other words, the second letter or letters after R indicate the "attractor" element.

RS most of the time are defined erroneously as "free radicals", and even though some of them are in this status, this is not the condition allowing them to be oxidants. In fact, any element of the Mendeleev table is defined as a "free radical" if it contains a single e^- instead of 2 e^- in one or more orbitals (usually the external orbitals). The most common RS are listed in Table 7.1.

The products containing the prefix *R* refer to compounds that are combined with a molecule of O_2, and the most frequent ones are the fat derivatives, but also proteins, saccharides, and nucleic acids. Therefore, the prefix R indicates different types of products with the exclusion of H.

All the ROOH (hydroperoxides) have the tendency to react with the transition metals (i.e., Fe, Cu) in the Fenton reaction (see further on) assuming the radical shape ($RO^{\bullet}$ or $ROO^{\bullet}$); therefore, they cumulatively have a considerable oxidant potential.

7.1.2.1 Reactive Oxygen Species (ROS)

The ROS represent the most important RS in the biological field, and their reactivity belongs to the O_2 characteristics. Atomic oxygen (*O*) in its most common conformation ($^{8}_{16}O$) consists of 8 protons and 16 neutrons in the nucleus, and 16 e^- in its 9 orbitals, being the two external orbitals (2πx and 2πy, red dotted lines in the Fig. 7.1) composed of a single e^- instead of 2 e^-. Because of this, O can be defined as "biradical" and maintains the same characteristics even when the orbitals are combined in the biatomic molecular configuration O_2.

This condition is the basis of its relative O_2 instability electrons in an attempt to capture electrons and reach the stable form of water (H_2O). O_2 undergoes some modifications to reach the stable condition of H_2O, following a 4 e^- capture in four different steps. However, each step ends up with an instable compound of both radical (i.e., with an unpaired electron in an orbital) and nonradical nature (i.e., with complete electronic orbitals), but still more oxidizing

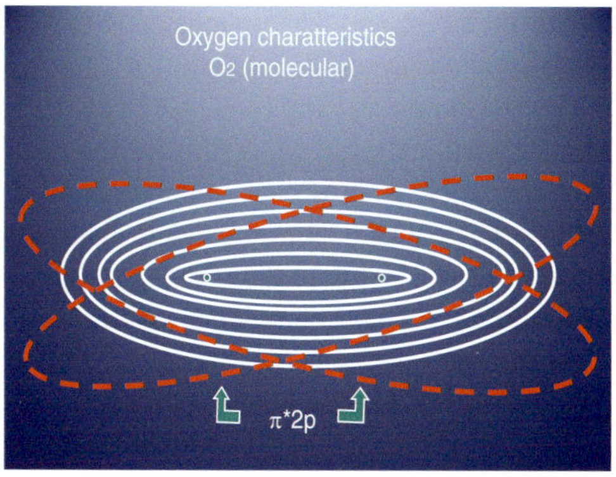

Fig. 7.1 Oxygen orbitals, with configuration π*2p orbitals (in *red*), are antibonding orbitals with unpaired parallel spins, and consequently O_2 is a "biradical"

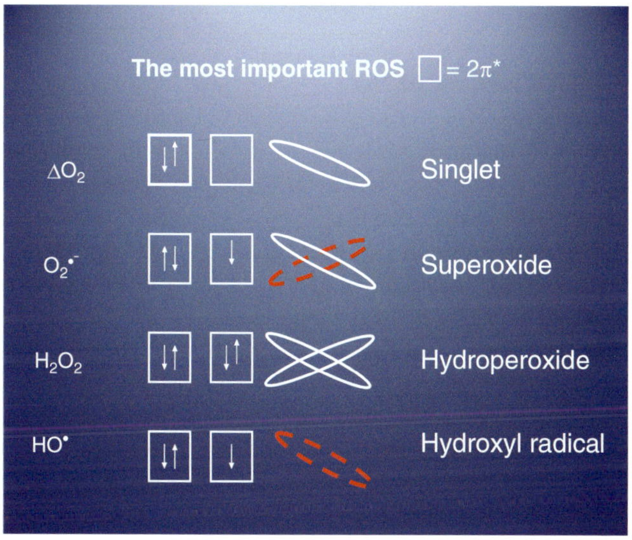

Fig. 7.2 The different ROS The unpaired orbitals (in *red*) determine the "free radical" status

than the original O_2. All these compounds formed before reaching the state of H_2O are called reactive oxygen species (ROS).

ROS in sequence are represented by: $O_2^{\bullet -}$ (superoxide, following 1 e−capture), H_2O_2 (hydrogen peroxide, following 2 e^- capture), •OH (hydroxyl radical, following 3 e^- capture). The fourth e^- capture will end up with H_2O, which, in essence, consists of O_2 that was picking up 4 e^- associated with 2 H+ (protons).

The radical nature of each of the ROS (see Fig. 7.2) is indicated by the point at the top right (or left); even though hydrogen peroxide (H_2O_2) is not a radical, it is nevertheless one of the most important oxidizing molecules of the human organism. An instable intermediate represented as $^{\bullet}O_2H$ is formed by the combination of $O_2^{\bullet -}$ with a H^+ and participates in many reactions. Other ROS exist in nature and are known as ΔO *and* ΣO (singlet oxygen, respectively, of nonradical and radical nature) which are formed in the atmosphere only, generated by the impact between a photon and O_2.

ΔO is not a radical because of the orbital "shift" of the e^- following the impact (as indicated in Fig. 7.2); ΣO on the other hand (not indicated in Fig. 7.2) is a radical, because the impact changes the electron spin.

$O_2^{\bullet -}$ is the primary radical, and once formed is immediately in equilibrium with its protonated form $H_2O^{\bullet}$, which is the main effector, and reacts with biological molecules forming $ROO^{\bullet}$ (peroxyl radicals) or $RO^{\bullet}$ (alcoxyl radicals) and also $HO^{\bullet}$ (hydroxyl radical), where R represents different types of structure (i.e., lipids, proteins, DNA, sugars). These molecules are much more complex than the direct ROS and have a similar reactivity.

7.1.2.2 Other Reactive Species Different from ROS

The most common RS are indicated in Table 7.1.

Among these, nitrogen monoxide ($NO^{\bullet}$, sometimes indicated as •NO) is the most important (see further on), since it is actively synthesized by different cellular systems (in particular, by the endothelial cells) called NO synthetases or NOS, in order to induce vasodilation, antiplatelet, and signaling functions. It can be defined as an RNS (Reactive Nitrogen Species) together with its most dangerous adduct $ONOO^-$ (peroxynitrite) deriving from the reaction with $O_2^{\bullet -}$ ($NO^{\bullet} + O_2^{\bullet -} \rightarrow ONOO$).

7.1.3 Modalities of ROS Formation

In terms of quantity, the mitochondria are the most important production sites of ROS (energetic formation) followed by the cell membranes (reactive formation) and finally by some metabolic processes (metabolic formation).

Energetic formation In the mitochondria, the presence of O_2 is fundamental for the production of ATP. There is a continuous generation of $O_2^{\bullet -}$ which flows both into the mitochondrial matrix and into the intermembrane space, where it immediately undergoes transformation into H_2O_2 (dismutation by the superoxide dismutase or SOD), which is capable of diffusing away from the place of production (the half-life is about 15 s.). For this reason, mitochondria (see Fig. 7.3) are the real producers/exporters of H_2O_2, which in case of overproduction can easily deplete both the mitochondrial and cytoplasmatic antioxidants reserve. The flow of e^- (red line) is indicated from complex I (CI) to complex IV (CIV). The $O_2^{\bullet -}$ produced can be directed either into the mitochondrial matrix or into the intermembrane space. The H_2O_2 is formed in complex IV (CIV), whereas the ATP production arises from complex V (CV).

Other enzymes (MAO or monoaminoxidase and Cb5R or cytochrome 5 reductase) are located in the outer mitochondrial membrane, whereas GPDH (glycerolphosphate dehydrogenase) and cytochrome p450 enzymes are located in the inner mitochondrial membrane [1].

Reactive formation This source of ROS belongs mainly to membranes.

A classic reactive formation is represented by neutrophils NAD(P)H (nicotinamide adenine dinucleotide phosphate) stimulation from bacteria as indicated in Fig. 7.4. NAD(P)H oxidases are a variegated family of enzymes (Nox_s) and cofactors (also see Fig. 7.8) that are located in mitochondria, endoplasmic reticulum, cellular particles such as cytochrome P450, and peroxisomes, and can be activated by many different stimuli. Immediately after $O_2^{\bullet-}$ production, SOD starts the dismutation to H_2O_2. NAD(P)H oxidase suddenly transforms O_2 into $O_2^{\bullet-}$, which is immediately dismutated into H_2O_2 by the SOD and then into the more aggressive $^{\bullet}OH$ (by Fenton reaction) or HClO (by myeloperoxidase).

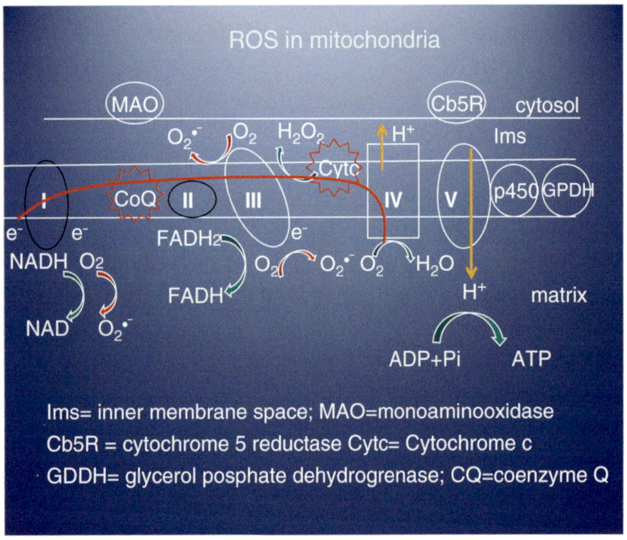

Fig. 7.3 Flow of $O_2^{\bullet-}$ and other ROS in the mitochondria

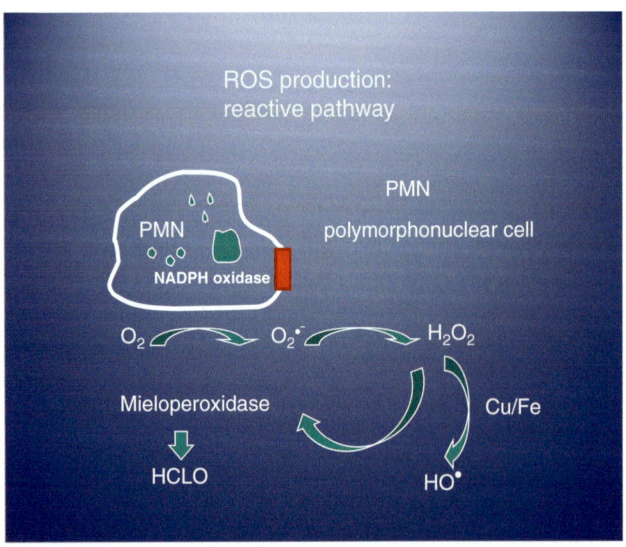

Fig. 7.4 ROS production in a polymorphonucleate (neutrophils). This process is known as "respiratory burst" or "oxidative burst"

Metabolic formation The metabolic source of ROS belongs to many different processes of transformation or activation of different molecules (i.e., prostaglandin synthesis from arachidonic acid, noradrenalin synthesis from dopamine, purine base metabolism up to the formation of uric acid). In this context, we will briefly describe $NO^{\bullet}$ and H_2O_2, which are produced both in the reactive and the metabolic processes.

7.1.3.1 The Case of $NO^{\bullet}$

The production of $NO^{\bullet}$ may be considered in a metabolic and a reactive way to produce RS, as it can fit both conditions and plays an important role in the regulation of redox signaling and cellular function [2].

$NO^{\bullet}$ can be generated by cellular nitric oxide synthases (NOS) or by reduction of nitrites (NO^{3-}) deriving from foods. The cellular $NO^{\bullet}$ is produced by conversion of L-arginine into L-citrulline in the presence of NADPH and tetrahydrobiopterin (BT_4). Three types of enzymes exist that can proceed with the synthesis represented respectively as eNOS (endothelial), nNOS (neuronal), and iNOS (induced). The latter operates exclusively during inflammatory processes. A well-controlled relationship exists between $NO^{\bullet}$ and O_2, since hypoxia and physical stimuli increase $NO^{\bullet}$ release, and the consequent vasodilatation facilitates a more efficient oxygen supply to the surrounding tissue [3]. In physiological conditions, an axis also exists between ROS and RNS. $NO^{\bullet}$ concentration is usually higher than $O_2^{\bullet-}$ concentration, which is immediately transformed into H_2O_2 by SOD. This condition of prevalence will favor the reaction between $NO^{\bullet}$ and the surrounding proteins in the process called "protein nitrosylation" that allows a normal transduction mechanism [4].

This is just an anticipation that some RS can govern normal physiological processes such that low levels of $NO^{\bullet}$ are prosurvival, whereas higher concentrations could be dangerous to the point of angiogenesis and tumor proliferation [5]. During stimulation (oxidative burst), cells of the immune system produce large amounts of both $NO^{\bullet}$ and $O_2^{\bullet-}$, and the reaction between the two molecules has one of the highest rate constants known (7x 10^9 $M^{-1}s^{-1}$). Despite the efficiency of SOD in distracting $O_2^{\bullet-}$, a large production of $NO^{\bullet}$ can bind $O_2^{\bullet-}$ forming $ONOO^-$. Thus, $NO^{\bullet}$ toxicity is predominantly linked to the ability to combine with superoxide anions, since

$ONOO^-$ is a powerful oxidizing agent that can cause DNA fragmentation and lipids oxidation. In particular environmental conditions (acidic pH), $ONOO^-$ tends to be transformed into $^{\bullet}OH$ (sometimes indicated as $HO^{\bullet}$), which is by far the most reactive oxidizer in the organism. Nitrosative modifications caused by $NO^{\bullet}$ (and also by other RNS) are addressed to many molecules, starting from protein with heme groups (either with Cu or Fe) that will be inactivated.

7.1.3.2 The Case of H_2O_2

H_2O_2 has a reactive half-life that enables it to cross the cell and then spread the OS condition. While $O_2^{\bullet-}$ and $^{\bullet}OH$ have an immediate reactivity and oxidize the substrates only in the place of their formation, H_2O_2 "carries" the oxidation far from the site of its generation. The consequence of this is that the cell needs specific apparatus that can protect against the possible damage due to H_2O_2 diffusion. As briefly mentioned before in the case of SOD, among the different ROS, H_2O_2 has a special role, because it can be directly produced by the cells as oxidant determinant for transduction mechanisms [6]. Mammalian cells produce H_2O_2 to mediate diverse physiological responses related to the mechanism of cellular defense, differentiation, and migration.

These activities are related to the impact that this molecule has on the cellular redox chemistry.

In neutrophils, the NAD(P)H oxidase complex generates H_2O_2 within a phagosome for microbial killing (see Fig. 7.5). The complex releases $O_2^{\bullet-}$ into the phagosome, and H_2O_2 is generated by dismutation with SOD.

The activation of surface receptors stimulates NAD(P)H oxidase that is located both on the cellular and internal organelle membranes. The diffusion of H_2O_2 both inside and outside the neutrophiles represents one of the most efficient mechanism against bacterial invasion.

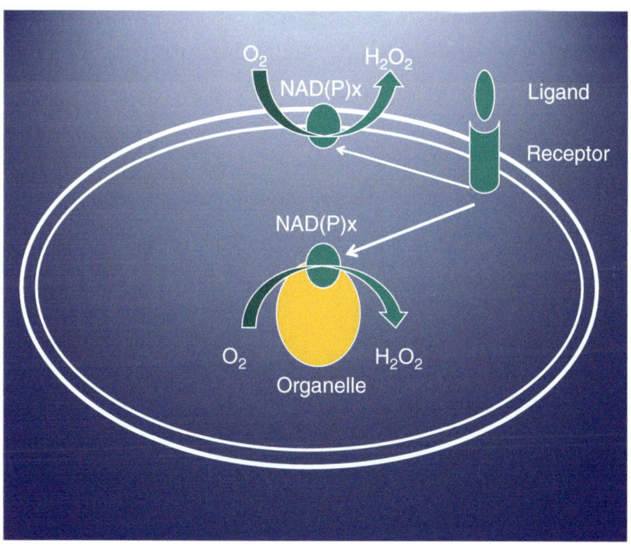

Fig. 7.5 Localization of the enzymes producing H_2O_2

However, in neutrophiles, NAD(P)H oxidase releases H_2O_2 directly into the phagosome (organelle in the Fig. 7.5) and can behave as an autocrine factor.

In nonphagocytic cells also, despite the mechanism is not fully understood, an active production of H_2O_2 takes place following stimulation with various growth factors such as PDGF (platelet-derived growth factor), EGF (epidermal growth factor), insulin, interleukin-1, and TNFα (tumor necrosis factor-α).

The biological redox activation catalyzed by H_2O_2 involves oxidation of cysteine residues on proteins, which may affect protein function. For example, in the TNF-α stimulated cells, the resulting H_2O_2 that is generated inactivates protein kinase phosphatases. The cytosolic H_2O_2 not only enhances protein tyrosine phosphorylation by inactivating the tyrosine phosphatase but at same time can activate the enzyme tyronine kinase. The following scheme can summarize the events (from [6] modified).

PTP (protein tyrosine phosphatase)		PTK (protein tyrosine kinase)	
Active protein	Inactive protein	Inactive protein	Active protein
$PTP\text{-}S_{reduced}$ + H_2O_2	→ $PTP\text{-}S_{oxidized}$	$PTK_{reduced}$	$PTK_{oxidised}$

It is important to underline that the above scheme has to be considered as an equilibrium between the two enzymes. To serve as a signal, the concentration of H_2O_2 must increase rapidly above a certain threshold and has to be protected from those enzymes that transform H_2O_2 into H_2O.

These enzymes are usually located in proximity of the production site. The most important are: thioredoxin (TRx), peroxiredoxin, and glutaredoxin (in relation to the GSH or glutathione), and finally the catalase [7].

During catalysis of H_2O_2 reduction by peroxiredoxin, the residue of the active site of the enzyme, Cys-SH, reacts with two molecules of H_2O_2 to form the hydroperoxide Cys-SOOH, and consequently peroxiredoxin will be inactivated. Another way to inactivate peroxiredoxin is through its phosphorylation. The protection of H_2O_2 is also derived also from sulfiredoxin, which is an adenosine triphosphate-dependent enzyme.

The following scheme reports the mechanism of H_2O_2 protection:

$$\text{Peroxiredoxin} + H_2O_2 \rightarrow \text{inactivation of } H_2O_2$$
$$\text{Sulfairedoxin} + \text{Peroxiredoxin} \rightarrow \text{inactivation of Peroxiredoxin}$$

7.1.4 RS/ROS Functions

The functions of RS are extremely important and are witnessed by the localization of their production (Fig. 7.6) that usually is very close to the structures they have to modify in order to avoid their dispersion which could generate uncontrolled effects.

All the cellular functions by definition are dynamic, which means that the cellular processes are "allostatic" more than "homeostatic," and consequently the components involved have to be reactive and coordinated.

To cope with this duty in the simplest way, it is necessary to make all the cellular components capable of reacting, minimizing the molecular structure modifications: this is the real duty of RS, since with the transfer of just one or a few electrons, they can rapidly modify every cellular function.

Energy production in the mitochondria depends on the production of ATP, which is accomplished using a series of e^- carriers localized in the inner mitochondrial membrane and creating a gradient of H^+ in the intermembrane space. The gradient energy accumulated during this process is used for the synthesis of ATP (oxidative phosphorylation) or partially dispersed as heat.

Part of the O_2 captures $4e^-$ and 2H+ to form H_2O. However, a part of O_2 and e^- is diverted from the process of oxidative phosphorylation and is dispersed both in the mitochondrial matrix and the membranes in the form of the simplest RS (ROS). This size dispersion (likeage) sets up the mitochondria as the main producer of H_2O_2.

The signaling results from RS production due to the action of some factors, such as the stimulation of MAP kinase receptors (mitogen-activated protein kinase, typical of innate immunity) and the release of NF-kB (nuclear factor kB), Nrf2 (nuclear factor-erythroid-2-related), ARE (antioxidant response element, preferably referred as EpRe or electrophile-responsive element), and AP-1 (activator protein 1). Among all these pathways, two have a particular relevance and concern the two most peripheral systems to produce RS located on the external cellular membrane: NAD(P) H oxidase and xanthine oxidase. In normal conditions, an equilibrium exists between Nox1 (the most common NAD(P)H oxidase) (Fig. 7.7) and protein kinase A (PKA) which behaves as a sensor for ROS, since Nox1 can generate a sufficient amount of ROS to enhance PKA activity [8]. If there is a high quantity of ROS (no matter how they are produced), PKA is inactivated and Nox1 starts working (positive feedback) producing ROS, and its synthesis creates a loop that ends up with a further increase in ROS. The activation of PKA maintains Nox1 quiescent (negative feedback), and consequently the synthesis of new Nox 1 does not take place, and ROS levels remain low (Fig. 7.7).

7.1.5 Xanthine Oxidase

Xanthine oxidase is a membrane enzyme belonging to the NAD(P)H oxidase family (capable of transforming purine bases into uric acid) and is responsible for the overproduction of $O_2^{\bullet-}$ following the ischemia/reperfusion process [9]. When tissues become ischemic, there is a depletion of cellular stores of high-energy adenine nucleotides (ATP, ADP, AMP). This leads to the build-up of hypoxanthine and xanthine, which serve as oxidizable purine substrates, and also to an increase in cytosolic Ca^{2+}concentration. The latter is due to inadequate ATP production to maintain the ion gradient across the cellular membrane. The Ca^{2+} increase activates proteases that irreversibly convert the xanthine hydrogenase (that usually reduces NADH to NAD^+) to xanthine oxidase. When reperfusion takes place, the restored O_2 availability occurs in an environment with a high concentration of xanthine and hypoxanthine, and with a converted enzyme (xanthine oxidase) that uses O_2 for the transformations of hypoxanthine into xanthine and to uric acid (Fig. 7.8). In both the reactions, $O_2^{\bullet-}$ is generated, and it will immediately be transformed into H_2O_2 by SOD. Such a large amount of ROS further damages the ischemic reperfused tissue. This process however does not pertain to cardiovascular diseases

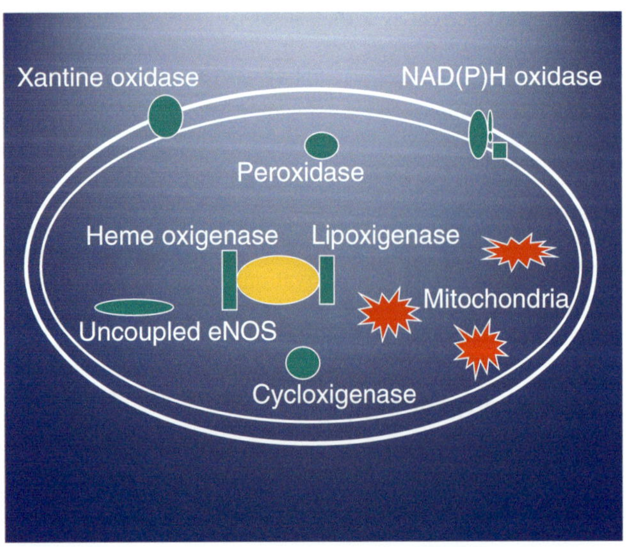

Fig. 7.6 Some localizations of structures generating ROS

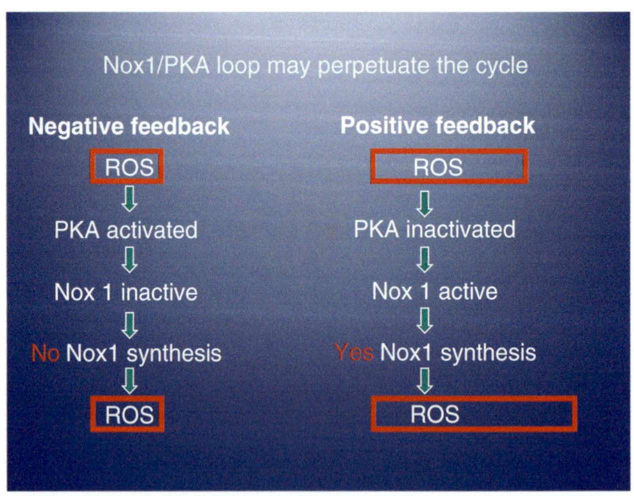

Fig. 7.7 Nox1/PKA/ROS interaction

only, but is common during endurance sport training as well as smoking. H_2O_2 can be transformed into H_2O and O_2 by some antioxidant enzymes (peroxidases) or by reaction with glutathione (GSH). In many instances, H_2O_2 undergoes a *nonenzymatic* reaction (Fenton reaction), which in the presence of Fe^{2+} transforms H_2O_2 into HO^- and $^{\bullet}OH$ as follows:

$$H_2O_2 + Fe^{2+} \rightarrow HO^- \text{ and } ^{\bullet}OH.$$

7.1.6 NAD(P)H Oxidase

Nicotinamide-adenine dinucleotide phosphate oxidase (NA(P)H oxidase) is one of the most important circulating mechanism of defense. The defense mechanism of lymphocytes (mainly neutrophils) and macrophages is specifically addressed to ROS production to attack the substances and microorganisms (bacteria, virus) considered harmful, activating the so-called respiratory burst (see Fig. 7.4). However, whereas this mechanism is addressed mainly to the external part of the cells, the internal mechanism of defense is such that RS are directed to the cytoplasm (Fig. 7.9). However,

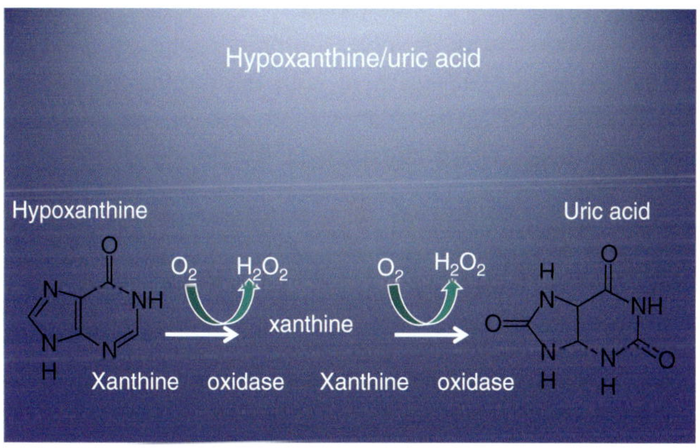

Fig. 7.8 Hypoxanthine modification to uric acid

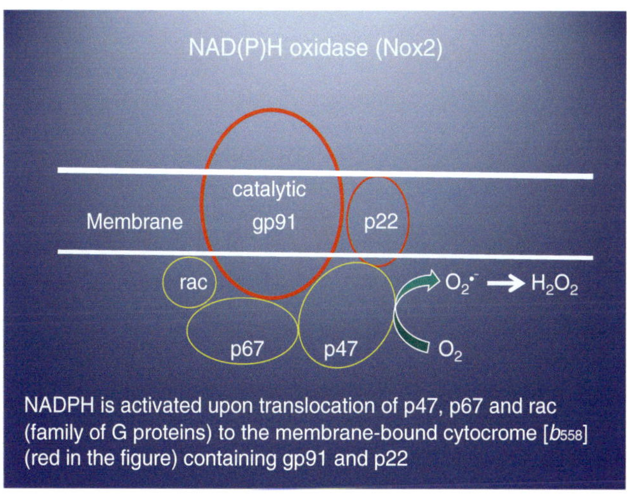

Fig. 7.9 NAD(P)H oxidase configuration

ROS can regulate the enzyme also in nonphagocytic cells by means of at least five different types of NAD(P)H oxidases called Nox_s (1–5).

One characteristic of Nox_s is that it can be stimulated either by components derived from the cytosol or by the external membrane through activation of different types of receptors [10]. They appear to mediate physiological functions, such as erythropoiesis and angiogenesis.

The structure in Fig. 7.9 is related to neutrophil NAD(P) oxidase [11]. The enzyme consists of the membrane-bound cytochrome b_{558}. Other forms in nonphagocitic cells exist and can have different configurations. An extremely important aspect related to reactivity is the immune function, which is triggered by ROS and can stimulate ROS production through Nox_s. An example can clarify the concept: ROOH that gets in contact with a macrophage can trigger its reactivity, as it is capable of activating a receptor of the innate immune reactivity, namely a Tall-like receptor.

7.1.6.1 Superoxide Dismutase (SOD) as Key for the ROS Reactions

As briefly mentioned before, the first reaction of $O_2^{\bullet-}$ is the formation of H_2O_2 through the superoxide dismutase (SOD). This reaction may be considered a real key for the ROS physiology, and for this reason is described in the part related to ROS functions. Dismutation is the biochemical reaction that modifies one substrate into two different products. In the case of SOD, 2 $O_2^{\bullet-}$ will be diverted into H_2O_2 and O_2 as indicated in Fig. 7.10. Usually, SODs are considered as antioxidant enzymes; however, their function does not correspond to the real duty of these enzymes because they produce H_2O_2 which is a powerful and diffusible oxidant. SODs have one of the largest K's (affinity constant) known in biology ($K \approx 10^9\ M^{-1}s^{-1}$) and prevent excessive formation of $ONOO^-$ derived from the reaction between $NO^{\bullet}$ and $O_2^{\bullet-}$, which is also an extremely fast reaction. It is clear that SOD represents the barycenter of the triangle $NO^{\bullet}/O_2^{\bullet-}/H_2O_2$, determining the initial orientation of ROS toward a pure oxidative environment or to the start of the transduction pathway.

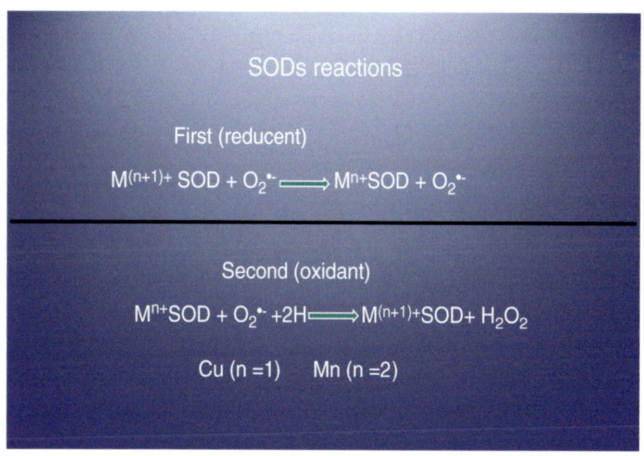

Fig. 7.10 Superoxide dismutase reactions

Three different SODs (SOD1, SOD2, and SOD3) are known in humans with different location. SOD1 has a large distribution; it is a dimer containing Cu-Zn and is located in the cytoplasm, nucleus, and intermembrane space of the mitochondria; SOD2 is a tetramer located in the mitochondrial matrix and contains Mn-Zn; SOD3 (or extracellular SOD) is a tetramer located in the extracellular matrix and contains Cu-Zn.

The reaction is divided into two parts: the first is the reduction of the metal pertinent to any given SOD (M represents Cu or Mn), and the second is the oxidation of the given metal.

In the mitochondria, SODs behave like a "rheostat" determining the shift between one e^- reaction (purely oxidative) and 2 e^- reaction forming H_2O_2 that can influence the transduction mechanisms [12].

$O_2^{\bullet -}$ is produced in proximity of aconitase which is the enzyme controlling the start of the Krebs cycle (energy production) which can be inactivated (by oxidation of the heme group). Following dismutation, $O_2^{\bullet -}$ can be transformed into H_2O_2 that needs to be carefully controlled because of its capability to diffuse within the cell. The H_2O_2 can be quenched through glutathione (GSH) consumption with the consequence of redox buffer modification.

The different types of SOD and the reason for the different metal content are still matters of speculation. As common characteristics, all SODs thousands of times accelerate the transformation into $O_2^{\bullet -}$ and H_2O_2 (the spontaneous reaction would occur too slowly). However, since H_2O_2 also has a high oxidizing power, the cells limit its diffusion through other enzymatic systems with antioxidant action (e.g., thioredoxin, glutathione, catalase, etc.) or using low molecular weight antioxidants (lipoic acid, coenzyme Q10, L-cysteine, ascorbic acid, vitamin E, polyphenols, etc.).

All the constitutive molecules of the living material (phospholipids, nucleic acids, proteins, etc.) are subject to oxidation determined by RS, even though at a different grade of sensitivity.

Despite the fact that allostasis is composed of many different biological variables that work together, each biological molecule can be modified by RS in a specific way and with a specific sensitivity to oxidation.

Lipids, proteins, DNA, and heme will be analyzed separately.

7.1.7 Lipids Oxidation

In general, lipids are the most ROS-sensitive molecules due to the linear structure, easy to be attacked. Among lipids, glycerophospholipids (PLs) have a structural importance, and they must be protected against oxidation in order to maintain their ability to form efficient membranes [13]. On the opposite, those lipids used for energy production (triglycerides, nonesterified fatty acids, or NEFA) must be actively oxidized to produce energy. PLs consist of a "phosphatidic head" (phosphoserine, phosphocoline, etc.) linked to almost two linear lipids: one is a saturated lipid and the other is unsaturated, with a different number of double C=C bonds (instaurations degree). The unsaturated lipids are the most sensitive to oxidative processes [14]. The first oxidative step (Fig. 7.13) is the transformation of the lipid (LH) into a hydroperoxide (LOOH) [13], which is a relatively stable molecule and may persist for a relatively long time in the blood. LOOH belong to the ROOH class and can act as an oxidant for thiol protein (Prot-S⁻), forming a protein sulfide (prot-SO⁻) and finally a less reactive hydroxide (LOH).

In case the thiol protein regulates a signaling pathway, its oxidation compromises the function. LOOH can be eliminated by the body via excretion (mainly but not exclusively renal), but while they are in the body, they can directly or indirectly damage the closer structures undergoing further metabolic transformations. In particular, PLs can follow three different ways.

The first way is the formation of oxidized phospholipids (OxPLs) with various combinations of functional groups (hydroperoxides, hydroxides, keto/epoxy groups).

The second way involves intramolecular cyclization which causes a rearrangement with the production of isoprostanes type F2-isoprostanes, and also of the so-called neuroprostanes, which are formed from long-chain lipids (e.g., DHA or docosahexaenoic) more properly brain-derived. This way also includes iso-levuglandin and isothromboxane which are then further oxidized.

The third way leads to the Fenton reaction (Fig. 7.11) where LOOH is transformed into LOO• or LO• that propagates oxidation to closer lipids and, after undergoing chain fragmentation, ends up with the formation of aldehydes, α,

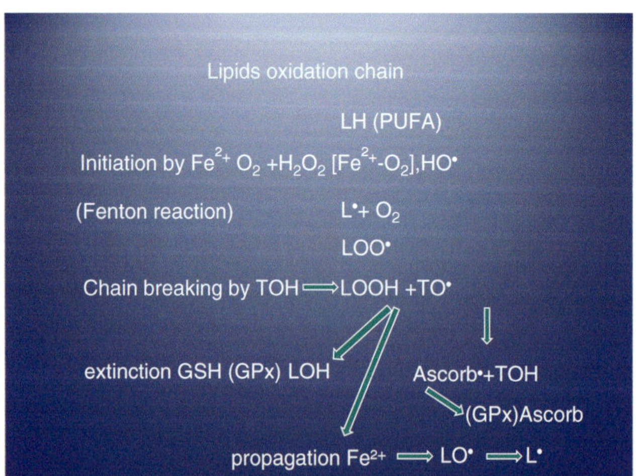

Fig. 7.11 Structural lipids oxidation

β-unsaturated, such as 4-hydroxynonenal (4-HNE), acrolein, and malondialdehyde (MDA) [14]. These latter aldehydes are formed to be rapidly eliminated in the urine. However, circulating in the blood, they form covalent bonds with proteins and nucleic acids, generating carbonylate proteins and oxidized DNA.

The lipid (LH), usually an unsaturated lipid, can be oxidized by a HO• (derived from a Fenton reaction with H_2O_2) and is transformed into a radical (L•) in the process defined as *initiation*. L• reacting with O_2 will become a peroxyl radical (LOO•) that, in the presence of a chain breaker antioxidant, such as Vitamin E (TOH), can be transformed into a hydroperoxide (LOOH). However, if vitamin E or other chain breakers (liposoluble antioxidants) are not available, LOOH can undergo the Fenton reaction (since it is an alkylperoxide) and start the *propagation* cycle. This reaction is quite common, since LOOH can freely move on the membrane (and outside the membrane), and its mobility allows the reaction with GSH getting to the *extinction* that will transform LOOH into the less reactive hydroxide (LOH). Vitamin E that has been oxidized to TO• through the reaction with LOO• can be reduced by Vitamin C (Ascorb), leaving behind the ascorbyl radical (Ascorb•) that can be regenerated by the glutathione peroxidase system (GPx).

Further oxidation process takes place with unsaturated lipids with •NO [15] that results in the formation of *cis* and *trans* nitro-alkanes, where the NO_2 group is present at the site of the double bond as well as nitrohydroxy and nitroperoxy lipids. Contrary to the initial belief that nitrofatty acids would be proinflammatory, accumulating evidence suggests that they have anti-inflammatory potential [28] and may be active on signaling mechanisms inhibiting platelet aggregation, cytokine release in monocytes, and also Nf-kB mediated gene expression (see further on) [16].

7.1.8 Protein Oxidation

Proteins can be oxidized in many different ways. The simplest is the oxidation of some of the amino acids either of the backbone or of the side chain (Fig. 7.12). Amino acid oxidation leads to hydroxylated derivatives [17], which can have the Fenton reaction as for ROOH, and it may be assumed that even for proteins the propagation can take place as for lipid oxidation. Oxidation of amino acid residue side chains allows the formation of protein-protein cross-linking and oxidation of protein backbone followed by protein fragmentation. A peculiar process of oxidation is represented by carbonylation (Fig. 7.13), which consists of a direct protein transformation in response to a metal-catalyzed formation of •OH or an indirect reaction with the products of lipid peroxidation.

This reaction is usually directed to proline, arginine, lysine, and threonine residues that are transformed into the relative aldehyde with the same or a smaller number of carbon atoms. It is a frequent oxidative process, since about 5 % of tissue proteins contain a carbonyl function [17]. Carbonyl groups can be introduced by the reaction with 4-HNE (or 4-hydroxynonenal) [18], MDA, ketoamine, and ketoaldehydes [19].

Reducing sugars or their oxidation products (glyoxal, arabinose) can also determine a similar process (Fig. 7.14) ending up with the so-called products of advanced glycosylation or AGEs (advanced glycosylated products) generated by the interaction of the primary aldehydic groups of the sugars with the amino groups of amino acids and proteins (Amadori's reaction).

Another aspect of protein oxidation regards the lipoproteins, since their oxidation occurs in both structures. Proteins can undergo nitrosative stress by the reaction with •NO or

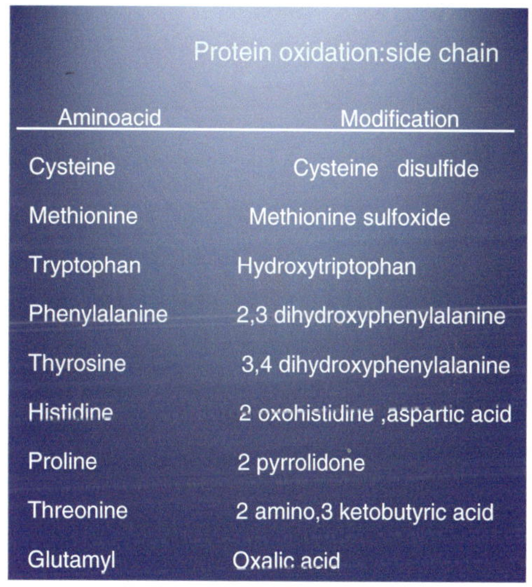
Protein oxidation:side chain

Aminoacid	Modification
Cysteine	Cysteine disulfide
Methionine	Methionine sulfoxide
Tryptophan	Hydroxytriptophan
Phenylalanine	2,3 dihydroxyphenylalanine
Thyrosine	3,4 dihydroxyphenylalanine
Histidine	2 oxohistidine ,aspartic acid
Proline	2 pyrrolidone
Threonine	2 amino,3 ketobutyric acid
Glutamyl	Oxalic acid

Fig. 7.12 Side chain amino acids oxidation

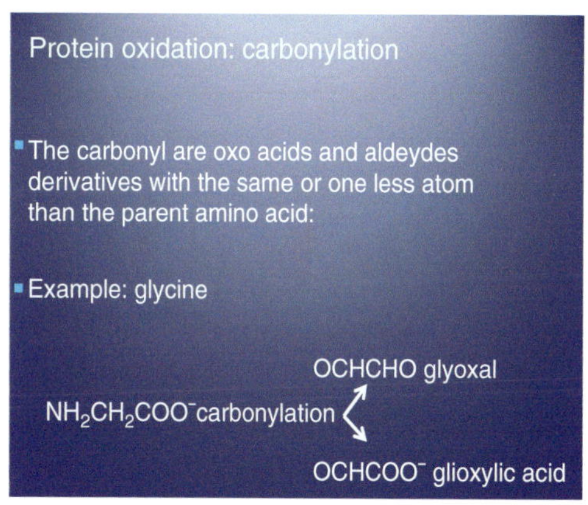

Fig. 7.13 Protein carbonylation of amino acids in the side chain of a protein

$ONOO^-$ (nitrosative stress), and this can manifest itself in two main forms: as S-nitrosylation of cysteine thiols [20] or as nitration of tyrosine residues that result from the covalent addition of a NO_2 to the phenolic ring of tyrosine residues [21].

7.1.9 DNA Oxidation

DNA oxidation can occur on all purine and pyrimidine bases (Figs. 7.15 and 7.16), as well as on deoxyribose sugar. It is believed that 1 out of 200 molecules of O_2, 10^{12} molecules of oxygen daily entering a cell, causes DNA damage [22]; therefore, very substantial oxidative damage takes place, which must be controlled with very efficient repairing systems. In particular, DNA oxidation shows the attack by •OH which leads to the formation of radicals centered on carbon. It is also possible that oxidation occurs on the deoxyribose, leaving the base intact but causing the loss of functionality. It is also noted that the amount of 8-oxo-dG is higher in mammals with a high basal metabolism [22] and more consistent in mitochondrial DNA than nuclear [23]. Unfortunately, the method of extraction from the cells may be due to the formation of 8-oxo-dG, and the data must hence be viewed with caution [24].

DNA is particularly sensitive to nitrosative stress. In particular, it was found that $ONOO^-$ reacts preferentially with guanine, forming 8-oxo-dG (8-idrossi guanine or 8OH-dG) which represents the type of base most studied as an OS marker. It is also noted that the amount of 8-oxo-dG is higher in mammals with high basal metabolism and [22] is more consistent in mitochondrial DNA than in nuclear DNA [23]. Unfortunately, the method of extraction from the cells may be due to the formation of 8-oxo-dG, and then the data must be viewed with caution [25].

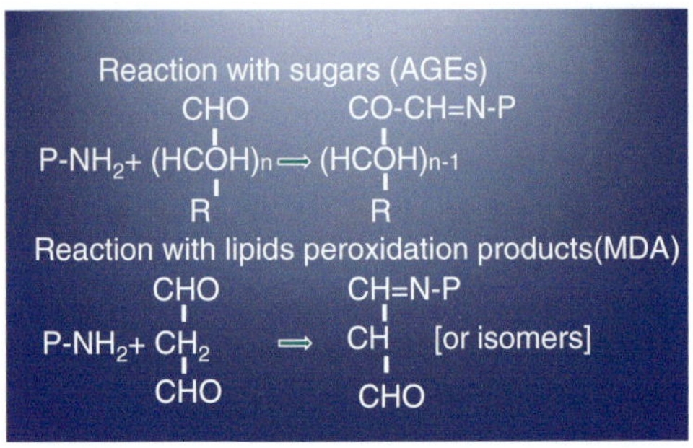

Fig. 7.14 AGE formation and carbonylation due to sugar or lipid peroxidation derivatives

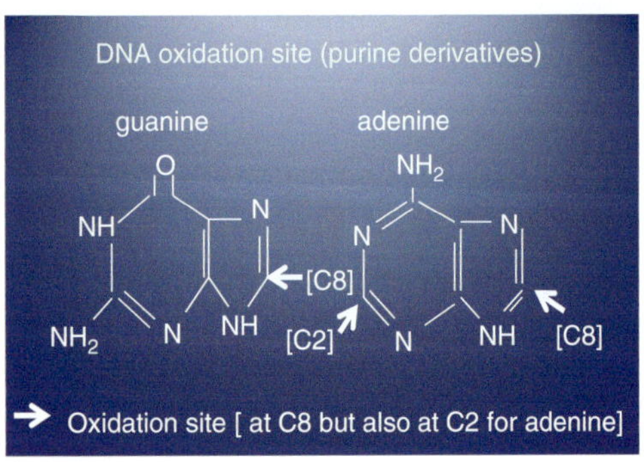

Fig. 7.15 Oxidation of purine bases

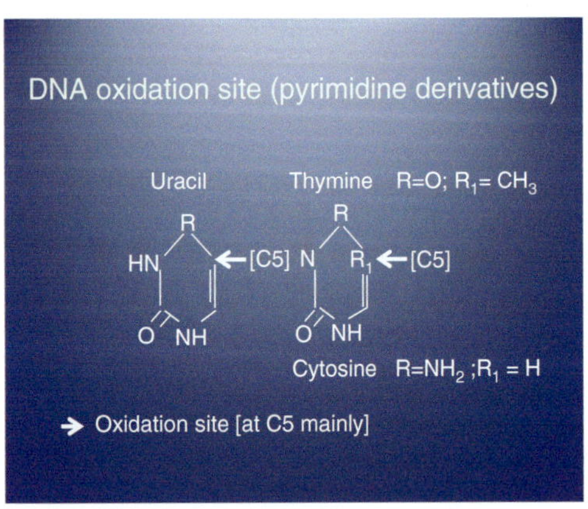

Fig. 7.16 Oxidation of pyrimidine bases

7.1.10 Heme Oxidation

The extremely high turnover of erythrocytes makes available a large quantity of hemoglobin containing Fe.

Each erythrocyte contains about 300 million hemoglobin molecules, and all the heme groups made available by them following their senescence make the availability of Fe-heme very high and potentially very critical. The heme group contains Fe^{2+} that may be released as Fe^{3+} during hemoglobin degradation and generating ROS; for this reason, it must be adequately controlled. Through the heme oxygenase enzyme (HO-1) [26], in the presence of NAPDH, heme is transformed into biliverdin, losing Fe^{2+} and a CO (Fig. 7.17). Biliverdin is transformed into bilirubin by the action of biliverdin reductase.

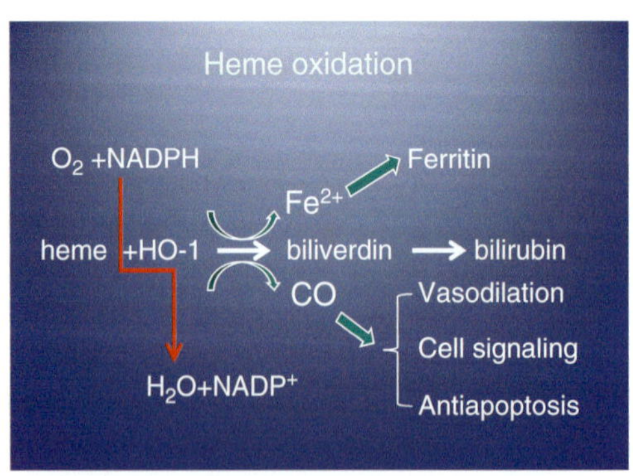

Fig. 7.17 Release of iron and CO by Heme

HO-1 through NADPH allows the release of Fe^{2+} that is collected by Ferritin, whereas CO can stimulate cell signaling, vasodilatation, and cellular apoptosis [27, 28]. Both ferritin and biliverdin, and subsequently bilirubin, have an antioxidant action, while CO exerts a relaxing action on vascular tone similar to, though less powerful than, •NO [29]. There are different types of heme oxygenases (HOs). The most important is HO-1, but other forms of HO emerged, such as HO-2 and HO-3, less active than HO-1.

Many diseases, from pulmonary to endocrine disorders, are characterized by an overproduction of HO-1 [29]. Several regulatory elements are capable of stimulating the production of HO-1. Among these, there are two important transcription factors, the nuclear factor NF-kB and the activator protein AP-1, which activate genes involved in OS. Identical stimuli can trigger both MAP kinase and HO-1 [26], resulting in the production of inflammatory mediators and protective factors, respectively.

Because the cellular response to OS is apoptosis, it is reasonable to consider HO-1 as an antiapoptotic enzyme. Indeed, experimental studies have confirmed that cell lines deficient in HO-1 are more vulnerable to toxic insults that generate apoptosis; the same was applied to animals (mice) lacking the HO-1 gene. It has been demonstrated that this antiapoptotic action is related to CO production [30]. HO-1 prevents the release of Fe^{3+} (strongly oxidizing) and implements the heme diversion which leads to Fe^{2+} (nonoxidizing) and CO (carbon monoxide) for the production of biliverdin/bilirubin. Both the final compounds (biliverdin and bilirubin) have an antioxidant capacity. This heme diversion process takes place not only in erythrocytes, because the HOs, though in different forms, are ubiquitous enzymes which are overregulated in almost every reactive condition, playing a protective role by increasing, in particular, the production of ferritin that binds Fe^{2+} [29, 31] and reduces its availability in the possible transformation of Fe^{2+}/Fe^{3+}.

7.1.11 The Propagation of Oxidation

Each biological molecule (proteins, lipids, nucleic acids, vitamins, antioxidants, etc.), once oxidized, has the ability to oxidize another molecule acting in the same way as a reactive species (RS).

This phenomenon of propagation is particularly harmful for cell membranes because of the contiguity of the phospholipids (PLs) in the membrane layers. In particular, lipoproteins (VLDL, LDL, HDL) that are very rich in PLs can form hydroperoxides (ROOH) which are very specific vehicles of the propagation process, because they circulate and can easily transfer the oxidative condition to the endothelial cells (and in general to all their receptors).

Even though the main source of *ROOH* is oxidized lipids or their isoprostane derivatives, ROOH can also be formed by proteins, DNA, and sugars; therefore, the prefix R indicates different types of products.

ROOH can directly oxidize other substrates containing SH groups (thiols) or trigger the propagation of the oxidative process, operating as multipliers of OS as classically represented by unsaturated lipids oxidation.

These ROOH have the tendency to react with the transition metals (see "Fenton reaction" below) assuming a radical shape (RO• or ROO•); therefore, they cumulatively have considerable oxidant potential.

The consequence of these processes is that the first sensors of the propagation of OS are the cell membranes, and consequently, as shown with appropriate investigations, the determination of plasma hydroperoxides (ROOH) can be considered the earliest markers of OS [32].

7.1.11.1 The Antioxidant Potential

The alternation of the oxidative and reductive processes is the basis of birth, growth, differentiation, and functionality of living organisms. It is therefore misleading to deal only with the oxidative process, but rather we should refer to an oxidative equilibrium or "oxidative balance." The potential danger of ROS implies the need for the cell to balance the potential harm with the antioxidant reserve in order to counteract the inevitable ROS diffusion and limit the propagation process. The antioxidant reserve is constituted primarily by enzymes with a ROS damping function (*quenching*) and by nonenzymatic antioxidants.

7.1.12 Main Endogenous Antioxidant Systems

7.1.12.1 Glutathione or GSH

Glutathione (GSH) consists of a tripeptide, γ-L-glutamyl-cysteinyl glycine (Fig. 7.18). It is produced in a substantial amount in each cell (1–11 mM) and represents the most important endogenous component to control oxidation. GSH is not only a prosthetic part of glutaredoxin, but is also produced as an essential water-soluble antioxidant. The difference between the nonenzymatic and the enzymatic product resides in cysteine, which is replaced by selenocysteine in the enzymatic system.

Each cell produces GSH in an autonomous way (including cells that lack the nucleus, such as erythrocytes and platelets) through a series of enzymes, of which the most

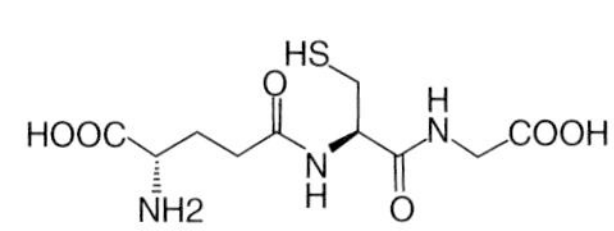

Fig. 7.18 Glutathione or GSH

important is γ-glutamyl cysteinyl synthetase (γGCS). GSH yields its hydrogen and is transformed into GSSG, which is then regenerated in GSH by the NADPH/NADP+ system. This is possible thanks to the energy supplied by the pentose phosphate cycle located in cytoplasm. The GSH/GSSG ratio is considered an index of antioxidant capacity. The process of detoxification that needs GSH for it to be accomplished is called S-glutathionylation, and it is particularly important for thiol proteins' protection. This process also involves inactivation and elimination of substances harmful to the body and is one of the main mechanisms of protection of exposed organs (lung) or involved in detoxification (liver) [33]. Another form of GSH exists, that is, the prosthetic part of the enzyme glutaredoxin (GRx – see further on) which contains selenocysteine (Se-cysteine) instead of cysteine.

7.1.12.2 Catalase

Also, this enzyme belongs to the peroxidase family, and is a ubiquitous, but mostly concentrated in peroxisomes, which are corpuscles located in the cellular cytoplasm. The structure consists of a tetramer which contains a heme group with Fe^{2+} in each of the polypeptide chains. It allows the enzyme to convert H_2O_2 into H_2O in the following reaction: $2H_2O_2 + O_2 \rightarrow 2H_2O$ [13], but it is also capable of binding •NO [34].

Since H_2O_2 is produced in every cell, catalase also has to be available to counterbalance the possible damage due to the powerful oxidation and diffusion capability of H_2O_2. Different concentrations can be produced in the tissue being very abundant in hepatocytes (between one and two orders of magnitude compared to other cells). In erythrocytes, the catalase concentration is between 1 and 2 μmol to protect hemoglobin molecules from oxidation.

7.1.12.3 Cysteine Biochemistry

Cysteine (SH) is probably the most important amino acid for the redox reaction [1]. It can be oxidized by H_2O_2 into a sulfenic acid (SOH), then into sulfinic acid (SOH_2), and finally into sulfonic acid (SO_3H). Whereas SOH is still a reversible form, SOH_2 and SO_3H are irreversible and stand for a definite inactivation of the proteins carrying them. This point raises an important consequence related to those proteins where cysteines have a structural role. For instance, in connexins, which are the proteins that form the intercellular hemi channels of the gap junctions (GJ), there are six cysteines in the external loop of the protein that make the connections with the other six cysteines of the opposite hemi channel. In this way, the complete channel is formed (connexon), allowing the flow of ions, sugars, and mediators (up to 1000 Da) [35]. In case of oxidation of these cysteines, the transfer of ions and other substances through the GJ will be compromised and could be the cause of impairment of muscle contraction coordination, which could be extremely threatening in the heart. This event has to be taken into consideration during the risk of ischemia/reperfusion damage.

7.1.12.4 Thioredoxin (Trx)

The thioredoxin system is considered a redox sensor: it is located both in the cytosol and the mitochondria. It is composed of thioredoxin reductase (TrxR) and proper thioredoxin (Trx) that acts in concert with the peroxiredoxin (Prx) to reduce H_2O_2 to H_2O (Fig. 7.19). Trx in the reduced form stimulates the production of hypoxic pulmonary factor (HIP). The latter is capable of overregulating an extremely consistent series of genes [36]: from those related to angiogenesis until the tumor development.

7.1.12.5 Peroxyredoxin (Prdx)

This enzyme exists in six different typologies (from Prdx1 to Prdx6) and belongs to the peroxidase family, which in addition to being directed to H_2O_2 detoxification may also protect against $ONOO^-$ and ROOH.

As shown in Fig. 7.21, Prdx acts in concert with the TrxR/Trx system as a terminal for the transformation of H_2O_2 in H_2O. There are, however, peroxyredoxins that act independently or in concert with other enzymatic systems different from TrxR/Trx, such as sulfiredoxin.

7.1.12.6 Glutaredoxin (GR)

This enzyme has similarity with thioredoxin, but instead of Prdx it uses GSH (glutathione) as prosthetic exchange terminal for the transformation of H_2O_2 into H_2O. The final enzyme of the system is glutathione peroxidase (GPx) that contains seleno-cysteine instead of cysteine. Seleno-cysteine (SeH) by oxidation due to H_2O_2 is transformed into selenenic acid (Se-OH) (Fig. 7.20).

GR (glutaredoxin) is reduced from NAPH, which in turn yields H to GSH (glutathione) which then yields it to GPx (glutathione peroxidase), which finally reduces H_2O_2 to H_2O. SeH represents a selenocysteine; Se-OH represents the

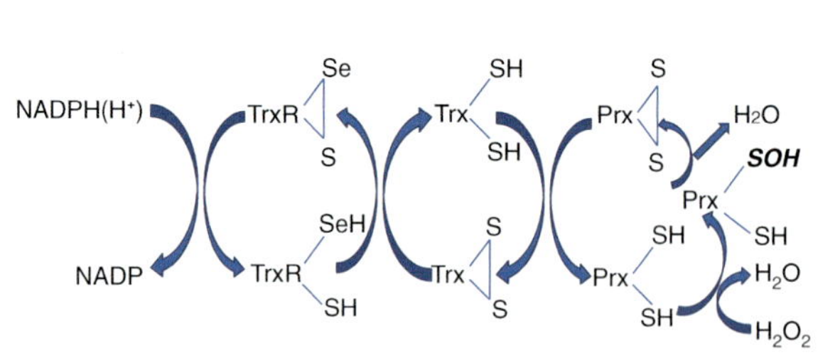

TrxR (reductase) is reduced by NAPH and transfers H toTrx that gives H to Prx (peroxiredoxine) that finally reduces H2O2 to H2O. SH is cysteine and Se is seleno-cysteine. SOH is a sulfenic residual produced by cysteine oxidation [15].

Fig. 7.19 Thioredoxin system cascade. TrxR (thioredoxin reductase) is reduced by NAPH, which in turn gives H to Trx (thioredoxin), which then transfers it to Prx (peroxiredoxin), which finally reduces H_2O_2 to H_2O. SH represents cysteine, while Se represents selenocysteine. SOH represents a sulfenic acid residue which is produced by oxidation of the thiol group of cysteine (Modified from [37])

selenenic residue products during selenocysteine oxidation (modified from [36]).

The presence of SeH allows the enzyme to operate in a broader pH range than it would with only cysteine; this may explain the presence of different peroxidase systems that are activated depending on the cellular conditions.

7.1.12.7 Paraoxonase (PON)

The paraoxonase (PON) family comprises three members of calcium-dependent hydrolytic enzymes, PON1, PON2, PON3, which takes its name from its ability to hydrolyze paraoxon (the active metabolite of the organophosphorous insecticide parathion). Considering that this activity is related to human-made chemicals, it seems to be an ancillary rather than a primary function of the enzymes [38], there also being a difference of some orders of magnitude among the three members (PON1 is much more active than PON2 and PON3). In contrast, lactonase activity that utilizes natural substrates (and also some drugs) is almost similar for all the members, and all three PONs efficiently metabolize lactons and hydroxy acid derivatives of arachidonic acid and docosahexaenoic acid, preventing the damage generated by these hydroperoxides.

The hydrolytic activity consists of protecting high-density lipoproteins (HDL) and other lipoproteins (LDL, VLDL, respectively, low density and very low density lipoproteins) from oxidative propagation by degrading lipid peroxides that are formed in membrane phospholipids [39].

In HDL, the estrogens have no antioxidant capacity, because the free phenolic groups required are present in the form of esters. PONs efficiently hydrolyze the estrogen esters of HDL, leading them to regain antioxidant activity [40]. The combination of the two hydrolytic processes, respectively, of phospholipid hydroperoxides and estrogen esters, seems to be responsible for the PONs activity in maintaining the HDL efficiency.

The ability of PON1 to prevent oxidative damage in tissues seems to be a reasonable hypothesis that emerges from atherosclerosis studies [41].

One important aspect of the PONs activity is the hydrolysis of homocysteine thiolactone (HCyTL) which is a toxic

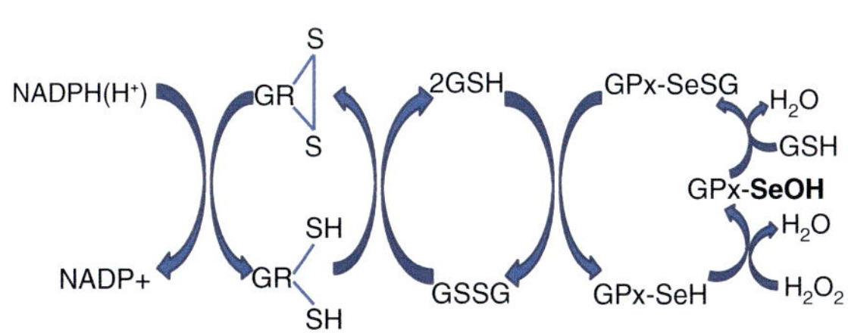

GR (glutaredoxin) is reduced by NAPH and transfers H to GSH (glutathione) that gives H to GPx (glutathione peroxidase), that finally reduces H_2O_2 to H_2O.SeH represents seleno-cysteine; Se-OH represents a selenenic residual deriving from seleno-cysteine oxidation [15].

Fig. 7.20 Glutaredoxin system cascade

metabolite of homocysteine. HcyTL can bind fibrinogen and make it resistant to lysis (thrombogenic) and bind proteins eliciting an inflammatory autoimmune response [42]. Hyperhomocysteinemic subjects have dysfunctional HDL particles with attenuated antiatherogenetic activity (reduced cholesterol efflux and anti-inflammatory effect) due to a parallel decrease of PON1 activity [43].

In humans, PON1 and PON3 are bound to HDL, and PON2 is an intracellular enzyme only.

The most characterized enzyme of the family is PON1, which is a protein of 43 kDA containing a cysteine (position 283) and has two amino acid polymorphisms (methionine/leucine [M/L] in position 55 and arginine/glutamine [R/Q] in position 192), such that individuals 192R/R and 55 L/L have greater hydrolytic capabilities and less risk of coronary heart diseases [41]. Many other single amino acid polymorphisms have been detected (about 200), some in the coding region, while others in the introns and regulatory regions that make PON1 a very complex full characterization of the enzyme [38]. There is at least a 40-fold variation in serum PON1 activity among individuals [42] due both to genetic reasons and exogenous factors (diet, smoking, environmental heavy metals). PON2 was shown to exert its antioxidant functions at the cellular level joining the host of the intracellular antioxidant enzymes [44].

PON1 is synthesized essentially in the liver with the aim of participating in oxidation by product elimination [45]. However, PON1 is just one of at least four enzymes (PON1, LCAT or lecithin cholesterol acyltransferase, PAF-AH or platelet-activating acetyl hydrolase, GSH peroxidases) and two lipoproteins (Apo a-1 and Apo-J, respectively, apolipoproteins a-1 and J) associated with HDL that can potentially modulate the formation or inactivation of the LDL-derived oxidized phospholipids [46]. In other words, more than a single enzyme is the combination of all these elements and can be the "antioxidant apparatus" affording the oxidative burden. During the acute phase of inflammation, some enzymes in the HDL decrease (PON, PAF-AH, LCAT), leading to the increase of hydroperoxides, and HDL becomes pro-oxidant. This means that this complex HDL antioxidant apparatus may have a "chameleon-like" behavior being anti-inflammatory in the basal state and proinflammatory during the acute-phase response [46] when losing the coordination of the antioxidant apparatus. There are different types of drugs (e.g., statins, fibrates, rosiglitazone, sulfonilureas, aspirin) and physiological modulators that seem to increase the PON1 activity and can prevent atherosclerotic disease [47].

7.1.12.8 Nonenzymatic Antioxidants

Nonenzymatic antioxidants can be derived from endogenous factors and food, and they represent a wide range of compounds as shown in Table 7.2.

Table 7.2 The antioxidant network

Function/structure	Type of product
Vitamin	Vitamin A, vitamin E, vitamin C, nicotinamide, riboflavin, niacin
Lipids	Omega 3, omega 6, squalene, cholesterol
Amino acids/thiol Metabolites	Taurine, L-arginine, histidine, glycine, cysteine, glutamine, methionine, N-acetyl cysteine, S-adenosil-L-methionine, lipoic acid, uric acid, bilirubin, squalene
Peptides	Carnosine, gamma-glutamyl-cysteinyl glycine (GSH)
Proteins	Albumin, thioredoxin, peroxiredoxin, lactoferrin, transferrin, ceruloplasmin
Plant derivatives	Polyphenols (hydroxycinnamic acid-derivated, hydroxybenzoic acid-derivated, flavonoids, stilbenes, lignans, tannins, ellagic acid), glucosinolates, carotenoids (α, β, γ, δ-carotene, lycopene, lutein, zeaxanthin, canthaxanthin, astaxanthin), phytic acid, allicin, policosanols
Minerals	Zinc, iron, copper, selenium, chromium

Most of the plant derivatives (from Goji berries, Garcinia fruits, curcumin, ginkgo biloba, berberine, etc.) proposed as antioxidants contain compounds included in Table 7.2.

Some compounds belonging to the vast category of polyphenols (>1000 different compounds) can be isolated as polymers. One example among many is procyanidins (flavan-3-ol polymers) considered to have many pharmacological activities that only partially can be linked to the antioxidant activity. This is the case of most antioxidants, which, given the minimal bioavailability (sometimes absent) [48], can be considered antioxidants only for the gut, whereas the systemic activity should be explained for other pharmacological actions. There are also compounds that show indirect antioxidant activity, such as fibers, phytates, polyglucosamine, and iron-chelating products that act in the gut only. This does not mean that they are systemically inactive, because protecting lipids against oxidation reduces the burden of oxidized lipoproteins that will trigger endothelial cell and macrophage reaction.

7.1.13 The Importance of the Oxidative Balance

Redox regulation is such a complex mechanism that it is impossible to fully understand the complete algorithm of its cascade of events on the basis of simplified routes. The potential of different redox couples (Ech mV) can be determined *in vitro* up to the definition of products that are highly oxidizing to highly reducing [49]. However, in biological conditions, many of the redox couples are present at the same time, and the evaluation of the final energy has to be measured in non-standard conditions. The redox potential has been measured considering those couples with the highest intracellular concentration (GSH, NADPH, and Ttx) using the Nernst equation and showing that the entity of the redox potential is directly correlated to the cellular functions (Fig. 7.21).

The same elements as Fig. 7.12 are shown with the relative values of Ehc mV that can determine cellular activity modification (see text).

In more biological terms, the oxidative process that takes place in the cellular environment can be divided into "passive" and "active" oxidation, where passive means easily reversible oxidation, and active means a more complex process characterized by cytokine release and cellular macrophage activation.

Passive oxidation is immediately compensated by the antioxidant mechanism, whereas active oxidation needs more energy availability and reducing capability by the antioxidant cellular systems. In case of insufficient antioxidant defense, the latter can precipitate into an inflammatory process that can be defined as "redox inflammatory condition" (RI).

7.1.13.1 The Coordinated Redox Signals

The evidence that oxidative allostasis is based on the balance between ROS production, reactivity, and protective mechanisms is clear, and it is also clear that the redox-responsive transcription system is a fundamental part of allostasis. At the present time, the best investigated redox-response mammalian transcription is represented by Keap 1/Nrf2 and NF-kB systems [50].

7.1.14 Nrf2/Keap-1 System

The Nrf2/Keap-1 transcription system plays a critical role in cellular defense against oxidative and electrophilic insults

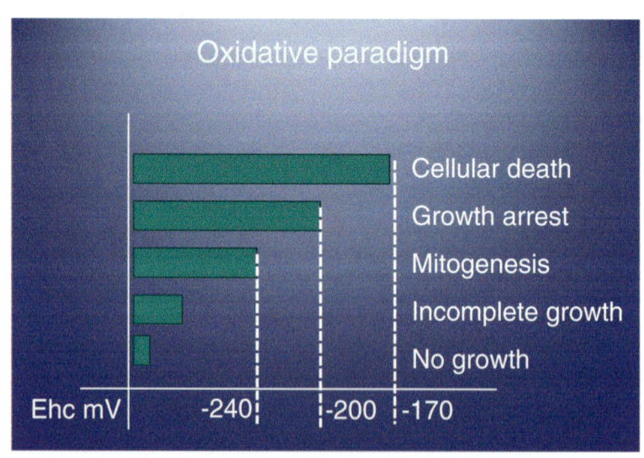

Fig. 7.21 The measure of standard redox potential (*Ech* mV) in relation to the cellular functions

[50, 51]. Nrf2 (nuclear factor erythroid 2-related transcription factor) is a 66.1kDa protein with a C-terminus containing repeats of leucine and N-terminus rich in glutamic and aspartic acid [46]. It is a powerful transcription factor that belongs to the family of basic leucine zipper proteins. They are a group of specialized factors known as xenobiotic-activated receptors (XRAs) that sense specific chemical changes in the cell and coordinate the transcription of an array of adaptive responses to the stimuli. Under basal conditions, Nrf2 protein is rapidly turned over with a half-life of about 20 min through a specific ubiquitin-26S proteasome (Fig. 7.22). In the cytoplasm, Nrf2 is bound to Keap-1. Keap-1 is a Kelch-like ECH-associated protein-1 (kelch indicates a protein produced by Drosophila kelch for detoxification gene expression, whereas ECH stands for epoxycyclohexenone which is an apoptosis inhibitor). Keap-1 is an adaptor protein with a ubiquitin ligase complex and a region (C-terminal Kelch domain) that binds Nrf2. This binding with Keap-1 allows the correct ubiquination of Nrf2. The protein Cul3 ligase (Cul3 of the Cullin family) targets Nrf2 within the Nrf2/Keap-1 complex. When the redox balance is tipped toward the oxidative side, Nrf2 translocates into the nucleus and activates the transcription of ARE (antioxidant-responsive element, also called EpRE or electrophile-responsive element). In this way, the expression of proteins is regulated and favors cell survival (enzymes with antioxidant function, GSH synthesis and regeneration, phase II detoxification and drug metabolism, recognition repair, removal of damaged protein, etc.) and inhibits cytokine-mediated inflammation and autophagy. Genes transcribed after Nrf2 activation are called "Nrf2 regulon" [53]. Within the nucleus, a balance between imported and exported Nrf2 exists, such that the normal condition is in favor of the import. Once Nrf2 is exported, it will be available for a cytoplasmatic binding with Keap-1 following proteasome degradation, unless Keap-1 is in the condition for binding.

OS may inactivate the Nrf2 binding site making it available again for its nuclear import. The phosphorylation cascade activated by pathogens or acute inflammation inhibits the reassociation to Keap-1 and triggers the nuclear import. Now, an important simple observation arises: all the processes mentioned need energy to be maintained in place efficiently, and the energy derives quite exclusively from mitochondria, and in case of reduced activity of malfunctioning of these organelles, the shortage of energy determines the shut-off of the Nrf2/Keap-1 system.

7.1.15 NF-kB

Nuclear factor kB (NF-kB) is a family of transcription factors which play a critical role in the immune, inflammatory, and apoptotic responses (Fig. 7.23), and are activated following ligation of many receptors including T-cell and B-cell, TNF receptors, and Tall-like/interleukin-1 receptors.

The family is composed of five members of homodimers or heterodimers: p65 (Re1A), Re1B, c-Re1, p50 (NF-kB), and p52 (NF-kB2) [kB stands for a k light chain of gene in a mature antibody-producing B cell; Re stands for "reticuloendotheliosis oncogen virus" of turkeys, showing a homology of 300 amino acids with p50 and also shared by c-Re1 also]. In theory, a total of 15 homodimers and heterodimers are possible from combinatorial dimerization of the five NF-kB units, and indeed, 12 have been detected *in vivo* [54], the dimer being composed of p50/p65, the most common, and p65, the only one that contains a transactivation domain (Fig. 7.25).

The canonical pathway to activate NK-kB belongs to IL-1R (interleukin-1 receptor) or the tall-like receptor (TLR), and is one of the three known modalities to start with the NF-KB cascade. The other two are via the tyrosine kinase receptor (RTK) known as "atypical pathway" or through the tumor necrosis factor receptor (TNFR) known as "alternative pathway". All three ways differ in many steps, but for all, the

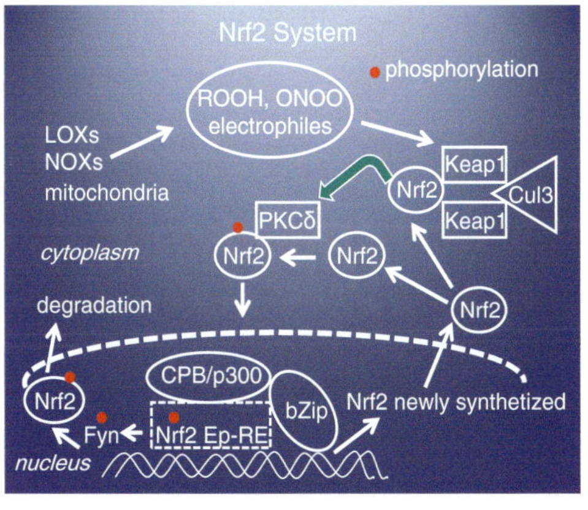

Fig. 7.22 The Nrf2 nuclear translocation

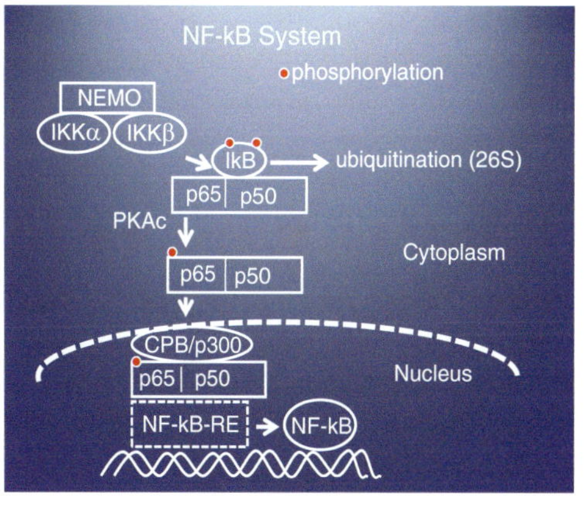

Fig. 7.23 Activation of NF-Kb via the canonical pathway

activation is regularly associated with the activation of NADPH oxidase (NOX) or lypoxigenase (LOX).

In an unstimulated cell, NF-kB is sequestered in the cytoplasm because of an interaction with a member of the inhibitory family IkB (or inhibitor of kB), and its activation occurs in response to extracellular stimuli that promote the dissociation of IkB. The release is possible only after the IkB phosphorylation that allows the IkB polyubiquitination via Lys 48 of ubiquitin, followed by degradation into 26S proteasome. However, this process has its bottleneck in IkB kinases (IKKs) which form a complex composed of IKKα, IKKβ, and IKKγ. Two molecules of IKKγ linked through sulfide bonds [Cys 54 and Cys 387] form the NF-kB essential modulator (NEMO) to which IKKα and IKKβ bind NF-kB in the resting state. The phosphorylation of IKKβ allows both the mobilization of NF-kB and the degradation of IkB. Phosphorylation of p65 by protein kinase A (PKAc) is also necessary to allow the dimer to enter the nucleus. There, it binds together with the coactivators CPB and p300 to the NF-kB responsive element.

All these complex mechanisms indicate a strong relation between NF-kB activation and redox phosphorylation. The overall outcome of NF-kB activation is an inflammatory response characterized by proinflammatory cytokines, macrophage inflammatory protein-1α (MIP-1α), adhesion molecules, and growth factors [50].

7.1.15.1 NF-kB/Nrf2…the Yin and the Yang

Occupation of receptors by the damage-associated molecular patterns (DAMPs), such as IL-1 or TNFα, leads to $O_2^{\bullet-}$ production through LOX or NOX. Immediately, H_2O_2 is formed by the SOD and favors the activation of NF-kB enhancing protein phosphorylation, but Keap-1 is also oxidized activating the Nrf2 system (Fig. 7.23). While NF-kB tends to enhance the inflammatory response through proinflammatory cytokines, Nrf2 dampens proinflammatory signaling by the expression of peroxidase and anti-inflammatory proteins.

Keap-1 also induces IKKβ degradation, thereby directly interfering with NF-kB.

In general, receptor activation and downstream signaling is immediate as it requires milliseconds (or at least far less than a minute); target gene expression extends its timing into hours or days; and the consequences of these processes, if cell recruitment and differentiation is involved, may take weeks.

Consequently, the persistence of DAMPs exposure is determinant for chronic inflammation, and any interruption of this event cascade, although for a short period of time, allows the system to regain equilibrium, like an athlete during a soccer game – he cannot run continuously, but with a few moments of endurance interruption, a well-trained athlete can play for hours. On the other hand, despite a protective activity, a persistent Nrf2 activation has to be considered a warning [50–55].

7.1.16 The "Sensors of Oxidation"

From the mechanistic point of view, aggressive radicals such as $^{\bullet}OH$, $O_2^{\bullet-}$ or any fast-reacting radical are not suitable to mediate redox regulation. This is because they react in a stochastic way with almost all kinds of biomolecules at a nearly constant diffusion-limited rate (about 2×10^{10} $M^{-1}s^{-1}$) and lack the ability to modify regulatory proteins with the mandatory selectivity [50]. Despite $^{\bullet}NO$ and $O_2^{\bullet-}$ having the potential to reversibly bind heme, the evidence on regulatory consequences of redox regulation is scarce.

The most prominent mechanism to modulate redox regulation is protein thiol modifications to sulfenic acid. This event does not result from any free radical attack, but from an electron pair transition from nonradical ROS such as H_2O_2, ROOH, or $ONOO^-$. The latter have to be considered the "*oxidant signals*," whereas the cysteine residues oxidized to sulfenic acid represent the "*sensor of oxidation*".

7.1.17 The Redox-Inflammatory Condition

It is clear that OS refers to an imbalance between factors that generate ROS and factors that oppose the potentially detrimental action of ROS impairing allostasis (Fig. 7.24). This impairment of the oxidative balance can be defined as *redox-inflammatory condition* (*RI*). The excessive presence of ROS causes a reduction of GSH and all the antioxidants in the extracellular fluid. At the cell membrane level, ROS triggers the transduction phenomena which lead to activation of the production of proinflammatory cytokines (TNF or tumor necrosis factor and IL-1 or interleukin 1). It also produces a stimulation of Nrf2 (nuclear factor-erythroid-2 related), which induces an antioxidant enzyme increase and synthesis for GSH production (γ-GCS or gamma-glutamylcysteine synthetase) as an example of all the antioxidant apparatus.

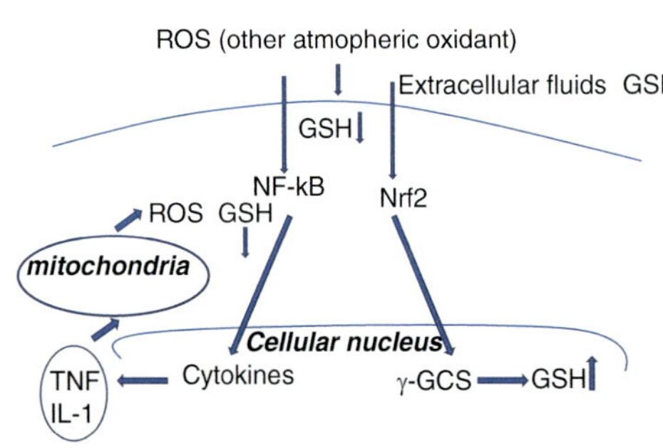

Fig. 7.24 Stimulation of NF-kB and Nrf2

However, a NF-kB stimulation excess can lead to inhibition of Nrf2 production [51].

A "vicious circle" is established for which the ROS production fuels the inflammatory process because of the shortage (depletion) of antioxidant defenses. This predisposition to inflammation allows the infiltration of reactive cells (lymphocytes, neutrophils, macrophages), as shown in Fig. 7.25 (modified from [56]) and determine an RI condition. From the mechanisms that have been described, it appears that the ideal conditions for correct functionality of a living organism is allostasis (dynamic equilibrium). The convergence of the two mechanisms' damage/protection at a particular time represents the "*physiological modulation*". Two important aspects of these processes have to be taken into consideration.

The first concerns the *dimension* of the oxidative stress in order to have an indication about the evolution into an RI condition.

The second is related to *localization*, since OS can specifically develop in one organ or apparatus. The latter concept is definable as "*compartition of OS*" and indicates that brain OS cannot be comparable to gastrointestinal or skin OS, and every apparatus may be characterized by peculiar pathways.

According to these concepts, methods to determine OS may differ for the type of markers they can detect.

7.1.18 Methods for OS Evaluation

For a very long time, researchers have tried to develop a method that would allow an assessment of the OS condition. The system that captures the reactive species is ESR (electric spin resonance), which for long time was considered a sort of golden standard, because it can detect $O_2^{\cdot-}$ and $^{\cdot}HO$ (and also $ONOO^-$) at the moment of their generation in the tissues. The use of resins that capture these two ROS (spin traps) are hardly applicable *in vivo*, because they should be administered parenterally to reach the blood and tissues. This is possible in experimental animals, but not in humans, because of their toxicity. Therefore, research has turned to *derivatization* systems that allow the determination of those endogenous substances that have been modified by reaction with RS and defined as adducts (Table 7.3).

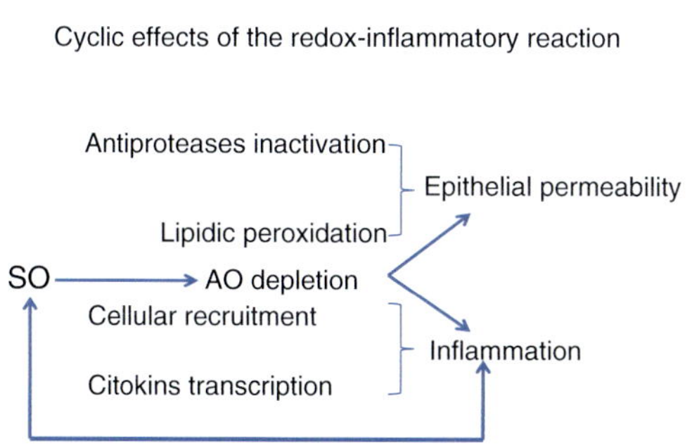

Fig. 7.25 Cyclical effects of redox-inflammatory reaction

An ideal method should be a reliable early indicator of OS, easy to be carried out, with limited costs.

Some of these tests are based on spin traps that are not permitted for human use. Other methods are extremely long and expensive, and for these reasons, they are used exclusively for research and not for monitoring diseases in humans. In medical literature, the most common methods are related to TBARS, MDA, 4-HNE, urinary/blood isoprostanes (F2), carbonylated proteins, DNA-oxidized, and hydroperoxides. Each method has some limitations. The analysis of TBARs, MDA, and 4-HNE are indicators that emerge when high levels of blood glucose (diabetes) undergo oxidation and escape the circulating AO reserve. They increase following inflammatory processes but cannot be considered early indicators, because the AO reserve creates a barrier to their formation. In other words, when these indicators are altered, a pathological state is clearly present, and they do not allow early diagnosis.

The same limitation is shared by isoprostanes, carbonylated proteins, and DNA, which do not help as early markers and lend themselves to monitoring the pathological condition signaling with their increase or decrease, respectively, the improvement or deterioration of a given disease. Despite the fact that they can be considered reliable markers, they suffer two important limitations: the first is a relatively high coefficient of variation (about 50–60 %) which makes it difficult to compare groups of data generated, unless they have large average differences; the second is that methods are quite complex, and data coming from different labs may carry a consistent amount of errors. A completely different

Table 7.3 Some of the main methods used for OS evaluation

Method	Derivate
oxDNA	Oxidized deoxyribonucleic acid
SPC	Carbonylated proteins
LPH	Lipids hydroperoxides
TBARS	Thiobarbituric acid-reactive substances
d-ROMs/FORT	Hydroperoxides
LNO_2	Nitrolinoleate
MDA	Malonyldialdehyde
4-HNE	4-hydroxynonenal
IsoPs	$F_2/D_2/E_2$/isoprostanes
NeuroPs	F_3/F_4 isoprostanes
H_2O_2	Hydrogen peroxides
BH	Respiratory hydrocarbons
$ONOO^{-}$[a]	Peroxynitrite
PTN[a]	Alfa-fenyl-N-tert-butylnitrone
AHS[a]	Aromatic hydroxylation of salicylate

[a]"Spin trap" methods which involve resins or potentially toxic substance administration

value has to be given to the hydroperoxide measurements (ROOH), which are direct markers of most of the derivatives that can modify redox signaling (lipids, proteins, and DNA). The ROOH measurement can be carried out using the d-ROMs or FORT test. The validity of these tests has been analyzed in comparison with the other most common tests used for the measurement of RS, such as isoprostanes, carbonylated proteins, oxidized DNA, and hydroperoxides. Furthermore, the values of all the tests were compared with C-reactive protein (hsCRP) as inflammation index. The experience [32] was conducted on healthy volunteers in conditions "mimicking" oxidative stress. In such conditions, the marker that changed in a more homogeneous way (with smaller interindividual variation) was considered the most reliable. The hydroperoxide determination showed the lowest coefficient of variation (CV < 15 %) compared to isoprostanes, carbonyl proteins, and ox DNA (CV between 50 and 60 %). The results were not unexpected, but confirmed that the ROOH are a derivatization of the oxidative modification of both PL (and lipids), proteins and DNA, while the other tests are unidirectional, and they only pick up their specific derivatization. In other clinical experiences, ROOH levels were shown to be correlated positively and significantly with isoprostane levels [32] and with hsCRP [50], and also with MDA levels in critical patients in intensive care [14], indicating that the d-ROMs test is ideal to determine the *redox inflammatory condition* (*RI*). Until now, at least 900 trials have used detecting ROOH to measure OS, which is one of most used by the clinical communities. Since the ROOH are detectable by the d-ROMs or FORT test only [57–60], it is believed that this test will be extremely valuable for monitoring various diseases and allows following the patient's clinical outcome to modulate the therapy.

7.2 Antimicrobial Peptide

Changlong Lu, MD, PhD and Xun Sun, MD, PhD

Antimicrobial peptides (AMPs) are evolutionarily conserved major contributors in host innate immune defense system. AMPs have been described in plants, insects, invertebrates, and vertebrates, which are of varying significance for each species' antimicrobial or innate immune response [61]. Antimicrobial peptides are polypeptides of fewer than 100 amino acids that are found in host defense settings, and that have antimicrobial activity at physiological concentrations [62]. The two main antimicrobial peptide families in humans and other mammals are defensins and cathelicidins [61]. Defensins are widely distributed at high concentration (up to millimolar) in mammalian epithelial cells and phagocytes. Cathelicidins are structurally and evolutionarily distinct antimicrobial peptides that are similar to defensins in abundance and distribution. There are other mammalian antimicrobial peptides, including histatins, dermcidin, and "anionic peptides." Defensins are prominent in humans, which are present in various forms in human tissues, and the ubiquitous occurrences in inflamed or infected human tissues [62] (Table 7.4).

Table 7.4 Major features of cathelicidins and β-defensins

	Cathelicidins	β-defensins
Structure	α-helix	β-sheet
	Cathelin prodomain	Six cysteine motifs
Source	Keratinocytes, neutrophils	Keratinocytes, sebocytes,
	mast cells, lymphocytes	sweat glands
	sweat glands	
Production	Constitutive and inducible	Constitutive and inducible
Antimicrobial properties	Broad spectrum	Broad spectrum

7.3 Cytokines and Eicosanoids

Jinyan Wang and Changlong Lu

Cytokines are small proteins (~5–20 kDa) that are released by cells and affect the biological behavior on either the cytokine-producing cells themselves (autocrine actions) or on other target cells (paracrine actions) [63]. Cytokines are often produced locally with rare limited biological half-lives and exert their functions via specific receptors. The functions of cytokines are diverse, including cell development, differentiation, growth, cytolytic activity, survival, apoptosis, and chemotaxis [64]. Cytokines are produced by diverse types of cells, such as immune cells including macrophages, B lymphocytes, T lymphocytes, and mast cells, as well as endothelial cells, fibroblasts, and epithelial cells. Basically, a particular type of cells may produce distinct cytokines in response to various environmental stimulatory factors, and a given cytokine may be produced by more than one type of cell [65].

It has been known that a cytokine binds with its receptor of high affinity. Upon binding to its corresponding receptor on target cells, cytokine can mediate a variety of different biological activities such as activation, proliferation, and differentiation of target cells [66]. For example, interleukin-2 (IL-2) secreted by activated Th1 cells can affect not only the producing cells themselves, but also the T cells nearby to promote their activation, proliferation, and differentiation. Furthermore, IL-2 can also act on B cells to promote the differentiation of B cell into plasma cells [67].

Cytokines can be produced by different cells; based on their structures and biological functions, cytokines can be classified as interleukins (ILs), interferons (IFNs), tumor necrosis factors (TNFs), colony-stimulating factors (CSFs), and chemokines [66]. ILs represent cytokines that mediate interactions among different source of cells, including leukocytes; these ILs exhibit diverse activities to modulate cell growth, differentiation, and activation during an immune response [68]. ILs can exert both proinflammatory and anti-inflammatory actions, and some are involved in the development of certain cutaneous diseases. For example, IL-6 is a classic proinflammatory cytokine critical in mounting an effective immune response. Elevated levels of IL-6 are found in patients with systemic sclerosis (SSc), and the level of IL-6 correlates with skin thickness, suggesting that IL-6 may be associated with the fibrotic process in SSc [69]. A recent study showed that IL-13 and its receptors, IL-13Rα1 and IL-13Rα2, showed positive expression by the tumor cells in the lesion of cutaneous T-cell lymphomas (CTCL), compared with specimens from normal skin, atopic dermatitis, and psoriasis. In vitro experiments revealed that IL-13 induces Sezary cells proliferation in a dose-dependent manner. Furthermore, IL-13 blocking showed an antiproliferative effects on cultured Sezary cells, suggesting that IL-13 may present a growth factor for CTCL and that inhibition of IL-13 or its signaling pathway may be potential therapeutic targets in the treatment of CTCL [70].

IFNs are mainly composed of two subtypes of IFNs with different structural and biological functions, type I- and type II IFNs. Both types of IFNs are known to mediate antiviral and immune modulatory effects. IFNs were found to be involved in the development of some autoimmune skin diseases, including psoriasis [71]. It has been proved that plasmacytoid dendritic cell derived IFN-α is essential for the development of psoriasis [72]. The importance of type I IFNs in the development of psoriasis has been well documented [73, 74]; it has been noted that the injection of IFN-α in the treatment of patients with hepatitis C can induce or exacerbate the preexisting psoriatic lesions, while blocking type I IFNs prevent the transformation of nonlesional to lesional skin in a xenograft model of psoriasis. However, anti-IFN-a treatment shows no effect on chronic plaque psoriasis, suggesting the complex roles played by type I IFNs in different types of psoriasis. Type II IFNs, such as IFN-γ, also was found to be involved in the development of psoriasis [75, 76]. Enhanced IFN-γ production secreted by cutaneous T cells was found in the psoriasis lesions. Administration of IFN-γ intradermally induce psoriatic lesions in the skin, indicating promoted effect of IFN-γ on psoriatic lesion; however, anti-IFN-γ therapy did not show preventive effect on psoriatic lesion, highlighting the complex network by IFN-γ on the pathogenesis of psoriasis.

TNFs are type II transmembrane proteins that are constituted by three homological domains, where the receptor-binding sites locate. TNFs are showed to orchestrate the development, homeostasis, and effector actions of immune cells [63]. It has been approved that TNFs function as mediators in both acute and chronic systemic inflammatory reactions. TNFs facilitate the production of other inflammatory cytokines and chemokines on target cells [77]. Controlling the secretion of TNFs by keratinocytes is essential for the maintenance of the skin immune homeostasis and is important to protect against spontaneous dermatitis [78]. TNFs also play a pitvotal role in the development of psoriasis [79]. Hidradenitis suppurativa (HS) is a disease difficult to treatment, with the pathogenesis remaining largely unknown; a recent study showed increased levels of IL-1β, TNF-α, and IL-10 in the HS lesions, and suggested potential therapies with biological agents targeting cytokines such as TNF-α and IL-1 [80].

Colony-stimulating factor (CSF) is a cytokine which can stimulate proliferation and differentiation of pluripotential hemopoietic stem cells and hematopoietic progenitor cells in different development stages; especially, CSF plays a critical role in the maintenance and function of macrophages [81]. Studies on a mouse model have shown that the development of Langerhans cells (LCs) is dependent on CSF-1 receptor signaling but independent of CSF-1 under physiological conditions, whereas inflammation-induced repopulation of LCs appears to be dependent on CSF-1; once inflammation resolved, LC survival is again CSF1-independent, suggesting that dependency of CSF on different situations regulate Langerhans cell dynamics and function [82]. Systemic increase in G-CSF contributed to the skin inflammatory response, characterized by massive dermal infiltration of neutrophils/macrophages. Deletion of the G-CSF gene prevents neutrophilia and partially ameliorates the inflamed skin [83]. TNF-α and IL-17 play a central role in the pathogenesis of psoriasis. IL-17 induces significant activation of Langerhans cells, while enhanced chemoattractant effect on epidermal LCs was found when in combination with TNF-α, supporting the interplay of cytokines on the Langerhans cells in the ongoing of the disease [84].

Chemokines constitute a large specialized family of cytokines that regulate immune response by activating specific G protein-coupled receptors (GPCRs) on leukocytes [85]. Chemokines are known to primarily attract leukocyte trafficking to certain areas of inflammation as well as to locations where primary immune responses initiate. There are four classes of chemokine molecules (C, CC, CXC, and CX3C) that are named after the number and location of cysteine residues at the amino terminus of the protein [86]. Interaction between chemokine and their receptors is characterized by considerable redundancy; a particular chemokine usually binds to more than one receptor, and a particular inflammatory chemokine receptor can recognize more than one chemokine [87]. Chemokines are likely to be primarily responsible for the infiltration of inflammatory cells in some skin diseases [88]. Basically, chemokines are responsible for the migration of activated T cells, NK cells, monocytes/macrophages, dendritic cells, and neutrophils, leading to the initiation of the inflammatory responses, or even acting as effector molecules to enhance the immune responses against self components. Abnormal production of chemokines may result in the development of some skin disorders. A recent study suggested that CXCR3 ligands CXCL9, CXCL10, and CXCL11 promote skin tumorigenesis by boosting inflammation, suggesting an established role in tumorigenesis of epithelial tumors [89]. Increased levels of CCL17 in the serum of atopic dermatitis patients correspond to the progression of atopic dermatitis (AD) and bullous pemphigoid (BP) [90]. Dysregulatory expression of CXCL12-CXCR4 axis was approved to be associated with the development of mycosis fungoides (MF), a chronic cutaneous disease that classically presents from patch stage to plaque stage over a number of years and finally progresses to tumor stage [91]; increased levels of CXCL12 in plaque stage was found in the pretumor stage, and the abundance of CXCL12 derived from the neoplastic T cells express CXCR4 in MF. These results suggested an important role of chemokine-chemokine receptor axis in the pathogenesis of cutaneous diseases.

Growth factors are cytokines that are specialized in promoting cellular growth, proliferation, differentiation, and healing [92]. Growth factors, such as transforming growth factor-β (TGF-β), vascular endothelial cell growth factor (VEGF), endothelial growth factors (EGF), and fibroblast growth factor (FGF), are important in regulating a variety of cellular processes. It has been well documented that growth factors are involved in the maintenance of the homeostasis of skin integrity [93]. Abnormal production of growth factors is responsible for the development of many skin diseases. For example, transforming growth factor beta (TGF-β) controls cell proliferation, cell differentiation, and acts as an antiproliferative factor in normal epithelial cells, while increased expression of TGF-β2 in skin wounds was found to promote keratinocyte proliferation and migration during wound healing via upregulation of microRNA-31 expression on keratinocytes [94], suggesting a role of TGF-β2 in restoring the integrity of the skin. VEGF is a signal protein that stimulates vasculogenesis and angiogenesis. VEGF released by follicular keratinocytes plays crucial roles in sustaining perifollicular angiogenesis resulting in an increase in follicle and hair size, and altered skin vasculature that can be found in some hair loss diseases such as androgenetic alopecia [95].

Eicosanoids are potent lipid mediators that play roles in many biological processes, including inflammation and immune function. These biological mediators are synthesized from phospholipase A2 that releases the polyunsaturated fatty acids from membrane phospholipids; oxidative enzymes, such as cyclooxygenases and lipoxygenase, are involved along with the synthases and hydrolases that carry out the final synthesis of the biologically active metabolites [96]. Two classes of eicosanoids, prostaglandins (PGs) and leukotrienes (LTs), have been increasingly studied in the context of respiratory viral infection [97]. Because of these effects, eicosanoids are likely to make significant contributions to the pathogenesis of respiratory virus infection. Eicosanoids are potent lipid mediators that involved in the inflammatory responses. Two classes of eicosanoids, the prostaglandins (PGs) and leukotrienes (LTs), are well-documented in the pathogenesis of some skin diseases. PGs are generated from arachidonic acid that catalyzed from membrane glycerophospholipids by phospholipase A2 (PLA2). PGE2 is one of the best known PGs and most well studied of regulatory mediators. PGE2 is mainly produced by leukocytes, mast cells, macrophage, and dendritic cells. PGE2 exerts its actions, in part, through G protein-coupled PGE receptors. Leukotrienes (LTs) are also generated from AA released from cell membranes. This process is regulated by a series of enzymes, such as 5-lipoxygenase (5-LO) [98].

In the type I hypersensitivity-mediated asthmatic response, PGEs and LTs, as important immune regulatory mediators, are released from mast cells by degranulation and phospholipase signaling that initiates the enzymatic breakdown of phospholipids in the plasma membrane. The contraction of human bronchial and tracheal smooth muscles is first initiated by histamine. Then LTs and PGEs contribute to the further contraction within 30–60 s. The LTs function as potent effectors at mediating bronchoconstriction and stimulator of vascular permeability and mucus secretion [99]. Accumulating data have suggested that PGEs and LTs are involved in the skin inflammation and wound healing. Leukotriene B4 (LTB4) receptor type 2 (BLT2) is a G protein-coulped receptor (GPCR) for LTB4 and 12(S)-hydroxyheptadeca-5Z,8E,10E-trienoic acid (12-HHT). BLT2 is highly expressed in murine epidermal keratinocytes, By using mouse skin wound healing model, Liu M et al. found that accumulation of 12-HHT in the wound fluid mice correlates with the skin wound healing processes. BLT2-deficiency in mice resulted in impaired re-epithelialization and delayed wound closure. Reduced 12-HHT production lead to delayed wound closure in wild-type mice, which was abrogated in BLT2-deficient mice, suggesting the involvement of the 12-HHT/BLT2 axis in epidermal keratinocytes, implicating the possibility that BLT2 may be a potential therapeutic target to accelerate wound healing [100]. In a murine imiquimod (IMQ) induced psoriasis model, a recent study found that CXCR2 and leukotriene B4 receptor BLT1 coordinate to drive the pathogenesis of psoriasis through the recruitment of neutrophils. CXCR2 ligands augment leukotriene B4 production from neutrophils and thus enhance the recruitment of neutrophil to the skin during the early phase of IMQ-induced inflammation; this study indicates that the interplay between chemokines and lipid eicosanoids might contribute to the pathogenesis of psoriasis; interference to this coordination of chemokines and lipid eicosanoids could be of a novel treatment for skin inflammatory skin disorders [101]. Neutrophil influx is associated with the scratching of human skin and tape-stripping of mouse skin. This influx was largely dependent on the formation of leukotriene B4 (LTB4) by neutrophils and their expression of the LTB4 receptor BLT1. LTB4R1 deficiency lead to impaired allergic skin inflammation mediated by effector CD4+T cells. Transfer of wild-type neutrophils restored the activation of effector CD4+T cells and initiate allergic skin inflammation to LTB4R1-deficient recipients [102]. These results indicated that LTB4-BLT1 interaction plays crucial role in the pathogenesis of allergic skin inflammation.

Taken together, cytokines and inflammatory lipid mediators play critical role in the maintenance of homeostasis and skin integrity. Abnormal production of certain cytokines and inflammatory lipid mediators correlate with skin inflammation and pathogenesis of certain skin disorders. The therapeutic targeting of these cytokines and lipid mediators might bring potential benefit to the clinical application.

7.4 Complement System

Roberto Perricone and Eleonora Ballanti

7.4.1 Introduction

The complement system is one component of the innate immune system. Traditionally, the main function of the complement system was believed to be restricted to the recognition and removal of pathogens through direct killing and/or stimulation of phagocytosis [103, 104]. However, in the past decades, the complement system was demonstrated to have immunoregulatory functions, and it was established that the complement proteins play an important role in modulating adaptive immunity and in bridging innate and adaptive responses [105]. A body of evidence demonstrated that the activation of the complement system is also critical to the development of B cell and T cell immunity [106]. Moreover, complement system is implicated in the pathogenesis of several diseases, from UV-mediated skin damage to autoimmune diseases.

This enzymatic system comprises more than 30 plasma and membrane-bound proteins [105, 107]. The activation of these proteins occurs through three possible pathways: the classical, the alternative, and the lectin pathway. All three pathways are activated according to a cascade system, with activation of one factor leading to the activation of the next [105].

7.4.2 Pathways of Complement System Activation and Regulation

Similar to the coagulation, fibrinolysis, and kinin pathways, complement activation occurs through enzymatic cascades. Most of the complement proteins are cleaved during activation of the system, and the fragments are generally indicated with suffixes "a" and "b". All three pathways converge at two main keypoints: the cleavage of C3 and C5 (Fig. 7.26). The activation of the classical pathway is dependent on antibodies forming immune complexes (IC) (IgM or IgG) and binding to the C1 complex [108]. The binding of C1q to the antibody leads to the activation of C4 and C2, inducing the formation of the C4bC2a complex, known as C3 convertase of the classical pathway [109]. In the alternative pathway, factor D, a serine protease, cleaves factor B, which is complexed with spontaneously hydrolyzed iC3b, leading to the formation of Ba and Bb. Bb and C3b form the C3 convertase of the alternative pathway, C3bBb. Properdin increases the stability of this enzyme [110]. The lectin pathway becomes activated, when either mannose-binding lectin (MBL) or ficolins recognize carbohydrate patterns on microbes and activate C2 and C4 through MBL-associated serine proteases (MASP), with the formation of C4bC2a (the same C3 convertase as the classical pathway) [109]. Similarly, the classical and lectin cascades form the same C5 convertase (C3bC4bC2a), whereas the alternative pathway generates a different C5 convertase (C3bBb3b). The activation of C5 generates C5a (a potent chemoattractant) and C5b that contribute to the formation of the membrane attack complex (MAC) C5b-9, capable of causing cell lysis. In addition to this function, complement system plays several roles, including: activation of neutrophils and endothelium by sublytic quantities of MAC; opsonization and enhanced phagocytosis through the deposition of C3 fragments (e.g., C3b, iC3b) on membranes and/or particles; immune complex clearance; clearance of apoptotic bodies; anaphylatoxin-mediated effects; modulation of cell adhesion, signal transduction, and cytokine production; [106]. The complement system is tightly controlled by proteins present in the fluid phase and on cell membranes in order to avoid host damage caused by excessive complement activation [111]. Interestingly, evidence shows that many pathogenic microorganisms interact with these complement regulators to elude the immune system [112]. Several complement regulators decrease the activity of C3 convertase, a crucial enzyme for the activation of the complement system, both in the classical and alternative pathways. Additionally, other control proteins act on C1 activity and MAC [111]. Overactivation of the complement system due to imbalance between activation triggers and regulatory mechanisms may cause damage, by induction and amplification of inflammatory pathways [105] (Fig. 7.26). The importance of the regulatory processes is evident in hereditary angioedema (HAE), characterized by the

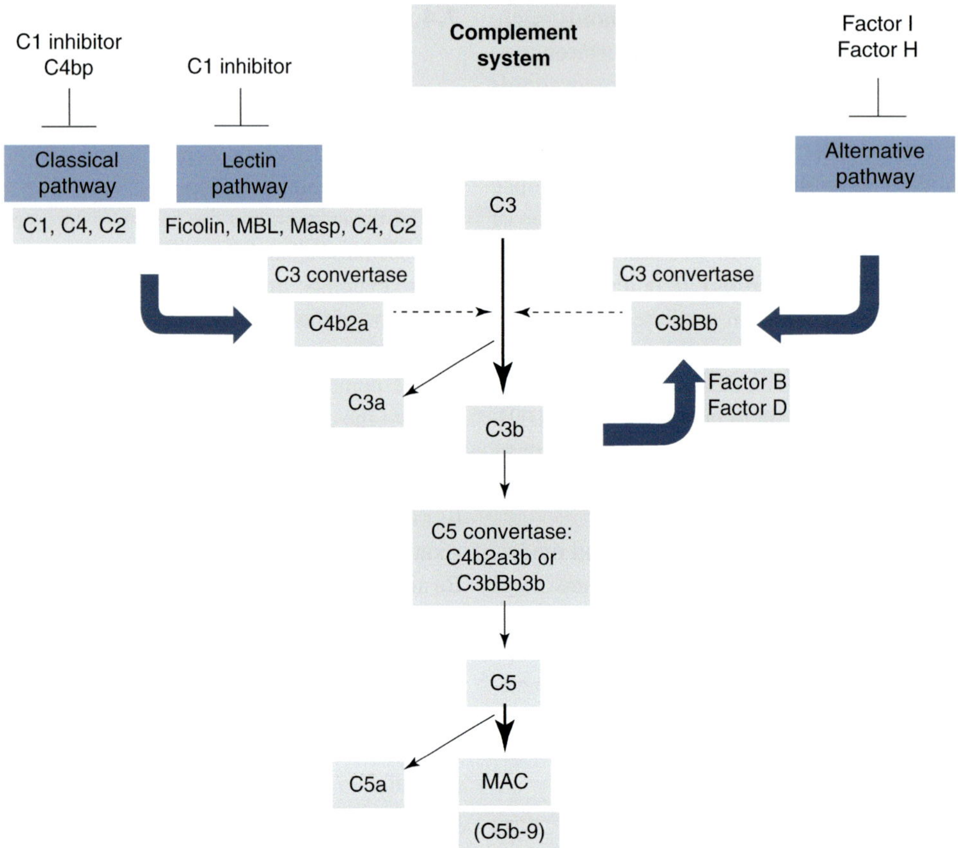

Fig. 7.26 Activation of the complement system. Activation of the complement system occurs through three possible pathways: the classical, the alternative, and the lectin pathway. All the pathways lead to the cleavage of C3 and finally converge at the activation of C5, with possible formation of the membrane attack complex (MAC). Activation of the cascades is tightly controlled by several regulatory proteins. C1 inhibitor, C4 binding protein, Factor I, and Factor H represent the most important regulators and act at different points of the pathways

deficiency of multifunctional serine protease C1 inhibitor (C1INH), causing inappropriate activation of the complement system as well as of the other plasma enzymatic systems (contact system, coagulation system). The defect results in recurrent episodes of angioedema involving the skin and the mucosa [113].

7.4.3 Complement System as Mediator of Tissue Damage and Diseases

Several studies demonstrated the involvement of complement system in inflammatory tissue damage. Its activation in the tissues mainly occurs through IC, which triggers the classical complement pathway [107]. Moreover, in ischemic tissues, phospholipids and mitochondrial proteins, normally enclosed within the cells, come out and activate the complement system either directly by binding C1q or MBL, or indirectly by binding natural antibodies or C-reactive protein (CRP) [107]. CRP can activate the classical pathway by binding C1q. Furthermore, necrotic cells and tissues lack the regulatory molecules that normally prevent the binding of complement proteins [107]. Inappropriate activation of the complement system causes the release of several proinflammatory mediators, including anaphylatoxins C3a and C5a. C5a is a potent chemoattractant for neutrophils, monocytes, and eosinophils [114]. In addition, C3a and C5a are able to stimulate the synthesis of other proinflammatory mediators [114]. The MAC can contribute to inflammation and tissue damage leading to cell death by necrosis or apoptosis [114].

Complement proteins are implicated in UV-mediated skin damage, and UV represents a trigger for complement synthesis in skin [115]. Moreover, this enzymatic system is involved in the pathogenesis of several autoimmune conditions such as systemic lupus erythematosus (SLE), antiglomerular basement membrane disease, vasculitides, Sjögren's syndrome (SS), antiphospholipid antibody syndrome (APS), systemic sclerosis (SSc), dermatomyositis (DM), and rheumatoid arthritis (RA) [116]. The relation between the complement system and autoimmunity could seem paradoxical. On one hand, the overactivation of complement system leads to tissue damage in autoimmune diseases, and on the other hand, deficiency of the complement proteins causes autoimmune diseases too, and it is difficult reconciling these two aspects.

Deficiencies of complement proteins may result in a large amount of clinical manifestations, including recurrent infections, HAE, leukocyte adhesion deficiency, hemolytic-uremic syndrome, and autoimmune disease, first of all SLE [117]. Several hypotheses have been proposed to explain the association between complement deficiencies and autoimmune diseases, mainly focusing on the inadequate clearance of IC in subjects with low levels of complement factors [118].

7.4.4 Immunological Roles for Complement Factors in Skin Diseases

A variety of skin cells, including mast cells [119], macrophages [120] keratinocytes [121], and fibroblasts [122] have been demonstrated to express complement proteins.

UV irradiation stimulates keratinocytes to produce C3 [115]. The complement pathway can be activated by oxidation-specific epitopes or damaged cells, which are typically generated by UV. Indeed, the activation of complement C3 into iC3b, probably through alternative pathway, leads to the differentiation of monocytic cells into activated macrophages [123]. Usually, macrophages infiltrating the epidermis after UV exposure are found next to damaged keratinocytes which are C3-positive [124]. Therefore, the complement bound-damaged keratinocytes seems to serve as a signal to recruit and activate macrophages, which later produce reactive oxygen species (ROS) able to exacerbate the oxidative damage.

Complement participates in the pathogenesis of autoimmune diseases involving the skin, including vasculitides, SLE, DM. In these diseases, skin biopsies often show deposits of complement fragments in the lesion area. Histological data indicate that the activation of the complement system substantially contributes to tissues damages in patients with SLE. Deposits of C3, C4, and associated complement fragments are easily detected in biopsies of inflamed skin from patients with SLE [125]. In these patients, the MAC is localized in the basement membrane zone of cutaneous lesions, and, compared with clinically normal tissues, more prominent MAC deposits have been observed in inflamed tissues [126]. Immunofluorescence studies in SLE patients show deposits of immunoglobulins and complement in skin and other inflamed tissues [127, 128]. Similarly, the deposition of MAC is found in a high proportion of biopsies from skin lesions of DM patients and is absent in unaffected skin, suggesting that the complement system is involved in the pathogenesis of skin lesions [129]. Among vasculitides, some small-medium vessel disorders show a prominent involvement of complement system, including urticarial vasculitis (UV), ANCA (antineutrophil cytoplasmic autoantibody)-associated vasculitides, cryoglobulinemia (CV), IgA vasculitis. In several cases, its activation occurs because of IC formation, and it predominantly happens through the classical pathway (UV, CV); in other cases, a prevalent activation of alternative (ANCA-associated vasculitides) or lectin (IgA vasculitis) pathway has been observed [130].

7.5 Neuropeptides

Yun-Feng Gao, Xun Sun, MD, PhD and Chang-Long Lu, MD, PhD

One way that neurons communicate with each other is via neuropeptides, which are small protein-like peptides. Neuropeptides are neuronal signaling molecules. They can affect the activity of the brain in specific ways. A wide range of brain functions can be effected by different types of neuropeptides, such as metabolism, learning and memory, reproduction, analgesia, reward, food intake, and social behaviors. The following is a list of important neuropeptides related to skin diseases.

7.5.1 Substance P

Substance P (SP) is a peptide composed of a chain of 11 amino acid residues; it belongs to the tachykinin neuropeptide family member. The major function of SP is acting as a neurotransmitter and neuromodulator. Substance P and its closely related neuropeptide neurokinin A (NKA) are produced by a polyprotein precursor after differential splicing of the preprotachykinin a gene.

7.5.1.1 The Functions of SP in Skin

SP can recognize nociception signal, convert the sensing of tissue damage to the sensation of pain, and then transmit information from peripheral receptors to the central nervous system. In other fields, SP has been known to stimulate cell growth in culture, and previous study shows that SP could promote wound healing of nonhealing ulcers in humans. Tissue injury may create a specific microenvironment to induce the systemic participation of stromal-like cells in the repair process. SP, as an injury-inducible factor, can mediate CD29+ stromal-like cell mobilization early in the wound-healing process [131].

7.5.1.2 SP in Skin Disease

Substance P and its receptor(R) neurokinin (NK)-1 may have a role in the pathogenesis of psoriasis and chronic stress. According to previous studies, stress has been reported to take part in the onset and exacerbation of psoriasis, which might mediate the substance P-NK-1 receptor(R) pathway. Pruritus, as a feature of psoriasis, has been correlated to the secretion of SP and severity of stress. The major immunoreactivity for SP is being found in inflammatory cells as a low number of SP-positive nerve fibers in involved and noninvolved skin. Compared to noninvolved psoriatic skin, the number of SP and NK-1R positive inflammatory cells was increased in involved psoriatic skin. Most of the SP-positive cells were lymphocytes, while most of the NK-1R positive cells were mast cells. Also, in the majority of patients, the immunoreactivity of NK-1R has been found as a reticular pattern in the upper part of the epidermis of involved skin. As an indicator of chronic stress, lower cortisol ratios in the patients were correlated to an increased number of SP- and NK-1R positive inflammatory cells in noninvolved psoriatic skin. Higher cortisol ratios to the presence of keratinocyte NK-1R immunoreactivity have been found in involved skin. But, the number of SP-positive fibers or cells could not be correlated to the severity of pruritus [132, 133].

7.5.2 Calcitonin Gene-Related Peptide

Calcitonin gene-related peptide (CGRP) is a member of the calcitonin family of peptides. There are two forms of CGRP in humans, α-CGRP and β-CGRP. α-CGRP is a peptide composed of 37-amino acid peptide, and it is created from the alternative splicing of the calcitonin/CGRP gene located on chromosome 11. Compared with α-CGRP,the β-CGRP differs in three amino acids (in humans), and is encoded in a separate gene in the same vicinity.

7.5.2.1 Functions of CGRP in Skin

CGRP enhances the sensitivity to sensory input at multiple levels in periphery and central nervous system [134]. Peripheral and central neurons can produce CGRP. It is a potent vasodilator peptide that can transmit the sensing of pain. The function and expression of CGRP in spinal cord may differ depending on the location of synthesis.

Most of CGRP is derived from the cell bodies of motor neurons when synthesized in the ventral horn of the spinal cord that play a role in regeneration of nervous tissue after injury. On the contrary, CGRP which derived from dorsal root ganglion may contribute to transmit the sensing of pain. The main source of CGRP in the trigeminal vascular system is the cell bodies on the trigeminal ganglion.

7.5.2.2 CGRP in Skin Diseases

Chronic spontaneous (idiopathic) urticaria: the mechanism for producing wheals in chronic spontaneous (idiopathic) urticaria (CSU) is still incompletely clear. Previously, the model of CSU proposed that leukocyte infiltration with vascular leakage and expression of the potent vasoactive agents, calcitonin gene-related peptide (CGRP) and vascular endothelial growth factor (VEGF), are features of late-phase allergic skin reactions. In CSU, lesional skin has more CGRP+ and VEGF+ cells than nonlesional skin. But, no significant differences were proved in CGRP and VEGF expression between nonlesional skin and controls. In lesional skin, CGRP and CGRP colocalize to UEA-1+ blood vessels. Neutrophils and eosinophils also produce CGRP, and less CGRP can be found in CD90+ fibroblasts, mast cells, CD3+, and CD68+ cells. The expressions of CGRP and VEGF were not related to the duration of the disease. The increased expression of CGRP and VEGF in lesion, but not in uninvolved skin, indicates that these potent vasoactive agents may play a role in tissue edema in CSU. So, it may be represent a novel target in therapy [135].

Atopic patients: Allergen-induced late-phase skin reactions are characterized by erythema and edema, but it is still incompletely clear how the vasoactive mediators are involved in atopic subjects. Limited evidence from human researches shows that infiltrating inflammatory cells in certain allergic tissue reactions, respectively, express calcitonin gene-related peptide (CGRP) and vascular endothelial growth factor (VEGF), potent vasodilator, and permeability factors. Compared with normal skin, the numbers of CGRP-immunoreactive and CGRP mRNA-positive cells were increased in biopsy specimens from sites of late-phase skin reactions; they paralleled the development and resolution of the edematous late-phase skin reaction. After 6 h after allergen challenge, they both have a peak. The majority of CGRP-immunoreactive cells were neutrophils and CD3+ cells, but eosinophils were CGRP-negative. VEGF-immunopositive cell numbers were also increased at 6 h after biopsy specimens from late-phase skin reactions compared with those at control sites, with a lesser but significant response at 24 h. Most of the VEGF+-positive cells were eosinophils, neutrophils, and CD68+ macrophages. Infiltration of inflammatory cells expressing CGRP and VEGF was associated with late-phase skin reactions in atopic subjects. It shows that these vasoactive factors may play a role in the erythema and edema, characteristic of allergic inflammation. So, they may represent novel target in allergic inflammation control [136].

7.5.3 Somatostatin

Somatostatin (SST) is a cyclic peptide composed of a chain of 14 amino acids; it is produced by pancreatic islets, the gastrointestinal tract, nervous system, and thyroid gland. One physiological function of SST is that it can inhibit adenyl cyclase and post-cAMP events in addition to fluid secretion stimulated by agents that do not generate cAMP [137]. Glucose-induced somatostatin secretion is primarily dependent on Ca^{2+}-induced Ca^{2+}-release (CICR) [138]. SST, also known as growth hormone-inhibiting hormone (GHIH), is a peptide hormone that regulates the endocrine system. By interacting with G protein-coupled somatostatin receptors, SST can affect neurotransmission and cell proliferation, and it can inhibit numerous secondary hormones release. And SST can inhibit insulin and glucagon secretion.

7.5.3.1 Functions of Somatostatin in Skin

SST is homologous with cortistatin. It can suppress the release of some other homologs.

7.5.3.2 SST in Skin Disease

Palmoplantar pustulosis (PPP) is one of the variant of psoriasis, which has a female predilection of 90%. PPP is commonest in women who smoke, and its characters are sterile pustules, erythema, and scaling. Palmoplantar skin is rich in eccrine sweat glands, which react in response to heat and mental stimuli, and many patients with PPP (46%) consider stress an obvious worsening factor for precipitation of new pustules.

The eccrine sweat duct has several differences from the interappendageal epidermis. No Langerhans cells are found, but the duct cells express interleukin (IL)1, IL-8, and tumor necrosis factor-α, and they are positive for human leukocyte antigen DR. In palmoplantar skin, the gland and duct also strongly express choline acetyltransferase and acetylcholinesterase (the acetylcholine synthesizing and degrading enzymes), β-adrenergic nicotinic and angiotensin receptors, and parathyroid hormone-related protein. The evidence shows that the gland and duct may be a hitherto neuroendocrine organ which has not been characterized.

SST immunoreactive cells are found in the central and peripheral nervous system, pancreas, intestine, thyroid gland, kidney, adrenals, and other organs. Evidence shows that in epidermis, Langerhans cells, nerve fibers, and Merkel cells are immunoreactive to SST. There are five receptor subtypes that induce SST effects (SSTRs 1–5). Studies showed that some of the receptors are functional, but the function of each receptor has not been clearly characterized in humans. Adams [139] found that proliferating endothelium expresses SSTRs 2 and 5 that may play a role in angiogenesis. In psoriasis, there is a vascular increase in papillary dermis. Expression of SSTRs 1–5 in healthy (hairy) human skin has been reported in psoriasis and atopic dermatitis.

Compared with healthy control skin, there are a number of significant differences in the expression of SSTRs in involved skin. Compared with healthy control skin, in PPP skin, SSTR1's expression has been decreased in a larger proportion of ducts in papillary and reticular dermis, but a larger proportion of ducts overexpress SSTRs 3 and 4; expression did not differ in the coils between PPP and control skin. Compared with healthy controls, the epidermis, in the stratum basale (SB), has weaker expression of SSTRs 1, 3, 4, and 5. The expression of SSTR3 also decreases in the stratum spinosum (SS), but compared with control group, there is stronger expression of SSTR4 in the upper part of vital epidermis in the palmar skin of patients with PPP. Compared with healthy palmar skin, the expression of SSTR1 in the endothelium of PPP skin also decreased, both in the papillary and reticular dermis. Compared with healthy skin, SSTR3 expression was more pronounced in the endothelium of the reticular dermis in PPP skin. Compared with healthy control skin, SSTR2 was expressed in inflammatory cells in PPP skin, and SSTRs 1 and 4 had stronger expression in PPP skin [140].

References

Oxidation and Antioxidants

1. Finkel T. Signal transduction by reactive oxygen species. J Cell Biol. 2011;194:7–15.
2. Hare JM, Stamler JS. NO/redox disequilibrium in the failing heart and cardiovascular system. J Clin Invest. 2005;115:509–17.
3. Shibata M, Ichioka S, Kamiya A. Nitric oxide modulates oxygen consumption by arteriolar walls in rat skeletal muscle. Am J Physiol Heart Circ Physiol. 2005;289:H2673–9.
4. White PJ, Charbonneau A, Cooney GJ, Marette A. Nitrosative modifications of protein and lipid signaling molecules by reactive nitrogen species. Am J Physiol Endocrinol Metab. 2010;299: E768–78.
5. Rindnour LA, Isemberg JS, Espey MG, et al. Nitric oxide regulates angiogenesis through a functional switch involving thrombospondin-1. Proc Natl Acad Sci. 2005;102:13147–52.
6. Rhee SG. Cell signaling. H2O2, a necessary evil for cell signaling. Science. 2006;30:1882–3.
7. Vlasits J, Jakopitsch C, Bernroitner M, et al. Mechanism of catalase activity of heme peroxidase. Arch Biochem Biophys. 2010;500:74–81.
8. Kroviarsky Y, Debbabi M, Bachoual R, et al. Phosphorylation of NADPH oxidase activator 1 (NOXA1) on serine 282 by MAP kinases and on serine 172 by protein kinase C and protein kinase A prevents NOX1 hyperactivation. FASEB J. 2010;24:2077–92.
9. Puig JG, Mateos FA, Diaz VD. Inhibition of xanthine oxidase by allopurinol: a therapeutic option for ischaemia induced pathological process? Ann Rheum Dis. 1989;48:883–8.
10. Maejima Y, Kuroda J, Matsushima S, Ago T, Sadoshima J. Regulation of myocardial growth and death by NAPH oxidase. J Mol Cell Cardiol. 2011;50:408.
11. Dröge W. Free radicals in the physiopathological control of cell function. Physiol Rev. 2002;82:47–95.
12. Buettner GR. Superoxide dismutase in redox biology: the roles of superoxide and hydrogen peroxide. Anticancer Agents Med Chem. 2011;11:341–6.
13. Bochkov VN, Oskolcova OV, Birukov KG, et al. Generation and biological activities of oxidized phospholipids. Antioxid Redox Signal. 2010;12:1009–59.
14. Valko M, Leibfritz D, Moncol J, et al. Free radicals and antioxidants in normal physiological functions and human diseases. Int J Biochem Cell Biol. 2007;39:44–84.
15. White PJ, Charbonneau A, Cooney GJ, Marette A. Nitrosative modifications of protein and lipid signaling molecules by reactive nitrogen species. Am J Physiol Endocrinol Metab. 2010;299:E868–78.
16. Baker PR, Schopfer FJ, O'Donnel VB, Freeman BA. Convergence of nitric oxide and lipids signaling: anti-inflammatory nitro-fatty acids. Free Radic Biol Med. 2009;15:989–1003.
17. Dean RT, Stocker R, Davies M. Biochemistry and pathology of radical-mediated protein oxidation. Biochem J. 1997;324:1–18.

18. Uchida K, Stadtman ER. Covalent attachment of 4-hydroxynonenal to glyceraldehydes-3-phosphate dehydrogenase. A possible involvement of intra-and intermolecular cross-linking reaction. J Biol Chem. 1993;268:6388–93.
19. Baynes JW, Thorpe SR. Role of stress in diabetic complications: a new perspective on an old paradigm. Diabetes. 1999;48:1–9.
20. Hess DT, Matsumoto A, Kim SO, et al. Protein S-nitrosylation: purview and parameters. Nat Rev Mol Cell Biol. 2005;6:150–66.
21. Ischiropèoulos H. Biological selectivity and functional aspects of protein tyrosine nitration. Biochem Biophys Res Commun. 2003;305:776–83.
22. Shigenaga MK, Gimeno CJ, Ames BN. Urinary 8-hydroxy-2'-deoxyguanosine as a biological marker of in vivo oxidative DNA damage. Proc Natl Acad Sci U S A. 1989;86:9697–701.
23. Richter C, Park JW, Ames BN. Normal oxidative damage to mitochondrial and nuclear DNA is extensive. Proc Natl Acad Sci U S A. 1988;85:6465–7.
24. Hara MR, Agrawal N, Kim SF, et al. S-nitrosylated GAPDH initiates apoptotic cell death by nuclear translocation following Siah1 binding. Nat Cell Biol. 2005;7:665–774.
25. Collins AR, Cadet J, Moller L, et al. Are we sure we know how to measure 8-oxo-7,8-dihydroguanine in DNA from human cells? Arch Biochem Biophys. 2004;423:57–65.
26. Morse D, Choi AMK. Heme oxygenase. The "emerging molecule" has arrived. Am J Respir Cell Mol Biol. 2002;27:8–16.
27. Slebos DJ, Ryter SW, Choi AM. Heme oxygenase-I and carbon monoxide in pulmonary medicine. Respir Res. 2003;4:7.
28. Nakao A, Kizimuka K, Stolz DB, et al. Carbon monoxide inhalation protects rat intestinal grafts from ischemia/perfusion injury. Am J Pathol. 2003;163:1587–98.
29. White KA, Marletta MA. Nitric oxide synthase is a cytochrome P-450 type hemoprotein. Biochemistry. 1992;31:6627–31.
30. Petrache I, Otterbein J, Alan GW, et al. Heme oxygenase 1 inhibits TNF-α-induced apoptosis in cultured fibroblasts. Am J Physiol Lung Cell Mol Physiol. 2000;278:L312–9.
31. Dohi K, Satoh K, Ohtaki H, et al. Elevated plasma levels of bilirubin in patients with neurotrauma reflect its pathophysiological role in free radical scavenging. In Vivo. 2005;19:855–60.
32. Cornelli U, Belcaro G, Finco A. The oxidative stress balance measured with different markers, following a single oral antioxidant supplement or a diet poor of antioxidants. JCDSA. 2011;1:64–70.
33. Kuipers I, Guala AS, Aesif SW, et al. Cigarette smoke targets glutaredoxin 1, increasing S-glutationylation and epithelial cell death. Am J Respir Cell Mol Biol. 2011;45:931–7.
34. Purwar N, McGarry J, Kostera J, et al. Interaction of nitric oxide with catalase: structural and kinetic analysis. Biochemistry. 2011;50:4491–503.
35. Figueroa XF, Duling BR. Gap junctions in the control of vascular function. Antioxid Redox Signal. 2009;11:251–66.
36. Manalo DJ, Rowan A, Lavoie T, et al. Transcriptional regulation of vascular endothelial cell response to hypoxia. Blood. 2005;105: 659–69.
37. Bindoli A, Fukuto JM, Forman HJ. Thiol chemistry in peroxidase catalysis and redox signaling. Antioxid Redox Signal. 2008;10: 1549–64.
38. Draganov DI, La Du BN. Pharmacogenetics of paroxonase: a brief review. Naunyn Schmiedebregs Arch Pharmacol. 2004;369:78–88.
39. Aviram M, Rosenblat M. Paraoxonase 1, 2, and 3, oxidative stress, and macrophage foam cell formation during atherosclerosis development. Free Radic Biol Med. 2004;37:1304–16.
40. Teiber JF, Billecke SS, La Du BN, et al. Estrogen esters substrates for human paraoxonase. Arch Biochem Biophys. 2007;461:24–9.
41. Durrington PN, Mackness B, Mackness MI. Paraoxonase and atherosclerosis. Arterioscler Thromb vasc Biol. 2001;21:473–80.
42. Yilmaz N. Relationship between paraoxonase and homocysteine: crossroad of oxidative diseases. Arch Med Sci. 2012;8:138–53.
43. Holven KB, Aukrust P, Retterstøl K, et al. The antiaterogenic function of HDL is impaired in hyperhomocysteinemic subjects. J Nutr. 2008;138:2070–5.
44. Ng CJ, Wadleigh DJ, Gangopadhyay A, et al. Paraoxonase-1 is ubiquitously expressed protein with antioxidant properties and is capable of preventing cell-mediated oxidative modification of low density lipoproteins. J Biol Chem. 2001;276:44444–9.
45. Camps J, Marsillach J, Joven J. Measurement of serum paraoxonase-1 activity in the evaluation of liver function. World J Gastroenterol. 2009;15:1923–33.
46. Navab M, Berliner JA, Subbanagounder G, et al. HDL and the inflammatory response induced by LDL-derived phospholipids. Arterioscler Thromb Vasc Biol. 2001;21:481–8.
47. Costa LG, Giodano G, Furlong CE. Pharmacological and dietary modulators of paraoxonase 1 (PON1) activity and expression: the hunt goes on. Biochem Pharmacol. 2011;81:337–44.
48. Williamson G, Manach C. Bioavailability and bioefficacy of polyphenols in humans. II. Review of 93 intervention studies. Am J Clin Nutr. 2005;81:243S–55.
49. Buettner GR. The pecking order of free radicals and antioxidants: lipid peroxidation, alpha tocopherol, and ascorbate. Arch Biochem Biophys. 1993;300:535–42.
50. Brigelius-Flohé R, Brigelius-Flohé L. Basic principles and emerging concepts in the redox control of transcription factors. Antioxid Redox Signal. 2011;15:2335–81.
51. He X, Ma Q. Nrf2 cysteine residues are critical for oxidant/electrophile-sensing, Kelch-like ECH-Associated Protein-1-dependent ubiquination-proteosomal degradation and transcription activation. Mol Pharmacol. 2009;76:1265–78.
52. Moi P, Chan K, Asunis I, et al. Isolation of NF-E2-related factor 2 (Nrf2), a NF-E2-like basic leucine zipper transcriptional activator that binds to the tandem NF-E2/AP1 repeat of the β-globin locus control region. Proc Natl Acad Sci U S A. 1994;91:9926–30.
53. Tufekci KU, Civi Bayin E, Genc S, Genc K. The Nrf2/ARE pathway: a promising target to counteract mitochondrial dysfunction in Parkinson's disease. SAGE-Hindawi Access to Res. 2011;article ID 314082.
54. Huxford T, Ghosh G. A structural guide to proteins of the NF-kB signaling molecule. Cold Spring Harbor Perspect Biol. 2009;1:a000075.
55. Garbin U, Fratta Pasini A, Stranieri C, et al. Cigarette smoking blocks the protective expression of Nrf2/ARE pathway in peripheral mononuclear cells of young heavy smokers favoring inflammation. PLoS One. 2009;4:e8225.
56. Mac NW. Oxidant/antioxidants and COPD. Chest. 2000;117: 303S–17.
57. Vassalle C, Boni C, Di Cecco P, et al. Automation and validation of a fast method for the assessment of in vivo oxidative stress level. Clin Chem Lab Med. 2006;44:1372–5.
58. Lubrano V, Vassalle C, L'Abbate A, Zucchelli GC. A new method to evaluate oxidative stress in humans. Immuno Anal Biologie Spécialisée. 2002;17:172–5.
59. Kamezaki F, Yamashita K, Kubara T, et al. Derivatives of reactive oxygen metabolites correlates with high-sensitivity C-Reactive protein. J Atheroscler Thromb. 2008;15:206–12.
60. Cighetti G, Paroni R, Marzorati S, et al. Evaluation of oxidative stress in critically ill patients by a commercial assay and gas chromatografic-mass spectrometry. Clin Chem. 2005;51:1515–7.

Antimicrobial Peptide

61. Afshar M, Gallo RL. Innate immune defense system of the skin. Vet Dermatol. 2013;24(1):32–8.
62. Ganz T. Defensins: antimicrobial peptides of innate immunity. Nat Rev Immunol. 2003;3(9):710–20.

Cytokines and Eicosanoids

63. Paul WE. Fundamental immunology. 7th ed. Wolters Kluwer health/Lippincott Williams & Wilkins; 2013.
64. "Cytokine". In: Lackie J. A dictionary of biomedicine. Oxford University Press; 2010. ISBN 9780199549351.
65. "Cytokine". In: Stedman's medical dictionary. 28th ed. Wolters Kluwer Health/Lippincott, Williams & Wilkins; 2006.
66. Owen JA, Jenni P, Stranford SA. Kuby immunology. 7th ed. Houndmills, Basingstoke: Macmillan Higher Education; New York 2012.
67. Ling NR, Brown B, Hardie D. Production of immunoglobulins by human sIgD+ and sIgD- human blood B lymphocytes in response to stimulation with activated T cells and agonistic antibodies; effect of IL-10, IL-2 and mode of activation of T cells. Clin Exp Immunol. 1995;101(2):369–75.
68. Feldmann M, Brennan FM, Maini RN. Role of cytokines in rheumatoid arthritis. Annu Rev Immunol. 1996;14:397–440.
69. O'Reilly S, Cant R, Ciechomska M, van Laar JM. Interleukin-6: a new therapeutic target in systemic sclerosis? Clin Translat Immunol. 2013;2(4):e4.
70. Geskin LJ, Viragova S, Stolz DB, Fuschiotti P. Interleukin-13 is over-expressed in cutaneous T-cell lymphoma cells and regulates their proliferation. Blood. 2015;125:2798–805, pii: blood-2014-07.
71. Choubey D, Moudgil KD. Interferons in autoimmune and inflammatory diseases: regulation and roles[J]. J Interferon Cytokine Res. 2011;31(12):857–65.
72. Nestle FO, Conrad C, Tun-Kyi A, Homey B, Gombert M, Boyman O, et al. Plasmacytoid predendritic cells initiate psoriasis through interferon-alpha production. J Exp Med. 2005;202:135–43.
73. Afshar M, Martinez AD, Gallo RL, Hata TR. Induction and exacerbation of psoriasis with interferon-alpha therapy for hepatitis C: a review and analysis of 36 cases. J Eur Acad Dermatol Venereol. 2013;27:771–8.
74. Bissonnette R, Papp K, Maari C, Yao Y, Robbie G, White WI, Le C, White B. A randomized, double-blind, placebo-controlled, phase I study of MEDI-545, an anti-interferon-alfa monoclonal antibody, in subjects with chronic psoriasis. J Am Acad Dermatol. 2010;62:427–36.
75. Fierlbeck G, Rassner G, Müller C. Psoriasis induced at the injection site of recombinant interferon gamma. Results of immunohistologic investigations. Arch Dermatol. 1990;126:351–5.
76. Johnson-Huang LM, Suárez-Fariñas M, Pierson KC, Fuentes-Duculan J, Cueto I, Lentini T, Sullivan-Whalen M, Gilleaudeau P, Krueger JG, Haider AS, Lowes M. A single intradermal injection of IFN-gamma induces an inflammatory state in both non-lesional psoriatic and healthy skin. J Invest Dermatol. 2012;132:1177–87.
77. Chu WM. Tumor necrosis factor. Cancer Lett. 2013;328(2):222–5.
78. Makris MP, Papadavid E, Zuberbier T. The use of biologicals in cutaneous allergies – present and future. Curr Opin Allergy Clin Immunol. 2014;14(5):409–16.
79. Arican O, Aral M, Sasmaz S, Ciragil P. Serum levels of TNF-alpha, IFN-gamma, IL-6, IL-8, IL-12, IL-17, and IL-18 in patients with active psoriasis and correlation with disease severity. Mediators Inflamm. 2005;5:273–9.
80. van der Zee HH, de Ruiter L, van den Broecke DG, Dik WA, Laman JD, Prens EP. Elevated levels of tumour necrosis factor (TNF)-α, interleukin (IL)-1β and IL-10 in hidradenitis suppurativa skin: a rationale for targeting TNF-α and IL-1β. Br J Dermatol. 2011;164(6):1292–8.
81. Akagawa KS. Functional heterogeneity of colony-stimulating factor-induced human monocyte-derived macrophages. Int J Hematol. 2002;76(1):27–34.
82. Greter M, Lelios I, Pelczar P, Hoeffel G, Price J, Leboeuf M, Kündig TM, Frei K, Ginhoux F, Merad M, Becher B. Stroma-derived interleukin-34 controls the development and maintenance of langerhans cells and the maintenance of microglia. Immunity. 2012;37(6):1050–60.
83. Chiang MF, Yang SY, Lin IY, Hong JB, Lin SJ, Ying HY, Chen CM, Wu SY, Liu FT, Lin KI. Inducible deletion of the Blimp-1 gene in adult epidermis causes granulocyte-dominated chronic skin inflammation in mice. Proc Natl Acad Sci U S A. 2013; 110(16):6476–81.
84. Prignano F, Arnaboldi F, Cornaghi L, Landoni F, Tripo L, Preis FW, Donetti E. Tumor necrosis factor-alpha and interleukin-17 differently affects Langerhans cell distribution and activation in an innovative three-dimensional model of normal human skin. Eur J Cell Biol. 2015;94(2):71–7.
85. Griffith JW, Sokol CL, Luster AD. Chemokines and chemokine receptors: positioning cells for host defense and immunity. Ann Rev Immunol Vol. 2014;32:659–702.
86. Dubinett SM, Lee J, Sharma S, et al. Chemokines: can effector cells be re-directed to the site of tumor? Cancer J. 2010;16(4):325.
87. Steen A, Larsen O, Thiele S, Rosenkilde MM. Biased and g protein-independent signaling of chemokine receptors. Front Immunol. 2014;5:277.
88. Sugaya M. Chemokines and skin diseases. Arch Immunol Ther Exp (Warsz). 2015;63(2):109–15. doi:10.1007/s00005-014-0313-y. Epub 2014 Sep 3.
89. Chung BM, Arutyunov A, Ilagan E, Yao N, Wills-Karp M, Coulombe PA. Regulation of C-X-C chemokine gene expression by keratin 17 and hnRNP K in skin tumor keratinocytes. J Cell Biol. 2015;208(5):613–27.
90. Miyagaki T, Sugaya M, Oka T, Fujita H, Sato S. Serum chemokine levels differentially regulated by vorinostat in a Sézary syndrome patient. Br J Dermatol. 2015;173:620–2. doi:10.1111/bjd.13696.
91. Daggett RN, Kurata M, Abe S, Onishi I, Miura K, Sawada Y, Tanizawa T, Kitagawa M. Expression dynamics of CXCL12 and CXCR4 during the progression of mycosis fungoides. Br J Dermatol. 2014;171(4):722–31.
92. Poniatowski LA, Wojdasiewicz P, Gasik R, Szukiewicz D. Transforming growth factor beta family: insight into the role of growth factors in regulation of fracture healing biology and potential clinical applications. Mediators Inflamm. 2015;2015:137823.
93. Wittmann M, McGonagle D, Werfel T. Cytokines as therapeutic targets in skin inflammation. Cytokine Growth Factor Rev. 2014;25(4):443–51.
94. Li D, Li X, Wang A, Meisgen F, Pivarcsi A, Sonkoly E, Ståhle M, Xu Landén N. MicroRNA-31 promotes skin wound healing by enhancing keratinocyte proliferation and migration. J Invest Dermatol. 2015;135:1676–85. doi:10.1038/jid.2015.48.
95. Bassino E, Gasparri F, Giannini V, Munaron L. Paracrine crosstalk between human hair follicle dermal papilla cells and microvascular endothelial cells. Exp Dermatol. 2015;24:388–90. doi:10.1111/exd.12670.
96. Capra V, Rovati GE, Mangano P, Buccellati C, Murphy RC, Sala A. Transcellular biosynthesis of eicosanoid lipid mediators. Biochim Biophys Acta. 2015;1851(4):377–82.
97. Funk CD. Prostaglandins and leukotrienes: advances in eicosanoid biology. Science. 2001;294(5548):1871–5.
98. Haeggström JZ, Rinaldo-Matthis A, Wheelock CE, Wetterholm A. Advances in eicosanoid research, novel therapeutic implications. Biochem Biophys Res Commun. 2010;396(1):135–9.
99. Serhan CN, Chiang N, Dalli J, Levy BD. Lipid mediators in the resolution of inflammation. Cold Spring Harb Perspect Biol. 2014;7(2):a016311.
100. Liu M, Saeki K, Matsunobu T, Okuno T, Koga T, Sugimoto Y, Yokoyama C, Nakamizo S, Kabashima K, Narumiya S, Shimizu T, Yokomizo T. 12-Hydroxyheptadecatrienoic acid promotes epidermal wound healing by accelerating keratinocyte migration via the BLT2 receptor. J Exp Med. 2014;211(6):1063–78.
101. Sumida H, Yanagida K, Kita Y, Abe J, Matsushima K, Nakamura M, Ishii S, Sato S, Shimizu T. Interplay between CXCR2 and

BLT1 facilitates neutrophil infiltration and resultant keratinocyte activation in a murine model of imiquimod-induced psoriasis. J Immunol. 2014;192(9):4361–9.
102. Oyoshi MK, He R, Li Y, Mondal S, Yoon J, Afshar R, Chen M, Lee DM, Luo HR, Luster AD, Cho JS, Miller LS, Larson A, Murphy GF, Geha RS. Leukotriene B4-driven neutrophil recruitment to the skin is essential for allergic skin inflammation. Immunity. 2012;37(4):747–58.

Complement System

103. Moffitt MC, Frank MM. Complement resistance in microbes. Springer Semin Immunopathol. 1994;15:327–44.
104. Morgan BP, Marchbank KJ, Longhi MP, Harris CL, Gallimore AM. Complement: central to innate immunity and bridging to adaptive responses. Immunol Lett. 2005;97:171–9.
105. Walport MJ. Complement. First of two parts. N Engl J Med. 2001;344:1058–66.
106. Hawlisch H, Köhl J. Complement and toll-like receptors: key regulators of adaptive immune responses. Mol Immunol. 2006;43:13–21.
107. Walport MJ. Complement. Second of two parts. N Engl J Med. 2001;344:1140–4.
108. Nauta AJ, Castellano G, Xu W, Woltman AM, Borrias MC, Daha MR, et al. Opsonization with C1q and mannose-binding lectin targets apoptotic cells to dendritic cells. J Immunol. 2004;173:3044–50.
109. Gál P, Dobó J, Závodszky P, Sim RB. Early complement proteases: C1r, C1s and MASPs. A structural insight into activation and functions. Mol Immunol. 2009;46:2745–52.
110. Rus H, Cudrici C, Niculescu F. The role of the complement system in innate immunity. Immunol Res. 2005;33:103–12.
111. Liszewski MK, Farries TC, Lublin DM, Rooney IA, Atkinson JP. Control of the complement system. Adv Immunol. 1996;61:201–83.
112. Lindahl G, Sjöbring U, Johnsson E. Human complement regulators: a major target for pathogenic microorganisms. Curr Opin Immunol. 2000;12:44–51.
113. Davis AE. The pathophysiology of hereditary angioedema. Clin Immunol. 2005;114:3–9.
114. Nauta AJ, Roos A, Daha MR. A regulatory role for complement in innate immunity and autoimmunity. Int Arch Allergy Immunol. 2004;134:310–23.
115. Rauterberg A, Jung EG, Rauterberg EW. Complement deposits in epidermal cells after ultraviolet B exposure. Photodermatol Photoimmunol Photomed. 1993;9(4):135–43.
116. Ballanti E, Perricone C, Greco E, Ballanti M, Di Muzio G, Chimenti MS, Perricone R. Complement and autoimmunity. Immunol Res. 2013;56(2–3):477–91.
117. Pettigrew HD, Teuber SS, Gershwin ME. Clinical significance of complement deficiencies. Ann N Y Acad Sci. 2009;1173:108–23.
118. Boackle SA. Complement and autoimmunity. Biomed Pharmacother. 2003;57:269–73.
119. Fukuoka Y, Hite MR, Dellinger AL, Schwartz LB. Human skin mast cells express complement factors C3 and C5. J Immunol. 2013;191(4):1827–34.
120. Colten HR, Strunk RC, Perlmutter DH, Cole FS. Regulation of complement protein biosynthesis in mononuclear phagocytes. Ciba Found Symp. 1986;118:141–54.
121. Pasch MC, Van Den Bosch NH, Daha MR, Bos JD, Asghar SS. Synthesis of complement components C3 and factor B in human keratinocytes is differentially regulated by cytokines. J Invest Dermatol. 2000;114(1):78–82.
122. Katz Y, Nadiv O, Rapoport MJ, Loos M. IL-17 regulates gene expression and protein synthesis of the complement system, C3 and factor B, in skin fibroblasts. Clin Exp Immunol. 2000;120(1):22–9.
123. Takahara M, Kang K, Liu L, Yoshida Y, McCormick TS, Cooper KD. iC3b arrests monocytic cell differentiation into CD1c-expressing dendritic cell precursors: a mechanism for transiently decreased dendritic cells in vivo after human skin injury by ultraviolet B. J Invest Dermatol. 2003;120(5):802–9.
124. Yoshida Y, Kang K, Berger M, Chen G, Gilliam AC, Moser A, Wu L, Hammerberg C, Cooper KD. Monocyte induction of IL-10 and down-regulation of IL-12 by iC3b deposited in ultraviolet-exposed human skin. J Immunol. 1998;161(11):5873–9.
125. Biesecker G, Lavin L, Ziskind M, Koffler D. Cutaneous localization of the membrane attack complex in discoid and systemic lupus erythematosus. N Engl J Med. 1982;306:264–70.
126. Helm KF, Peters MS. Deposition of membrane attack complex in cutaneous lesions of lupus erythematosus. J Am Acad Dermatol. 1993;28:687–91.
127. Paronetto F, Koffler D. Immunofluorescent localization of immunoglobulins, complement, and fibrinogen in human diseases. I. Systemic lupus erythematosus. J Clin Invest. 1965;44:1657–64.
128. Lachmann PJ, Muller-Eberhard HJ, Kunkel HG, Paronetto F. The localization of in vivo bound complement in tissue section. J Exp Med. 1962;115:63–82.
129. Mascaró Jr JM, Hausmann G, Herrero C, Grau JM, Cid MC, Palou J, et al. Membrane attack complex deposits in cutaneous lesions of dermatomyositis. Arch Dermatol. 1995;131:1386–92.
130. Chimenti MS, Ballanti E, Triggianese P, Perricone R. Vasculitides and the complement system: a comprehensive review. Clin Rev Allergy Immunol. 2014;49:333–46.

Neuropeptides

131. Hong HS, et al. A new role of substance P as an injury-inducible messenger for mobilization of CD29+ stromal-like cells. Nat Med. 2009;15(4):425–35.
132. Remröd C, et al. Study of substance P and its receptor neurokinin-1 in psoriasis and their relation to chronic stress and pruritus. Arch Dermatol Res. 2007;299(2):85–91.
133. Snider RM, et al. A potent nonpeptide antagonist of the substance P (NK1) receptor. Science. 1991;251(4992):435–7.
134. Russo AF, et al. Calcitonin gene-related peptide (CGRP): a New target for migraine. Annu Rev Pharmacol Toxicol. 2015;55:533–52.
135. Kay AB, et al. Calcitonin gene-related peptide and vascular endothelial growth factor are expressed in lesional but not uninvolved skin in chronic spontaneous urticarial. Clin Exp Allergy. 2014;44(8):1053–60.
136. Kay AB. Calcitonin gene-related peptide and vascular endothelial growth factor–positive inflammatory cells in late-phase allergic skin reactions in atopic subjects. J Allergy Clin Immunol. 2011;127(1):232–7.
137. Caroli A, et al. Effect of longacting somatostatin analogue on kidney and cyst growth in autosomal dominant polycystic kidney disease (ALADIN): a randomised, placebo-controlled, multicentre trial. Lancet. 2013;382(9903):1485–95.
138. Zhang Q, et al. R-type Ca(2+)-channel-evoked CICR regulates glucose-induced somatostatin secretion. Nat Cell Biol. 2007;9(4):453–60.
139. Adams RL, Adams IP, Lindow SW, et al. Somatostatin receptors 2 and 5 are preferentially expressed in proliferating endothelium. Br J Cancer. 2005;92:1493–8.
140. Hagforsen E. Somatostatin receptors are strongly expresssed in palmoplantar sweat glands and ducts: studies of normal and palmoplantar pustulosis skin. Clin Exp Dermatol. 2011;36(5):521–7.

Part III

Immunodermatological Conditions

1.1 Overview

It has been estimated that about 40% of skin diseases are immune-related. Immunological responses may work either at the initiation, progression, or ending of certain skin diseases. In this part of the book, we categorized dozens of immune related skin diseases according to their etiologies, immnopathogenesis, and that of immuno-activities involved. Chapter 8 describes a group of conditions with clear etiology, for example, bacterial or viral skin infection, that often evoke a well elucidated immune response in the skin. Changes in general conditions may also induce immunological responses in the skin, and typical conditions as such are described in chapter 9. It is often the case in dermatology that a skin condition starts through the immunological reactions of an array of classified or unknown factors. More than a dozen of such typical conditions are described in chapter 10, in the aim to understand the involvement of immune responses in them, and the subsequent strategies to manage these frustrating conditions. Genetic defects of the human immune system often lead to manifestations in the skin. Chapter 11 describes a couple of skin conditions of primary Immunodeficiency or hereditary autoinflammatary reactions. It is of great significance that these model diseases open insights into the mechanistics of the immune system as a whole. Tumor immunology is a fast growing field in modern medicine, inspired by successful reports on tumor immunotherapy. Chapter 12 covers several benign and malignant skin tumors, especially the in focus tumor model of melanoma, immunological study and management of which give hope to control of tumors. Lastly, chapter 13 describes several skin specific or non-specific autoimmune conditions, their etiologies, immunopathogenesis and immune-based management.

Skin Diseases Caused by Factors from the Environment

8

Lei Ma, Min Chen, Zhenzong Fa, Weihua Pan, Wanqing Liao, Xing-Hua Gao, Wei Huo, Yang Yang, Hong-Duo Chen, H.M. Holahan, A.C. Laureano, R.A. Schwartz, Xiao-ying Chen, Alex Anstey, Joachim Bugert, Tsu-Man Chiu, Yi-Giien Tsai, Shivani Nanda, Henry W. Lim, Wen-Hui Wang, Lin-Feng Li, Yong-Hu Sun, and Fu-Ren Zhang

L. Ma (✉)
Department of Dermatology, Binzhou Medical University Hospital, Yantai, China
e-mail: iwf50@sina.com

M. Chen • Z. Fa • W. Pan • W. Liao (✉)
Shanghai Key Laboratory of Molecular Medical Mycology, Department of Dermatology, Shanghai ChangZheng Hospital, Second Military Medical University, Shanghai 200003, China
e-mail: liaowanqing@sohu.com

X.-H. Gao (✉) • W. Huo • Y. Yang • H. D. Chen
Department of Dermatology, No.1 Hospital of China Medical University, Shenyang 110001, China
e-mail: gaobarry@hotmail.com

H.M. Holahan • A.C. Laureano • R.A. Schwartz (✉)
Departments of Dermatology, Pediatrics, and Pathology, Rutgers-New Jersey Medical School and Rutgers University School of Public Affairs and Administration, Newark, NJ, USA
e-mail: raschwartz@gmail.com

X.-y. Chen (✉)
Department of Dermatology, Ruijin Hospital, School of Medicine, Shanghai Jiaotong University, Shanghai 200025, China
e-mail: endophasia@163.com

A. Anstey
Royal Gwent Hospital, Aneurin Bevan Health Board, Newport NP20 4SZ, UK

Dermatology and Wound Healing Department, Cardiff University, School of Medicine, Cardiff CF14 4XN, UK
e-mail: Alex.Anstey@wales.nhs.uk

J. Bugert
Institut für Mikrobiologie der Bundeswehr, Neuherbergstr. 11, 80937 München, Germany
e-mail: joachim1bugert@bundeswehr.org

T.-M. Chiu
Department of Dermatology, Changhua Christian Hospital, Changhua, Taiwan
e-mail: 68003@cch.org.tw

Y.-G. Tsai (✉)
Department of Pediatrics, Changhua Christian Hospital, Changhua, Taiwan
e-mail: 107239@cch.org.tw

S. Nanda, MD
Department of Dermatology, Henry Ford Hospital, Detroit, MI, USA

H.W. Lim, MD (✉)
Department of Dermatology, Henry Ford Hospital, Detroit, MI, USA

Department of Dermatology, Henry Ford Medical Center – New Center One, 3031 West Grand Blvd, Suite 800, Detroit, MI 48202, USA
e-mail: hlim1@hfhs.org

W.-H. Wang
Department of Dermatology, Peking University Third Hospital, Beijing 100191, China

L.-F. Li (✉)
Department of Dermatology, Allergy and Clinical Immunology Center, Capital Medical University Beijing Friendship Hospital, Beijing 100050, China
e-mail: zoonli@sina.com

Y.-H. Sun, MD, PhD • F.-R. Zhang, MD, PhD (✉)
Shandong Provincial Institute of Dermatology and Venereology, Shandong Academy of Medical Science, 27397, Jingshi Road, Jinan, Shandong 250022, China
e-mail: zhangfuren@hotmail.com

X.-H. Gao, H.-D. Chen (eds.), *Practical Immunodermatology*, DOI 10.1007/978-94-024-0902-4_8

Contents

8.1 Bacterial Infectious Skin Diseases

Lei Ma, MD, PhD

Normal bacterial flora on the skin can be divided into two categories, namely, resident and transient. *Staphylococcus epidermidis* is the dominant species of resident bacteria [1]. Other resident bacteria include *Staphylococcus hominis*, other coagulase-negative *Staphylococci*, and coryneform bacteria (*Propionibacteria*, *Corynebacteria*, *Dermobacteria*, and *Micrococci*) [2]. In general, resident flora is less likely to be associated with skin infections but may cause infections on non-intact skin [3]. *Staphylococcus aureus*, *Streptococcus*, and Gram-negative bacilli are the dominant pathogenic flora of transient bacteria [4]. Their transmissibility depends on the species present, the number of microorganisms on skin surface, and the degree of skin moisture [5, 6]. There is a close relationship between bacteria and skin diseases. Infection by bacteria can cause erysipelas; toxin-mediated diseases, such as staphylococcal scalded skin syndrome (SSSS); as well as immune-mediated disease, such as acute guttate psoriasis [7–9].

8.1.1 Erysipelas

8.1.1.1 Introduction

Erysipelas, also called superficial cellulitis, is a rapidly spreading bacterial skin infection involving the upper dermis that characteristically extends into the superficial cutaneous lymphatics [10]. The lesion classically exhibits a sharply raised border with abrupt demarcation from healthy skin and with advancing margins. More severe lesions can exhibit vesicles and bullae, along with petechiae and even frank necrosis. The infection may rapidly invade and spread through the lymphatic vessels, then cause regional lymph node enlargement and tenderness. Some systemic symptoms such as fever, chills, and malaise are usually accompanied [11]. Erysipelas has been reported in all age groups, but it does appear that the peak incidence is 60–80 years old. The face and lower extremities are the most easily affected area, which account for 5–20% and 70–80% of patients, respectively [12]. Bacterial inoculation into an area of skin trauma is the initial event in developing erysipelas. Thus, infections of the nasopharynx as well as venous insufficiency, inflammatory dermatoses, dermatophyte infections, and surgical incisions of the lower extremities are the common incentive for erysipelas [13–15]. Cultures together with other available evidence such as serological data indicate that the group A streptococci strain is the most prevalent pathogen [16, 17].

8.1.1.2 Genetic Susceptibility to Erysipelas

Host genetics is a significant factor in determining susceptibility to severe group A streptococcal sepsis in mouse and humans [18, 19]. Mouse susceptibility loci for group A streptococcal infection have been mapped to chromosome 17, including the mouse MHC region (syntenic to human 6p21); chromosome 7, which is also linked with susceptibility to *Streptococcus pneumoniae* infection (syntenic to human 19q13.1–13.3); chromosome 2, including genes of the interleukin 1 alpha; and prostaglandin E synthetase pathways (syntenic to human 2q14 and 9q33–34) [20–22]. In human, the HLA system has been found to take part in the formation of predisposition to erysipelas and its clinical forms. HLA-A2, B5, B12, and Bw35 are associated with erysipelas infection, while HLA-A10, Aw12, B7, and B8 have, seemingly, a protective character [23]. Additionally, several SNPs in the promoter of AGTR1 (angiotensin II receptor type I) has also been associated with susceptibility to erysipelas [24].

8.1.1.3 Pathogenesis

The human contact system is composed of three enzymatic factors (coagulation factor XI and XII, plasma kallikrein, and the nonenzymatic cofactor high-molecular-weight kininogen (HK)) and activated with three potential consequences (the initiation of the intrinsic pathway of coagulation, the generation of antibacterial peptides, and the release of bradykinin) (Fig. 8.1) [11, 25, 26]. The human contact system interacts with the cell surface of many bacterial pathogens, including group A streptococci [27, 28]. In group A streptococci, HK is bound to the bacteria by the cell-wall-attached M protein, which activates neutrophils by binding to β2 integrins and then leads to the secretion of the heparin-binding protein (HBP) and the induction of vascular leakage [29, 30]. On the other hand, when HK is associated to the cell surface of group A streptococci, HK is cleaved and bradykinin is released, which further increases vascular permeability and induces fever and pain [31].

In erysipelas, group A streptococcal is confirmed by positive bacterial cultures, immunohistochemical stain and electron micrographs in inflamed skin tissue, and specific streptococcal antibodies in convalescent sera [11]. Moreover, in the inflamed skin tissues, the phenomenon of a limited solubilization of the surface-attached M protein, degradation of HK, upregulation of bradykinin-1 receptor, and increased levels of HBP also demonstrate the activation of the contact system and neutrophils [11]. These support the notion that the inflammation of erysipelas is induced close to the bacterial surfaces and not only as a distant effect of streptococcal toxins [11].

8.1.1.4 Clinical Presentation

Erysipelas begins as a small erythematous patch that progresses to a fiery-red, indurated, tense, and shiny plaque. As abovementioned, the classical lesion exhibits a sharply raised border with abrupt demarcation from healthy skin and with advancing margins. Numerous vesicles and bullae, along with petechiae and even frank necrosis, can be found in more severe situation. Local signs of inflammation include warmth, edema, and tenderness. Lymphatic involvement often is manifested by overlying skin streaking and regional lymphadenopathy.

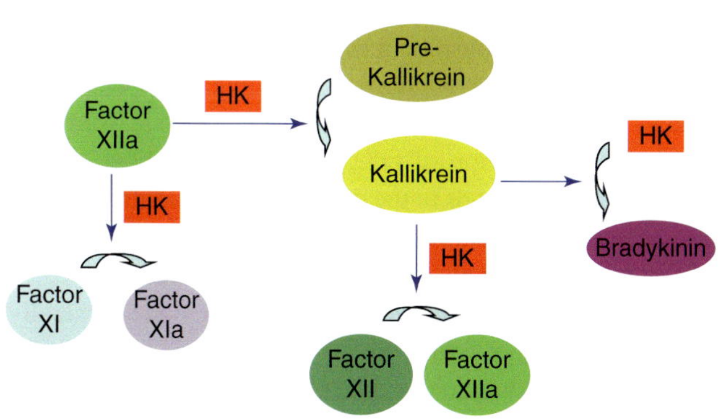

Fig. 8.1 The composition and activation of the contact system

8.1.1.5 Management

Erysipelas may be severe, especially in the elderly with comorbidities, but, unlike necrotizing infections, is generally not life-threatening [32]. As group A streptococci stain is the most prevalent pathogen of erysipelas, penicillin has remained as a first-line therapy [33, 34]. If the patient has an allergy to penicillin, the first-generation cephalosporin or macrolide, such as erythromycin or azithromycin, can be used. In addition to antibiotic treatment, it is also important that patients with acute infections involving the lower legs should limit their activity and keep affected limbs elevated to decrease swelling. Coverage for staphylococcus aureus is not usually necessary for typical infections, but it should be considered in patients who do not improve with penicillin or who present with atypical forms of erysipelas, including bullous erysipelas.

Recurrence is the major complication of erysipelas, which occurs in 10–50 % of the patients [35, 36]. Long-term antibiotic prophylaxis has the potential benefit of preventing recurrences [37]. As the research reported that through antibiotic prophylaxis taking for 30.6 months, 84 and 72 % of the patients were recurrence-free after 1 and 2 years, respectively [36]. Patients with recurrent erysipelas should be educated regarding local antisepsis and general wound care. Predisposing lower extremity skin lesions should be treated aggressively to prevent superinfection.

8.1.2 Staphylococcal Scalded Skin Syndrome (SSSS)

8.1.2.1 Introduction

SSSS is a potentially life-threatening disorder caused mainly by a phage group II *Staphylococcus aureus*. *Staphylococcus aureus* can release serine protease exfoliate toxins and cleave desmosomal cadherins, specifically desmoglein-1 (Dsg1) in the superficial epidermis, and then result in destruction of cell–cell adhesion and cause blistering and denuding of the skin. SSSS is more common in newborns, infants, and children less than 5 years old than in adults [38, 39].

8.1.2.2 Pathogenesis

Staphylococcus aureus is usually regarded as a transient, pathogenic organism in the skin, and approximately 20 % of the general population always harbors it on the nasal mucosa without any pathogenic event [40]. However, in certain situations, *Staphylococcus aureus* can express a wide array of potential virulence factors, which are involved in disruption of the epithelial barrier, inhibition of opsonization by antibody and complement, interference with neutrophil chemotaxis, cytolysis of neutrophils, and inactivation of antimicrobial peptides [41]. The involvement of exfoliative toxins (ETs) in the pathogenesis of SSSS was first speculated by the injection of organisms isolated from SSSS patients into neonatal mice causing intraepidermal splitting resembling the human disease [42]. There are three serological forms of staphylococcal ETs (ETA, ETB, and ETD), among which only ETA and ETB have been firmly linked to human SSSS, and ETB is more frequently isolated than ETA in children with generalized SSSS [43]. Staphylococcal ETs can cleave Dsg1, a desmosomal cadherin involved in keratinocyte cell-to-cell adhesion, resulting in a deterioration of keratinocyte-to-keratinocyte adhesivity in the stratum granulosum, as well as bullae formation and denudation [44–46]. As the relative quantity of Dsg1 differs with age, it may partially explain the elevated frequency of SSSS in children younger than 5 years old. Additionally, children are more at risk because of the lack of immunity and immature renal clearance capability [43]. Maternal antibodies transferred to infants through breast milk are believed to be partially protective, but a neonate can still suffer from SSSS, which may be a result of inadequate immunity or immature renal clearance of exotoxin [47–50]. On the other hand, the presence of antibodies specific for exotoxins and improved renal clearance may partially contribute to the reduced frequency of SSSS in adults.

The superantigen theory was once speculated to explore the possible mechanisms of intraepidermal separation caused by staphylococcal ETs [46, 51]. However, the following observations argues about this superantigen theory [46]: there is no finding of obviously intense T-cell recruitment into the epidermis in the location of blisters; there is no finding of keratinocyte necrosis as being expected with superantigen-stimulated T cells; and purified recombinant ETA fails to stimulate T cells of both human and murine.

Staphylococcal ETA and ETB share significant homology with other known trypsin-like serine proteases, including the catalytic triad, and their three-dimensional structures resemble those of glutamate-specific serine proteases [46, 52, 53]. ETA and ETB can cleave human and mouse Dsg1 at one position after glutamic acid residue 381, which is located in the putative calcium-binding site of Dsg1. The removal of calcium ions can also block the cleavage reaction of Dsg1 by both ETA and ETB [54]. In addition, ETA and ETB may completely lose their Dsg1-cleaving activities if the predicted catalytic serine is substituted [45]. So, in SSSS, staphylococcal ETA and ETB function as glutamate-specific serine proteases to specifically recognize and cleave the single peptide bond within the calcium-binding site of Dsg1 and result in the epidermal exfoliation [51].

8.1.2.3 Clinical Presentation

Severity of SSSS varies from a few blisters localized to the site of infection to a severe exfoliation affecting almost the entire body. SSSS may firstly present a prodrome of irritability, malaise, and fever. Abrupt, faint, erythematous, tender patches may be the initial skin damage, and then the patches become well demarcated and coalesce into a confluent scarlatiniform erythema. Fragile bullae develop within the erythematous areas that can extend to large sheets of epidermal exfoliation [38]. Positive Nikolsky's sign is often observed.

8.1.2.4 Treatment

SSSS will continue to progress until circulating exotoxin has been neutralized by antibodies or excreted via the kidneys, so it is important to start antibiotics as early as possible [55]. Penicillinase-resistant penicillins are recommended. If a patient has a penicillin allergy, clarithromycin or cefuroxime may be used. If a patient is not improving, it is necessary to consider ET produced by methicillin-resistant *Staphylococcus aureus* and switch to vancomycin [56]. And in severe cases, IVIG treatment is strongly recommended [57].

8.2 Human Immune Responses to Invasive Fungal Pathogen

Min Chen, Zhenzong Fa, Weihua Pan, and Wanqing Liao

Approximately 1.5 million of fungal species exist in the environment, and approximately 400 species are documented as human pathogens [58]. The threat of fungal pathogens to human health has steadily risen over the past several decades, primarily in hosts with impaired immunity as a consequence of medical interventions and HIV infection [59–61]. The main fungal pathogens that exhibit the potential to cause invasive infections, including *Candida albicans*, *Aspergillus fumigatus*, *Cryptococcus neoformans*, and *Histoplasma capsulatum* are defined as invasive fungal pathogens. These fungal pathogens are considered as opportunistic pathogens, but they also cause invasive infections in immunocompetent individuals [61, 62]. Invasive fungal pathogens are primarily acquired by inhalation of infectious particles under normal conditions, which leads to the development of serious pulmonary infections that can spread systemically. The mechanisms of the human immune system that defend against invasive fungal pathogens are complicated, but they are generally divided into innate and adaptive mechanisms [63]. Innate immunity is the first line of defense, and it also mediates the mechanisms of adaptive immunity, with the support of specific signals. Antifungal defense serves direct antifungal effectors by performing fungal pathogen destruction using either phagocytic processes or regulation of the adaptive immune system [63–65]. The latter immune response generally occurs via production of pro-inflammatory mediators, including chemokines and cytokines, the induction of costimulatory activity by phagocytic cells, and antigen uptake and followed by antigen presentation [64, 65]. Infection induces most innate mechanisms, which requires an interaction between pathogen recognition receptors (PRRs) and conserved pathogen-associated molecular structures, namely, the pathogen-associated molecular patterns (PAMPs). Therefore, activation of these receptors leads to the recognition and effective elimination of fungal pathogens. Host defensive capacity is defined by the sum of resistance and tolerance. Resistance normally manifests as the ability to limit fungal burden and eliminate pathogens, and tolerance means the ability to limit host damage caused by the immune response. Notably, T-cell activation is crucial for the development of optimal immune responses in fungal infections [64, 65]. Both $CD4^+$ (T helper cell, TH) and $CD8^+$ T cells are required for the clearance of invasive fungal pathogens [64, 65]. For example, $CD4^+$ T cells produce essential lymphokines that activate and recruit phagocytic cells to sites of fungal pathogen [64, 65]. Therefore, the presence of $CD4^+$ T cells is essential to the outcome of invasive fungal infection. The role of $CD8^+$ T cells is yet not clearly defined, but recent data demonstrated an essential role of T cells played in memory response to fungal pathogens [64, 65]. Our understanding of human immune responses to invasive infection caused by fungal pathogens lags behind better-studied microorganisms such as bacteria and viruses, but antifungal immunity has advanced significantly during last decade. Hence, this chapter focuses on human immune responses that are important for the eradication of fungal pathogens during the period of invasive infection.

8.2.1 Recognition of Fungal Pathogens: The First Line of Defense

To the best of our knowledge, host PRRs are likely stimulated by fungal PAMPs in different combinations that rely on the fungal morphology and on the host cell types during the course of invasive fungal infection [63]. Therefore, the final immune response is associated with the relative degree of stimulation of the individual receptors and/or the level of receptor cooperativity and cellular localization [65]. Invasive fungal pathogens lead to the stimulation of multiple PRRs via interaction with conserved structures, the PAMPs, which are present on the surface of fungi. PAMP stimulation of PRRs triggers phagocytosis and respiratory bursts (via the NADPH oxidase) and mediates intracellular signaling pathways that lead to the production of several pro-inflammatory cytokines and chemokines, which are important for host defense against fungi. Two main families of innate receptors are clearly shown to be involved in recognition of fungal pathogens, including toll-like receptors (TLRs) and C-type lectins (CLR), which is the first line of defense of the human immune system to invasive fungal pathogens [64].

Certain members of the TLR family (e.g., TLR2/1, TLR4, and TLR3) are involved with the initial recognition of fungal PAMPs on the cell surface and inside phagosomes of innate immune cells [66–69]. However, the precise molecular mechanism of fungal PAMPs that activate specific TLRs is difficult to elucidate because TLR recognition and the plasticity of the fungal cell wall are frequently orchestrated. For example, TLR2 recognizes the fungal β-glucans of several fungal species and phospholipo-mannans (PLMs), which are linear beta-1,2-oligomannoside structures that are unique to *C. albicans* [67], and TLR4 is activated upon ligation of O-linked mannans of *C. albicans* and GXM of *C. neoformans* [70, 71]. Certain TLRs also recognize nucleic acids that are liberated from fungi.

The C-type lectins are one of the PRRs with lectin-like carbohydrate recognition domains (CRDs) in their extracellular carboxy-terminal domains. TLRs recognize various PAMPs, such as lipopolysaccharides, proteoglycans, DNAs, and RNAs, but C-type lectins mostly recognize carbohydrate structures in pathogens. Dectin-1 recognizes the 1-3-β-glucans that are present in the cell wall of most fungi and contributes to antifungal defense in multiple ways [72, 73]. The presence of a functional, tyrosine-based, activation-like motif in the cytoplasmic tail of dectin-1 distinguishes it from other non-TLR PRRs. Receptor engagement leads to tyrosine phosphorylation by Src family kinases, which provide docking sites for Syk kinases. Syk activation is followed by the assembly of the CARD9/BCL10/MALT1 complex, which leads to the activation of NFAT and the canonical NF-κb pathway, and then induces the production of pro- and anti-inflammatory cytokines and chemokines, such as TNF, IL-6, IL-23, and IL1b [74–76]. The recognition of β-glucan by dectin-1 induces phagocytosis and the production of reactive oxygen species (ROS) by NADPH oxidase, and NADPH-dependent production of ROS is a crucial factor in the containment of fungal pathogens [64].

The first evidence for a role of dectin-1 in fungal infection used blockade dectin-1 during intratracheal *A. fumigates* infection [65]. Several blocking agents reduced alveolar macrophage inflammatory responses, including the production of TNF and MIP-2, blockade correlated with reduced inflammatory cell recruitment, and modest increases in fungal burden. Dectin-1-deficient mice were more susceptible than wild-type mice in a *C. albicans* IV infection model, which initiated innate and adaptive responses. Both arms of the immune system contribute to infection control in this system [77]. However, studies in $CARD9^{-/-}$ mice indicate that fungal infection is more severe in the absence of CARD9 than single dectin-1 deficiency [78, 79]. Despite the significance of dectin-1 as the most important β-glucan receptor, it appears that the recognition of other fungal components by innate receptors can compensate the impaired function of dectin-1 in antifungal defense [77, 80].

CARD9 is a downstream of other CLRs including dectin-2, dectin-3, and mincle, which suggests the integration of various CLR signals by CARD9 [81, 82]. Dectin-2 and dectin-3 recognizing fungal pathogens leads to the production of multiple cytokines, and these proteins are crucial for the induction of Th17 responses during *Candida* infection [83].

CLRs and TLRs mediate distinct signaling cascades and independently contribute to antifungal immunity, but these receptors modulate antifungal responses synergistically and antagonistically [84]. Dectin-1 and TLR-2 have been found to synergize in the production of cytokines and chemokines such as TNF and CCL3 [85, 86]. In contrast, dectin-1 has been shown to inhibit specific TLR responses. The triggering of both TLR4 and dectin-1 leads to diminished CXCL9 and CXCL10 expression but unaltered TNF and IFN-b production [87]. Innate receptors mediate a crucial function in the elicitation of direct antifungal mediators by innate cells and coordinate the activation of adaptive immunity. In our opinion, infection caused by invasively fungal pathogens leads to the stimulation of multiple innate receptors. Future studies are likely to delineate how complex interactions of multiple innate receptors regulate immunity to invasively fungal pathogens.

8.2.2 Innate Immune Responses to Fungal Pathogens

Phagocytes utilize numerous oxidative and non-oxidative mechanisms that act synergistically to kill extracellular and internalized fungi. Phagocytes vary in their ability to kill fungi or restrict fungi growth, and these activities are dependent on the fungal species involved. Macrophages and neutrophils have been found to confer important direct antifungal effects against numerous fungal pathogens [88]. NK cells and iNKT cells are also protective against fungal pathogens.

The mechanisms of innate-mediated pathogen eradication are diverse, and they are divided into oxidative antifungal mechanisms and non-oxidative antifungal mechanisms. The production of reactive oxygen intermediates (ROI) is particularly significant in the fight against fungal pathogens. This reaction is also termed as respiratory burst, and it is mediated through a multicomponent protein complex, the phagocyte NADPH oxidase (phox), which results in the production of superoxide that exhibits limited toxicity. The superoxides are converted to hydroxyl radicals and hydrogen peroxide, which are termed as toxic reactive oxygen intermediates [89], through several reactions. Other enzymes located in the azurophilic granules of neutrophils and in lysosomes of monocytes, such as myeloperoxidase (MPO), produce other types of effective fungicidal oxidants like hypochlorous and hypoiodous acid [90]. Patients with the defects in ROS generation (e.g., mutations in NADPH oxidase that lead to impaired ROS production) are susceptible to fungal infections especially *Aspergillus* species [91]. Several soluble and membrane-bound PRRs are capable of triggering the respiratory burst, including dectin-1, Fcγ receptors, and the TLRs. TLRs can directly induce the respiratory burst in leukocytes via a MyD88- and Vav-dependent pathway. Dectin-1 induced in this response may be restricted to specific subset(s) of phagocytes through their cytoplasmic ITAM sequences and intracellular signaling via Syk kinase [92]. A variety of innate cells produce nitric oxide (NO), but its fungicidal activity in humans is still uncertain. Several pathogenic fungi are capable of detoxifying NO via the production of enzymes and the inhibition of NO production of innate cells [93–95]. There was no significant difference between $iNOS^{-/-}$ mice and the control group when challenged with *Coccidioides* infection [96]. However, NO can be effective against *Candida* in vitro [97], and it contributes to the priming of protective $CD8^{+}$ T cells during *Histoplasma* infection [98]. These results suggest a protective function of NO against at least some fungal pathogens.

Phagocytic cells, particularly neutrophils, possess several non-oxidative mechanisms that are very effective at killing intra- and extracellular fungi or restricting their growth, including antimicrobial peptides (AMP), hydrolases, and components designed to restrict access to essential nutrients. LL-37 and other cathelicidins can kill *Candida* and *Cryptococcus* by disrupting their cellular membranes. But these factors are not effective against filamentous fungi such as *Aspergillus* [99]. Lysozymes also exhibit activity against fungi and have been shown to kill or inhibit the growth of *Candida*, *Cryptococcus*, *Histoplasma*, and *Aspergillus*, which are mostly found in the granules and lysosomes of granulocytes, monocytes, and macrophages [100]. Serprocidins are a family of serine proteases that are stored within neutrophil granules including proteinase-3, cathepsin G, and elastase in numerous pathogens, such as *Histoplasma*, *Aspergillus*, and *Candida* [101]. Neutrophil extracellular traps (NETs) are composed of DNA and represent a variety of enzymes and antimicrobial peptides with antifungal activity that may be an important mechanism of fungal containment [102]. Innate cells contribute to defense via the production of protective cytokines that coordinate the activities of other immune cells, including TNF-α, IFN-γ, IL-12, and GM-CSF, which are associated with the Th1 response [103]. However, recent studies in mice have suggested that the IL-17 axis contributes to the defense against diverse fungal pathogens, including *Histoplasma*, *Aspergillus*, and

Blastomyces [104–106]. Cytokines, including IL-17A, IL-17 F, and IL-22, are produced by innate cells such as iNKT cells and neutrophils. And IL-17-mediated protection is due at least in part to enhanced recruitment of neutrophils [107]. Mice defective in IL-17 responsiveness are more susceptible to *Candida* infection, and patients with defects in the production of IL-17 family members often suffer from recurrent fungal infections.

8.2.3 Inflammatory Monocytes

A variety of innate cells are implicated in antifungal defense [63, 64]. Neutrophils, macrophages, and dendritic cells (DCs) are important cellular mediators of innate immune defense. However, circulating monocytes are increasingly implicated as essential players in the defense against numerous fungal pathogens. Circulating blood monocytes supply peripheral tissues with macrophages and DCs, and these cells also directly contribute to immune defense against fungal pathogens [108]. The recruitment of monocytes to sites of fungal infection was demonstrated in vivo [109]. Purified murine and human monocytes or cultured macrophages were studied in vitro to characterize the induction of inflammatory and fungicidal mediators, rates of fungal killing, and host cell and fungal transcriptional responses [110, 111]. The performance of in vitro-defined mechanisms of fungal inactivation is operative in vivo and its contribution to fungal clearance. Inflammatory monocytes ($CCR^{2+}Ly^{6C+}CD^{11b+}$ myeloid cells) are important precursors to inflammatory DCs that are crucial for the initiation of antifungal $CD4^+$ T-cell responses in the context of pulmonary infections with fungal pathogens. Recent studies indicate that inflammatory monocyte recruitment to sites of infection is complex and involves $CCR2^-$-mediated emigration of monocytes from the bone marrow into the bloodstream, followed by the trafficking into infected tissue. $CCR2^{-/-}$ mice demonstrate a defective emigration of monocytes from the bone marrow and thus limited recruitment of these cells to the sites of infection [112]. Recent studies in $CCR2^-$-deficient mice indicate that inflammation-induced monocyte recruitment contributes to host antifungal immune responses. In murine pulmonary cryptococcosis, $CCR2^{-/-}$ mice cannot control fungal growth due to diminished pulmonary macrophage recruitment and the induction of maladaptive Th2-biased T-cell responses [113]. These defects are likely related to the impaired recruitment of inflammatory monocytes to sites of *C. neoformans* infection. In a murine model of allergic disease associated with *A. fumigatus* antigen exposure, $CCR2^{-/-}$ mice exhibit prolonged pulmonary allergic responses, airway inflammation, and delayed clearance of fungal antigens in a murine model of allergic disease associated with *A. fumigatus* antigen exposure, which suggests that CCR2 signaling restricts the development of fungus-associated asthmatic disease [114]. One hypothesis to explain this finding is the $CCR2^{-/-}$-mediated recruitment of monocytes sways *A. fumigates*-specific $CD4^+$ T-cell responses toward a Th1 as opposed to a Th2 phenotype. CCR2-mediated recruitment of cells other than inflammatory monocytes may be critical in the defense against *A. fumigatus* infection. Similarly, the depletion of $CCR2^+$ inflammatory monocytes prior to infection leads to increased fungal burden in the kidney during systemic *Candida* infection and mortality, and the adoptive transfer of bone marrow monocytes reconstituted fungal growth restriction [115]. These studies support evidence for $CCR2^+$ inflammatory monocytes as crucial innate effectors of fungal growth restriction.

8.2.4 Adaptive Immune Responses to Fungal Pathogens

The significant contributions of $CD4^+$ T cells in defense against fungal pathogens are clearly illustrated by the susceptibility of patients with AIDS to cryptococcal infections, *Pneumocystis* and *Histoplasma* among others [63]. The role of $CD4^+$ T cells was further studied in mouse models of fungal infection in which depletion of $CD4^+$ T cells often leads to uncontrolled fungal growth and mortality [116]. Multiple studies highlight the importance of Th1 $CD4^+$ T cells in the defense against fungal pathogens [63, 64, 116]. Recent studies further suggest a protective role for Th17 cells, and Th2 responses appear to be uniformly detrimental against most clinically relevant fungi [117, 118]. The differentiation of fungus-specific $CD4^+$ T cell is thus tightly linked to protection, and it is clearly shaped by innate responses. The development of fungus-specific $CD4^+$TCR-tg mice specific for *A. fumigates* and *B. dermatitidis* has facilitated the dissection of the early steps that are required for fungus-specific $CD4^+$ T-cell activation and differentiation [119]. $CD4^+$ T cells response to a pulmonary infection with live *A. fumigatus* spores, and proliferative responses are evident 3 and 4 days after infection [73]. The majority of *A. fumigatus*-specific $CD4^+$ T cells differentiate into IFN-c^+Th1 cells with a small fraction of the cells becoming IL-17-producing Th17 cells. The differentiation of *A. fumigatus*-specific Th1 cells was partly dependent on MyD88 signals with the frequency of IFN-c + cell was reduced in $MyD88^{-/-}$ mice. Dectin-1 signals favored Th17 differentiation via the suppression of T-bet induction and the Th1 program, which primes *A. fumigatus*-specific $CD4^+$ T cells in dectin-$1^{-/-}$ mice and results in an absence of Th17 cells and enhanced frequency of IFN-c + Th1 cells [73, 119, 120]. In contrast, Th17 differentiation following vaccination with *B. dermatitidis* is dependent on MyD88 and independent of dectin-1 [121]. These findings highlight the diversity of immune responses against fungal pathogens and the need for a better understanding of the early steps of immune activation to each clinically relevant fungal pathogen, which will in turn facilitate the development of vaccination strategies that are optimal to each pathogen. Whether Th17 cells are similarly protective against other fungi is currently debated [122, 123]. Some studies suggest a protective role for Th17 against *Candida*, but other studies demonstrated a detrimental effect of these responses to both *Candida* and *Aspergillus*. Further studies are required to decipher the diverse contributions of Th17 cells against fungal pathogens, but clinical observations suggest that Th17-derived products can be clearly protective against *Candida* [124, 125]. Whether the protection is dependent on $CD4^+$ T cells or innate cells as found in mouse models must be determined [126].

Various studies clearly demonstrate that CD8 T cells and antibodies are protective against fungal pathogens [127–129]. CD8 T cells protect against *B. dermatitidis* in the absence of CD4 T cells [130]. CD8 T-cell responses are elicited against *H. capsulatum* that are protective especially in the absence of CD4 T cells [130, 131]. Recent studies reveal that $CD8^+$ T cells are part of the immune response that is generated to *A. fumigates*, and these cells contribute to vaccine-dependent protection [131, 132]. In vitro studies with human CD8 T-cell clones further demonstrate the possibility of $CD8^+$ T cells as cytolytic agents against fungal pathogens [132, 133]. These studies provide a clear evidence for a role of $CD8^+$ T cells in the immunological armament that is responsible for antifungal defense.

Although lack of B cells does not in generally lead to enhanced susceptibility to fungal pathogens, there is clear evidence of the capacity of fungus-specific antibodies to eliminate pathogens [134–137]. There is evidence of the possibility to exploit antibodies for protection via passive transfer and vaccination strategies that are centered on humoral immunity [136]. The importance of antibodies was demonstrated in which antibodies are protective via a combination of direct and indirect mechanisms [136]. Proof of principle studies demonstrated the possibility of developing antibody-based vaccines with broad protection against fungal pathogens [136, 137], which is similar to the concept of cross-protective CD4 T-cell responses. Therefore, the development of vaccine strategies should target multiple fungi via both cellular and humoral mechanisms of protection.

8.2.5 Summary

Invasive fungal pathogens remain a clinical challenge, and better therapeutic interventions are urgently needed. Recent studies in the field of fungal immunology significantly have improved our understanding of the distinct immune components that mediate protective immunity against invasively fungal pathogens. The foremost understanding of human immune responses to invasive fungal pathogens is that host susceptibility determines the morphological form, antigenic structure, and physical location of the fungus. Innate immunity was traditionally considered as the first defense line, which activates adaptive immune mechanisms via the provision of specific signals; innate and adaptive immune responses are intimately linked.

8.3 Viral Diseases

8.3.1 HPV Infection of the Skin

Xing-Hua Gao, Wei Huo, Yang Yang, and Hong-Duo Chen

Human papillomavirus (HPV), belonging to the family *Papillomaviridae*, is a circular double-stranded DNA virus of about 8000 base pairs (Fig. 8.2 The genomic organization of HPV). At present, more than 170 HPV types have been identified, based on nucleotide sequencing (refer to Papillomavirus Episteme (PaVE); http://pave.niaid.nih.gov/#home). A new HPV isolate is recognized as such when the following conditions are met: (1) the complete genome has been cloned and (2) the DA sequence of the L1 ORF differs by more than 10 % from the closest known HPV type. An isolate is defined as a subtype when there are homology differences of between 2 and 10 % and as a variant when the differences are less than 2 % [138, 139]. A confirmed HPV type is numbered, as exemplified by HPV 2, HPV 6, HPV 16, etc. Nucleotide sequence information can be accessed in the general GenBank and EMBL databases and relatively more specifically at the website http://hpv-web.lanl.gov/stdgen/virus/hpv/compendium/htdocs/ (established by Myers et al.1994 and described by Farmer et al. 1995) [138].

Papillomaviruses are species specific. HPV infects keratinocytes in human skin and/or mucosal epithelia. Infections can be productive, subclinical, or latent in both the skin and mucosa. Productive infections can be seen clinically, where there is full viral gene expression and production of mature virus particles. Subclinical infections need additional tools or agents to help in making the diagnosis. These include microscopic examination with the aid of topically applied acetic acid, colposcopic examination of the cervix, or anoscopy of the anal canal. Latent papillomavirus infections are detectable only through the demonstration of HPV DNA in clinically and histologically normal-looking skin and mucosal surfaces [140]. Because a wide variety of different types of HPV can be detected in healthy human skin, it has been suggested that HPVs occur mostly in a latent life cycle form. Immune suppression in humans leads to activation of latent infections or increases susceptibility to reinoculation.

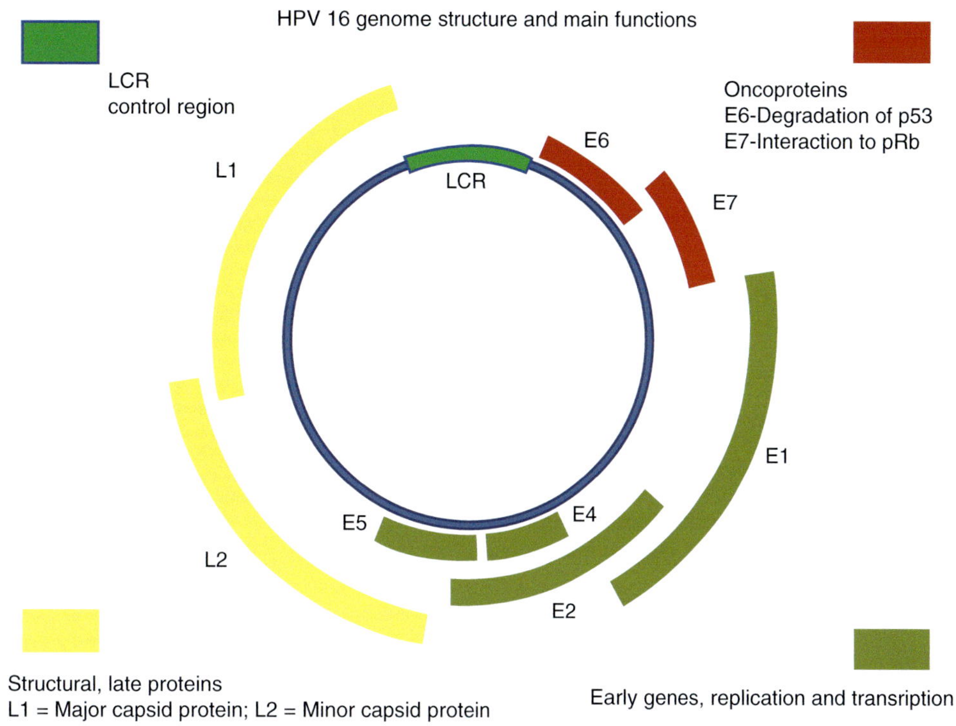

Fig. 8.2 Genomic structure of HPV (Reprint with permission from: Immune escape and immunotherapy of HPV-related oropharyngeal cancer: has the future arrived? 2015). Three oncogenes, *E5*, *E6*, and *E7*, modulate the transformation process; two regulatory proteins, *E1* and *E2*, modulate transcription and replication; and two structural proteins, *L1* and *L2*, compose the viral capsid. The *E1*, *E2*, *L1*, and *L2* ORFs are particularly well conserved among all members of the family. Most *cis*-responsive elements are in the long control region (*LCR*) between *L1* and *E6*. The *L1* ORF is the most conserved gene within the genome and has therefore been used for the identification of new PV types

8.3.1.1 Entry into the Skin

The first event during infection by HPV occurs via lacerations or minor abrasions that reveal the basal skin layer. Prior to entry into basal cells, which is a slow process (about 14 h half-time for uptake), virions first must attach to heparan sulfate moieties in the basement membrane, followed by interaction with the elusive uptake receptor [141]. After entering a host cell, the virus sheds its protein coat, and the double-stranded DNA infects cellular nuclei. Two genes, E6 and E7, are expressed first, and they have the capacity to inhibit normal cellular apoptosis and to inhibit cell growth regulation. As keratinocytes infected with HPV DNA replicate and transit upward toward more superficial layers of the skin, E1, E2, E4, and E5 genes are activated. As these cells continue to replicate, the final two structural genes, L1 and L2, are expressed to synthesize the capsid proteins. The fully enclosed icosahedral virus particle has at that point reached the skin surface. The particles can then be shed, allowing reinfection of the host and infection of other hosts [142].

8.3.1.2 Clinical Spectrum of HPV Infection

Most HPV infections are subclinical. Progression from subclinical to clinical infection may take months or years. When infection reaches the clinical phase, it manifests as benign papillomas or cancer of the cervix, vulva, vagina, penis, anus, and oropharynx. HPV types generally correlate with three categories of infections seen clinically, namely, nongenital cutaneous disease, nongenital mucosal disease, and anogenital disease (Table 8.1 and Fig. 8.4). In addition, HPV is suspected to be a cause of (or being harbored in) some several skin diseases, including keratoacanthoma, Bowen's disease, Bowenoid papulosis, actinic keratosis, nonmelanoma skin cancers, and seborrheic keratoses [143]. Seventy percent of clinical HPV infections, in young men and women, may regress to subclinical in 1 year and 90 % in 2 years. However, when subclinical infections persist, there is high risk of developing precancerous lesions or invasive cancer.

8.3.1.3 HPV Infection and Immunity

The first line of defense against HPV infection is the innate immune response at its early stages. The infected keratinocytes aberrantly express an array of cytokines, chemokines, and adhesion molecules. LCs, cells that neighbor keratinocytes in the epidermis, also begin to express immune-related molecules in the presence of HPV infection [139] (Fig. 8.3). The innate immune system strives to create a pro-inflammatory microenvironment by recruiting innate immune cells to eliminate the infected cells, including dendritic (DC), Langerhans (LC), natural killer (NK), and natural killer T (NKT) cells. Most of these cell types can promote a cytokine-mediated pro-inflammatory process, which links the innate with the adaptive immune response. NK cells can directly eliminate the virus-infected cells [139]. However, HPV exhibits a wide range of strategies for evading immune surveillance, generating an anti-inflammatory microenvironment. The viral mechanisms of immune evasion are complex. The life cycle of HPV is non-lytical and thus renders its limited production of antigens required for processing and presentation to the adaptive immune system. Some viral proteins share sequence

Table 8.1 HPV types associated with particular disease

Disease		Most frequently associated HPV types
Common warts		HPV 2, 4, 7; occasionally other types in immunosuppressed (e.g., HPV 75–77)
Flat plane warts		HPV 3, 10; occasionally HPV 26–29 and 41
Plantar warts		HPV 1, 2, 4
Epidermodysplasia verruciformis	Plane warts	HPV 3, 10
	Pityriasis-like plaques	HPV 5, 8; less commonly 9, 12, 14, 15, 17, 19, 20, 21–25, 36–39, 47, 49
	Squamous cell carcinomas of sun-exposed skin	HPV 5, 8, less commonly 14, 17, 20, and 47
Anogenital warts	External warts	HPV 6, 11, 40, 42, 43, 44, 54, 61, 72, 81, 89
	Buschke–Lowenstein tumor	HPV 6
	Bowenoid papulosis	HPV 16, 55
Anogenital cancers and precancers	Group 1: carcinogenic to humans	HPV 16, 18, 31, 33, 45, 51, 52
	Group 2A: probably carcinogenic to humans	HPV 68
	Group 2B: possibly carcinogenic to humans	HPV 26, 53, 64, 65, 66, 67, 69, 70, 73, 82
Oral lesions	Oral papillomas	HPV 2, 6, 7, 11, 16, 18, 32, 57
	Laryngeal papillomas	HPV 6, 11
	Focal hyperplasia (Heck's disease)	HPV 13, 32
	Oropharyngeal carcinoma	HPV 16 predominantly, 18

Adapted from several sources and compiled in Cubie [140]

similarities to host cell proteins, such that HPV16 E7 with xeroderma pigmentosum group G complementing proteins and the retinoblastoma binding protein-1, a mechanism that HPV has evolved to escape immune recognition. HPV develops machinery to modulate antigen presentation, to avoid the effects of type I IFN, and to inhibit or skew the production of pro-inflammatory cytokines, chemoattractants, and adhesion molecules. At a cellular level, HPV-infected cells inhibit the migration of APCs, and they inhibit apoptosis of infected cells [144, 145]. High-risk types of HPV maintain persistent infection, and immunodeficiency in the affected individual may lead to tumors, such as cervical cancer, head and neck SCC, and others. Tumors also may possess escape mechanisms, possibly through downregulation of tumor antigen expression, aberrant regulation of members of the signal transducer and activator of transcription (STAT) family, creation of an immunosuppressive cytokine milieu, and dysregulation of immune effector cells [146].

Understanding mechanisms of interplay between HPV and immune responses helps investigators in their efforts to develop interventional strategies to eliminate infection. Immunoadjuvants, such as TLR agonists (imiquimod as one example) and alpha-galactosylceramide, have been demonstrated to reverse an anti-inflammatory microenvironment by downregulating a number of adhesion molecules and chemoattractants and by activating keratinocytes, dendritic cells, Langerhans cells, natural killer cells, and natural killer T cells, thus promoting a strong specific cytotoxic T-cell response [139, 147]. The use of local hyperthermia on warty lesions accelerates the migration and maturation of LCs [148], and it increases the production of IFNs, most possibly from infected keratinocytes [149]. In the complicated battle between HPV and human immunity, the development of adaptive cellular immunity against HPV antigen emerges as the prime mechanism to clear the infection, largely by the destruction of virus-infected cells [150], whereas humoral responses lead to the production of neutralizing antibodies, which will prevent the virus from entering epithelial cells. Humoral responses that follow natural infection are inefficient, although the newly developed vaccines against HPV capsid protein antigen dramatically reduce the incidences of cervical cancer and genital warts. HPV vaccines boost stronger serological responses (one to four logs higher) than the responses that follow natural infections, which is likely due to the absence of specific adjuvants and different routes of administration (exposure) [151, 152].

Detection of HPV

Because there are no in vitro systems to culture HPV, the detection of HPV infection is based primarily on finding evidence of the viral genome. For cutaneous warts, HPV detection is seldom performed, as clinical and/or histological manifestation are commonly sufficient to make a diagnosis. In the case of screening against cervical cancer or other suspected cancers, especially for lesions found on mucous membranes, the detection of HPV is of great value.

Molecular methods for HPV detection include signal amplification (liquid phase hybridization) and target

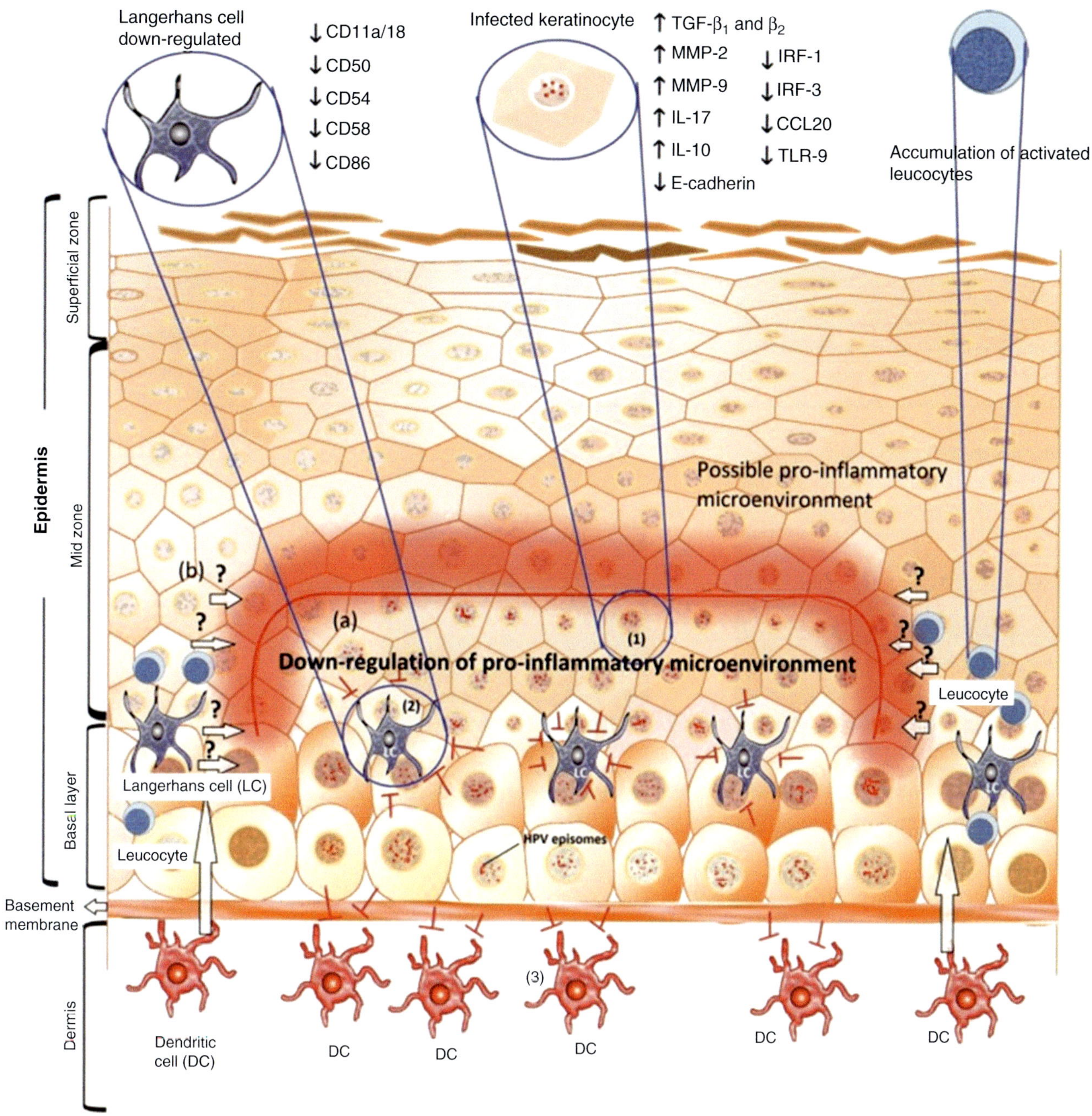

Fig. 8.3 Schematic representation of the role of the innate immune response following adjuvant stimulation during HPV infection (Reprint from role of innate immunity against human papillomavirus (HPV) infections and effect of adjuvants in promoting specific immune response, 2015)

amplification (gene amplification by polymerase chain reaction). Subsequently, genotyping and quantification of viral DNA are also employed. Another approach has been the detection of mRNA of HPV E6 and E7 oncogenes [153].

8.3.1.4 Prevention and Management of HPV Infection

There are two main tasks in preventing HPV infection: (1) preventing the acquisition of HPV infection and (2) preventing carcinogenesis, which may follow HPV infection. Typical cutaneous infection is usually caused by benign types of HPV, and it manifests most often as warts (e.g., common warts, plantar warts, and plane warts). The chance to malignant transformation is very low for these types of clinical lesions. Thus, the major task is to avoid skin injury, to avoid direct and close contact with warty lesions in other patients, and to avoid of self-inoculation through scratching and rubbing. There is, as yet, no vaccine for the HPV types that cause these diseases. For several types of anogenital HPV, however, the efficacy of (HPV types 6, 11, 16, and 18)

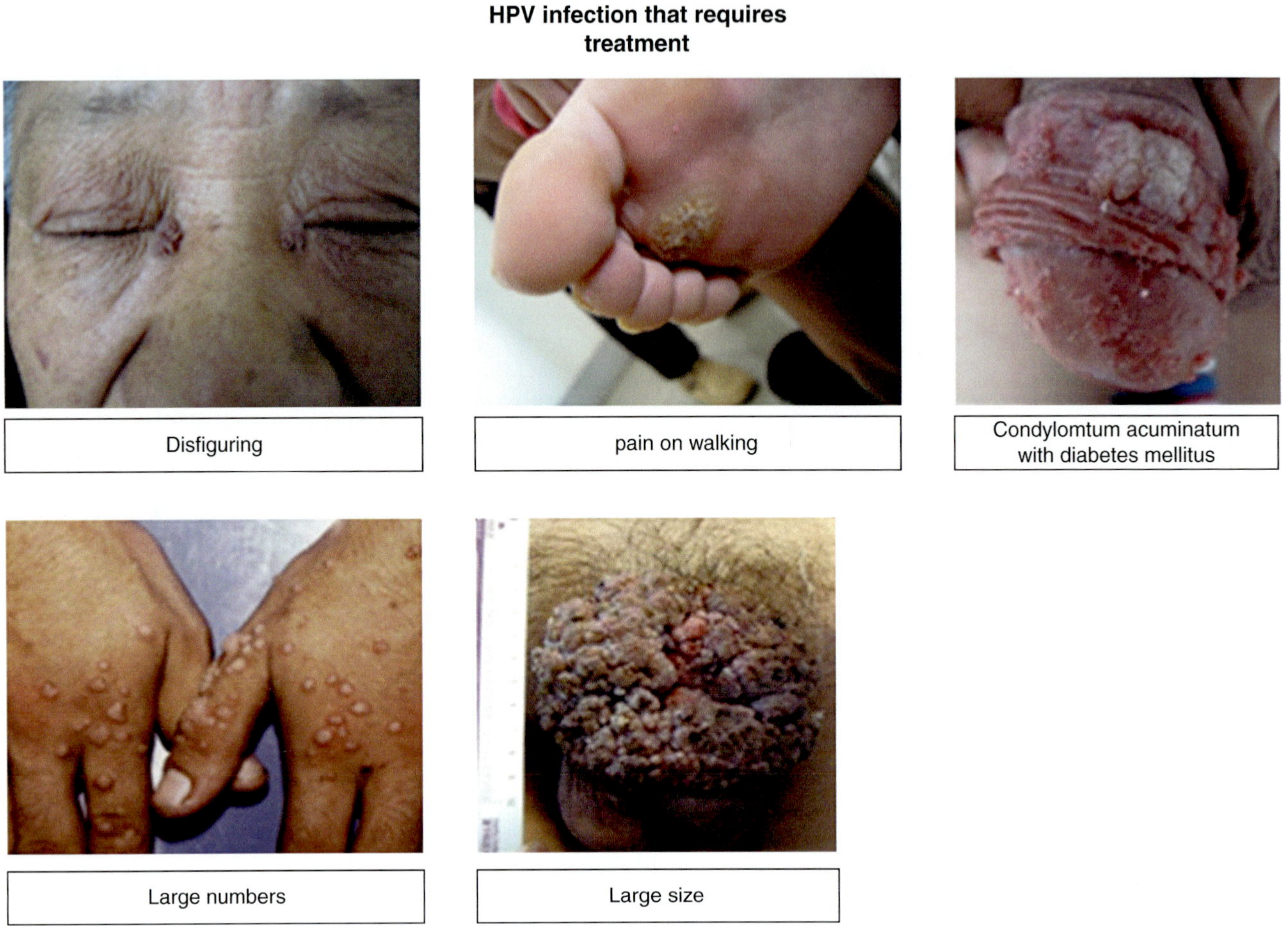

Fig. 8.4 HPV infection that requires treatment

vaccine in the prevention of preinvasive lesions and infection with these HPV types has been well documented [154]. In cases of anogenital acquisition and carcinogenesis of HPV infection, multiple risk factors should be avoided, such as early-age sexual activities, high numbers of sexual partners, suppression and alteration of the immune status, and long-term use of oral contraceptives and other hormonal influences [155]. Condom use offers good protection against these HPV infections and the associated cervical neoplasia [156].

The majority of patients with warts have a benign and self-limited course, and, thus, it is not necessary for all warts to be treated. The American Academy of Dermatology Committee on Guidelines of Care has established the following indications for the treatment of warts: (1) the patient's desire for therapy, (2) symptoms of pain, bleeding, itching, or burning, (3) disabling or disfiguring lesions, (4) large numbers or large sizes of lesions, (5) the patient's desire to prevent the spread of warts to unblemished skin of self or others, and (6) immunocompromised conditions [157]. Figure 8.4 illustrates cases of patients with warts that need active treatment.

The ideal treatment for warts would be the following: (1) effective in eliminating warts in all or a large percentage of treated patients, (2) painless, (3) effective for all warts on a patient when only one or part of one is treated, (4) effective after no more than three treatments, (5) produce no scars, (6) provide lifelong HPV immunity to prevent recurrences and reinfection, and (7) be available for all patients [158, 159]. In clinical practice, the choices of treatment often depend on factors such as size, shape, number, anatomical location, and previous treatments. It is common for combination therapies to be employed.

Traditional local therapies rely on destructive, cytotoxic methods or agents. Specific methods include treatment with cryotherapy, trichloroacetic acid, electrosurgery, curettage, laser vaporization, topical cytotoxic agents, podophyllin, podophyllotoxin, 5-FU, and many others. In recent years, 15 % sinecatechins (green tea extract) ointment was approved for genital and perianal warts. It is applied three times a day for up to 16 weeks, and more than 50 % of patients have been cleared of their warts [160]. The mechanisms of action have not been fully elucidated for this drug. Photodynamic therapy with 5-amnolevulinic acid (5-ALA) is also an emerging option for genital warts. Twenty percent 5-ALA was applied to the lesion followed by irradiation with a 635-nm laser (or other red-light source) with an energy fluence of 100 J/cm^2 for 20–30 min. The procedure could be repeated on a weekly basis [161]. The efficacy of this method was rather high, and it seems especially useful for genital warts found in reclusive locations; this would include cervical, urethral, or anal warts [160].

Immunotherapies are applied either topically, intralesionally, or systemically.

Topical immunomodifiers are usually are self-applied. A 3.75 % imiquimod cream once a day for 8 weeks achieved a clearance rate of 36.6 % in genital warts [162]. Sensitization with diphenylcyclopropenone has been employed for both children and adults, and the reported clearance rate has been as high as high as 88 %. Children seem to respond earlier than the adults [163]. This method was claimed to be more suitable and quite effective for periungual warts [164] and recalcitrant palmar–plantar warts [165]. Other topical sensitizers, such as squaric acid dibutylester, have also been used to treat warts, through its impact on the balance of T-cell patterns [166].

Intralesional delivery of an antigen combination – mumps, measles, and rubella (MMR) vaccine – has been used to treat plantar warts and recalcitrant or multiple warts. The MMR vaccine was injected into single lesions or the largest wart for patients with multiple lesions at 3-week intervals until there was complete clearance. The complete clearance of the warts was reported to occur in 82–87 % of patients [167, 168]. Other antigen combinations, including mumps, *Candida*, and *Trichophyton* skin test antigens, have shown effects that are superior to that seen in control populations [169].

Intralesional injection of *Candida* antigen one time every 3 weeks for three sessions cleared 56 % of resistant or recalcitrant warts [170]. A phase I trial of *Candida* antigen reached clearance of warts in 9 of the 11 patients who completed the study (82 %) [171]. Weekly intralesional injections of Mycobacterium w vaccine cleared genital warts in 8 out of 9 patients, maximum treatment session was 10 [172]. There are also other different antigens or antigen combinations being tried or developed.

Cyclophosphamide is a conventional chemotherapy drug. Low-dose cyclophosphamide showed effects on genital warts. Its mechanism of action may be through selective targeting of Treg cells, thereby enhancing the function of HPV-specific T cells and NK cells [173].

Local hyperthermia is emerging as an easy and patient-friendly noninvasive, immune-modulatory method to treat warts. It is usually conducted such that local heating to 44° C for 30 min on a target lesion, once a day for 3 consecutive days, followed by treatment in a similar fashion for 2 days after an interval of 2 weeks. In patients with numerous warts, resolution of the target lesions often results in clearance of untargeted lesions. Local hyperthermia is safe with negligible side effects such as burning sensations, heat-induced transient bullae, and postinflammatory hyperpigmentation [174, 175]. For recalcitrant warts, repeated hyperthermia treatments may increase the cure rates.

Patients with inherited or acquired immunodeficiencies, autoimmune disorders, and organ or bone marrow transplantation are especially susceptible to developing persistent and extensive cutaneous wart infections. No large-scale clinical trials have been performed in these rare conditions. Single or combined treatment strategies including acitretin, cidofovir, *Candida* antigen, cimetidine, imiquimod, isotretinoin, fluorouracil, selenium, podophyllotoxin, photodynamic therapy, mammalian target of rapamycin inhibitors, and the quadrivalent HPV vaccine have all been used successfully [176].

Warts that develop during pregnancy usually grow rapidly. Ablative treatments, such as cryotherapy and laser therapy, are applicable, but the methods are not well accepted by patients. Repeated intradermal PPD achieved 47.5 % clearance [177]. Local hyperthermia at 44° C for 30 min a day for 3 consecutive days plus 2 additional days 1 week later and then on a once-a-week protocol cleared giant warts in less than 2 months [178]. Warts that develop in patients with diabetes mellitus also grow rapidly, and this may make patients desperate. Local hyperthermia has also showed remarkable effects, in the protocol as applied to patients in pregnancy [178, 179].

8.3.2 HSV Infection

H.M. Holahan, A.C. Laureano, and R.A. Schwartz

8.3.2.1 Introduction

The herpes viruses are members of the herpesviridae family and characteristically all share a genome of encapsulated, linear, double-stranded DNA composed of 152-k base pairs (kbp) [180–183]. Structurally, the DNA is housed within a capsid or protein covering that is shielded by tegument and an envelope decorated with glycoproteins [180, 182–184]. Among the more than 100 known herpes viruses, only eight are able to infect the human: herpes simplex virus 1 (HSV-1), herpes simplex virus 2 (HSV-2), Kaposi's sarcoma-associated herpesvirus (type 8), Epstein–Barr virus, varicella zoster virus, cytomegalovirus, and herpesviruses 6 and 7 [180, 182]. Although modest in number, seroprevalence of the above eight diseases is ubiquitous, ranging from 60 to 95 % worldwide [180, 185]. Infection is incurable and lifelong, principally due to the virus's ability to elude host immune detection, and remain latent in sensory ganglia until optimal conditions are met for reactivation [180, 182].

Herpes simplex infection rates vary widely according to age, socioeconomic status, race, and geographical region

[180, 182, 183, 186]. In 2003, the World Health Organization estimated that approximately 536 million people aged 15–49 years old were seropositive for HSV-2 infection worldwide, with a yearly incidence of 23.6 million cases in this age group [186]. Latency, mode of entry, and degree of host immune competency all impact the disease's presentation, which varies from asymptomatic to life-threatening [187]. The array of clinical disease includes gingivostomatitis, herpes labialis, eczema herpeticum, herpetic whitlow, keratoconjunctivitis, herpes gladiatorium, neonatal HSV, HSV encephalitis, an association with erythema multiforme, and genital HSV infections [180, 182].

8.3.2.2 Viral Entry

Infection initiates the attachment of HSV virus to cell membrane receptors, whereby the viral envelope fuses with the plasma membrane [183, 188]. Both attachment and fusion are mediated through conformational changes in viral glycoprotein structure and creation of a multi-glycoprotein complex [181, 183]. Microtubule transport of the de-enveloped viral capsid through the cytoplasm and into the nucleus then occurs [181, 183]. In the nucleus, viral proteins are expressed in a synchronized manner dependent on timing and necessity. Alpha gene expression occurs first, beta gene expression follows as it uses alpha gene products for DNA replication, and gamma expression is last, using replicated viral DNA to synthesize its structural proteins [182, 184].

8.3.2.3 Clinical Spectrum of HSV Infection

Following primary infection, the virus moves by retrograde transport intra-axonally to the sensory ganglia. Here, the viral genome replicates, followed by either host neuronal destruction or viral latency [183]. During a host's lifetime, HSV reactivation can result after inducement from internal or environmental sources such as emotional stress, ultraviolet light exposure, fever, tissue injury, or immunosuppression [180, 182, 188, 189]. At that time, the genome will travel anterograde into the epithelial cell where replication will occur, and mucocutaneous lesions may develop. Disease often recurs in the area of primary infection [190]. The reactivated state may present as either asymptomatic or symptomatic infection [180, 181, 190].

HSV reactivation rates vary by virus type and site of infection [191]. Overall, genital infections recurred six times more frequently than orolabial infections. Persons with concurrent HSV-2 oropharyngeal and HSV-2 genital disease reported more frequent recurrences with genital infection rather than orolabial disease (.33 vs. .001 recurrences per month) [191]. Reactivation rates are also increased when HSV-1 causes orolabial disease, 0.12 recurrences per month, and when HSV-2 produces genital disease, 0.33 recurrences per month. Individuals with concurrent oropharyngeal and genital infections caused by HSV-1 had more recurrences with orolabial rather than genital disease (0.12 vs. .020 recurrences per month). HSV-2 genital infections more frequently recurred than HSV-1 orolabial infections (.33 vs. .02), but HSV-1 genital infection recurrences were more often than HSV-2 orolabial infections (0.02 vs. .001 per month) [188, 191]. Similarly, an increase in genital infections caused by HSV-1 has been noted in reproductive-aged women, but recurrence rates still remain higher by a rate of three to one when HSV-2 is the pathogen [189].

8.3.2.4 Demographics

HSV-1 infection rates are largely influenced by demographic elements such as socioeconomic status, age, race, and geographic region [180, 182, 183]. Seroconversion in HSV-1 happens earlier in developing countries, lower socioeconomic class, and in the African-American population [182]. In lower socioeconomic groups, HSV seroconversion occurs in 33 % of children by 5 years old, with a rate of 70–80 % by adolescence, while middle-class groups have HSV-1 seroconversion rates of 20 % by 5 years of age without significant alteration until 30–40 years of age [182].

Similar to HSV-1, HSV-2 figures are impacted by age, race, and geographic region but also by gender, marital status, and number of sexual partners [180, 182]. Specifically, HSV-2 seroprevalence rises from approximately 10 % in 15–29 years old to 35 % by age 60. African-Americans have three to four times higher seroprevalence rates than Caucasians. Infectivity is higher in women than men, with an 80 % risk of contraction in females having one-time intercourse with HSV-2-infected males [180, 182]. Due to the venereal mechanism of infection, seroconversion prior to puberty is uncommon [180, 182].

8.3.2.5 Transmission

HSV infection is primarily transmitted through direct contact of mucous membranes or skin with mucosal secretions or lesions from a person with active infection [180, 182, 192]. Of note, the presence of symptomatic infection is not necessary to transmit disease, as virus can be spread via contact with respiratory droplets or mucocutaneous secretions from asymptomatic persons if they are shedding virus [180]. Experimental investigation has retrieved virus from the saliva and hands of greater than 60 % of patients with active herpes labialis. Additionally, virus can be located on plastic and cloth surfaces for up to 3–4 h [180, 193]. Recovery of virus from the skin, saliva, and external surfaces demonstrates the manner in which the virus can be spread by close, direct contact [180, 193, 194].

Although serotypes HSV-1 and HSV-2 share approximately 82 % sequence homology, critical differences in glycoprotein structure have been identified and led to facilitating serological distinction [180, 181, 189, 195]. HSV-1 exposure and infection frequently happen in childhood through nonvenereal mechanisms. Latency is most often established in the trigeminal ganglia. Conversely, HSV-2 is spread sexually and develops latency in the lumbosacral ganglia [180, 187, 189, 190]. Generally, these serotypes infect different anatomical regions of the body with HSV-1 causing orolabial and ocular lesions, herpesvirus labialis, and conjunctivitis, respectively, while HSV-2 commonly infects the perineal and anal regions producing genital herpes [180, 181, 196]. In spite of this, both viruses can infect area interchangeably [180, 182, 197].

8.3.2.6 HSV-1 and HSV-2 Infections

Primary Herpetic Gingivostomatitis (PHGS)

Primary HSV-1 orolabial infection most commonly presents as PHGS in children. Symptomatic infection renders painful, vesiculo-ulcerative lesions both inside and around the oral cavity (Fig. 8.5) [180, 182, 190]. Accompanying symptoms may include fever, fatigue, cervical, and submandibular lymphadenopathy [180, 188]. Great discomfort can result from vesicle ulceration with subsequent avoidance of food and drink; severe cases may require hospitalization for hydration [187]. Healing of lesions usually occurs in 10–14 days; however, a majority of PGHS cases are not recognized due to the mild nature of infection [180, 188, 190]. Viral shedding will continue for several weeks after clinical disease resolves [180]. Infections presenting in later adolescence can include pharyngitis and an illness clinically resembling mononucleosis [180, 182].

Treatment may mainly rely on symptomatic relief using over the counter agents such as anesthetic oral washes prior to eating. When infections are more severe, oral acyclovir suspension, administered within 3 days of symptom presentation, has increased healing, decreased viral shedding, and increased nutritional intake [180].

Human Herpes Simplex Labialis (HSL)

HSL is the most common manifestation of recurrent HSV-1 orolabial infection. Infection is usually mild, with less symptoms than primary infection (Fig. 8.6) [187]. In 60% of recurrent infections, tingling, burning, pain, itching, and paresthesias may present a few hours prior to lesion formation [188]. The vermillion border is commonly the site of vesicular formation. After approximately 72–96 h, vesicles enter the pustular and crusting phase with healing occurring in 8–10 days [188]. Patients should be cautioned against kissing and sharing utensils or towels and reminded to wash hands after topical medication administration [180, 188]. Recurrent intraoral herpes infection is less common in individuals who are immunocompetent [180, 192].

Treatment includes antiviral agents that ameliorate disease by decreasing both symptomatology and illness duration. Such agents are docosanol 10% cream, which blocks viral entrance into the host cell, and penciclovir 1% cream, which prevents DNA polymerase from functioning [180, 192]. Idoxuridine 15% solution has also been shown to decrease pain and hasten healing if used early in the treatment of the disease [180, 187, 192]. Acyclovir use has provided mixed results in the acute episodic treatment of HSL but has demonstrated effectiveness in the prevention of reactivation in immunosuppressed patients [180, 187, 192]. Oral valacyclovir and famciclovir have increased bioavailability, require less frequent dosing, and result in improved compliance. Both have demonstrated reduced outbreak duration in immunocompetent as well as immunosuppressed patients [180, 192]. Foscarnet and cidofovir are agents dispensed

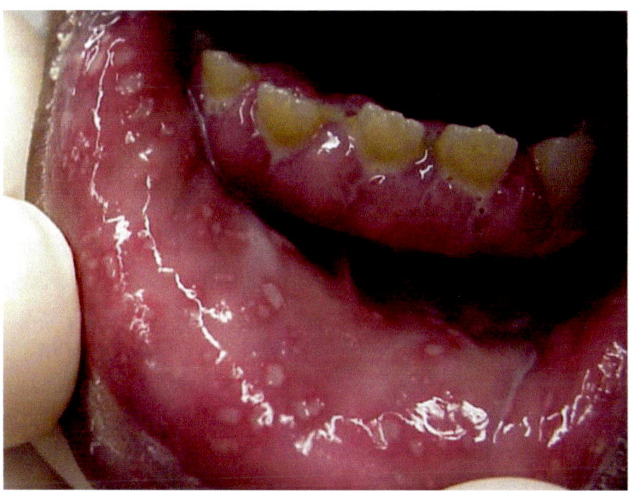

Fig. 8.5 Primary herpetic gingivostomatitis in a pediatric patient. Note intense gingival inflammation and multiple, round ulcers on labial mucosa (Reprinted from Fatahzadeh and Schwartz [198], Copyright (2007), with permission from Elsevier)

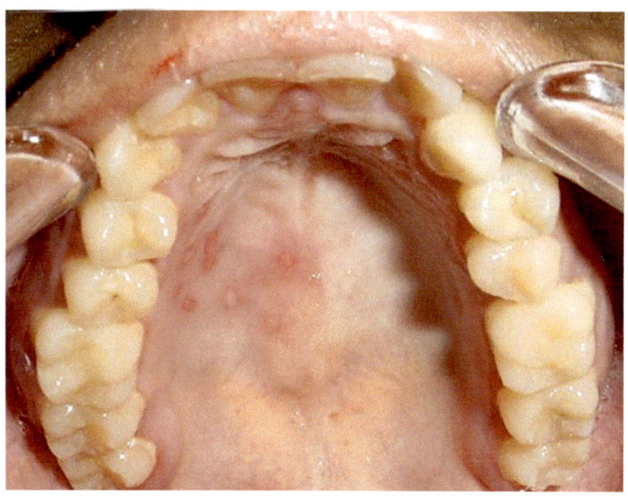

Fig. 8.6 Recurrent intraoral herpes in an adult. Note cluster of small, symptomatic ulcers caused by the rupture of transient vesicles of keratinized tissue of the right palate (Reprinted from Fatahzadeh and Schwartz [198], Copyright (2007), with permission from Elsevier)

intravenously and are saved for acyclovir-resistant HSV infections in immunosuppressed patients.

Eczema Herpeticum

Eczema herpeticum, also known as Kaposi's varicelliform eruption, commonly occurs in children with preexisting atopic dermatitis [180, 199–201]. However, the infection can also occur in cutaneous burns, Darier's disease, and Wiskott–Aldrich syndrome. Both HSV-1 and HSV-2 can cause infection, but HSV-1 is the more common pathogen [202]. Infection causes vesicle formation within the eczematous regions, and over the next 10 days, the eruption may spread to normal skin (Fig. 8.7) [199, 203]. Fever, malaise, and lymphadenopathy may also be presented [199, 203]. Clinical diseases can range from mild to life-threatening when infection includes visceral organs [199]. Additionally, bacterial superinfection can occur with *Staphylococcus aureus*, *Pseudomonas aeruginosa*, and *Streptococcus pyogenes* [203].

Transmission may occur through autoinoculation in children with concurrent herpes labialis and herpetic whitlow infections or through hetero-inoculation from parents or family members with herpes labialis infections [199, 203]. It has been postulated that the application of corticosteroid agents may increase disease dissemination. However, current data has not demonstrated a link between EH and these agents but has shown a relationship concerning EH, early-onset of AD, and increased total serum IgE levels [199, 203, 204]. Increased viral penetration into these areas is likely due to vulnerability from injured cell immunity, skin barrier compromise, and open excoriations [180, 204].

Diagnosis is made clinically and can be confirmed with viral culture or viral PCR [180, 203]. In the pediatric population, acyclovir is the treatment of choice. Route of administration varies by severity of presentation and thus whether management is inpatient versus outpatient. Specifically, oral acyclovir is reserved for milder presentations due to its low bioavailability, while IV acyclovir can be used for more serious cases. Antibiotics are used to treat superinfection. Clear guidelines for hospitalization have not been established, but a study of 79 pediatric patients with EH determined such predictors of hospitalization to be age less than 1 year, the presence of fever and systemic symptoms, and the male sex [203]. Additionally, hospitalization was associated with an increased risk of recurrent episodes. However, recurrent episodes were not associated with length of hospital stay, age, sex, or type of treatment [203].

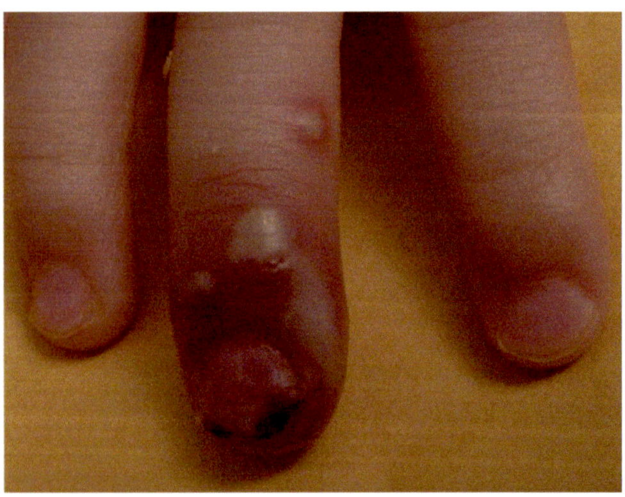

Fig. 8.7 Primary herpetic whitlow of a 2-year-old child with concurrent primary oral herpes. Note erythema, vesicular eruptions, and crusted ulceration on the involved digit (Reprinted from Fatahzadeh and Schwartz [198], Copyright (2007), with permission from Elsevier)

Herpetic Whitlow

Herpetic whitlow is a rare manifestation of HSV-1 and HSV-2 infection [180, 205–207]. Viral inoculation occurs directly through breaks in the skin or cuticle and produces vesicular eruptions on the fingers and toes [180, 206–208]. The finger pulp is often involved, but paronychial, eponychial, and subungual areas may also be affected [180, 206, 209]. Infection incidence is bimodal, affecting young adults between the ages of 20–30 years and children under the age of 10 [208]. Within the pediatric population, a peak is observed in children during the first 2 years of life [180, 205, 206, 208]. Autoinoculation from HSV-1 infection such as herpes labialis and gingivostomatitis, through such acts as thumb sucking and fingernail biting, are the primary means of infection in children [180, 205, 206, 208, 210]. Hetero-inoculation occurred when parents and others family members infected with herpes labialis kiss a child's fingers and toes [205, 206]. In adults older than age 20, infection primarily resulted from autoinoculation with HSV-2. Healthcare workers are also at elevated risk for disease contraction due to direct contact with oral secretions if universal health precautions such as hand washing and glove wearing are not followed [180, 206–208].

Burning, tingling, itching, edema, erythema, pain, fever, and regional lymphadenopathy can all result prior to the formation of deep, clear vesicles (Fig. 8.8) [180, 206, 207]. Later, vesicles can become clouded from a leukocyte infiltration [205]. Amalgamation of the vesicles may mirror a bacterial pyogenic infection and render misdiagnosis [184, 206, 207]. Complicating features include superinfection with *Staphylococcus aureus* or other bacteria and permanent forfeiture of the nail plate [180, 206, 207].

Immunocompetent patients generally experience resolution in 2–3 weeks with a recurrence rate of 20 %, increased when HSV-2 is the pathogen [209]. Primary infection tends to be generally more symptomatic than recurrent disease. Infection in immunocompromised patients can become severe with longer disease course, more progressive infection, prompt recurrence, and frequent bacterial infection

[206, 209]. Significant destruction from necrosis and microbial superinfection can obscure the clinical picture and complicate diagnosis in these patients [208]. In cases in which lesions are chronic or significantly atypical, a biopsy may be necessary to help in diagnosis [209].

Diagnosis is centered on the clinical presentation of painful vesicles on the fingers or toes. If this is the first infection, the patient might report HSV infection in self or a near contact. If it is a recurrent infection, the patient will commonly recall a prior episode in the same area. History information might also note trauma to the nail, which imparts a route for viral inoculation [206, 207]. The diagnosis can then be confirmed with a Tzanck test, viral culture, or PCR. It is important to note that the differential diagnosis includes both felon and paronychia. Of note, the vesicles in paronychia are purulent upon formation unlike the initial, clear vesicular fluid in herpetic whitlow. Administration of proper treatment requires clinical differentiation between all three diseases [180, 206, 207].

Incision and drainage is not advisable, as adverse events such as viremia and superinfection can result. The infected area should be covered so as to prevent exposure to viral shedding. In immunocompetent patients treatment is primarily symptomatic with analgesics to lessen pain, and antibiotics to treat superinfection [180, 206, 207]. Limited data has been provided regarding the efficacy of antivirals in immunocompetent patients and remains unclear if there is a role in decreasing the severity of infection. Longer courses of systemic antivirals such as acyclovir are used in the treatment of herpes infection in immunocompromised patients. The use of suppressive therapy in these patients is controversial, as acyclovir-resistant strains can develop. It remains to be seen if antiviral implementation shortly after reactivation provides appreciable benefit [206, 209].

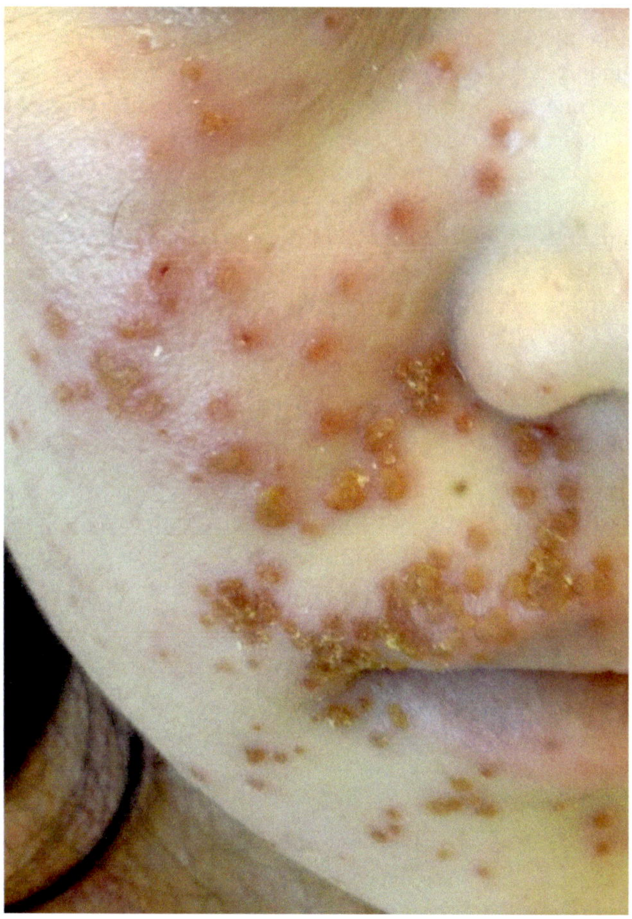

Fig. 8.8 Eczema herpeticum on the face in an adult. Note several, umbilicated vesiculopustules with hemorrhagic crusting and punched out erosions on the face (Reprinted from Fatahzadeh and Schwartz [198], Copyright (2007), with permission from Elsevier)

Ocular Herpes

Herpes simplex virus can produce unilateral or bilateral keratoconjunctivitis, most often causing epithelial keratitis [180, 183, 211]. HSV remains a major cause of blindness worldwide owing to viral cytolytic and immune-mediated damage that result in corneal scarring worsened with repeated infection [190, 212]. Ocular presentations of HSV infection occur at a prevalence of 140 per 100,000 person-years [213]. Sensitivity to light, blurry vision, discharges, and pain are common presenting symptoms [180, 183, 189]. Recurrent disease is common and associated with shorter intervals between episodes as recurrence rate increases [213]. Immunocompromised patients, notably organ transplant recipients, can develop serious infection of the respiratory and gastrointestinal tracts [183].

Infection can occur after autoinoculation from an active oral HSV infection with 22 % of patients reporting a concomitant HSV orolabial infection at the time of presentation [180]. Alternatively, virus can also be reactivated in the trigeminal ganglia and travel anterograde along the ophthalmic division of the trigeminal nerve [212]. After a lesion has formed, the virus may remain latent in the stroma of the cornea [212, 214].

Diagnosis is largely based on clinical presentation and can be confirmed with PCR, viral culture, and Tzanck test. Demonstration of dendritic ulcers can also be seen under fluorescein staining [184]. A meta-analysis of therapeutic regimens concluded that topical agents trifluridine, acyclovir, and vidarabine were more efficacious than idoxuridine but that all three had equivalent efficacy in treating dendritic epithelial keratitis [211]. Keratoplasty can also be performed in severe and chronic disease with importance placed on concurrent antiviral therapy for 6 months post-surgery to prevent recrudescence [211, 212].

Herpes Gladiatorum

HSV-1 infection can result from inoculation via abraded skin, in such sports as rugby and wrestling, in which close, repetitive, skin-to-skin contact occurs [180, 215]. Scattered vesicles can commonly present on the face, ears, neck, and back with concurrent lymphadenopathy, fever, and malaise. Additionally, infection can include the eye, which may be due to autoinoculation. Infections may recur without systemic symptoms or adenopathy. Importance is placed on early recognition and sequestration of infected players with the potential administration of prophylactic antiviral agents for the duration of the athletic season [180, 187, 215].

Neonatal Herpes

Genital HSV infection can be caused by both serotypes, and infectivity during pregnancy can result in intrauterine growth restriction, spontaneous abortion, prematurity, and congenital and neonatal HSV infection [189]. Incidence rates of neonatal herpes infection range from 1 case in 2 to 5000 deliveries annually [182]. Infection route in order of frequency is peripartum, postnatal, and intrauterine, with more than 95 % of babies obtaining infection during the first two time periods [180, 216]. Infectivity results from viral shedding at delivery, direct contact from family members and hospital workers with orolabial herpes, and transplacental viral transmission [180, 182, 187].

Neonatal HSV can present with localized disease in the skin, eyes, and mouth; with disseminated illness; and with CNS infection [180, 189, 216]. In localized disease, vesicles and keratoconjunctivitis are first evident at approximately 10 days (Fig. 8.9). If cutaneous lesions are present, recurrence will most likely result during the first 6 months of life. Disseminated disease can involve encephalitis, liver failure, and coagulopathy and carries significant mortality (Fig. 8.10) [180, 216]. Without treatment, mortality approaches 80 %, and even with treatment, survivors may sustain permanent disability. Encephalitis is occurs in 33 % of infants with HSV infection and presents with seizures, lethargy, poor oral intake, and irritability [180, 189, 216]. Cultured virus from CSF samples can be retrieved in 25–40 % of patients. If treatment is not rendered, 50 % of infants will not survive and those that do will have long-term neurological deficits [180, 182].

Peripartum infection is achieved when the mother is shedding virus at delivery, regardless of whether the infection is symptomatic [180, 216]. Sixty to eighty percent of women who give birth to an HSV-infected infant do not have active infection at birth, history of HSV infection, or a partner claiming a history of HSV infection [180, 216]. Several variables affect transmission from mother to fetus such as infection type, maternal antibody levels, use of fetal scalp monitors, rupture of membrane duration, and route of delivery. In recurrent infection, transmission rates are less than 3 % but increase to 30–50 % in maternal primary infection [182, 216].

Intrauterine HSV disease is extremely rare with rates of 1 in 300,000 deliveries. Neonates display various cutaneous findings such as hyper- and hypopigmentation, aplasia cutis, scarring, and lesions; ophthalmologic features like microphthalmia, retinal dysplasia, and chorioretinitis; and neurological manifestations such as microcephaly, encephalomalacia, and cerebral calcifications [180, 216]. Identification of infants born with congenital HSV is paramount as morbidity and mortality are very high, and prompt administration of antiviral therapy is required [180, 182].

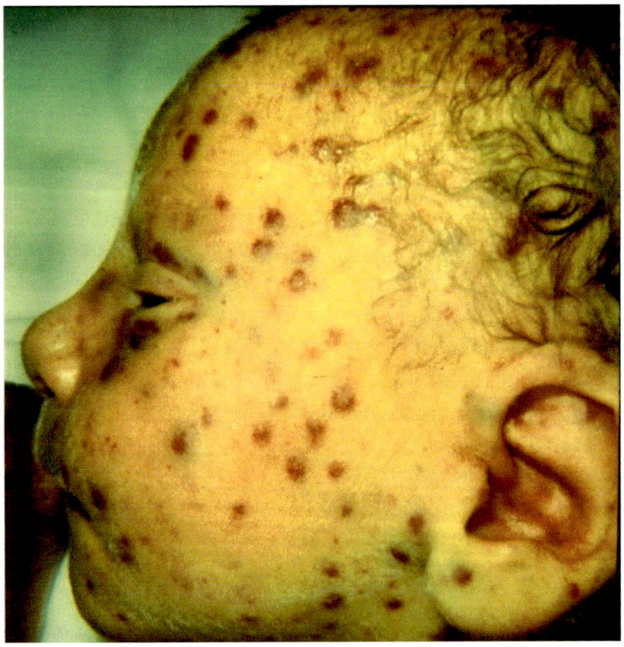

Fig. 8.9 Localized HSV disease in a neonate. Note the scattered, hemorrhagic pustules on the face

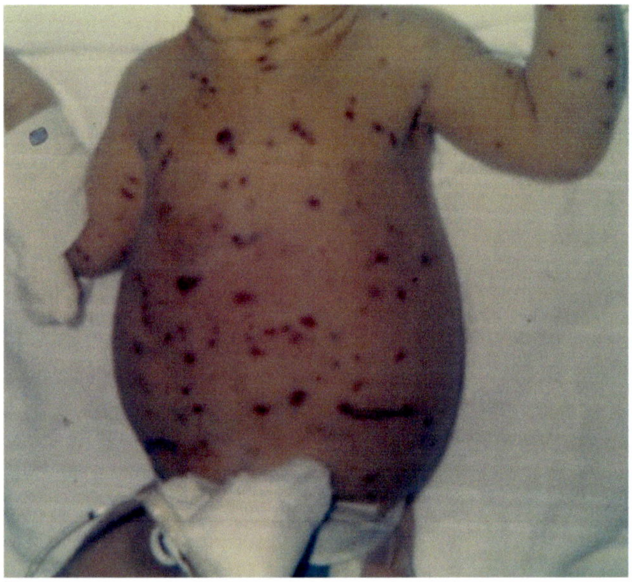

Fig. 8.10 Disseminated HSV disease in a neonate. Note the hepatosplenomegaly

HSV Encephalitis

HSV is the primary infectious cause of sporadic HSV encephalitis worldwide [180, 182, 188]. Without treatment, the mortality rate is greater than 70 %, and only 2.5 % of survivors sustain normal neurological functioning. Unlike neonatal encephalitis, HSV-1 is the common pathogen in adults and children and is often produced by recurrent infection [180]. Symptoms can include fever, altered consciousness, disordered thinking, and localized neurological deficits. Suspicion for the diagnosis should be raised with the following constellation of findings: altered consciousness, fever, CSF abnormalities, and focal neurological findings, with exclusion of other pathogenic cause [180]. Prompt diagnosis and antiviral administration are paramount for effective management of the disease [180].

Immunocompromised State

HSV infection in an immunocompromised host can be severe due to increased illness duration and delayed treatment response (Fig. 8.11) [180, 188]. Increased frequency and degree and length of immunosuppression are all correlated with advanced HSV disease, and extensive antiviral therapy poses the risk for therapeutic resistance [182, 187, 217, 218]. Intraoral disease can decrease nutritional intake due to pain from ulcerations on the palate. Fungal and bacterial superinfection may present in large mucocutaneous lesions in the nasolabial and genital areas with concern for subsequent bacteremia [218, 219].

Apart from severity, clinical patterns of disease presentation are also unique, and sites of infection may include the gastrointestinal tract, esophagus, and respiratory tract [180, 182]. Reactivation can occur at sites of manipulation including where nasogastric and tracheal intubation devices were located.

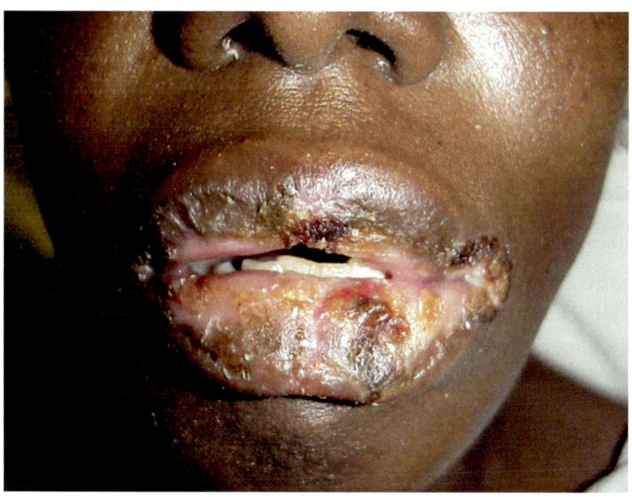

Fig. 8.11 Recurrent herpes labialis in an immunocompromised individual. Extensive disease affecting the vermilion border of both the upper and lower lip (Reprinted from Fatahzadeh and Schwartz [198], Copyright (2007), with permission from Elsevier)

Anogenital disease may manifest atypically, as painful, persistent verrucous lesions and ulcers, mimicking condyloma acuminatum and verrucous carcinoma [220–222]. Verrucous papules may form on the vulva, penis, scrotum, and intergluteal region. A case of a pregnant woman with severe combined immunodeficiency presenting with recurrent vegetations encasing the vulva has been described [223]. Verrucous varicella can also occur in HIV/AIDS patients and may present difficulty in distinguishing between herpes zoster and herpes simplex infection [192].

Herpes-Associated Erythema Multiforme (HAEM)

Erythema multiforme (EM) presents clinically as circular, targetoid lesions, commonly located on the extensor surface of the acral extremities [224, 225]. Herpes simplex infection, mycoplasma infection, and drug reactions are the primary causative agents [224, 225]. A variant of EM infections are recurrent, of which HSV reactivation accounts for at least 80 % of cases [180, 192, 219]. HSV viral shedding may occur with clinically apparent or asymptomatic disease, and viral exposure is approximately 2–17 days prior to HAEM formation [180, 224–226].

HAEM eruption is believed to result from a hypersensitivity reaction in the host. Viral antigen trapping within host immune cells in the keratinocyte layer provokes the subsequent release of interferon gamma and causes an inflammatory response by host T cells [180, 225].

Most acute infections are self-limited, and treatment is usually symptomatic using topical corticosteroids and oral antihistamines [227]. HSV antiviral therapy for at least 6 months is advised in order to decrease recurrence in HAEM [227]. If patients do not respond appropriately to antiviral therapy, dapsone and azathioprine have showed some efficacy in HAEM [226, 227].

Genital Herpes

Genital herpes is one of the most common sexually transmitted infections worldwide. HSV-2 still remains the culprit for the majority of these infections [180] However, HSV-1 can also be responsible for this infection with recent studies showing an increase of HSV-1 genital herpes in the USA, Canada, and the UK [181].

Primary and non-primary genital herpes outbreaks are frequently asymptomatic, accounting for 80 % with positive HSV serology never having clinical symptoms or a previous diagnosis of genital HSV infection [181]. However, a primary presentation can be very painful with a patient experiencing erosive balanitis, vulvitis, or vaginitis. Lesions in men typically occur on the glans or shaft of the penis and/or buttock. In contrast, women have a more complicated course with lesions involving the cervix, buttocks, and perineum with accompanied inguinal adenopathy and dysuria (Fig. 8.12). In addition, systemic complaints and complica-

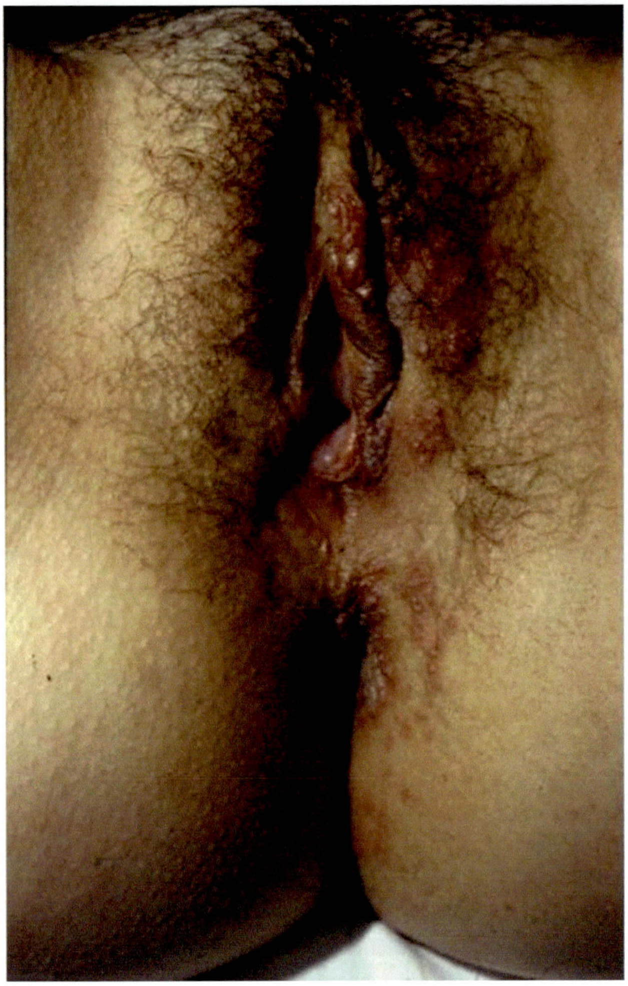

Fig. 8.12 Genital herpes in an immunocompetent female

tions are more common in women [182]. Females tend to experience such complications as extragenital lesions, urinary retention, and aseptic meningitis.

Subclinical shedding and clinically evident recurrences are common. Recurrences tend to be mild and occur more often with HSV-2 infection. Vesicles reappear on the genitalia and/or buttock and resolve in about 1 week. The frequency and time interval between recurrences varies greatly, with an average of 4–7 outbreaks annually [182].

Synergy of HSV-2 with HIV

Epidemiologic data has demonstrated that infection with mycobacterium, hepatitis, and HSV-2 facilitates the acquisition, replication, and transmission of HIV [217, 228]. The association between HSV-2 and HIV infection was recognized in the late 1980s, as HSV-2 infection often preceded detection of HIV [215, 228, 229]. Results of a meta-analysis showed that patients who were seropositive to HSV-2 had three times the risk of infection with HIV than those who were seronegative [230]. Studies have demonstrated that HSV-2 enhances HIV viral shedding and hence replication, as large amounts of HSV-2 DNA correlated with elevated amounts of concurrent HIV-1 RNA in cervical secretions. Parallel shedding occurred regardless of whether or not the HSV-2 infection was symptomatic [231]. The most compelling support for these observations comes from treatment of HSV-2 infection with valacyclovir and the subsequent decrease in genital and plasma HIV RNA levels [217, 232].

Immune mechanisms employed by HSV-2 enhance HIV infection [215, 228, 232]. During HSV-2 reactivation, CD4 + T cells infiltrate into the mucosa and skin, which readily provides the main target cell for HIV infection and replication. Additionally, HSV-2 proteins are able to activate latent HIV infection [228]. HSV-2's impact on HIV progression and transmission provides additional treatment aims when managing HIV infection [228].

8.3.2.7 Immune Response

Cell-mediated responses via CD8+ T cells and CD4+ T cells are vital to the destruction of herpes simplex virus through interferon gamma production. The value of host cell-mediated responses can best be appreciated in mouse knockout models and in the immunodeficient state [181, 184]. Mice deficient in lymphocytic populations and interferon gamma signaling show increased viral penetration, replication, and decreased survival [233]. The exact role of antibody-mediated defense is still controversial, as the presence of an antibody response to herpes simplex virus does not yield immunity in humans. However, antibody-treatment prior to viral inoculation has decreased viral load and clinical disease recurrence rate in mouse models [182].

Equally as impressive are HSV's mechanisms to evade immune system surveillance [183]. HSV blocks its peptide transport to the endoplasmic reticulum and subsequent MHC class presentation by inhibiting TAP-1 and TAP-2 transport. HSV also inhibits programmed cell death by itself and the host and synthesizes proteins to dephosphorylate host translation factors, which keeps protein synthesis constitutively turned on [183].

Interestingly, human herpes simplex virus infection has been postulated to perhaps play a role in autoimmune disease development through the activation of human endogenous retrovirus elements [234]. Human endogenous retroviruses (HERVs) consist of approximately 8 % of the human genome and are surrounded by long terminal repeats. Most of the HERVs have been inactivated by mutations and rarely remain active to produce protein. HERVs and antibodies against HERVs are elevated in several autoimmune diseases such as psoriasis, scleroderma, and systemic lupus erythematous. In vitro investigation has detected that HSV can activate expression of HERV elements, and further, the inflammatory response produced against HSV infection may uncover these antigens and expose them to the immune system [234].

8.3.2.8 Detection/Diagnosis

Diagnosis is usually rendered from visualization of clinical lesions and patient history [188]. If diagnosis is unclear, PCR, viral culture, serology, Tzanck test, and direct fluorescent antibody testing can be used. The "gold standard" for diagnosis is HSV isolation in tissue culture. A period of 2–7 days is necessary before cytopathic changes are appreciated [180, 187]. Viral culture should be sampled from the fluid of unroofed blisters as vesicles contain the greatest virus titer in the first 24–48 h; however, culture only yields a sensitivity of 50 % [180, 188]. PCR allows for more precise detection of virus in asymptomatic shedding and is the best test for isolating HSV in cerebrospinal fluid [187]. Tzanck smear involves scraping the floor of a vesicle, staining it, and identifying multinucleated giant cells. However, the Tzanck smear cannot distinguish between herpes simplex and herpes zoster infection. Direct fluorescent antibody testing is useful in air-dried samples and has a sensitivity of 80 %. Lastly, serological tests can distinguish serotype-specific antibodies [180].

Treatment Resistance

Resistance to antiviral therapy has been growing increasingly more common in immunocomprised patients, while immunocompetent populations have not seen similar frequencies [180, 217, 235, 236]. Resistant strains of HSV may be explained by the lengthened course of antiviral therapies in suppressive therapy, and in the treatment of chronic, persistent lesions in immunocompromised individuals [217].

Acyclovir is a guanosine analogue that requires phosphorylation by viral thymidine kinase (TK) for activation [217, 236]. Incorporation of the triphosphate form of acyclovir into viral DNA obstructs DNA polymerase and causes DNA synthesis to stop. Resistance to acyclovir, a mainstay of treatment for both HSV-1 and HSV-2, has resulted when mutations are acquired in viral TK and DNA polymerase genes. 95 % of resistant strains are due to either a decreased function of TK or complete absence of the gene. The three main variants in mutation of TK are *viral TK partial* which has decreased TK activity, *viral TK altered* with reduced phosphorylation efficiency, and *TK negative* with deletion of the gene [236]. Because penciclovir employs a similar mechanism of action as acyclovir, substitution to treat acyclovir-resistant strains is not advised. Replacement with valacyclovir or famciclovir is equally as unsuitable as both drugs rely on TK for activation [180, 217, 236].

Preventing treatment resistance relies both on selecting the correct antiviral dose in order to avoid suboptimal concentrations and on determining the viral genotype to ensure appropriate treatment selection [217, 236]. The use of multiple agents simultaneously can also be employed when infections are life-threatening, intractable, or presenting with varied drug susceptibilities. Both foscarnet and cidofovir can be used in acyclovir-resistant infections, but they must be intravenously administered and carry serious risk of renal toxicity. Unfortunately, resistance to foscarnet has been described due to mutations in viral DNA polymerase, and strains resistant to acyclovir can have cross-resistance to foscarnet. Further, strains carrying mutations in both DNA polymerase and TK have also been documented. Cidofovir does not rely on viral TK for activation, and strains resistant to acyclovir and foscarnet are still sensitive to this agent [217, 236].

Drug development aims to produce medications that have an effect on viral targets distinct from DNA polymerase, in order to combat emerging avenues of resistance. The helicase-primase inhibitor, AIC136, completed a phase II trial and was successful in decreasing both viral shedding and duration of genital herpes infection [236, 237]. Other potential targets are directed at viral proteins and peptides and hence would inhibit viral attachment and entry. In the interim, intralesional cidofovir and imiquimod have been used as alternatives in patients with acyclovir-resistant infections [217, 235, 236].

Vaccine Development

HSV infection carries significant morbidity and mortality worldwide, especially in neonates and immunocompromised patients [238]. Vaccine development has focused on HSV-2, and aims have been twofold: to produce a robust antibody response upon primary infection and to generate cell-mediated responses in order to prevent the transmission and recurrent attacks in genital herpes [238, 239]. Some HSV-2 vaccines aimed at producing antibody responses to viral glycoproteins have been successful in animal models but have not carried over into human models. This may be attributed to alterations in viral glycoprotein structure over time, as well as discordant immune cells in animals and humans. Unfortunately, patients can be infected with multiple strains of HSV-2, and complete immunity from the virus may not be possible. A current phase II study in Europe is investigating a compound, Immunovex, deficient in HSV immune evasion genes, as a candidate vaccine. Investigation into safe, replication-deficient vaccines and inactivated virus vaccines or alternatively, a safe live vaccine, is still in progress. No matter the vehicle, primary importance is placed on invoking a strong immune response [238].

8.3.3 Molluscum Contagiosum Virus Infection of the Human Skin

Xiao-ying Chen, Alex Anstey, and Joachim Bugert

Molluscum contagiosum (MC) is a benign viral infection of the skin, which presents clinically as skin-colored, waxy, dome-shaped papules with a dimpled center, averaging

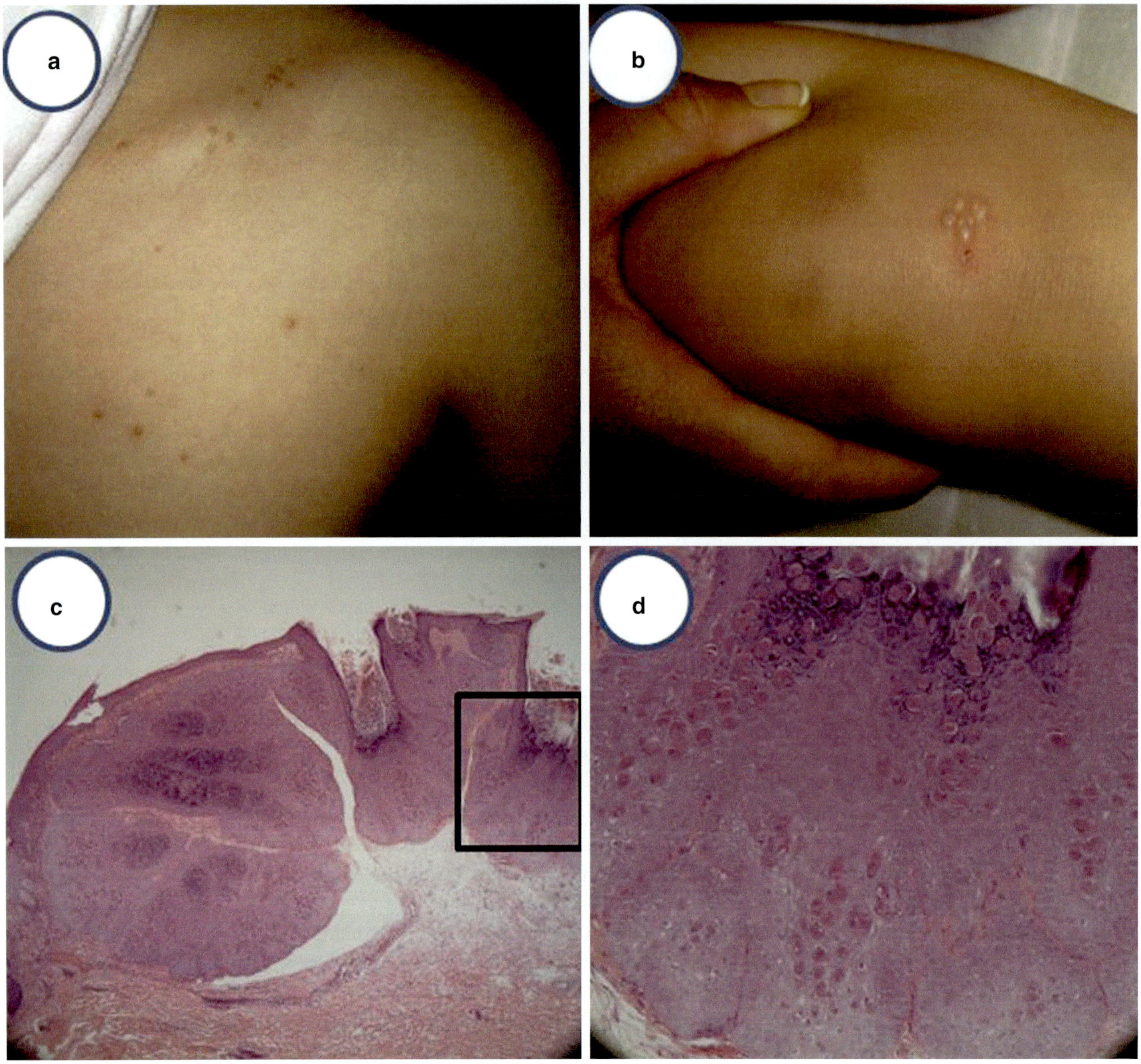

Fig. 8.13 Clinical, histological, and electron microscopy pictures of MC. Bland MC lesions on the chest of a 10-year-old girl (**a**). A cluster of lesions on the right knee of a 13-year-old boy (**b**). Hematoxylin and eosin stained section (5×) of an MC lesion reveals inverted lobules of hyperplastic, acanthotic squamous epithelium forming a central crater filled with keratin fragments and molluscum bodies (**c**). Hematoxylin and eosin stained section (20×) of above sample showed large, eosinophilic, intracytoplasmic inclusion bodies (**d**) (**a–d** taken by Xiaoying Chen (2014) with permission from patients seen in the Department of Dermatology, Rui Jin Hospital, School of Medicine, Shanghai Jiao Tong University, Shanghai, China)

3–5 mm in diameter [240] (Fig. 8.13a, b). MC often affects children and young people but may also arise in immunosuppressed individuals, either due to HIV infection, drug-induced immunosuppression, or genetic defects affecting the innate immune response [241]. The lesions may propagate via autoinoculation or spread directly by skin contact. Although MC lesions can involve any anatomic site, it usually affects the trunk, axillae, extremities, and sometimes the genital area, especially in sexually active individuals [242].

8.3.3.1 Histopathology

The clinical diagnosis of MC can usually be made by observing the typical lesions. When necessary, biopsy samples can be taken either with a shave, punch biopsy, or by excision. The histopathology of MC is characterized by inverted lobules of hyperplastic, acanthotic squamous epithelium (acanthoma), forming a central crater filled with keratin fragments. Henderson-Paterson bodies are seen above the basal layer of the epidermis, consisting of large cells with abundant eosinophilic cytoplasm (accumulated virions), and a small peripheral nucleus (Fig. 8.13c, d).

In electron microscopy (EM), the virions of MCV appear as enveloped, pleomorphic, generally ovoid to brick-shaped, with a dumbbell-shaped central core and lateral bodies, measuring approximately 320×250×200 nm [243]. Membrane fragments often loosely attach to virions, which indicate a noncontinuous lipid envelope wrapping the core [244].

8.3.3.2 MCV Genetics and Epidemiology

MCV is classified as a member of the family *Poxviridae*, genus *Molluscipoxvirus*. The linear double-stranded DNA genome of MCV type I (MCV 1/80) has been cloned into 18 recombinant bacterial plasmid clones, representing overlapping EcoRI, BamHI, and HindIII restriction fragment libraries [245]. The overlapping genome fragment library was sequenced and found to comprise 190,289 bp (GenBank accession U60315: MCV type 1/80) [246]. The MCV genome was described to encode 182 genes, with 154 that were highly likely to be coding genes [247], among which 105 hypothetical proteins have homologues to smallpox virus and other poxviruses. The remaining ORFs are unique to MCV; some are involved in the suppression of the host response to infection, whereas others affect nucleotide biosynthesis and cell proliferation [247, 248].

MCV DNA restriction fragment patterns reveal four main genetic types, MCV-I, MCV-II, MCV-III, and MCV-IV, and a number of variants with single restriction site variations [249–251]. MCV-I is the most prevalent and MCV-II is usually seen in adults. The molecular epidemiology of MCV infection showed geographical variations in the distribution of the MCV. It was reported that the ratios of MCV-I/MCV-II/MCV-III (previously designated MCV-II variant) were 32:1:0 in Germany [252], 174:7:2 [253] and 80:25:1 [250] in the UK, 44:22:2 in Australia [254], and 61:0:0 in Turkey [255]. A large molecular epidemiological study of MCV in Japan revealed the ratio of MCV-I/MCV-II/MCV-III/MCV-IV as 436:13:24:4, in which MCV-IV was a new subtype not previously detected [251].

A comprehensive study on MCV serum prevalence using a virion ELISA was reported by Konya and Thompson from Australia in 1999. MCV antibody was identified in 77 % of persons with MC lesions: in 17 of 24 HIV-1-negative persons and in 10 of 11 who were HIV-1-positive. The population survey revealed an overall seropositivity rate of 23 % (81/357) [256]. The most recent study, using a novel ELISA, found MC084-specific antibodies in 100 % (12/12) of individuals with clinical MC and determined the overall seroprevalence of MC in German and UK populations as 14.8 % (43/289) and 30.3 % (10/33), respectively [257].

8.3.3.3 MCV Lifecycle

A schematic drawing of the MCV life cycle is shown in Fig. 8.14. MCV, like all poxviruses, is a cytoplasmically replicating virus. MCV reaches basal epidermal cells, likely through minor trauma cracking the epidermal surface layers. After attachment, viral cores penetrate into the cytoplasm of the basal cells by endocytosis/macropinocytosis [258]. MCV induces an enhanced rate of mitosis in infected keratinocytes, possibly by means of EGFR upregulation and interferes with the normal epidermal cell differentiation process [259]. The early genes of MCV are thought to be expressed in basal cells, while the virus particles are uncoated, and the late gene products follow upon progression to the spinous cell layer. Henderson-Paterson bodies, the viral inclusion bodies, appear about 3–4 layers above the basal cell layer and grow in size as they progress toward the higher cell layers. These granular epidermal cells are found in uninfected epidermis, as cell differentiation is modulated by viral gene expression, and keratin granules are replaced by viral inclusion bodies. The later represent the typical cytoplasmic poxviral assembly site, or "factories," where virus is assembled en masse, pushing the cellular organelles, including the cell nucleus, to the periphery of the cell [258]. The "factories" are surrounded by a collagen and lipid-rich saclike structure which has only been observed by EM [244] and may be a cellular organelle used by MCV for assembly. The maturation of MCV in vivo has been demonstrated to take 5 days using electron microscopic autoradiography [260]. The upper layers of infected epidermal cells are ultimately transformed into an amorphous mass of cellular debris and molluscum bodies with large quantities of MCV virions and extruded into the dimpled lesion center. Thus MC contagious debris is passed on to others through smear infections [258, 261].

8.3.3.4 MCV Local Immune Response in the Skin

The MCV viral colony sac [244] surrounding viral inclusion bodies provides a layer of invisibility to the immune system, by physically separating MCV antigen from all pathways of presentation to the immune system. Ku et al. revealed that in MC lesions, toll-like receptor (TLR)3 and TLR9 were strongly expressed in endosomal vesicles of epidermal keratinocytes, inducing local IFN-α and TNF-β responses [262]. A homozygous mutation of tyrosine kinase 2 (Tyk2) in a hyper-IgE syndrome patient leads to the deficiency of Tyk2 and downstream cytokine signals involved in innate and acquired immunity and explained susceptibility to various microorganisms including MCV [263].

There are two major types of MCV lesions with regards to immunological activity: lesions with immune cells absent and lesions with strong immunological activity. Initial, dense polymorphic lymphocyte infiltration was

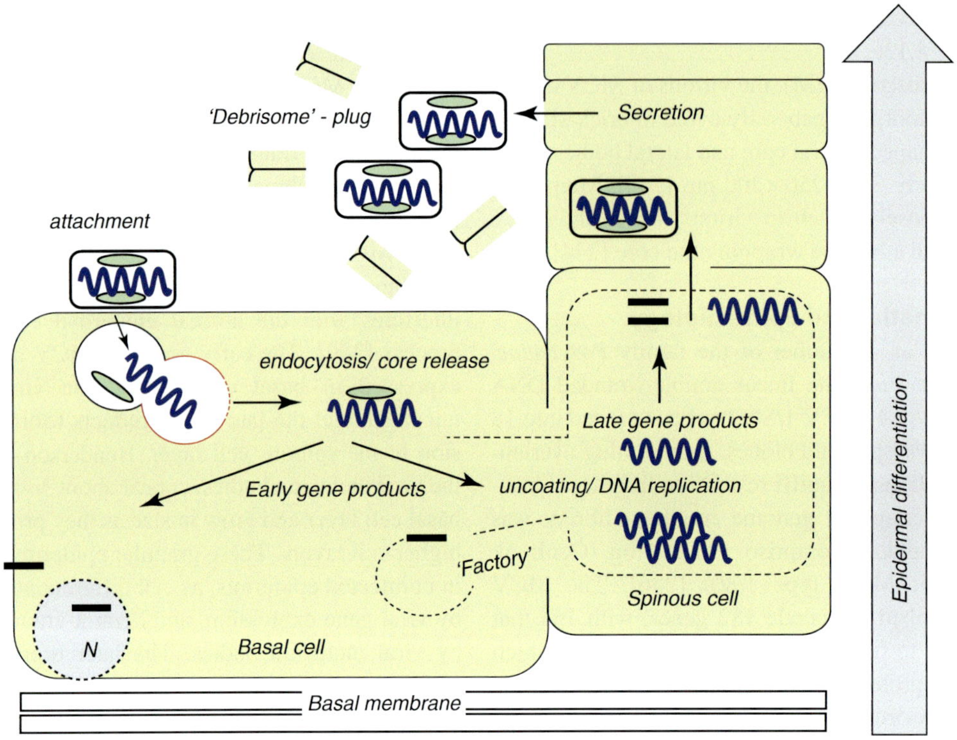

Fig. 8.14 MCV life cycle in the epidermis. After attachment, MCV viral cores penetrate into the cytoplasm of the basal cells, where the early genes of the MCV are expressed. Early viral proteins inhibit innate immune responses leading to apoptosis and the tissue interferon response (mc159, mc160). Virus particles are then uncoated in transit between the basal layer and spinous layers of the epidermis, the step believed to be blocked in standard cell culture. Late genes are expressed following genome replication in the spinous cell layer. Virions are assembled en masse in cytoplasmatic assembly sites, inclusion bodies also known as poxvirus "factories," containing "molluscum bodies." As the "factories" grow, the cellular organelles, including the cell nucleus, are pushed aside, forming a thin crescent at the periphery of the cell. The stratum corneum ultimately disintegrates as the inclusions enlarge, releasing the "molluscum bodies" with large numbers of infectious MCV virions into the typical central indentation of the mature molluscum lesion along with cellular debris. This "debrisome plug" extrudes upon pressure, and MC is transmitted via smear infection

described in MC skin biopsies [264]. However, other studies showed that dendritic cells (DC) were absent in MC lesions but were normal or increasing in the perilesional normal skin [265]. Benign MC with lesions cleared by strong local immune responses may be typical for the immunocompetent host. Patients with immune disorders, especially those affecting the innate immune response, are likely to have more extensive manifestations of MC. In atopic dermatitis, characterized by a T helper 2 (Th2) cytokine switching pattern, more extensive MC lesions remain undetected for longer and may be resistant to immune therapy.

The above considerations suggest that MCV in an uninflamed lesion is hidden from the immune system, through active (immune evasive gene products) and passive (viral colony sac) defenses. A recent study by Vermi et al. shed light on the mechanism for spontaneous regression of MC, once the immune system has identified MCV infection [266]. MCV virions, once exposed, are apparently highly immunogenic; a vigorous immune response leads to complete viral clearance from the human skin. Swiecki et al. speculated that in inflamed MC lesions, the activated dendritic cells produce type I interferon (IFN) and other cytokines which induce the differentiation of monocytes into IFN-DCs ($CD123^{+}CD11c^{+}CD16^{+}CD14^{+}MxA^{+}$). These novel tissue DCs may secrete IFN-I, kill virus-infected cells via granzyme B (GrB) and/or TNF-related apoptosis-inducing ligand (TRAIL), and promote natural killer cell, DC, T-cell, and B-cell function [267]. MCV-induced skin immunity may prove to be a valuable tool to study skin-specific immune defenses.

Due to the lack of a MCV cell culture model or animal models, to date, no study has clearly characterized the interaction between immune cells, keratinocytes, and MCV. The process of "uncloaking" of MC virions in infected tissue, leading to spontaneous regression is still not clearly elucidated. MCV appears to be a powerful immunogen in the human skin and, due to non-neutralizing immunity in the population, could be considered as a potent vaccine vector if further genetically modified in cell culture. Growing the virus in standard cell culture must therefore be a priority for MCV research.

8.3.3.5 MCV Genes Implicated in Immune Evasion

In MCV-infected skin, there is little or no inflammatory cell infiltration of the epidermis or surrounding dermis in undisturbed lesions. This changes, when the MCV lesion is exposed to the immune system, and a full immune response is mounted [266]. It has been proposed that the initial lack of immune responses to MCV in situ is due to the activity of a number of host-response evasion genes present in the MCV genome and the absence of others [268]. A ligand inhibitor encoded by MCV, MC54, binds to interleukin-18 and inhibits IFN-γ production [269, 270]. MC66L-mediated antiapoptotic activity may also explain the increased survival time of MCV-infected cells in the UV-exposed epidermis, allowing MCV a longer productive cycle [271]. MC148, expressed early in the MCV lifecycle, encodes a human macrophage inflammatory protein (MIP)-1β and may provide an anti-inflammatory activity gradient in the transition zone between epidermal and dermal tissue as a form of standoff defensive device for the virus before other mechanisms engage [272]. MC159 and MC160 belong to intracellular inhibitors of NF-κB and are members of viral FLICE-inhibitory proteins (vFLIPs). MC159 protein was shown to inhibit apoptosis induced by Fas and TNF [273–275].

8.3.3.6 Prevention and Management of MCV Infection

Molluscum contagiosum is benign and generally undergoes a self-limiting nature history; watchful waiting is always recommended in immunocompetent individuals. The average duration of a single lesion is about 2 months [276]. However, since the lesions spread easily by autoinoculation from scratching or trauma, the mean duration of MC is about 8 months; some may even persist for 1 year or longer [277].

Treatment of MC is not usually necessary, and no consensus has yet been established concerning the management of this condition. The age of the patient, the number and position of the lesions, and complications such as inflammation, pruritus, dermatitis, and secondary infection should all be taken into account when considering treatment. When therapy is required, options include physical ablative methods, chemical agents, immune modulators, and antiviral drugs. Patients with HIV or those with immune incompetency may suffer from extensive and severe MC lesion. The aim of the treatments is to directly destroy or remove the virus itself, by destroying the infected epidermal cells or by stimulating an immunological response.

Current treatment options for immunocompetent patients include curettage [278], cryotherapy [279], pulsed dye laser [280], phenol [281], cantharidin [282], podophyllotoxin cream [283], salicylic acid [284], benzoyl peroxide cream [285], retinoic acid cream [285], potassium hydroxide (KOH) [286, 287], oral cimetidine [288], intralesional *Candida* antigen injection [289], and measles, mumps, and rubella (MMR) vaccine intralesional injection [290].

Unfortunately, the few published randomized, controlled trials for the treatment of MC have limited utility due to small sample sizes or failure to include the mast common interventions, such as cryotherapy [291]. A number of common treatments for MC are still widely used in primary healthcare despite the lack of evidence for their efficacy. For example, curettage may be used for sparse MC [292]. Pain is the most common side effect and can be minimized by local anesthetic. Two recent descriptive studies showed that the effectiveness of curettage was 34 % (22/64) and 38.7 % (29/75), respectively [278, 293].

Cantharidin, an extract from the blister beetle, is widely used in the USA for treating MC with a quoted efficacy of 90–96 % [294, 295]. The widely reported side effect of cantharidin is blister formation and secondary infection. In a recent study on 10 % KOH solution and salicylic and lactic acid combination in the treatment of MC, 83.3 % (10/12) of KOH group and all the 14 patients of salicylic and lactic acid group demonstrated complete remission at the end of a 6 week study in Turkey [296].

Imiquimod, a toll-like receptor 7 (TLR7) agonist, activates the innate immune system through TLR7 and has been prescribed as a medical treatment for MC [292, 297]. However, two large randomized controlled trials in the USA both demonstrated that imiquimod 5 % cream, applied three times per week for up to 16 weeks, was no more effective than placebo cream in treating MC in a total of 702 children aged 2–12 years old [298].

MC in HIV may be extensive and include giant lesions in unusual locations such as the face, neck, and genital area. In patients with known HIV infection, the presence of MC may signify advancing immunosuppression [299]. The increase in incidence and difficulty in management correlate with depletion of T-helper lymphocytes typical for the late stages of AIDS when CD4 counts are below 100–200/mm^3 [300, 301]. Anecdotal reports of treatments for HIV-related MC indicate that antiviral and immune-modulating medications (imiquimod) appear to be more effective than local ablative therapies [302].

In conclusion, no single intervention has been shown to be effective for all patients with MC [303]. In clinical practice, most doctors encourage their patients to wait for spontaneous remission. Curettage and shave ablation are commonly practiced in China and in continental Europe but are best restricted to adults with very localized and limited MC.

8.4 Mosquito Bite Allergy

Tsu-Man Chiu and Yi-Giien Tsai

8.4.1 Introduction

Members of the order Diptera, the family Culicidae, mosquitoes are vectors for the transmission of many diseases worldwide. There are over 3000 different species of mosquitoes, which grouped into more than 40 genera [304]. Mosquitoes transmit many infectious diseases. Several genera of mosquito, including *Anopheles*, *Culex*, and *Aedes*, serve as vectors of malaria, yellow fever, dengue fever, filariasis, and encephalitis viruses, West Nile virus. The last pathogen causes the largest arboviral meningoencephalitis outbreak has ever recorded in North America. Because only female mosquitoes have piercing mouthparts, they inflict all human bites. CO_2-, odor-, and estrogen-surrounded skin can help mosquitoes to find and bite human [305].

8.4.2 Mosquito Allergy

Sensitization to mosquito bites occurs commonly in childhood, and bite reactivity often persists for years [306]. Sensitization is induced by salivary proteins which cause mosquito bite allergic reactions [307]. The saliva of mosquitoes contains a number of pharmacologically active compounds which inhibit the body's protective innate immune responses and cause anticoagulation, impairing platelet formation, vasodilation, and anti-inflammatory activities. Additionally, allergic reactions are also caused by saliva-induced bacterial or parasitic transmission, initial colonization, and allergens [308, 309]. Mosquito saliva-specific immunoglobulin E (IgE) and immunoglobulin G (IgG) antibodies and T-cell-mediated delayed hypersensitivity reaction appear to be involved in the pathogenesis [307, 310, 311]. Common cutaneous manifestations include immediate wheals and flares with a peak within 20 min and delayed itchy indurated erythematous papules with a peak at 24 ~ 36 h and then gradually resolving within days or weeks [310, 312]. The skin reaction patterns of mosquito bite had been classified into five stages in the process of sensitization and desensitization: stage 1, the bites do not induce a reaction; stage 2, delayed type of reaction (erythematous papules develop >4 mm during 3 ~ 4 h after bite with a peak at 24 ~ 36 h); stage 3, both immediate and delayed type of reaction (wheals develop >4 mm within a peak ≤20 min after bite); stage 4, only immediate wheals; and stage 5, the persons who have been repeated bitten eventually lose the reactions. The younger population (less than 20 years old) is mainly in stages 2 or 3. The older population (more than 20 years old) is mainly in stages 3 or 4 [313, 314]. In the prospective experimental study, an individual who had received mosquito bites developed immediate and delayed skin reactions at week 3 with a peak at 5 ~ 19 weeks. Reactions disappeared by week 26. However, natural desensitization may be different from the experimental study in real life. Peng et al. studied 401 infants, children, and adolescents and reported that both saliva-specific IgE and IgG declined with age. They suggested that "natural desensitization probably occurs during childhood and adolescence" [315].

Other reactions include vesicles, bullae, ecchymosis, Skeeter syndrome (large cellulitis-like local inflammatory reaction and low-grade fever), generalized urticaria, angioedema, and anaphylaxis [307, 316]. Wongkamchai et al. studied the serum from Thai patients who were allergic to mosquitoes bites; the specific IgE antibodies were not only bound to saliva allergens of the three human biting species but also bound to the allergens of Anopheles minimus, which is a zoophilic strain, suggesting that sensitization of allergic subjects by mosquito bites from one species can confer reactivity against another species [317].

8.4.3 Histopathology of Mosquito Allergy

In the acute phase, there is a superficial or deep perivascular or interstitial inflammatory infiltrate, which is characteristically wedge shaped. The infiltrate is usually mixed in composition with an abundance of lymphocytes and eosinophils, although neutrophils and histiocytes can also be seen. Neutrophils may predominate in reactions to mosquitoes. Over the most prominent superficial infiltrates, spongiosis can be seen, sometimes with progression to vesicle formation or epidermal necrosis. At last, excoriated areas are usually altered by the effect of scratching, with the development of parakeratosis, serum exudates, and a dermal infiltrate with neutrophils and more abundant lymphocytes [318].

8.4.4 Hypersensitivity to Mosquito Bite

In severely allergic patients, hypersensitivity to mosquito bite (HMB) may occur. HMB is a unique feature characterized by bullae formation with intense erythema on mosquito-bitten sites and subsequently develops into necrosis, ulcers, or eschars, healing with residual scarring in the end (Fig. 8.15). In addition to these local skin reactions, patients exhibit various systemic manifestations like fever, malaise,

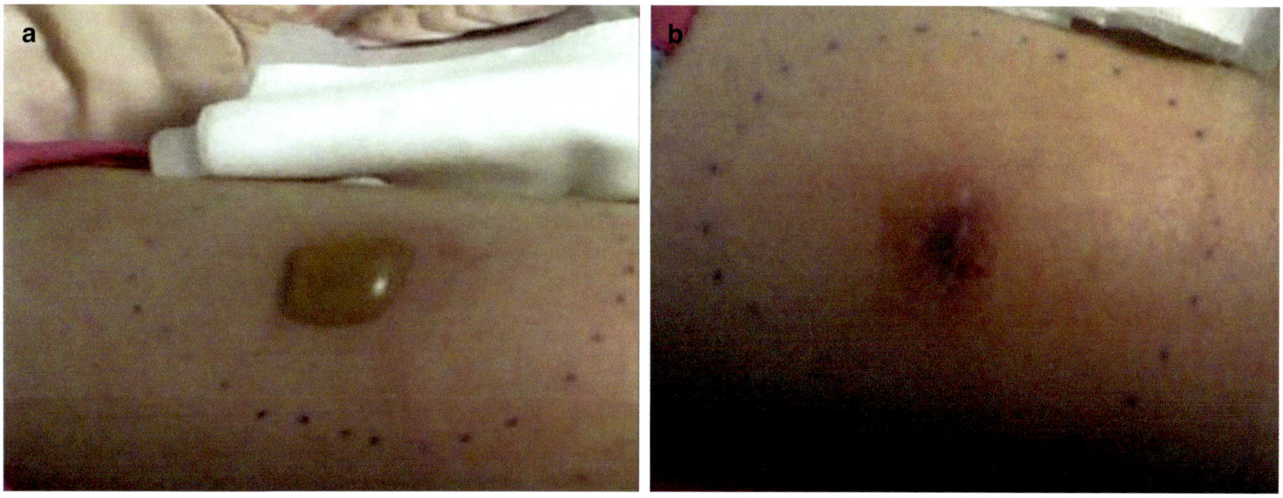

Fig. 8.15 Skin lesion at a mosquito bite site on the left forearm shows (**a**) erythema, swelling, bullae, and (**b**) subsequent necrosis formation [322] (Used by permission of *Journal of Microbiology*, Immunology and infection)

lymphadenopathy, hepatic dysfunction, and hepatosplenomegaly [319–322].

HMB is mainly reported in Japanese patients in the first two decades of life, with a median age of 6.7 years old, although the first case of HMB was reported in Florida, USA, in 1938 [323]. More than 50 cases of HMB have been reported in Japan [321, 324–329], and several cases reported in Taiwan [330, 331] and Mexico [332]. After recovering from these severe conditions, they are symptomatically free until the next mosquito bite. Therefore, the patients usually have repeated episodes of local and systemic symptoms induced by mosquito bites. Exaggerated reactions to mosquito bites were reported in lymphoproliferative disorders such as chronic lymphocytic leukemia (CLL) and natural killer (NK) cell leukemia/lymphoma related to chronic Epstein–Barr virus (EBV) infection [329, 333]. Tokura et al. reported that "the triad of hypersensitivity to mosquito bites, chronic EBV infection and NK cell leukemia/lymphoma is a clinical entity seen mostly in Asians" [321]. Davis et al. studied eight patients with CLL (aged 51–69 years old), and one patient had exaggerated arthropod-bite lesions 10 years prior to the diagnosis of CLL [329]. Seven patients had CLL before developing skin lesions. Ohshima et al. demonstrated that EBV-carrying NK cells in patients with HMB had overexpressed Fas ligand or soluble Fas ligand [334].

EBV is a human herpes virus that causes infectious mononucleosis as the primary infection [335]. Over the last 20 years, researchers have revealed that EBV is associated with various cases of lymphoproliferative diseases of NK or T-cell origin and is occasionally implicated in the pathogenesis of leukocytoclastic vasculitis, granulomatous vasculitis, lymphocytic vasculitis, and granulomatous vasculitis [336, 337]. Several reports have demonstrated that EBV-infected NK cell or T-cell proliferative disorders show characteristic cutaneous manifestations, such as HMB, hydroa vacciniforme, and severe hydroa vacciniforme-like eruption. It became apparent that up to 33% of HMB patients have been associated with chronic active EBV infection (CAEBV) [319]. Major NK cell type of CAEBV infection is characterized by higher EBV DNA loads, high titer of IgE, and hypersensitivity to mosquito bites [334]. These suggested that enhanced Fas ligand might be related to tissue damage. Asada et al. reported that CD4+ T cells in these patients could have reactive latent EBV infection in NK cells that might be involved in the pathogenesis of HMB [338].

8.4.5 Histopathology of Hypersensitivity to Mosquito Bite

Different from common histopathologic appearance in mosquito allergy, we can see epidermal necrosis, interstitial and perivascular eosinophilic, lymphocytic infiltrate, and sometimes small vessels with fibrinoid necrosis (Fig. 8.16a). In situ, hybridization for EBV-encoded RNA (EBER) could be positive (Fig. 8.16b), and NK cell marker (CD56) was variable in the mosquito bite site.

Pathogenic mechanisms linking oncogenesis of EBV-infected NK cells in HMB patients is due to mosquito salivary gland extracts that could induce reactivation of latent EBV infection in NK cells [339]. Mosquito antigen markedly increased expression of the EBV oncogenes, such as latent membrane protein 1 (LMP-1) in NK cells, which induced proliferation of NK cells and led to NK cell neoplasm [319]. Asada et al. demonstrated that adding corticosteroids to the culture of PBMC from the HMB patient inhibited the enhancement of LMP1 expression and NK cell growth. It suggests that topical and systemic corticosteroid to HMB patients immediately after mosquito bites may provide an approach to prevention of oncogenesis of EBV-infected NK Cells [319].

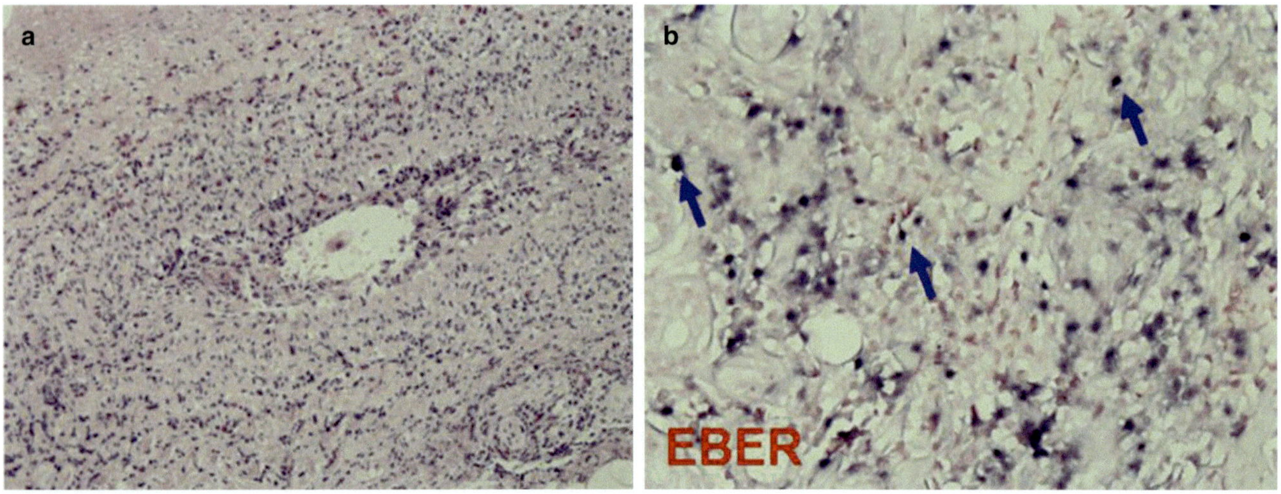

Fig. 8.16 (**a**) Histology of the HMB skin lesion shows necrosis, interstitial and perivascular eosinophilic, lymphocytic infiltrate, and small vessels with fibrinoid necrosis (H&E 200×). (**b**) In situ, hybridization analysis for EBER may demonstrate that EBV is present within the perivascular inflammatory infiltrates (400×) [322] (Used by permission of *Journal of Microbiology*, Immunology and infection)

Penneys et al. studied seven patients with AIDS, five of whom had chronic nonspecific-appearing skin eruption that could not be explained by definable cause and could be suggested of insect bite reaction. The reaction increased antibody titer to mosquito salivary glands of *Aedes taeniorhynchus*, a mosquito commonly found in Southern Florida, USA [340]. Resneck et al. studied 102 patients with pruritic papular eruption (PPE) in HIV infection, and 84 % had biopsy findings of characteristic arthropod bites. These patients had significantly higher peripheral eosinophil counts and low CD4 cell counts in general [341].

8.4.6 Treatment Principles

Discomfort of patients should be addressed, and the treatments can involve numerous modalities, including the use of ice packs and application of topical corticosteroids and antipruritics. Oral antihistamines may also minimize cutaneous reactions [342]. Prednisolone is effective in reducing itchy or severe local reactions to mosquito bites. Supportive measures for systemic toxic and allergic reactions should be instituted when necessary. Secondary infection should be treated with appropriate antibiotics. In patients with HMB, topical and systemic corticosteroid use immediately after mosquito bites may not only alleviate clinical symptoms but also prevent oncogenesis of EBV-infected NK Cells [319].

8.4.7 Prevention

Several simple steps can be taken to minimize the occurrence of mosquito bites. Clothing in bright color and artificial scents like perfume, which are attractants for mosquitoes, are best avoided on warm summer nights. Chemical repellents are also useful in preventing mosquito bites. Several different chemical compounds have been studied, including *N,N*-diethyl-3-methylbenzamide (DEET, previously diethyltoluamide), picaridin (KBR 3203), and *p*-menthane-3,8-diol (eucalyptus oil). The most effective repellent for all mosquitoes is DEET. Generally, a product that contains 10–30 % DEET provides adequate protection for most outdoor activities, and higher concentrations of DEET provide longer protection times. Although DEET has an excellent safety record, there are reports of encephalopathy after exposure to this chemical particularly in children. For this reason, only products with DEET concentrations less than 10 % should be used on children.

8.5 Immunologically Mediated Photodermatoses

Shivani Nanda, MD and Henry W. Lim, MD

8.5.1 Introduction

Photodermatoses are classified into four general categories: immunologically mediated, chemical- or drug-induced, DNA repair-deficient, and photoaggravated (Table 8.2). This chapter will focus on immunologically mediated photodermatoses.

8.5.2 Polymorphous Light Eruption

8.5.2.1 Introduction

First reported in 1942 by Epstein, polymorphous light eruption (PMLE), also known as polymorphic light eruption, is the most common photodermatosis. The action spectrum ranges from broadband ultraviolet (UV)-B to UVA and rarely visible light. Its prevalence is inversely related to latitude, with the highest prevalence reported at 22 % in Scandinavia and the lowest prevalence reported at 1 % in Singapore [343]. While PMLE can affect all skin types, it is more commonly seen in people with Fitzpatrick skin type I [344].

Table 8.2 Classification of photodermatoses

Immunologically mediated
Polymorphous light eruption
Actinic prurigo
Hydroa vacciniforme
Solar urticaria
Chronic actinic dermatitis
Chemical or drug-induced photosensitivity
Topical agents (sunscreens, fragrances, nonsteroidal anti-inflammatory drugs)
Systemic agents (nonsteroidal anti-inflammatory drugs, diuretics, quinolones, tetracyclines, sulfonamides, phenothiazines)
Cutaneous porphyrias
Defective DNA repair disorders
Xeroderma pigmentosum
Cockayne syndrome
Trichothiodystrophy
Bloom syndrome
UV-sensitive syndrome
Rothmund–Thomson syndrome
Photoaggravated dermatoses
Atopic dermatitis
Darier disease
Dermatomyositis
Lichen planus
Lupus erythematosus
Pityriasis rubra pilaris
Reticular erythematous mucinosis
Rosacea

8.5.2.2 Clinical Features

PMLE presents with symmetric, monomorphic, erythematous to flesh-colored papules that frequently coalesce into plaques over sun-exposed areas such as the extensor arms, upper chest, and neck. However, cutaneous manifestations can take on variable morphologies including papules, vesicles, bullae, or confluent edematous plaques (Fig. 8.17). In darker-skinned individuals, the lesions are more often monomorphic pinpoint papules [345]. A variant of PMLE termed juvenile spring eruption is typically seen in young boys and manifests as papulovesicles on the helices of the ears. PMLE develops minutes to hours after exposure to UV radiation (UVR) and can last for days. Very rarely, systemic symptoms such as headaches, nausea, and fevers can occur [346]. The eruption diminishes in frequency as summer progresses due to a phenomenon known as "hardening," in which the skin acclimatizes to graduated UVR exposure.

8.5.2.3 Immunological Factors (Table 8.3)

In genetically predisposed individuals, PMLE is thought to be a result of an immunological response to UVR-induced cutaneous antigens. Support for this hypothesis is evidenced by a study which found that peripheral blood mononuclear cells from PMLE patients had an increased proliferative response to irradiated skin biopsy samples when compared with healthy subjects, suggesting an immune sensitization against ultraviolet light-induced skin antigens [347]. However, the putative photoantigen has not been identified at this time. Heat-shock protein 65 (HSP65) has been suggested as a possibility. McFadden et al. identified that PMLE lesions showed an increase in HSP65 expression in keratinocytes 1 h after exposure to ultraviolet radiation. Similar findings were not observed in healthy patients [348].

The specific immunological response triggered in PMLE is thought to be a delayed-type hypersensitivity (DTH) response similar to that seen in allergic contact dermatitis.

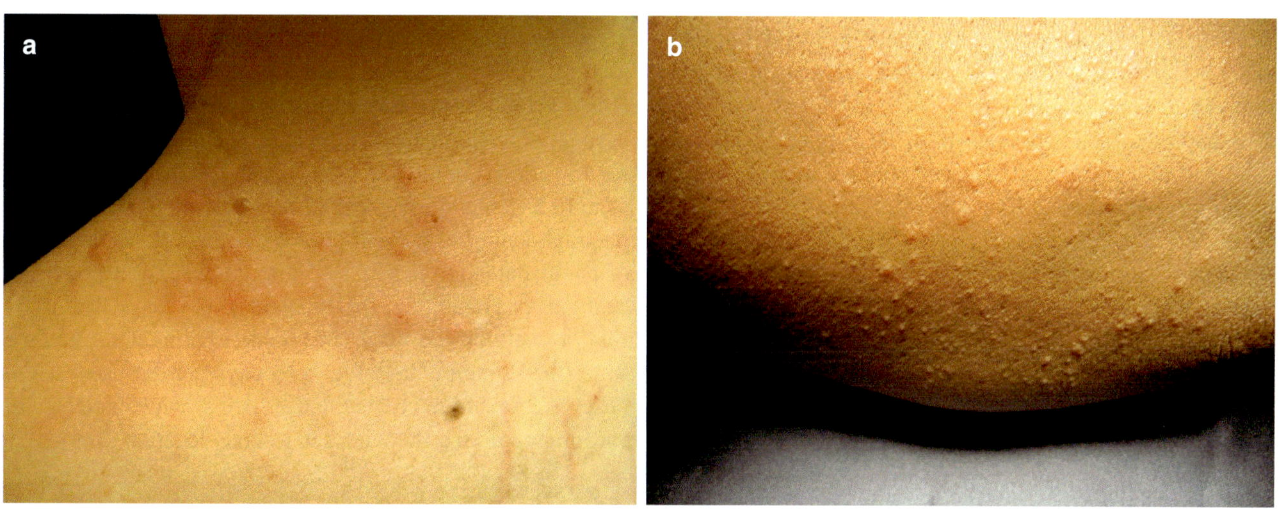

Fig. 8.17 Variability in clinical manifestations of polymorphous light eruption with a papular eruption on the extensor forearm (**b**) and papules, vesicles, and excoriation on the upper back (**a**)

Table 8.3 Immunological mechanisms proposed for the pathogenesis of polymorphous light eruption

Delayed-type hypersensitivity response to a photo-induced antigen
Aberrant ultraviolet radiation-induced immunosuppression
17β-estradiol-mediated resistance to ultraviolet radiation-induced immunosuppression
Decreased serum 25-hydroxy-vitamin D levels

An immunohistochemical study conducted on skin biopsies from PMLE lesions demonstrated a prominent perivascular T-cell infiltrate that was initially composed of CD4+ T cells. At 72 h, a CD8+ T-cell infiltrate predominated with dermal macrophages and Langerhans cells [349].

In addition, a reduction in the normal immunosuppressive response induced by UVR in PMLE patients results in an exaggerated immune reaction to UVR-induced photoantigens. In healthy skin, exposure to UVR results in decreased cell-mediated immunity through various mechanisms. Firstly, UVB induces migration of epidermal Langerhans cells to draining lymph nodes, thus inducing immunologic tolerance [350]. This phenomenon fails to occur in PMLE [351]. Furthermore, IL-4+ neutrophils appear in normal skin after UVR exposure. IL-4 tends to favor the development of a Th2 response and subsequent suppression of delayed-type hypersensitivity reactions [352]. In PMLE, a decreased infiltrate of IL-4+ neutrophils was seen following UVR exposure [353]. Further, mast cells play an integral role in UV-induced immune suppression [354]. UVB induces mast cell infiltration and then upregulates regulatory T cells, which decrease autoimmunity [355, 356]. In PMLE, a decreased infiltrate of both mast cells [357] and regulatory T cells [358] was seen after UVR exposure, further supporting an aberrant UVR-induced immunosuppressive response in these patients.

Interestingly, PMLE is observed two to three times more frequently in women compared with men [346] and may be due to 17-β-estradiol, a predominantly female hormone, which prevents UVR-induced suppression by inhibiting release of IL-10, an immunosuppressive cytokine [359]. Thus, increased susceptibility to PMLE in women may be due to a propensity for a decreased immunosuppressive response to UVR exposure.

It has also been proposed that PMLE patients have an increased susceptibility to autoimmunity because of reduced serum vitamin D levels. Vitamin D increases concentrations of regulatory T cells and suppresses T-cell activation [360]. Decreased serum vitamin D levels have been reported in various autoimmune disorders, suggesting a role in inducing autoimmunity [361]. PMLE patients have reduced serum vitamin D levels compared with healthy controls [362]. However, as vitamin D is synthesized after sunlight exposure, it is unclear whether decreased vitamin D levels are due to increased photoprotective measures followed by these individuals or truly due to an inherent deficiency in vitamin D.

8.5.2.4 Diagnosis

The diagnosis of PMLE is primarily based on history and clinical findings. Determination of the minimal erythema dose (MED) to UVA or UVB is typically not helpful as most patients have a normal value [363]. Further support of the diagnosis can be made via a cutaneous biopsy. Typical findings include a superficial and deep perivascular lymphoid infiltrate with subepidermal edema. While the histology of PMLE is characteristic, it is nonspecific. Further diagnostic confirmation can be obtained through photo provocation, which is the most reliable procedure for reproducing PMLE. The test involves repeated exposure of two symmetrically located test sites daily for 4–8 days to increased doses of UVA and UVB radiation. It is positive if typical PMLE patient's lesions are induced. Testing should be performed in late spring as patients can develop natural hardening as the summer months progress. A practical method to induce lesions is to ask the patient to deliberately expose him/herself to sunlight that is known to precipitate lesions and schedule the patient to return for evaluation a day later.

8.5.2.5 Prevention and Management

Education on basic photoprotective measures is paramount. Patients should avoid sun exposure between the hours of 10 AM and 2 PM, wear photoprotective clothing, and use high SPF, broad-spectrum sunscreen [364]. For mild cases of PMLE, basic photoprotective measures are sufficient, especially when combined with topical corticosteroids and oral antihistamines to shorten the duration of flares [365].

In contrast, patients with more severe condition require aggressive treatment as the condition can significantly affect their quality of life [366]. They often benefit from prophylactic photohardening to induce photoadaptation through exposure to gradually increasing doses of UVR. Photohardening is able to restore UV-induced immunosuppression via normalization of Langerhans cell migration and neutrophil influx [367]. Narrowband UVB (NB-UVB) is commonly used for photohardening, delivered two to three times weekly for 15 sessions in the late spring/early summer. Oral prednisone (0.5–1 mg/kg/day) can be used for the first 7 days of photohardening to prevent photoexacerbation. Maintenance of photoadaptation is achieved through weekly exposure to sunlight for 20–30 min; for the most severe cases, cyclosporine or azathioprine [368] are viable options. Oral prednisone (0.5–1 mg/kg/day) for 7–10 days can be used at the onset of a flare or to prevent flares, such as while patients are vacationing during the winter in a sunny location [369].

8.5.3 Actinic Prurigo

8.5.3.1 Introduction

Actinic prurigo (AP) is a chronic photodermatosis with a prevalence ranging from 0.1 [370] to 8 % [371]. Although most commonly observed in the mestizo population of Latin America [372], cases occur worldwide. Women are two to four times more likely to develop AP than men [373]. AP usually occurs in childhood but may appear at any age. The early-onset form can spontaneously remit, but adult-onset AP tends to be chronic [374]. A strong association with HLA-DR4, subtype DRB1*0407 is present [375].

8.5.3.2 Clinical Features

AP manifests with pruritic, erythematous papules or nodules associated with hemorrhagic crusting, excoriation, or even lichenification (Fig. 8.18). Lesions appear in sun-exposed areas, particularly the face, chest, extensor arms, and dorsal hands. Covered sites such as the buttocks and back may also be affected, especially in patients reported from the UK [372]. Cheilitis is seen in up to 85 % of cases and can present with fissuring, ulceration, and crusting [376]. Conjunctivitis is seen in 62 % of Latin Americans but less commonly in Caucasians [377]. Symptoms appear in the summer but may be seen throughout the year in warmer climates.

8.5.3.3 Immunological Factors

Similar to the PMLE, it is postulated that in those who are genetically predisposed, AP results from an immunologic response to an unidentified UVR-induced autoantigen [378]. This suggestion has been supported by the presence of clonal populations of T cells in AP biopsies [379]. Further, the induction of an inflammatory response to UVR-induced antigens likely is a result of a lack of UVR-induced depletion of Langerhans cells [380]. The role of TNF-α in AP has also been elucidated. Arrese et al. found that AP biopsy specimens obtained after UVR exposure contained elevated levels of TNF-α within keratinocytes. They hypothesized that TNF-α may then propagate an inflammatory response in AP [381].

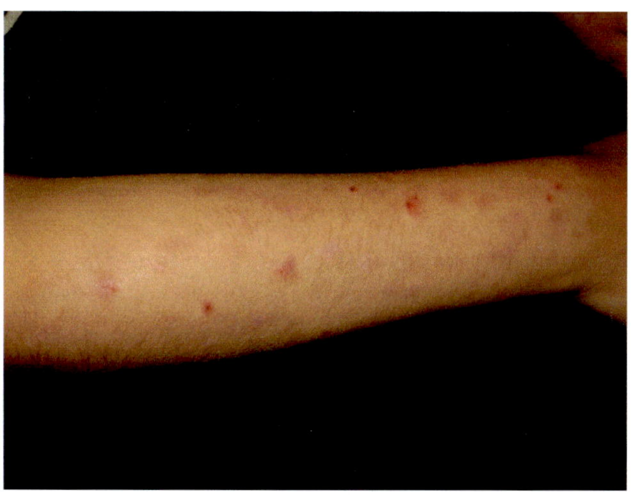

Fig. 8.18 Clinical findings of actinic prurigo. Papules and excoriation on the forearm (Courtesy of Tor Shwayder M.D.)

8.5.3.4 Diagnosis

While the clinical history and physical examination may initially suggest the diagnosis, phototesting can provide further support. Lowered MED to UVA is seen in up to 60 % of cases. Lowered MED to UVB is also sometimes observed [382]. Photoprovocation to UVA induces AP lesions in up to 90 % of cases and can be diagnostic [373]. Further, HLA typing can suggest a diagnosis if HLA-DR4 is present.

Skin biopsy is often not helpful as histologic findings tend to be nonspecific. Typically hyperkeratosis, regular acanthosis, and a perivascular lymphocytic infiltrate are seen in the superficial dermis. Spongiosis and papillary dermal edema can also be seen. However, a characteristic histological finding is the presence of lymphoid follicles, which is commonly observed in biopsies of the lip and conjunctiva [374].

8.5.3.5 Prevention and Management

Photoprotection with broad-spectrum sunscreens, photoprotective clothing, lip balm, and sunglasses is paramount. Photoprotective films on window glass can also decrease UVA exposure. In addition, patients often require topical corticosteroids and oral antihistamines to reduce pruritus. Phototherapy, especially NB-UVB, three times weekly for 5 weeks can provide further relief, albeit temporary [383]. Short courses of oral corticosteroids (0.5–1 mg/kg/day) can be added to the treatment regimen for acute flares. If ocular involvement is present, cyclosporine 2 % ophthalmic solution applied for 3 months has been shown to result in rapid clearance of ocular symptoms [384]. To date, however, the most effective treatment is thalidomide. At a dose of 50–200 mg weekly, it results in rapid clearance by inhibiting TNF-α synthesis [385]. Unfortunately, concern for teratogenicity and peripheral neuropathy has limited its availability. Other systemic therapies used for severe AP include oral cyclosporine and azathioprine [374].

8.5.4 Hydroa Vacciniforme

8.5.4.1 Introduction

Hydroa vacciniforme (HV) is a rare photodermatosis with a prevalence of 0.34 cases per 100,000 [386]. It is typically seen in children with onset between the ages of 1 and 16, but cases of adult-onset HV have been reported [387, 388]. While most cases occur sporadically, rare familial cases are reported [389]. Similar to other photodermatoses, HV does significantly affect the quality of life of patients [390].

8.5.4.2 Clinical Features

Within hours of summer sun exposure, patients experience an itching or stinging sensation in sun-exposed areas, especially the face and dorsal hands. Subsequently, erythematous macules develop and progress into painful papules that undergo vesiculation or form large hemorrhagic bullae (Fig. 8.19). These lesions can then umbilicate and crust. Healing occurs over weeks, leaving behind varioliform scars.

Atypical cases of HV, usually among adults, present with more diffuse cutaneous lesions, occurring at times in sun-protected sites. Facial edema and disfigurements of the ear, nose, and fingers can be seen [391, 392]. These patients are more likely to develop Epstein–Barr virus-associated hematologic malignancies [393]. Systemic complications are not seen in classic HV. However, atypical cases and a clinical entity known as hydroa-vacciniforme-like lymphoma present with HV-like cutaneous lesions and systemic symptoms, including gastrointestinal erosions, lymphadenopathy, fever, and hepatosplenomegaly [394].

8.5.4.3 Immunological Factors

While the exact immunologic basis for HV is unknown, exposure to summer sunlight elicits the characteristic lesions. The role of UVR exposure in HV has been validated in studies that have exposed HV patients to repetitive doses of UVA radiation and reproduced clinical lesions [395]. Epstein–Barr virus (EBV), a member of the herpes virus family, has been implicated as an important pathogenic factor in HV and HV-like eruptions. In particular, when biopsy specimens taken from HV lesions were analyzed, studies confirmed the presence of EBV DNA sequences [396]. When the cutaneous infiltrate of biopsy specimens were analyzed, a large number of cytotoxic T cells were identified and outnumbered the T cells which contained EBV-encoded small nuclear ribonucleic acid. Thus, the response of cytotoxic T cells to EBV-infected cells may lead to the development of HV lesions. Similar findings were observed in biopsy specimens of severe HV-like eruptions. However, in these cases, an increased quantity of EBV DNA was detected [393]. Given these findings, classic HV and HV-like eruptions are thought to be pathogenically related and that should be considered as a disease spectrum.

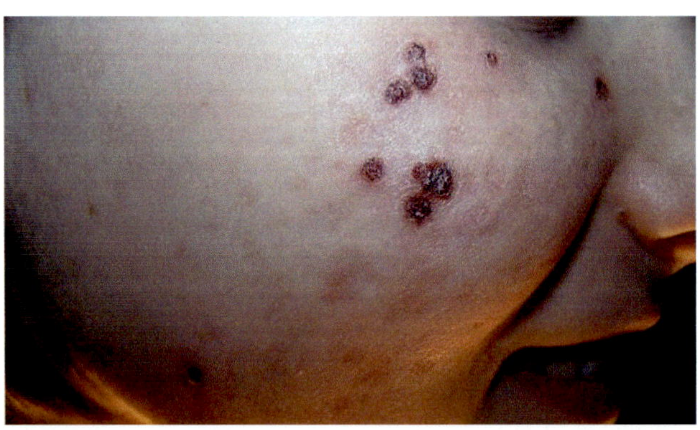

Fig. 8.19 Clinical findings in hydroa vacciniforme. Crusted erosions on the face

8.5.4.4 Diagnosis

HV is diagnosed based on a combination of clinical and histologic findings. Biopsies will reveal the characteristic presence of focal keratinocyte degeneration in association with intraepidermal vesicles, confluent epidermal and upper dermal necrosis, and a perivascular lymphohistiocytic infiltrate. Further confirmation can be obtained by phototesting with administration of repetitive doses of UVA [395].

8.5.4.5 Prevention and Management

Strict photoprotection is crucial as treatment is otherwise unsatisfactory. Hardening with NB-UVB has been shown to increase sunlight tolerance and decrease disease severity in a small number of patients [386]. Systemic agents including β-carotene, thalidomide [397], hydroxychloroquine [398], cyclosporine, azathioprine [399], and dietary fish oils [400] have been effective in select cases.

8.5.5 Solar Urticaria

8.5.5.1 Introduction

Solar urticaria (SU) is rare, with its prevalence among other photosensitivity disorders ranging from 0.08 to 17 % [344, 401, 402]. It occurs most commonly in women in the third decade of life, but cases presenting in infancy [403] and childhood [404] have been reported. The action spectrum for SU includes visible light, UVA, and rarely UVB, all of which can trigger the characteristic wheal–flare response.

8.5.5.2 Clinical Features

SU presents with erythematous, edematous pruritic plaques within 5–10 min of sun exposure, typically on the arms and upper chest with a decreased propensity of development in regularly sun-exposed sites such as the face and hands. Symptoms can even occur at covered sites if thin clothing is worn [405] or, if severe, on mucosal surfaces leading to angioedema [406]. Resolution of symptoms generally occurs within 1–2 h but can take up to 24 h. The severity of symptoms varies depending on geography, exposure time, and light intensity. For instance, very short periods of sun exposure may only elicit an itching/burning sensation at sun-exposed sites, while prolonged exposure could result in a dramatic wheal–flare response [407]. Associated systemic symptoms include nausea, wheezing, syncope, dizziness, and even anaphylactic shock [408].

8.5.5.3 Immunological Factors

It is hypothesized that after exposure to UVR, inactive chromophores in SU are converted into immunologically active photoallergens in the dermis and serum [409]. Subsequent production of IgE to this photoallergen results in the production of classic wheals through a type I hypersensitivity reaction. The theory that UV-induced serum photoallergens resulted in SU was tested through a series of passive transfer tests. These involved extracting serum from patients with SU, transferring the serum into healthy subjects, and then irradiating with the causative wavelengths of UVR. Many healthy subjects developed SU after serum transfer from affected individuals, although some did not [410, 411]. Reverse transfer tests involved irradiation of the skin of healthy subjects with subsequent serum transfer to SU patients. To explain the variability in the results of the transfer tests, Leenutaphong et al. [412] proposed the classification of SU into two types. Type I SU is caused by an abnormal chromophore found only in SU patients to which IgE antibodies react. Passive transfer tests will be variable, while reverse transfer tests will be negative. Type II SU is caused by an abnormal IgE antibody against normal chromophores present in all individuals. Passive transfer tests will always be positive, and reverse transfer tests will be variable. For ethical reasons, these tests are no longer performed.

8.5.5.4 Diagnosis

Due to the transient nature of SU, patients often have no clinical findings on physical exam. While the clinical history can help in establishing the diagnosis, confirmation can be made via phototesting (Fig. 8.20). Due to the diversity in the action spectra for SU, phototesting to UVA, UVB, and visible light is preformed. Assessment for a wheal–flare response is conducted every 10 min for up to 1 h after irradiation [413]. Repeat phototesting may be needed as the action spectrum can change over time [414].

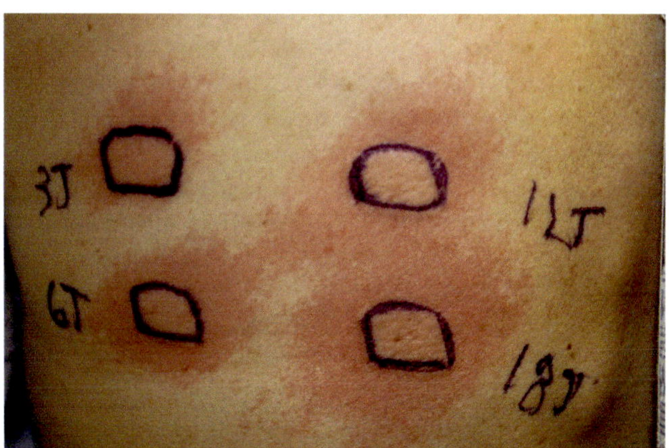

Fig. 8.20 Positive phototesting results in solar urticaria immediately after UVA exposure

Histology is similar to that seen in other forms of urticaria and includes dermal edema with a perivascular dermal infiltrate composed of eosinophils and neutrophils. Major basic protein, which results in histamine release from mast cells, can be present [415]. Features of leukocytoclastic vasculitis are rarely seen [416].

8.5.5.5 Prevention and Management

While photoprotection is important, sunscreens are often not effective given that the action spectrum for SU can include visible light. Oral H_1-antihistamines, including hydroxyzine, cetirizine, fexofenadine, loratidine, and doxepin, are first-line therapy. Another oral antihistamine, terfenadine, was found to be effective but had been withdrawn from the US market due to associated cardiotoxicity [417]. Higher doses of antihistamines are needed in SU than those used conventionally [418].

Artificial hardening can be achieved through the use of UVB, UVA, or PUVA. Currently, in many centers, UVA, or UVA1 if available, is the most commonly used light source. Treatment protocols vary, but generally doses begin below the minimal urticarial dose (MUD) and increase by 10–20 % per session. Treatments are received three times weekly for 10 weeks with subsequent tapering. Maintenance therapy is often needed, although effects with PUVA are longer lasting than with other forms of phototherapy [419].

Systemic therapies reported to be successful for SU include cyclosporine [420], intravenous immunoglobulin (IVIg) [421], and oral corticosteroids [422]. Omalizumab, a monoclonal IgE antibody, has resulted in partial and complete [423] remission in patients who had failed with other conventional therapies and demonstrated elevated serum IgE levels. Afamelanotide, an α-melanocyte-stimulating hormone analogue, has been shown to be beneficial in five patients by increasing the MUD and decreasing the frequency of the wheal–flare response [424]. Plasmapheresis has been successfully used, but relapse is often short-lived [425].

8.5.6 Chronic Actinic Dermatitis

8.5.6.1 Introduction

Chronic actinic dermatitis (CAD), previously referred to as actinic reticuloid, persistent light reaction, or photosensitive eczema, is an immunologically mediated photodermatosis. Cases have been reported worldwide, with the highest number reported in northern Europe [426]. Although the condition is most often seen in males over 50 years old, cases in females and younger patients are also seen [427]. All skin types can be affected, but patients with Fitzpatrick skin type V or VI are more commonly affected in the USA [428]. CAD can be associated with HIV and is often the presenting sign of AIDS [429].

8.5.6.2 Clinical Features

CAD presents with erythematous papules, some excoriated, that over time become lichenified in sun-exposed areas. Importantly, the condition spares sun-protected sites including the nasolabial folds, retroauricular areas, upper eyelids, base of body folds, and submental chin (Fig. 8.21). Severe cases may result in erythroderma [430]. Symptoms worsen in the summer but can present year-round. CAD is generally chronic but remission is attained in 35 % of cases in 10 years [431].

8.5.6.3 Immunologic Factors

The predominance of CD8+ T cells and Langerhans cells in biopsy specimens from CAD resembles findings seen in allergic contact dermatitis. In addition, studies have revealed increased expression of ICAM-1, VCAM-1, and E-selectin on dermal vessels in CAD, suggesting that CAD may represent a DTH response [432]. Unfortunately, while it has been postulated that the immunologic response seen in CAD is likely due to a photo-induced endogenous antigen, the antigen has not yet been identified.

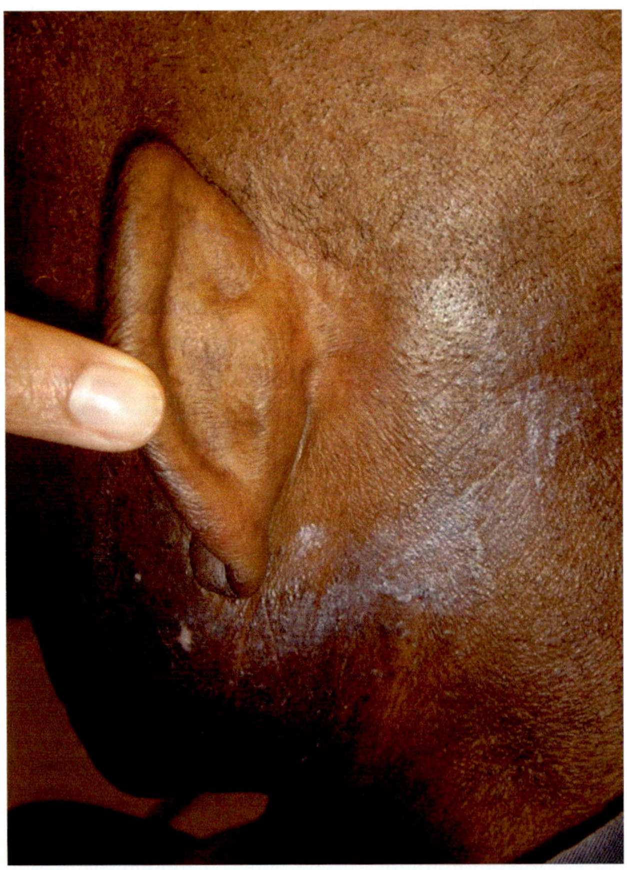

Fig. 8.21 Lichenification and hyperpigmentation on sun-exposed sites, with sparing of postauricular areas

Further, given the propensity of preceding contact allergy in CAD, mostly seen in patients reported from the UK, the persistence of an immune response to environmental contact allergens may heighten the ability to mount an immune response against a photo-induced endogenous antigen in these patients [433]. This combined with an aberrant UVR-induced immunosuppressive response likely results in the cutaneous manifestations of CAD [434].

8.5.6.4 Diagnosis

Confirmation of the diagnosis via phototesting to UVB, UVA, and visible light is recommended. Phototesting will reveal a decreased MED to UVA and/or UVB [427]. Patch testing and photopatch testing is also recommended in patients with the appropriate clinical history. Coexisting allergic contact dermatitis or photocontact dermatitis to allergens in Compositae plants as well as avobenzone and oxybenzone in sunscreens is often seen [435, 436]. Interestingly, while the coexistence of contact and photocontact dermatitis is seen in studies from the UK, similar associations were not seen in the USA or Japan [428].

Histological features can be nonspecific and similar to that seen in allergic contact dermatitis with the presence of epidermal spongiosis with a lymphohistiocytic infiltrate, focal parakeratosis, and acanthosis. The presence of atypical lymphocytes and lymphocyte exostosis in some cases resembles histologic features of cutaneous T-cell lymphoma (CTCL). The predominance of CD8 cells and the absence of a T-cell receptor gene arrangement in CAD can help in distinguishing this condition from CTCL [437].

8.5.6.5 Prevention and Management

Photoprotection is essential in all patients. Those with positive patch or photopatch test results should avoid known contact allergens. Mild cases may be treated with topical corticosteroids or topical calcineurin inhibitors [438]. Severe or refractory cases can be treated with systemic therapies. Oral prednisone (0.5–1 mg/kg/day) can be used at the time of flares. For long-term systemic therapies, azathioprine [439], cyclosporine [440], and mycophenolate mofetil [441] are beneficial. In a small number of patients, low-dose PUVA [442] or UVB therapy [443] has been reported to be effective.

8.6 Contact Dermatitis

Wen-Hui Wang and Lin-Feng Li

Contact dermatitis, also known as environmental and occupational dermatitis, is an inflammatory skin reaction resulting from exposure to various external substances. At least six types of contact dermatitis have been classified so far including irritant contact dermatitis (ICD), allergic contact dermatitis (ACD), immediate contact reactions, phototoxic and photoallergic reactions, systemic contact dermatitis (SCD), and noneczematous contact reactions. ICD and ACD are the main types, and contact dermatitis, in most circumstance, incorrectly refers to ACD. There are two major societies on contact dermatitis: http://www.contactderm.org by American Contact Dermatitis Society (ACDS) and http://www.dermis.net/org/ESCD by European Society of Contact Dermatitis (ESCD).

8.6.1 Clinical Spectrum of Contact Dermatitis

Typical contact dermatitis is an eczematous skin reaction that varies according to the severity, location, and duration of the inflammation. In acute ACD, the lesions present with a well-demarcated erythema, edema with or without closely grouped papules and/or vesicles, or oozing; in subacute form, slight oozing with crust and scaling can be seen; and in chronic form, scaling and lichenification manifest. Itch predominates in ACD. The lesion is usually localized to the contact site; however, patchy or diffuse disease can also occur, depending on the nature of the allergen, secondary transfer, or the development of autosensitization. Acute ICD ranges from mild erythema, with or without vesiculation or bullae, to caustic burns and necrosis. Chronic ICD predominates with dryness, hyperkeratosis, scaling, and fissures. The lesions of ICD are usually painful.

Noneczematous contact dermatitis refers to dermatitis that resembles other skin diseases, such as erythema multiforme (the most common of all noneczematous types), purpura, urticaria, angioedema, lichen planus, exanthema, erythroderma, vasculitis, pustules, granuloma, psoriasis, bullous epidermal necrolysis, change in pigmentation, photosensitivity, etc. It is reported that noneczematous forms are even slightly more common (52 %) than the classic eczematous one (48 %) in an over 30,000 patch-tested individuals for contact dermatitis [444]. Factors determining the peculiar polymorphic clinical features of ACD include causative agent, patient sensitizing level, way of exposure (cutaneous, systemic), means of exposure (cutaneous direct, airborne), tissue structures targeted by the causative agent, anatomical sites involved, possible concomitant irritation, environmental factors (UV, temperature, humidity), itching intensity variability, preexisting dermatitis underlying the overlapping contact allergy, etc [444]. Systemic symptoms may also occur, e.g., systemic nickel allergy syndrome may have extracutaneous signs and symptoms (gastrointestinal, respiratory, neurological, etc.). Fatal anaphylactic shock could be seen in contact urticaria syndrome.

Certain allergens are known to produce clinically atypical reactions. For example, hair dye dermatitis by paraphenylenediamine (PPD) presents as acute and dramatic facial swelling with scalp sparing that may be mistaken for a type I reaction; the optical whiteners in washing powder and the fragrances and chemicals in cosmetics (e.g., aniline dyes in face powder) can cause pigmented contact dermatitis (PCD), which is a subtype of ACD, characterized by reticulate brown or gray hyperpigmentation with little or no signs of dermatitis [445]. Woods and plants frequently elicit erythema multiforme-like eruption [444]. Nitrofurazone [446], minoxidil [447, 448], and black rubber [449] are known to cause allergic pustular reactions. In these conditions, the clinical findings are similar with the original diseases, but the distribution of the lesions can give a clue to contact dermatitis. For example, in erythema multiforme-like contact dermatitis, the eruption develops only on the allergen-contacted skin.

Table 8.4 gives the common causative agents of contact dermatitis on different human body sites.

Table 8.4 Common causative agents of contact dermatitis on different human body sites

Body site	Common causative agents
Scalp	Hair dye, shampoo, hair spray, topical medication
Face	Hair dye, cosmetics, cosmetic applicators and tools, glasses, eye drops, hat, nail varnishes and acrylic nails (particularly periocular dermatitis), topical medication, airborne allergens
Lip	Food, drug, lipstick, things bitten in the mouth habitually or occasionally, such as pencil, hairpin
Ear	Earring, cosmetics, topical medication, glasses frame
Neck and shoulder	Jewelry, clothes, shoulder straps
Trunk	Cosmetics, clothes, accessories, elastic band
Umbilical region	Buckle
Axilla	Deodorant, depilatory, shower lotion, topical medication, clothes
Waist	Underwear, swimsuit, elastic band
Perineum	Stool, urine, sanitary pad, cosmetics, topical medication
Buttocks	Cushion, clothes, chair, underwear
Hand	Water, detergent, plant, food, occupation contacts
Leg	Clothes, shower lotion, chair
Foot	Shoes, socks, topical medication
Widespread	Clothes, shower lotion, topical medication, massage lotion

Airborne contact dermatitis is induced by chemicals disseminated in the air. Both ACD and ICD can occur; the lesions commonly affect the face, neck, and other exposed sites. The clinical findings of airborne contact dermatitis and phototoxic or photoallergic dermatitis may look almost identical, because they both affect exposed sites. However, the sparing of Wilkinson's triangle (i.e., the area behind the ears), the nasolabial folds, and the area under the chin are the significant features for photodermatitis [450].

Connubial or consort dermatitis is caused by the products that his or her partner is using; this should have more attention during history taking. Connubial dermatitis caused by cosmetics typically presents with a unilateral facial dermatitis; disseminated dermatitis could also occur in patients with profound sensitivity to fragrance [451].

SCD is a condition occurring in previously sensitized individuals after systemic absorption of the same or cross-reacting substance. The most typical presentation of SCD includes diffuse erythema in the major flexures and the anogenital area, also known as baboon syndrome. Other manifestations include a flare of eczema and/or a patch-test reaction, vasculitis-like lesions, pompholyx, or a generalized eczematous dermatitis [452].

8.6.2 Contact Dermatitis and Immunity

ICD occurs as a result of direct damage to the stratum corneum by external chemicals or physical stimuli that occur faster than the skin is able to repair itself [450]. It involves a combination of endogenous and exogenous factors. Antigen-specific acquired immunologic mechanisms are not involved, but skin's innate immune system is activated. ICD can occur after a single episode of exposure to a strong irritant (e.g., strong acids or alkalis) or repeated exposure to weak irritants. Multiple interlinked pathways are now considered to be involved in ICD, including pathophysiologic changes of skin barrier disruption which results in increased skin permeability and transepidermal water loss, epidermal cellular damage, pro-inflammatory mediators released from keratinocytes, and the activation of innate immunity.

In experimental ICD studies, acute skin barrier disruption from exposure to surfactants (e.g., sodium lauryl sulfate) induces the release of cytokines (e.g., IL-1α, IL-1β, IL-1α, IL-6) and TNF-α from keratinocytes. These cytokines then act as signals for the release of further pro-inflammatory chemokines, which attract mononuclear and polymorphonuclear cells at the injury site. Anti-inflammatory cytokines are also released in response to irritant exposure and may be involved in the resolution of the inflammatory process.

ACD results primarily from type IV hypersensitivity, that is, the delayed-type cell-mediated immunity. Two important factors are involved: allergen and susceptible individual. Deeper investigation of ACD has found the reaction is not limited to type IV hypersensitivity, for example, persistence of ACD induced by a nickel can mimic a Th2-dominant immune response.

The development of ACD can be divided into three stages: sensitization phase, elicitation phase, and resolution phase. Sensitization starts when the contact allergen, usually small molecular (less than 500 days) hapten, penetrates the stratum corneum. Skin barrier defects such as filaggrin mutations and/or skin irritation facilitate the process. Then the allergen is uptaken by skin antigen-presenting dendritic cells, i.e., Langerhans cells or other APCs. This process involves members of the organic anion transport polypeptide (OATP) family and may be relevant for prohaptens that must be metabolically activated to become protein reactive haptens. The metabolic activation of prohaptens involves xenobiotic metabolizing enzymes (XMEs) of the cytochrome P450 (CYP) system. The targeting of skin proteins and of residues within these proteins by contact allergens is selectively modified. Allergen capturing APCs migrates from skin to draining lymph nodes, and T cells there recognize specifically allergen-MHC II complex and are activated.

Sensitization phase refers to the period from the first contact of allergen to the activation of hapten-specific T cells, which include TH1, TH2, TH17, and regulatory T (Treg) cells. It takes at least 3 days, typically 10–15 days in human and 5–7 days in mice, respectively, for sensitization [453]. In this phase, allergens also activate innate immunity through keratinocyte release of IL-1α, IL-1β, TNF-α, GM-CSF, IL-8, and IL-18, inducing vasodilation, cellular recruitment, and infiltration. Specific T lymphocytes proliferate in the lymph nodes, differentiate into CD4+ effector T helper cells and CD8+ cytotoxic T cells, and propagate all over the body including skin homing, along with mast cells and eosinophils.

In elicitation phase, reexposure to the allergen results in the activation of allergen-specific T lymphocytes, along with other inflammatory cells, entering the exposure site and, through release of cytokines and consequent stimulation of keratinocytes, induce an inflammatory cascade. The peak inflammatory reactions are at 72 and 24 h for human and mice, respectively [454, 455]. The reaction is often more severe and rapid in onset with subsequent episodes of reexposure.

The regulation or resolution phase starts upon activation of CD4+ regulatory T cells (IL-10-producing Treg1, TH2, or CD4+ CD25+ FoxP3+ T cells). Others cells, γδT cells and B cells, also have potential participation in the downregulation process [450]. If the allergen is removed, this process can turn the dermatitis into normal skin.

There are two animal models on type IV hypersensitivity: contact hypersensitivity reaction (CHS), which is sensitized by skin contact, and delayed-type hypersensitivity (DTH), which is sensitized by subcutaneous injection. The former is more like the human ACD in real life and is more popularly used in ACD research. CD4+ and CD8+ T cells have distinct roles in normal CHS responses to potent haptens, with primarily CD8+ T cells being pathogenic and promoting the killing of haptenic skin cells and CD4+ T cells, mainly CD4+ CD25+ Treg cell population, being predominately downregulatory. However, in some instances, especially those where there is a deficient CD8+ T-cell pool, CD4+ T cells can be effector cells of CHS [456]. CD4+ T cells may also contribute to CHS by the generation of pro-inflammatory cytokines, and in some settings being essential for the mobilization of CD8+ T cells to the skin [457].

CHS model is usually induced by potent sensitizers (e.g., dinitrofluorobenzene), but common human ACD is induced by weak-to-moderate sensitizers (e.g., nickel, fragrance), which cannot induce reactions in mice. It is considered that there was one major difference between the two types of ACD. In ACD induced by potent haptens, the CD4+ Treg cells do not prevent priming but participate in the resolution of skin inflammation, whereas in ACD due to weak haptens, the presence of CD4+ Treg cells totally abrogates the CD8+ T-cell priming [453]. Gene arrays in human demonstrate that individual allergens selectively induce polar immune responses. Nickel significantly increased TH1/IFN and innate immune responses and induced significant TH17 skewing. Fragrance, and to a lesser extent rubber, showed a strong TH2 bias and some TH22 polarization, with much smaller TH1/TH17 contributions. Dust mite induced TH2-polarized responses [454].

8.6.3 Detection of Allergens

All dermatitis without a clear cause should be suspected for ACD. Patch testing is the gold standard in diagnosing of ACD [458]. Allergens in chambers are applied to the upper back for 2 days, and test results are read at day 2 and at day 3 or 4. An extra reading at day 7 could detect the possible late positive reactions. The reported incidences of late positive reactions in patch-tested patients ranged between 8.2 and 21 % [459–462]. These allergens include metals, corticosteroids, antibiotics, preservatives, fragrances, acrylic and methacrylic monomers, mercury, colophony, PPD, and fabric dye [459–462]. The guideline for grading scale of the patch-test results is in Table 8.5.

Unlike these delayed reactions at around day 7, patch test-induced sensitization usually develops at least 10 days after patch-test application and is regarded as an extremely infrequent adverse event of patch testing [463]. No matter what the positive tests are, the results of sensitization and of a late reaction in an allergic individual both indicate a present allergy [464].

Table 8.5 Recording of patch test reactions according to the International Contact Dermatitis Research Group (ICDRG)

+?	Doubtful reaction	Faint erythema only
+	Weak positive reaction	Erythema, infiltration, possibly papules
++	Strong positive reaction	Erythema, infiltration, papules, vesicles
+++	Extreme positive reaction	Intense erythema and infiltration and coalescing vesicles

The reading of + ? and + reactions from some irritant reactions may cause difficulties. This argument also occurs in pustular and follicular patch-test reactions, which is generally accepted as irritant, yet true relevant allergy could also be found [464]. The hallmarks of ICD are perturbation of the skin barrier, and the epidermal regenerative hyperproliferation and that in acute ACD is spongiosis [465]. It has been reported that reflectance confocal microscopy [466] and high-definition optical coherence tomography [467] provide useful noninvasive tools for the differentiation in patch-test reading, with increased epidermal thickness significant in irritant reactions. However, utilizing these instruments would not be very popular in most clinics considering the feasibility.

The clinical relevance of the positive patch-test reactions must be analyzed. The positive results may be relevant to present dermatitis, i.e., the primary cause or an aggravating factor, or may be relevant to a dermatitis that happened in the past. No result is unrelevant, it is just unknown or "unexplained positive" currently, but allergy may be noticed in the future [468].

The most common clinically relevant sensitizers in occupational and nonoccupational exposure include metals (particularly nickel), fragrance, preservatives, and rubber. Among the cosmetic-related allergens, fragrance mixes, balsam of Peru (BOP), methylchloroisothiazolinone/methylisothiazolinone (MCI/MI), and lanolin alcohols are principal allergens in Europe. MCI/MI was by far the leading one; moist cleansing wipes are a well-known source of MCI/MI, and other sources of exposure include shampoo, dishwashing liquid, and cosmetics. Sensitization to other widely used compounds like parabens or phenoxyethanol was rare [472]. The common cosmetic-related allergens in China are fragrance mix, thimerosal, parabens, imidazolidinylurea, formaldehyde, and shellac [473, 474] and that in India are gallate mix, cetrimide, and thiomersal [475].

The most common causes of an airborne contact dermatitis are plants, particularly those of the family Compositae. Woods, plastics, rubbers, glues, natural resins, pharmaceutical chemicals, insecticides, and pesticides have also been implicated. The sources of the reactions are multiple: drugs; plants, natural resins, and wood allergens; plastics, rubbers, and glues; preservatives and other chemicals; and metals. Drugs and preservatives have recently become more important causes [476].

The most common photoallergens in sunscreen include benzophenone-3, benzophenone-4, butylmethoxydibenzoylmethane, and octyl triazone (octocrylene).

Well-described food allergens that can trigger SCD include BOP, nickel, propylene glycol, chamomile, and formaldehyde. Major related foods to BOP are citrus fruits, tomatoes, and certain spices, e.g., cinnamon, vanilla, and cloves [469]. Foods that are rich in nickel include certain grains, including whole wheat bread and oatmeal, beans, lentils, peas, soybeans, soy products, shellfish, processed meats with fillers, and canned meats or fish. Other sources of dietary nickel include chocolate, nuts, seeds, black tea, cocoa, and canned foods in general [469–471].

8.6.4 Prevention and Management of Contact Dermatitis

In order to prevent and cure a contact dermatitis, it is essential to identify and avoid the underlying cause. Management of ICD is helpful for treatment of ACD. ICD is known to be the most common type of contact dermatitis; it represents approximately 80 % of occupational contact dermatitis cases, and it is considered the most common cause of hand eczema [477, 478]. ICD has an adjuvant-like effect on contact allergy, so it is important to protect the skin from irritation for both ICD and ACD. The regular use of emollients enhances the barrier function of the skin. Barrier creams containing dimethicone [479] or perfluoropolyethers [480], cotton liners [481], and softened fabrics [482] can prevent ICD. Lipid-rich moisturizers (e.g., 5 % urea, 5 % hydrogenated canola oil [483]) prevent and treat ICD [484]. Creams containing ceramides, rhamnosoft, and isoleucine may help restore and protect skin barrier function [485, 486]. However, a barrier cream containing aluminum chlorohydrate as the active ingredient was ineffective in preventing ICD and in fact was worse than a vehicle control on capacitance measures [487]. Glove occlusive has a significant negative effect on skin barrier function [481]. Topical skin protectant [488] and quaternium-18 bentonite [489] prevent *Rhus* dermatitis.

Thorough history investigation, physical examination, patch test, and repeated open application test help detect and identify the allergens. Patient education should be made on substances that they are allergic to and how to avoid further exposure. An informational leaflet is useful if the name of the chemical, its synonyms, its common uses, and examples of the types of products in which it may be found is supplied. Patients should be advised to check the lists of ingredients of all of the products before applying them. It is also important to inform patients about the risk of cross-reactivity to other related chemicals. Alternative choice to replace the allergic material should also be provided if possible. There is a Contact Allergen Replacement Database (CARD) in ACDS website, which is a members-only page, to provide a lot of allergen replacement information.

In addition, for a patient with an ACD due to nickel, balsam of Peru, or other well-recognized dietary allergens without improvement upon avoidance of cutaneous contact, dietary avoidance would be recommended for a period of 6–8 weeks [469].

The surveillance of irritants and allergens can promote public health. Measures should be taken (e.g., the use of personal protective equipment in the workplace, appeal to legislation on limiting the potent allergen use in manufacturer) to reduce the risk of exposure in wider population. Consumers should be reminded that products with "organic," "natural," "dermatologist recommended," or "safe" in labels can also be allergenic.

Topical treatment: Topical corticosteroids are the mainstay of topical treatment, with the strength of the topical corticosteroid appropriate to the body site. Topical macrolide immunomodulators (tacrolimus or pimecrolimus) or Chinese medicine, Qingpeng ointment [490], has also been shown to be effective. Diethylenetriamine pentaacetic acid (chelator) cream prevents nickel, chrome, and copper dermatitis [484]. Symptomatic cool wet compresses are helpful for acute vesicular dermatitis. Patients should avoid using topical antihistamines, including topical doxepin, because of the high risk of iatrogenic allergy and/or systemic contact dermatitis [491–493].

Systemic treatment: Sedating oral antihistamines may help diminish pruritus via a central effect. Systemic corticosteroids may be required for a short term during an acute phase of an extensive or severe contact dermatitis. If left untreated, contact dermatitis can develop into chronic dermatitis. PUVA treatment, narrow-band UVB treatment, or systemic treatment with immunomodulators (e.g., methotrexate, cyclosporine, mycophenolate, azathioprine) and targeted biologic therapy may be considered for recalcitrant cases of severe chronic widespread allergic contact dermatitis or severe hand dermatitis that prevents the individual from working or performing daily activities. The treatment of any underlying skin conditions (e.g., atopic dermatitis, psoriasis) should also be optimized.

Oral disulfiram, a nickel-chelating agent and low nickel diet has been considered an option for the control of chronic hand eczema in nickel-sensitive individuals; however, recurrence is common. The reported regimens are 50–400 mg per day for 4–56 weeks [494] or 125 mg/day after starting with low nickel diet for 2 weeks and then increased to 250 mg/day from the second week to the fourth week of treatment [495].

If patients develop chronic severe allergic reactions to their home or workplace, they may require a temporary change of environment until the cause of the dermatitis is identified and avoided. Hospital admission might be a choice.

8.7 Drug Eruption

Yong-Hu Sun, MD, PhD and Fu-Ren Zhang, MD, PhD

Drug eruptions are common adverse reactions that occur following the administration of medications and that are not characteristic of the desired pharmacodynamics effects, with clinical manifestations ranging from local skin changes to life-threatening diseases. Due to the lack of standardized coding for drug reactions and the method of data collection may be biased, it is difficult to acquire reliable and exact information on the incidence of drug reactions. However, it is estimated that about 1 of every 1000 hospitalized patients has a consequence of adverse drug reactions [496].

8.7.1 Drug Eruptions and Immunology

Hypersensitivity reactions can result from allergic sensitization to a drug by previous exposure to the same drug or a chemically related substance. Once sensitization has occurred, a hypersensitivity reaction may occur within minutes or even seconds, but always within 24 h. Prolonged therapy with certain drugs can cause a cumulative toxicity effect, while allergic reactions can even occur with very small doses of the drug, far below the therapeutic level of the drug. There are certain factors responsible for the development of hypersensitivity. Immunosuppression may increase the risk of obtaining hypersensitivity by inhibiting the regulatory functions of suppressor T lymphocytes [497]. In addition, the administration route may also be relevant to the possibility of sensitization, regarding to topical administration or oral administration of a certain drug. The duration of hypersensitivity is unpredictable. The level of antibodies falls if the patient is not exposed to the primary allergen or a related substance.

Four types of immunologically mediated reactions were proposed by Coombs and Gell [498]: Type I is IgE-dependent reactions, which can result in angioedema, urticaria, and anaphylaxis. Immediate reactions appear within minutes of administration of the drug, while accelerated ones appear within hours or days. Penicillins are the commonest cause. Type II is cytotoxic reactions; hemolysis and purpura are the manifestations. Penicillin, cephalosporins, sulfonamides, quinine, and rifampicin can cause such reactions. Type III is immune complex reactions, resulting from the binding of antigens to antibodies, which may result in urticaria, vasculitis, and serum sickness. They can be caused by quinine, salicylates, chlorpromazine, and sulfonamides. Type IV is delayed-type cell-mediated reactions, usually takes 2–3 days after exposure, which may result in contact dermatitis, exanthematous reactions, fixed drug reactions, lichenoid reactions, LE-like reactions, and photoallergic reactions.

8.7.2 Pharmacogenetic Mechanisms

Besides of the immunology aspects, there are several predisposing factors that may increase the risk of drug eruptions, such as viral infections, past history of medicament allergies, and polymorphisms in human leukocyte antigen (HLA). Recently, there is increasing evidence of the important role played by T cells in drug-induced skin disease. Analysis of drug-specific T cell has revealed that a drug can be recognized by αβ T-cell receptors, not only if bound covalently to peptides but also if the drug binds in a rather labile way to the histocompatibility complex peptide [499]. On initial exposure of the drug, T cells are primed, and on repeated exposure, the memory pool is restimulated. The key proteins that mediate T-cell immune responses are the HLA molecules encoded within the major histocompatibility complex (MHC) gene family. HLA molecules have a direct role in the pathogenesis of drug hypersensitivity because they are the primary elements in T-cell stimulation. The MHC is extremely polymorphic, and there are specific HLA alleles. Significant ones include hypersensitivity to abacavir and HLA-B*5701 [500], SJS induced by carbamazepine in Han Chinese [501] and European [502], and drug-induced hypersensitivity by dapsone [503]. There are numerous other HLA alleles implicated in drug-induced SCARs (severe cutaneous adverse reaction to drugs) (Table 8.6).

8.7.3 Clinical Type and Treatment of Drug Eruption

8.7.3.1 Morbilliform

The most common type of adverse drug reaction pattern affecting the skin is morbilliform eruptions. Erythematous maculopapules classically develop 3–14 days after exposure to a new medication. The rash can even sustain several days after the drug has been withdrawal. The lesion usually begins from the trunk and chest and may progressively become confluent mucosae, and the face is usually spared. Skin biopsy usually shows nonspecific changes for the morbilliform eruptions. Regarding the differential diagnosis of morbilliform drug eruptions, the major entity is a viral exanthem, such as early HIV, EBV, HHV-6, and parvovirus B19. Moreover, the risk of developing a drug eruption may be enhanced by the viral infections.

The common culprits which can induce morbilliform eruption include the following classes of drugs: ACE inhibitors, anticonvulsants, aminopenicillins, sulfonamides, and cephalosporins. The treatment for morbilliform eruptions begins with the withdrawal of suspect drug. The treatment method is mainly supportive. It is useful to treat itch with emollients and antihistamines. Topical corticosteroids may sometimes be help to the alleviate pruritus.

8.7.3.2 Urticaria and Angioedema

Urticaria is the second most common cutaneous manifestation of drug allergy. Drug-induced urticaria may be caused by several different mechanisms: acute urticaria usually representing an immediate hypersensitivity reaction (i) mediated by immunoglobulin (Ig) E antibodies; (ii) mediated by circulating immune complexes (serum sickness) and antigen-antibody formation with deposition of immune complexes

Table 8.6 Drugs could induce severe cutaneous adverse drug reaction and associated HLA alleles

Agents	Syndrome	Alleles	Ethic
Abacavir	HSS/DIHS/DRESS (rash, fever, gastrointestinal, respiratory symptoms)	HLA-B*5701	White
			Black
			Australian
Allopurinol	SJS/TEN	HLA-B*5801	Han Chinese
			Thai
			Korean
Carbamazepine	SJS/TEN	HLA-B*1502	Han Chinese
		HLA-B*1502	Canadian
		HLA-B*1502	Han Chinese
		HLA-B*1511	Korean
		HLA-B*1511	Japanese
		HLA-A*3101	Northern European
		HLA-A*3101	Japanese
	HSS/DIHS/DRESS	HLA-A*3101	European
			Canadian
			Northern European
	Delayed rash (MPE)	HLA-B*3101	European
			Canadian
			Northern European
Dapsone	DIHS	HLA-B*1301	Chinese
Minocycline	DIHS (lupus-like)	HLA-DR4/HLA-DR2	European
Nevirapine	HSS/DIHS/DRESS (skin rash, fever, hepatitis)	HLA-B*3505	Thai
		HLA-Cw*04	Han Chinese
Salazosulfapyridine	DRESS	HLA-B*1301	Han Chinese

within postcapillary venules; and (iii) mediated by non-immunologic activation of effector pathways [504].

Drug-induced urticaria is indistinguishable with those caused by other factors. The lesions vary in size and can be developed anywhere on the body. The lesions are usually short-lived, lasting a few hours to 24 h, and the skin is normal in appearance after the urticaria resolves. Hypotension, breathing difficulties, shock, and even death can occur in the severe type of urticaria. A number of medications can induce chronic and acute urticaria, and the major responsible one is antibiotics. Sulfonamides, tetracycline, and even monoclonal antibodies for tumors will be the cause of urticaria. Immunological test for specific IgE antibodies may be useful in confirming the diagnosis, but rarely helpful in confirming the inducing drugs.

Drug-induced angioedema is characterized by transient edema of the deep dermal, subcutaneous, and submucosal tissues. It usually affects the face with an acute pale or pink subcutaneous selling, but not often limbs or genitalia. Gastrointestinal symptoms, including abdominal pain, vomiting, and nausea, can be occasionally seen due to the edema of the gastrointestinal wall. ACE inhibitors are the main cause that induces the angioedema [505].

The key step in the treatment of urticaria and angioedema is withdrawal of the most likely causative agents. The treatment that consists primarily of H1 antihistamines is sufficient for the majority of moderate drug-induced urticaria. For those patients who have a systemic reaction, systemic corticosteroids are helpful [506].

8.7.3.3 Fixed Drug Eruptions (FDE)

Fixed drug eruption describes the development of one or more annular or oval erythematous patches as a result of systemic exposure to a drug. These reactions normally may recur at the same site upon readministration of the drug. The lesions can develop from 30 min to 8 h and longer after ingestion of the drugs, which are usually round, sharply demarcated erythematous and edematous plaques or coin shaped and may vary from one to a few in number. FDE recur at the same site following the administration of the offending drug or occasionally a member of the same group of drugs. Based on the clinical features and distribution of the lesions, there are many variants of fixed drug eruption as the following: pigmenting fixed drug eruption, bullous fixed drug eruption, eczematous fixed drug eruption, vulvitis, psoriasiform, etc. FDE can occur on any part of the body but frequently involve the glans penis, oral mucosa, hands, and feet.

More than 100 drugs have been implicated in causing FDE, and the list is steadily growing. The most frequently associated with FDE are sulfonamides, barbiturates, and carbamazepine. In adults the active ingredient of laxatives (phenolphthalein) is commonly implicated.

Treatment consists of removal of the suspected drugs. It also highlights that removal of unnecessary polypharmacy. Therapy of the acute lesions is disappointing. Neither topical nor systemic steroids seem to have any significant effect on the natural history of the lesions.

8.7.3.4 Drug-Induced Erythroderma

It is characterized by widespread, generalized erythema and desquamation extending to >90% of BSA (body surface area). Compared to other causes of erythroderma, the drug-induced cases are sudden in onset, rapidly progressive, and resolve fast. Drug-induced erythroderma usually begins as erythema and exudation in the flexures and progresses to generalized scaling. Several manifestations, such as pruritus; lymphadenopathy; hepatosplenomegaly; pedal and facial edema; hypothermia; pneumonia; fluid, protein, and electrolyte loss; and infection, can occur during the disease period. Basal metabolic rate is usually high with increased catabolism. It takes 4–6 weeks for the rash to resolve even after withdrawal of drug.

Drugs commonly incriminated are sulfonamides, penicillin, isoniazid, antimalarials, allopurinol, phenytoin, omeprazole, captopril, and vancomycin. Drug-induced erythroderma is seen twice more often in males than in females and is definitely more common among elderly [507].

Common lab abnormalities are anemia, leukocytosis with eosinophilia, increased erythrocyte sedimentation rate, decreased serum albumin levels, and increased uric acid levels. IgE levels may increase. Biopsy reports are nonspecific including hyperkeratosis, parakeratosis, and acanthosis along with a chronic mainly perivascular inflammatory infiltrate with few eosinophils.

For the treatment of erythroderma, emollients, maintenance of fluid and electrolyte balance, nutritious protein-rich diet, and antihistamines for pruritus are advised. Local skin care such as starch baths and wet dressings for crusted sites followed by the application of bland emollients and low-potency corticosteroids are in order. Secondary infections should be treated with antibiotics. The patient should be placed in a regulated environmental temperature to avoid cooling and overheating. Systemic steroids are required when conservative therapy is ineffective.

8.7.3.5 Acute Generalized Exanthematous Pustulosis (AGEP)

AGEP was firstly described as a widespread pustular eruption resembling pustular psoriasis in 1980, but it is usually seen as a drug reaction in patients without a history of psoriasis. Main manifestation is high fever and numerous small and primarily non-follicular sterile pustules arising on a large area of edematous erythema that develops within 2 weeks of starting a medication. The pustules usually begin on the face or the major intertriginous zones and can locate in the trunk and upper extremities. Confluence of pustules may result in superficial detachment, not rarely misdiagnosed clinically as TEN [507]. Edema of the face and hands, purpura, vesicles, bullae, erythema multiforme-like lesions, and mucous membrane involvement are additionally present. Mucosal involvement occurs in about 25 % of AGEP patients. Approximately 87 % of AGEP cases are associated with drug exposure, but viral infections and contact dermatitis have also been implicated [508]. Antibiotics are the primary drugs implicated in AGEP. Calcium channel blockers, NSAIDs, anticonvulsants, aminoglycosides, and macrolides are the drugs most frequently implicated.

It is difficult to differentiate AGEP from acute pustular psoriasis. The pustules in both diseases are clinically indistinguishable. The skin biopsy can be helpful with spongiform pustules in the superficial layers of the epidermis, beneath the stratum corneum. Edema of the papillary dermis and a perivascular mixed infiltrate with neutrophils and some eosinophils are usually present and helpful for the diagnosis. The diagnosis criteria of AGEP include: (1) an acute pustular eruption, (2) fever above 38 °C, (3) neutrophilia with or without a mild eosinophilia, (4) subcorneal or intraepidermal pustules on skin biopsy, and (5) spontaneous resolution in less than 15 days [509].

The causative drug has to be withdrawn, and antibiotics are not given unless there is a clear and well-documented associated infection. Treatment consists of topical corticosteroids and antipyretics. Usually, AGEP is benign and self-limited course, while systemic corticosteroid treatment is often not taken into consideration.

8.7.3.6 Drug Rash with Eosinophilia and Systemic Symptoms (DRESS), Drug-Induced Hypersensitivity Syndrome (DIHS)

DRESS is a severe idiosyncratic drug reaction associated with multi-organ involvement, which is further strictly named as drug-induced hypersensitivity syndrome (DIHS) or drug-induced delayed multi-organ hypersensitivity syndrome (DIDMOHS). The exact mechanisms for DRESS remain unclear but has suggested that a specific alteration in the metabolism of particular drugs. Moreover, HHV-6 and HHV-7 may play a role in the pathogenesis of DRESS. Clinically, DRESS is characterized by drug reaction with eosinophilia and systemic symptoms. The most common cause of DRESS is anticonvulsants. Allopurinol, dapsone, salazosulfapyridine, minocycline, and mexiletine can also be the causative medication. The syndrome typically develops 2–6 weeks after the initiation of drug administration, and the initial symptoms are fever and maculopapular eruption that may progress to exfoliative dermatitis. The hallmark of the disease is a striking facial edema. Lymphadenopathy, hepatitis, renal dysfunction, atypical lymphocytosis, and hematologic abnormalities, such as leukocytosis and eosinophilia, are observed to varying degrees.

There are mainly two diagnostic criteria for DIHS, the RegiSCAR and the Japanese. For the RegiSCAR criteria, three out of five criteria are required:

1. Acute skin rash
2. At least one internal organ involvement
3. Lymph node enlargement of at least two sites
4. One of the following blood count abnormalities: (a) lymphocytosis/lymphopenia, (b) eosinophilia, and (c) thrombocytopenia
5. Fever > 38° C

The Japanese scale have the following criteria:

1. Maculopapular rash at least 3 weeks after starting drug
2. Clinical symptoms lasting for more than 2 weeks after discontinuation of drug
3. Fever > 38
4. Raised LFT (Serum ALT > 100 IU/L)
5. Abnormal blood counts, at least one of: (a) WBC count > 11,000/mm^3, (b) atypical lymphocytes > 5 %, and (c) eosinophilia > 1500/mm^3
6. Lymphadenopathy
7. HHV-6/EBV/CMV reactivation

If all seven criteria are present, it is a classical DHS, and if at least five criteria are present, it is an atypical DHS.

The causative drugs need to be removed immediately. Besides, systemic corticosteroids (0.5–1 mg/kg/day) have been advocated for the treatment. However, due to the involvement of HHV-6 infection in DIHS pathogenesis and recovery without systemic corticosteroids of some patients, only severe DIHS cases are recommended with high doses of systemic corticosteroids or steroid pulse therapy. In addition, combined systemic corticosteroids and high-dose intravenous immunoglobulin will be effective but remains controversial and requires further RCT investigations.

References

Bacterial Infectious Skin Diseases

1. Rayan GM, Flournoy DJ. Microbiologic flora of human fingernails. J Hand Surg (America). 1987;12:605–7.
2. Evans CA, Smith WM, Johnston EA, Giblett ER. Bacterial flora of the normal human skin. J Invest Dermatol. 1950;15:305–24.
3. Lark RL, VanderHyde K, Deeb GM, Dietrich S, Massey JP, Chenoweth C. An outbreak of coagulase-negative staphylococcal surgical-site infections following aortic valve replacement. Infect Control Hosp Epidemiol. 2001;22:618–23.
4. Adams BG, Marrie TJ. Hand carriage of aerobic gram-negative rods may not be transient. J Hyg (London). 1982;89:33–46.
5. Marples RR, Towers AG. A laboratory model for the investigation of contact transfer of micro-organisms. J Hy (London). 1979;82:237–48.
6. Patrick DR, Findon G, Miller TE. Residual moisture determines the level of touch-contact-associated bacterial transfer following hand washing. Epidemiol Infect. 1997;119:319–25.
7. Gunderson CG, Martinello RA. A systematic review of bacteremias in cellulitis and erysipelas. J Infect. 2012;64:148–55.
8. Machida K. Immunological investigations on pathogenesis of staphylococcal scalded skin syndrome. Rinsho Byori. 1995;43:547–56.
9. Leung DY, Travers JB, Giorno R, Norris DA, Skinner R, Aelion J, et al. Evidence for a streptococcal superantigen-driven process in acute guttate psoriasis. J Clin Invest. 1995;96:2106–12.
10. Swartz MN. Clinical practice. Cellulitis. N Engl J Med. 2004;350(9):904–12.
11. Linder A, Johansson L, Thulin P, Hertzén E, Mörgelin M, Christensson B, et al. Erysipelas caused by group a streptococcus activates the contact system and induces the release of heparin-binding protein. J Invest Dermatol. 2010;130:1365–72.
12. Morris AD. Cellulitis and erysipelas. BMJ Clin Evid. 2008; pii: 1708.
13. Pavlotsky F, Amrani S, Trau H. Recurrent erysipelas: risk factors. J Dtsch Dermatol Ges. 2004;2:89–95.
14. Björnsdóttir S, Gottfredsson M, Thórisdóttir AS, Gunnarsson GB, Ríkardsdóttir H, Kristjánsson M, et al. Risk factors for acute cellulitis of the lower limb: a prospective case–control study. Clin Infect Dis. 2005;41:1416–22.
15. Karppelin M, Siljander T, Vuopio-Varkila J, Kere J, Huhtala H, Vuento R, et al. Factors predisposing to acute and recurrent bacterial non-necrotizing cellulitis in hospitalized patients: a prospective case–control study. Clin Microbiol Infect. 2010;16:729–34.
16. Eriksson B, Jorup-Rönström C, Karkkonen K, Sjöblom AC, Holm SE. Erysipelas: clinical and bacteriologic spectrum and serological aspects. Clin Infect Dis. 1996;23:1091–8.
17. Rantala S, Vuopio-Varkila J, Vuento R, Huhtala H, Syrjänen J. Clinical presentations and epidemiology of beta-haemolytic streptococcal bacteraemia: a population-based study. Clin Microbiol Infect. 2009;15:286–8.
18. Chatellier S, Ihendyane N, Kansal RG, Khambaty F, Basma H, Norrby-Teglund A, et al. Genetic relatedness and superantigen expression in group a streptococcus serotype M1 isolates from patients with severe and nonsevere invasive diseases. Infect Immun. 2000;68:3523–34.
19. Aziz RK, Kansal R, Abdeltawab NF, Rowe SL, Su Y, Carrigan D, et al. Susceptibility to severe Streptococcal sepsis: use of a large set of isogenic mouse lines to study genetic and environmental factors. Genes Immun. 2007;8:404–15.
20. Medina E, Lengeling A. Genetic regulation of host responses to group a streptococcus in mice. Brief Funct Genomic Proteomic. 2005;4:248–57.
21. Goldmann O, Lengeling A, Böse J, Bloecker H, Geffers R, Chhatwal GS, et al. The role of the MHC on resistance to group a streptococci in mice. J Immunol. 2005;175:3862–72.
22. Abdeltawab NF, Aziz RK, Kansal R, Rowe SL, Su Y, Gardner L, et al. An unbiased systems genetics approach to mapping genetic loci modulating susceptibility to severe streptococcal sepsis. PLoS Pathog. 2008;4:e1000042.
23. Iushchuk ND, Frolov VM, Gaĭdash IS, Peresadin NA. The immunogenetic aspects of erysipelas infection. Zh Mikrobiol Epidemiol Immunobiol. 1991;3:57–9.
24. Hannula-Jouppi K, Massinen S, Siljander T, Mäkelä S, Kivinen K, Leinonen R, et al. Genetic susceptibility to non-necrotizing erysipelas/cellulitis. PLoS One. 2013;8:e56225.
25. Joseph K, Kaplan AP. Formation of bradykinin: a major contributor to the innate inflammatory response. Adv Immunol. 2005;86:159–208.

26. Colman RW, Schmaier AH. Contact system: vascular biology modulator with anticoagulant, profibrinolytic, antiadhesive, and proinflammatory attributes. Blood. 1997;90:3819–43.
27. Oehmcke S, Mörgelin M, Herwald H. Activation of the human contact system on neutrophil extracellular traps. J Innate Immun. 2009;1:225–30.
28. Mattsson E, Herwald H, Cramer H, Persson K, Sjöbring U, Björck L. Staphylococcus aureus induces release of bradykinin in human plasma. Infect Immun. 2001;69:3877–82.
29. Herwald H, Cramer H, Mörgelin M, Russell W, Sollenberg U, Norrby-Teglund A, et al. M protein, classical bacterial virulence determinant, forms complexes with fibrinogen that inducevascular leakage. Cell. 2004;116:367–79.
30. Gautam N, Olofsson AM, Herwald H, Iversen LF, Lundgren-Akerlund E, Hedqvist P, et al. Heparin-binding protein (HBP/CAP37): a missing link in neutrophil-evoked alteration of vascular permeability. Nat Med. 2001;7:1123–7.
31. Herwald H, Collin M, Müller-Esterl W, Björck L. Streptococcal cysteine proteinase releases kinins: a virulence mechanism. J Exp Med. 1996;184:665–73.
32. Chosidow O, Le Cleach L. Prophylactic antibiotics for the prevention of cellulites (erysipelas) of the leg. A commentary. Br J Dermatol. 2012;166:6.
33. Bishara J, Golan-Cohen A, Robenshtok E, Leibovici L, Pitlik S. Antibiotic use in patients with erysipelas: a retrospective study. Isr Med Assoc J. 2001;3:722–4.
34. Vos MD, Bos RR, Vissink A. A sudden redness and swelling of the face. Ned Tijdschr Tandheelkd. 2009;116:383–6.
35. Cox NH. Oedema as a risk factor for multiple episodes of cellulitis/erysipelas of the lower leg: a series with community follow-up. Br J Dermatol. 2006;155:947–50.
36. Leclerc S, Teixeira A, Mahé E, Descamps V, Crickx B, Chosidow O. Recurrent erysipelas: 47 cases. Dermatology. 2007;214:52–7.
37. Oh CC, Ko HC, Lee HY, Safdar N, Maki DG, Chlebicki MP. Antibiotic prophylaxis for preventing recurrent cellulites: systematic review and meta-analysis. J Infect. 2014;69:26–34.
38. Handler MZ, Schwartz RA. Staphylococcal scalded skin syndrome: diagnosis and management in children and adults. J Eur Acad Dermatol Venereol. 2014;28:1418–23.
39. Patel NN, Patel DN. Staphylococcal scalded skin syndrome. Am J Med. 2010;123:505–7.
40. Resnick SD, Elias PM. Staphylococcal scalded skin syndrome. In: Freedberg IM, Eisen AZ, Wolff K, Frans-Austen K, Goldsmith LA, Katz SI, editors. Fitzpatrick's dermatology in general medicine. 6th ed. New York: McGraw-Hill; 2003. p. 878–1883.
41. Iwatsuki K, Yamasaki O, Morizane S, Oono T. Staphylococcal cutaneous infections: invasion, evasion and aggression. J Dermatol Sci. 2006;42:203–14.
42. Melish ME, Glasgow LA. The staphylococcal scalded skin syndrome: development of an experimental model. N Engl J Med. 1970;282:1114–9.
43. Ladhani S. Understanding the mechanism of action of the exfoliative toxins of Staphylococcus aureus. FEMS Immunol Med Microbiol. 2003;39:181–9.
44. Amagai M, Matsuyoshi N, Wang ZH, Andl C, Stanley JR. Toxin in bullous impetigo and staphylococcal scalded-skin syndrome targets desmoglein 1. Nat Med. 2000;6:1275–7.
45. Hanakawa Y, Schecter NM, Lin C, Garza L, Li H, Yamaguchi T, et al. Molecular mechanisms of blister formation in bullous impetigo and staphylococcal scalded skin syndrome. J Clin Invest. 2002;110:53–60.
46. Ladhani S, Joannou CL, Lochrie DP, Evans RW, Poston SM. Clinical, microbia, and biochemical aspects of the exfoliative toxins causing staphylococcal scalded-skin syndrome. Clin Microbiol Rev. 1999;12:224–42.
47. Norbury WB, Gallagher JJ, Herndon DN, Branski LK, Oehring PE, Jeschke MG. Neonate twin with staphylococcal scalded skin syndrome from a renal source. Pediatr Crit Care Med. 2010;11:e20–3.
48. Kadam S, Tagare A, Deodhar J, Tawade Y, Pandit A. Staphylococcal scalded skin syndrome in a neonate. Indian J Pediatr. 2009;76:1074.
49. Kapoor V, Travadi J, Braye S. Staphylococcal scalded skin syndrome in an extremely premature neonate: a case report with a brief review of literature. J Paediatr Child Health. 2008;44:374–6.
50. O'Connell NH, Mannix M, Philip RK, MacDonagh-White C, Slevin B, Monahan R, et al. Infant Staphylococcal scalded skin syndrome, Ireland, 2007 – preliminary outbreak report. Euro Surveill. 2007;12:E070614.5.
51. Nishifuji K, Sugai M, Amagai M. Staphylococcal exfoliative toxins: "molecular scissors" of bacteria that attack the cutaneous defense barrier in mammals. J Dermatol Sci. 2008;49:21–31.
52. Yamaguchi T, Nishifuji K, Sasaki M, Fudaba Y, Aepfelbacher M, Takata T, et al. Identification of the Staphylococcus aureus etd pathogenicity island which encodes a novel exfoliative toxin, ETD, and EDIN-B. Infect Immun. 2002;70(2):5835–45.
53. Vath GM, Earhart CA, Rago JV, Kim MH, Bohach GA, Schlievert PM, et al. The structure of the superantigen exfoliative toxin a suggests a novel regulation as a serine protease. Biochemistry. 1997;36:1559–66.
54. Hanakawa Y, Selwood T, Woo D, Lin C, Schechter NM, Stanley JR. Calcium-dependent conformation of desmoglein 1 is required for its cleavage by exfoliative toxin. J Invest Dermatol. 2003;121:383–9.
55. Blyth M, Estela C, Young AE. Severe staphylococcal scalded skin syndrome in children. Burns. 2008;34:98–103.
56. Ladhani S, Joannou CL. Difficulties in diagnosis and management of the staphylococcal scalded skin syndrome. Pediatr Infect Dis J. 2000;19:819–21.
57. Li MY, Hua Y, Wei GH, Qui L. Staphylococcal scalded skin syndrome in neonates: an 8-year retrospective study in a single institution. Pediatr Dermatol. 2013;31:1–5.

Human Immune Responses to Invasive Fungal Pathogen

58. Hube B. Fungal adaptation to the host environment. Curr Opin Microbiol, 2009;12(4):347–49.
59. Garcia-Solache MA, Casadevall A. Global warming will bring new fungal diseases for mammals. mBio, 2010;1(1):e00061–10.
60. Fisher MC, Henk DA, Briggs CJ, Brownstein JS, Madoff LC, McCraw SL, Gurr SJ. Emerging fungal threats to animal, plant and ecosystem health. Nature, 2012;484(7393):186–94.
61. Fauci AS, Morens DM. The perpetual challenge of infectious diseases. N Engl J Med. 2012;366(5):454–61.
62. Underhill DM, Iliev ID. The mycobiota: interactions between commensal fungi and the host immune system. Nat Rev Immunol, 2014; 14(6):405–16.
63. Romani L. Immunity to fungal infections. Nat Rev Immunol. 2011; 11(4):275–88.
64. Rivera A. Protective immune responses to fungal infections. Parasite Immunol. 2014;36(9):453–62.
65. Lass-Flörl C, Roilides E, Löffler J, Wilflingseder D, Romani L. Minireview: host defence in invasive aspergillosis. Mycoses. 2013; 56(4):403–13.
66. Bourgeois C, Kuchler K. Fungal pathogens-a sweet and sour treat for toll-like receptors. Front Cell Infect Microbiol. 2012; 22(2):142.

67. Biondo C, Signorino G, Costa A, Midiri A, Gerace E, Galbo R, Bellantoni A, Malara A, Beninati C, Teti G, Mancuso G. Recognition of yeast nucleic acids triggers a host-protective type I interferon response. Eur J Immunol, 2011;41(7):1969–79.
68. Chai LY, Kullberg BJ, Vonk AG, Warris A, Cambi A, Latgé JP, Joosten LA, van der Meer JW, Netea MG. Modulation of Toll-like receptor 2 (TLR2) and TLR4 responses by Aspergillus fumigatus. Infect Immun, 2009;77(5):2184–92.
69. Kasperkovitz PV, Cardenas ML, Vyas JM. TLR9 is actively recruited to Aspergillus fumigatus phagosomes and requires the N-terminal proteolytic cleavage domain for proper intracellular trafficking. J Immunol, 2010;185(12):7614–22.
70. Jouault T, Ibata-Ombetta S, Takeuchi O, Trinel PA, Sacchetti P, Lefebvre P, Akira S, Poulain D. Candida albicans phospholipomannan is sensed through toll-like receptors. J Infect Dis 2003;188(1):165–72.
71. Shoham S, Huang C, Chen JM, Golenbock DT, Levitz SM. Toll-like receptor 4 mediates intracellular signaling without TNFalpha release in response to Cryptococcus neoformans polysaccharide capsule. J Immunol, 2001;166:4620–6.
72. Rivera A, Hohl TM, Collins N, et al. Dectin-1 diversifies Aspergillus fumigatus-specific T cell responses by inhibiting T helper type 1 CD4 T cell differentiation. J Exp Med 2011;208:369–81.
73. Rivera A, Ro G, Van Epps HL, et al. Innate immune activation and CD4+ T cell priming during respiratory fungal infection. Immunity 2006;25:665–75.
74. Goodridge HS, Shimada T, Wolf AJ, et al. Differential use of CARD9 by dectin-1 in macrophages and dendritic cells. J Immunol 2009;182:1146–54.
75. Gross O, Gewies A, Finger K, et al. Card9 controls a non-TLR signalling pathway for innate anti-fungal immunity. Nature 2006;442:651–6.
76. Fric J, Zelante T, Wong AY, Mertes A, Yu HB & Ricciardi-Castagnoli P. NFAT control of innate immunity. Blood, 2012;120:1380–9.
77. Rosentul DC, Plantinga TS, Oosting M, et al. Genetic variation in the dectin-1/CARD9 recognition pathway and susceptibility to candidemia. J Infect Dis 2011;204:1138–45.
78. Drewniak A, Gazendam RP, Tool AT, et al. Invasive fungal infection and impaired neutrophil killing in human CARD9 deficiency. Blood 2013;121: 2385–92.
79. Jhingran A, Mar KB, Kumasaka DK, et al. Tracing conidial fate and measuring host cell antifungal activity using a reporter of microbial viability in the lung. Cell Rep 2012;2:1762–73.
80. Chai LY, de Boer MG, van der Velden WJ, et al. The Y238X stop codon polymorphism in the human beta-glucan receptor dectin-1 and susceptibility to invasive aspergillosis. J Infect Dis, 2011;203:736–43.
81. Hara H, Ishihara C, Takeuchi A, et al. The adaptor protein CARD9 is essential for the of myeloid cells through ITAM associated and Toll-like receptors. Nat Immunol, 2007;8:619–29.
82. Robinson MJ, Osorio F, Rosas M, et al. Dectin-2 is a Syk-coupled pattern recognition receptor crucial for Th17 responses to fungal infection. J Exp Med 2009;206:2037–51.
83. Saijo S, Ikeda S, Yamabe K, et al. Dectin-2 recognition of alpha-mannans and induction of Th17 cell differentiation is essential for host defense against Candida albicans. Immunity, 2010;32: 681–91.
84. ONeill LA. When signaling pathways collide: positive and negative regulation of toll-like receptor signal transduction. Immunity 2008;29:12–20.
85. Gantner BN, Simmons RM, Canavera SJ, Akira S & Underhill DM. Collaborative induction of inflammatory responses by dectin-1 and Toll-like receptor 2. J Exp Med, 2003;197:1107–17.
86. Dennehy KM, Ferwerda G, Faro-TrindadeI, et al. Syk kinase is required for collaborative cytokine production induced through Dectin-1 and Toll-like receptors. Eur J Immunol 2008;38:500–6.
87. Huynh L, Wang L, Shi C, Park-Min KH & Ivashkiv LB. ITAM-coupled receptors inhibit IFNAR signaling and alter macrophage responses to TLR4 and Listeria monocytogenes. J Immunol 2012;188:3447–57.
88. Brown GD. Innate antifungal immunity: the key role of phagocytes. Annual review of immunology 2011;29:1–21.
89. Vazquez-Torres A, Balish E. Macrophages in resistance to candidiasis. Microbiology and molecular biology reviews. MMBR, 1997;61(2):170–92.
90. Levitz SM, Diamond RD. Killing of Aspergillus fumigatus spores and Candida albicans yeast phase by the iron-hydrogen peroxide-iodide cytotoxic system: comparison with the myeloperoxidase-hydrogen peroxide-halide system. Infection and immunity, 1984;43(3):1100–2.
91. Henriet S, Verweij PE, Holland SM, Warris A. Invasive fungal infections in patients with chronic granulomatous disease. Advances in experimental medicine and biology, 2013;764:27–55.
92. Miletic AV, Graham DB, Montgrain V, et al. Vav proteins control MyD88-dependent oxidative burst. Blood 2007;109(8):3360–8.
93. Rocco NM, Carmen JC, Klein BS. Blastomyces dermatitidis yeast cells inhibit nitric oxide production by alveolar macrophage inducible nitric oxide synthase. Infection and immunity, 2011;79(6):2385–95.
94. Youseff BH, Holbrook ED, Smolnycki KA, Rappleye CA. Extracellular superoxide dismutase protects Histoplasma yeast cells from host-derived oxidative stress. PLoS pathogens 2012;8(5):e1002713.
95. Collette JR, Lorenz MC. Mechanisms of immune evasion in fungal pathogens. Current opinion in microbiology, 2011;14(6): 668–75.
96. Gonzalez A, Hung CY, Cole GT. Nitric oxide synthase activity has limited influence on the control of Coccidioides infection in mice. Microbial pathogenesis 2011;51(3):161–8.
97. Miramon P, Dunker C, Windecker H, et al. Cellular responses of Candida albicans to phagocytosis and the extracellular activities of neutrophils are critical to counteract carbohydrate starvation, oxidative and nitrosative stress. PloS one 2012;7(12):p.e52850.
98. Hsieh SH, Lin JS, Huang JH, et al. Immunization with apoptotic phagocytes containing Histoplasma capsulatum activates functional CD8(+)T cells to protect against histoplasmosis. Infection and immunity, 2011;79(11):4493–502.
99. Den Hertog AL, van Marle J, Veerman EC, et al. The human cathelicidin peptide LL-37 and truncated variants induce segregation of lipids and proteins in the plasma membrane of Candida albicans. Biological chemistry 2006;387(10):1495–502.
100. Lopera D, Aristizabal BH, Restrepo A, Cano LE, Gonzalez A. Lysozyme plays a dual role against the dimorphic fungus Paracoccidioides brasiliensis. Revista do Instituto de Medicina Tropical de Sao Paulo 2008;50(3):169–75.
101. Pham CT. Neutrophil serine proteases: specific regulators of inflammation. Nature reviews Immunology, 2006;6(7):541–50.
102. Kaplan MJ, Radic M. Neutrophil extracellular traps: double-edged swords of innate immunity. Journal of immunology, 2012;189(6):2689–95.
103. Espinosa V, Rivera A. Cytokines and the regulation of fungus-specific CD4 T cell differentiation. Cytokine 2012;58(1):100–6.
104. Werner JL, Metz AE, Horn D, et al. Requisite role for the dectin-1 beta-glucan receptor in pulmonary defense against Aspergillus fumigatus. Journal of immunology, 2009;182(8):4938–46.
105. Deepe GS, Gibbons RS. Interleukins 17 and 23 influence the host response to Histoplasma capsulatum. The Journal of infectious diseases, 2009;200(1):142–51.

106. Rudner XL, Happel KI, Young EA, Shellito JE. Interleukin-23 (IL-23)-IL-17 cytokine axis in murine Pneumocystis carinii infection. Infection and immunity, 2007;75(6):3055–61.
107. Ye P, Rodriguez FH, Kanaly S, et al. Requirement of interleukin 17 receptor signaling for lung CXC chemokine and granulocyte colony-stimulating factor expression, neutrophil recruitment, and host defense. The Journal of experimental medicine, 2001;194(4):519–27.
108. Serbina NV, Jia T, Hohl TM, Pamer EG. Monocyte-mediated defense against microbial pathogens. Annual review of immunology, 2008;26:421–52.
109. Duong M, Ouellet N, Simard M, Bergeron Y, Olivier M, Bergeron MG. Kinetic study of host defense and inflammatory response to Aspergillus fumigatus in steroid-induced immunosuppressed mice. The Journal of infectious diseases, 1998;178(5):1472–82.
110. Schaffner A, Douglas H, Braude AI, Davis CE. Killing of Aspergillus spores depends on the anatomical source of the macrophage. Infection and immunity, 1983;42(3):1109–15.
111. Ibrahim-Granet O, Philippe B, Boleti H, et al. Phagocytosis and intracellular fate of Aspergillus fumigatus conidia in alveolar macrophages. Infection and immunity, 2003;71(2):891–903.
112. Serbina NV, Pamer EG. Monocyte emigration from bone marrow during bacterial infection requires signals mediated by chemokine receptor CCR2. Nature immunology, 2006;7(3):311–7.
113. Traynor TR, Herring AC, Dorf ME, Kuziel WA, Toews GB, Huffnagle GB. Differential roles of CC chemokine ligand 2/ monocyte chemotactic protein-1 and CCR2 in the development of T1 immunity. Journal of immunology, 2002;168(9):4659–66.
114. Blease K, Mehrad B, Lukacs NW, Kunkel SL, Standiford TJ, Hogaboam CM. Antifungal and airway remodeling roles for murine monocyte chemoattractant protein-1/CCL2 during pulmonary exposure to Asperigillus fumigatus conidia. Journal of immunology, 2001;166(3):1832–42.
115. Ngo LY, Kasahara S, Kumasaka DK, Knoblaugh SE, Jhingran A, Hohl TM. Inflammatory monocytes mediate early and organ-specific innate defense during systemic candidiasis. The Journal of infectious diseases, 2014;209(1):109–19.
116. Espinosa V & Rivera A. Cytokines and the regulation of fungus-specific CD4 T cell differentiation. Cytokine, 2012;58:100–6.
117. Hernandez-Santos N & Gaffen SL. Th17 cells in immunity to Candida albicans. Cell Host Microbe, 2012;11:425–35.
118. Jones SA, Sutton CE, Cua D & Mills KH. Therapeutic potential of targeting IL-17. Nat Immunol 2012;13:1022–25.
119. Wuthrich M, Hung CY, Gern BH, et al. A TCR transgenic mouse reactive with multiple systemic dimorphic fungi. J Immunol 2011;187:1421–31.
120. Rivera A, Hohl TM, Collins N, et al. Dectin-1 diversifies Aspergillus fumigatus-specific T cell responses by inhibiting T helper type 1 CD4 T cell differentiation. J Exp Med, 2011;208:369–81.
121. Wuthrich M, Gern B, Hung CY, et al. Vaccine-induced protection against 3 systemic mycoses endemic to North America requires Th17 cells in mice. J Clin Invest, 2011;121:554–68.
122. Conti HR, Shen F, Nayyar N, et al. Th17 cells and IL-17 receptor signaling are essential for mucosal host defense against oral candidiasis. J Exp Med, 2009;206:299–311.
123. Zelante T, De Luca A, Bonifazi P, et al. IL-23 and the Th17 pathway promote inflammation and impair antifungal immune resistance. Eur J Immunol 2007;37:2695–2706.
124. Cua DJ & Tato CM. Innate IL-17-producing cells: the sentinels of the immune system. Nat Rev Immunol 2010;10:479–89.
125. Cypowyj S, Picard C, Marodi L, Casanova JL & Puel A. Immunity to infection in IL-17-deficient mice and humans. Eur J Immunol 2012;42:2246–54.
126. Gladiator A, Wangler N, Trautwein-Weidner K & LeibundGut-Landmann S. Cutting edge: IL-17-secreting innate lymphoid cells are essential for host defense against fungal infection. J Immunol, 2013;190:521–25.
127. Allen HL & Deepe GS Jr. B cells and CD4–CD8- T cells are key regulators of the severity of reactivation histoplasmosis. J Immunol 2006;177:1763–71.
128. Carvalho A, De Luca A, Bozza S, et al. TLR3 essentially promotes protective class I-restricted memory CD8(+) T-cell responses to Aspergillus fumigatus in hematopoietic transplanted patients. Blood 2012;119:967–77.
129. Lindell DM, Moore TA, McDonald RA, Toews GB & Huffnagle GB. Generation of antifungal effector CD8+ T cells in the absence of CD4+ T cells during Cryptococcus neoformans infection. J Immunol 2005;174:7920–7928.
130. Wuthrich M, Filutowicz HI, Warner T, Deepe GS Jr & Klein BS. Vaccine immunity to pathogenic fungi overcomes the requirement for CD4 help in exogenous antigen presentation to CD8+ T cells: implications for vaccine development in immune-deficient hosts. J Exp Med, 2003;197:1405–16.
131. Nanjappa SG, Heninger E, Wuthrich M, Gasper DJ & Klein BS. Tc17 cells mediate vaccine immunity against lethal fungal pneumonia in immune deficient hosts lacking CD4+ T cells. PLoS Pathog, 2012;8:e1002771.
132. Khanna N, Stuehler C, Conrad B, et al. Generation of a multipathogen-specific T-cell product for adoptive immunotherapy based on activation-dependent expression of CD154. Blood, 2011;118:1121–31.
133. Ramadan G, Davies B, Kurup VP & Keever-Taylor CA. Generation of cytotoxic T-cell responses directed to human leucocyte antigen Class I restricted epitopes from the Aspergillus f16 allergen. Clin Exp Immunol 2005;140:81–91.
134. Rivera J, Zaragoza O & Casadevall A. Antibody-mediated protection against Cryptococcus neoformans pulmonary infection is dependent on B cells. Infect Immun 2005;73:1141–50.
135. Lund FE, Hollifield M, Schuer K, Lines JL, Randall TD & Garvy BA. B cells are required for generation of protective effector and memory CD4 cells in response to Pneumocystis lung infection. J Immunol 2006;176:6147–54.
136. Casadevall A & Pirofski LA. Immunoglobulins in defense, pathogenesis, and therapy of fungal diseases. Cell Host Microbe 2012;11:447–56.
137. Torosantucci A, Bromuro C, Chiani P, et al. A novel glyco-conjugate vaccine against fungal pathogens. J Exp Med, 2005;202: 597–606.

Viral Diseases: HPV Infection of the Skin

138. Bernard HU, Burk R, Chen Z, van Doorslaer K, zur Hausen H, de Villiers EM. Classification of papillomaviruses (PVs) based on 189 PV types and proposal of taxonomic amendments. Virology. 2010;401(1):70–9.
139. Amador-Molina A, et al. Role of innate immunity against human papillomavirus (HPV) infections and effect of adjuvants in promoting specific immune response. Viruses. 2013;5(11):2624–42.
140. Cubie HA. Diseases associated with human papillomavirus infection. Virology. 2013;445(1–2):21–34.
141. Sapp M, Bienkowska-Haba M. Viral entry mechanisms: human papillomavirus and a long journey from extracellular matrix to the nucleus. FEBS J. 2009;276(24):7206.
142. Patel RK. Molecular anatomy project: human papillomavirus. http://maptest.rutgers.edu/drupal/?q=node/444, 2011. Spring2011_ Projects 2.
143. Davit B, Guan P, Franceschib S, Dillnera J, Clifford G. A systematic review of the prevalence of mucosal and cutaneous human papillomavirus types. Virology. 2013;445(1–2):224–31.

144. Kanodia S, Fahey LM, Kast WM. Mechanisms used by human papillomaviruses to escape the host immune response. Curr Cancer Drug Targets. 2007;7(1):79–89.
145. Frazer IH. Interaction of human papillomaviruses with the host immune system: a well evolved relationship. Virology. 2009;384(2):410–4.
146. Gildener-Leapman N, Ferris RL, Bauman JE. Promising systemic immunotherapies in head and neck squamous cell carcinoma. Oral Oncol. 2013;49(12):1089–96.
147. Sun S, et al. TLR7/9 antagonists as therapeutics for immune-mediated inflammatory disorders. Inflamm Allergy Drug Targets. 2007;6(4):223–35.
148. Li X, et al. Local hyperthermia could induce migrational maturation of Langerhans cells in condyloma acuminatum. J Dermatol Sci. 2009;54(2):121–3.
149. Zhu LL, et al. Local hyperthermia could induce antiviral activity by endogenous interferon-dependent pathway in condyloma acuminata. Antiviral Res. 2010;88(2):187–92.
150. Hausen HZ. Infections causing human cancer. Weinheim: Wiley-Blackwell; 2011.
151. Dochez C, et al. HPV vaccines to prevent cervical cancer and genital warts: an update. Vaccine. 2014;32(14):1595–601.
152. Deligeoroglou E, et al. HPV infection: immunological aspects and their utility in future therapy. Infect Dis Obstet Gynecol. 2013;2013:540850.
153. Eide ML, Debaque H. HPV detection methods and genotyping techniques in screening for cervical cancer. Ann Pathol. 2012;32(6):e15–23, 401–9.
154. Erickson BK, Landers EE, Huh WK. Update on vaccination clinical trials for HPV-related disease. Clin Ther. 2014;36(1):8–16.
155. Asiaf A, et al. Review of the current knowledge on the epidemiology, pathogenesis, and prevention of human papillomavirus infection. Eur J Cancer Prev. 2014;23(3):206–24.
156. Lam JU, et al. Condom use in prevention of Human Papillomavirus infections and cervical neoplasia: systematic review of longitudinal studies. J Med Screen. 2014;21(1):38–50.
157. Drake LA, et al. Guidelines of care for warts: human papillomavirus. Committee on guidelines of care. J Am Acad Dermatol. 1995;32(1):98–103.
158. Micali G, et al. Management of cutaneous warts: an evidence-based approach. Am J Clin Dermatol. 2004;5(5):311–7.
159. Kuykendall-Ivy TD, Johnson SM. Evidence-based review of management of nongenital cutaneous warts. Cutis. 2003;71(3):213–22.
160. Scheinfeld N. Update on the treatment of genital warts. Dermatol Online J. 2013;19(6):18559.
161. Sun Y, et al. Topical photodynamic therapy with 5-aminolaevulinic acid for condylomata acuminata on the distal urethra. Clin Exp Dermatol. 2012;37(3):302–3.
162. Baker DA, et al. Imiquimod 3.75% cream applied daily to treat anogenital warts: combined results from women in two randomized, placebo-controlled studies. Infect Dis Obstet Gynecol. 2011;2011:806105.
163. Kang HS, et al. Comparison of cure rates and durations of treatment with diphenylcyclopropenone immunotherapy for warts in children/adolescents and adults. Int J Dermatol. 2014;53: 1293–8.
164. Choi Y, et al. Topical immunotherapy with diphenylcyclopropenone is effective and preferred in the treatment of periungual warts. Ann Dermatol. 2013;25(4):434–9.
165. Buckley DA, et al. Recalcitrant viral warts treated by diphencyprone immunotherapy. Br J Dermatol. 1999;141(2):292–6.
166. Park HJ, et al. Change in cytokines in patients with warts after contact immunotherapy with squaric acid dibutylester. Clin Exp Dermatol. 2013;38(7):775–81.
167. Gamil H, et al. Intralesional immunotherapy of plantar warts: report of a new antigen combination. J Am Acad Dermatol. 2010;63(1):40–3.
168. Nofal A, Nofal E. Intralesional immunotherapy of common warts: successful treatment with mumps, measles and rubella vaccine. J Eur Acad Dermatol Venereol. 2010;24(10):1166–70.
169. Horn TD, et al. Intralesional immunotherapy of warts with mumps, Candida, and Trichophyton skin test antigens: a single-blinded, randomized, and controlled trial. Arch Dermatol. 2005;141(5):589–94.
170. Majid I, Imran S. Immunotherapy with intralesional Candida albicans antigen in resistant or recurrent warts: a study. Indian J Dermatol. 2013;58(5):360–5.
171. Kim KH, et al. Phase 1 clinical trial of intralesional injection of Candida antigen for the treatment of warts. Arch Dermatol. 2010;146(12):1431–3.
172. Gupta S, et al. Intralesional immunotherapy with killed Mycobacterium w vaccine for the treatment of ano-genital warts: an open label pilot study. J Eur Acad Dermatol Venereol. 2008;22(9):1089–93.
173. Zhao J, et al. Immunotherapy of HPV infection-caused genital warts using low dose cyclophosphamide. Expert Rev Clin Immunol. 2014;10(6):791–9.
174. Huo W, et al. Local hyperthermia at 44 degrees C for the treatment of plantar warts: a randomized, patient-blinded, placebo-controlled trial. J Infect Dis. 2010;201(8):1169–72.
175. Gao XH, et al. Non-ablative controlled local hyperthermia for common warts. Chin Med J (Engl). 2009;122(17):2061–3.
176. Varada S, et al. Management of cutaneous human papillomavirus infection in immunocompromised patients. Curr Probl Dermatol. 2014;45:197–215.
177. Eassa BI, Abou-Bakr AA, El-Khalawany MA. Intradermal injection of PPD as a novel approach of immunotherapy in anogenital warts in pregnant women. Dermatol Ther. 2011;24(1):137–43.
178. Huo W, et al. Clearance of genital warts in pregnant women by mild local hyperthermia: a pilot report. Dermatol Ther. 2014;27(2):109–12.
179. Huo W, et al. Clinical and immunologic results of local hyperthermia at 44 degrees C for extensive genital warts in patients with diabetes mellitus. Int J Hyperthermia. 2013;29(1):17–20.

Viral Diseases: HSV Infection

180. Fatahzadeh M, Schwartz RA. Human herpes simplex virus infections: epidemiology, pathogenesis, symptomatology, diagnosis, and management. J Am Acad Dermatol. 2007;57(5):737–63; quiz 764–6.
181. Akhtar J, Shukla D. Viral entry mechanisms: cellular and viral mediators of herpes simplex virus entry. FEBS J. 2009;276(24):7228–36.
182. Whitley RJ, Kimberlin DW, Roizman B. Herpes simplex viruses. Clin Infect Dis. 1998;26(3):541–53; quiz 554–5.
183. Whitley RJ, Roizman B. Herpes simplex virus infections. Lancet. 2001;357(9267):1513–8.
184. Corey L, Spear PG. Infections with herpes simplex viruses (1). N Engl J Med. 1986;314(11):686–91.
185. Prevention and control of herpesvirus diseases. Part 1. Clinical and laboratory diagnosis and chemotherapy. A WHO meeting. Bull World Health Organ. 1985;63(2):185–201 contd.
186. Looker KJ, Garnett GP, Schmid GP. An estimate of the global prevalence and incidence of herpes simplex virus type 2 infection. Bull World Health Organ. 2008;86(10):805–12, A.

187. Brady RC, Bernstein DI. Treatment of herpes simplex virus infections. Antiviral Res. 2004;61(2):73–81.
188. Usatine RP, Tinitigan R. Nongenital herpes simplex virus. Am Fam Physician. 2010;82(9):1075–82.
189. Miranda CA, et al. Genital infection with herpes simplex virus types 1 and 2 in women from natal, Brazil. ISRN Obstet Gynecol. 2014;2014:323657.
190. Simmons A. Clinical manifestations and treatment considerations of herpes simplex virus infection. J Infect Dis. 2002;186 Suppl 1:S71–7.
191. Lafferty WE, et al. Recurrences after oral and genital herpes simplex virus infection. Influence of site of infection and viral type. N Engl J Med. 1987;316(23):1444–9.
192. Fatahzadeh M, Schwartz RA. Human herpes simplex labialis. Clin Exp Dermatol. 2007;32(6):625–30.
193. Turner R, et al. Shedding and survival of herpes simplex virus from 'fever blisters'. Pediatrics. 1982;70(4):547–9.
194. Nerurkar LS, et al. Survival of herpes simplex virus in water specimens collected from hot tubs in spa facilities and on plastic surfaces. JAMA. 1983;250(22):3081–3.
195. Marsden HS, et al. Characterization of the 92,000-dalton glycoprotein induced by herpes simplex virus type 2. J Virol. 1984;50(2):547–54.
196. Ohana B, et al. Novel approach for specific detection of herpes simplex virus type 1 and 2 antibodies and immunoglobulin G and M antibodies. Clin Diagn Lab Immunol. 2000;7(6):904–8.
197. Beauman JG. Genital herpes: a review. Am Fam Physician. 2005;72(8):1527–34.
198. Fatahzadeh M, Schwartz RA. Human Herpes Simplex virus infections: epidemiology, pathogenesis, symptomatology, diagnosis, and management. Am Acad Dermatol. 2007;57(5):737–63.
199. Novelli VM, Atherton DJ, Marshall WC. Eczema herpeticum. Clinical and laboratory features. Clin Pediatr (Phila). 1988;27(5):231–3.
200. Kramer SC, et al. Kaposi's varicelliform eruption: a case report and review of the literature. Cutis. 2004;73(2):115–22.
201. Mooney MA, Janniger CK, Schwartz RA. Kaposi's varicelliform eruption. Cutis. 1994;53(5):243–5.
202. Liaw FY, et al. Eczema herpeticum: a medical emergency. Can Fam Physician. 2012;58(12):1358–61.
203. Luca NJ, Lara-Corrales I, Pope E. Eczema herpeticum in children: clinical features and factors predictive of hospitalization. J Pediatr. 2012;161(4):671–5.
204. Segura S, et al. Eczema herpeticum during treatment of atopic dermatitis with 1% pimecrolimus cream. Acta Derm Venereol. 2005;85(6):524–5.
205. Szinnai G, Schaad UB, Heininger U. Multiple herpetic whitlow lesions in a 4-year-old girl: case report and review of the literature. Eur J Pediatr. 2001;160(9):528–33.
206. Wu IB, Schwartz RA. Herpetic whitlow. Cutis. 2007;79(3):193–6.
207. Clark DC. Common acute hand infections. Am Fam Physician. 2003;68(11):2167–76.
208. Gill MJ, Arlette J, Buchan K. Herpes simplex virus infection of the hand. A profile of 79 cases. Am J Med. 1988;84(1):89–93.
209. Robayna MG, et al. Destructive herpetic whitlow in AIDS: report of three cases. Br J Dermatol. 1997;137(5):812–5.
210. Scott TF, et al. Some comments on herpetic infection in children with special emphasis on unusual clinical manifestations. J Pediatr. 1952;41(6):835–43.
211. Wilhelmus KR. The treatment of herpes simplex virus epithelial keratitis. Trans Am Ophthalmol Soc. 2000;98:505–32.
212. Tullo A. Pathogenesis and management of herpes simplex virus keratitis. Eye (Lond). 2003;17(8):919–22.
213. Liesegang TJ. Herpes simplex virus epidemiology and ocular importance. Cornea. 2001;20(1):1–13.
214. Kennedy DP, et al. Ocular herpes simplex virus type 1: is the cornea a reservoir for viral latency or a fast pit stop? Cornea. 2011;30(3):251–9.
215. White WB, Grant-Kels JM. Transmission of herpes simplex virus type 1 infection in rugby players. JAMA. 1984;252(4):533–5.
216. Kimberlin DW. Neonatal herpes simplex infection. Clin Microbiol Rev. 2004;17(1):1–13.
217. Lolis MS, et al. Drug-resistant herpes simplex virus in HIV infected patients. Acta Dermatovenerol Croat. 2008;16(4):204–8.
218. Bustamante CI, Wade JC. Herpes simplex virus infection in the immunocompromised cancer patient. J Clin Oncol. 1991;9(10):1903–15.
219. Sokumbi O, Wetter DA. Clinical features, diagnosis, and treatment of erythema multiforme: a review for the practicing dermatologist. Int J Dermatol. 2012;51(8):889–902.
220. Schwartz RA. Giant verrucous penile tumor. J Am Acad Dermatol. 2009;63(6):e107.
221. Nadal SR, et al. Hypertrophic herpes simplex simulating anal neoplasia in AIDS patients: report of five cases. Dis Colon Rectum. 2005;48(12):2289–93.
222. Carrasco DA, et al. Verrucous herpes of the scrotum in a human immunodeficiency virus-positive man: case report and review of the literature. J Eur Acad Dermatol Venereol. 2002;16(5):511–5.
223. Beasley KL, et al. Herpes simplex vegetans: atypical genital herpes infection in a patient with common variable immunodeficiency. J Am Acad Dermatol. 1997;37(5 Pt 2):860–3.
224. Lamoreux MR, Sternbach MR, Hsu WT. Erythema multiforme. Am Fam Physician. 2006;74(11):1883–8.
225. Stampien TM, Schwartz RA. Erythema multiforme. Am Fam Physician. 1992;46(4):1171–6.
226. Schofield JK, Tatnall FM, Leigh IM. Recurrent erythema multiforme: clinical features and treatment in a large series of patients. Br J Dermatol. 1993;128(5):542–5.
227. Levin J, Hofstra T. Recurrent erythema multiforme. JAMA. 2014;312(4):426–7.
228. Corey L. Synergistic copathogens – HIV-1 and HSV-2. N Engl J Med. 2007;356(8):854–6.
229. Stamm WE, et al. The association between genital ulcer disease and acquisition of HIV infection in homosexual men. JAMA. 1988;260(10):1429–33.
230. Freeman EE, et al. Herpes simplex virus 2 infection increases HIV acquisition in men and women: systematic review and meta-analysis of longitudinal studies. AIDS. 2006;20(1):73–83.
231. McClelland RS, et al. Association between cervical shedding of herpes simplex virus and HIV-1. AIDS. 2002;16(18):2425–30.
232. Nagot N, et al. Reduction of HIV-1 RNA levels with therapy to suppress herpes simplex virus. N Engl J Med. 2007;356(8):790–9.
233. Chew T, Taylor KE, Mossman KL. Innate and adaptive immune responses to herpes simplex virus. Viruses. 2009;1(3):979–1002.
234. Rapala-Larek A, Zaba R, Kowalczyk MJ, Pawlak-Szramka B, Schwartz RA. Herpes simplex virus infection as a possible modulator of autoimmune diseases facilitated by human endogenous retroviruses. Post Dermatol Alergol. 2011;28(4): 313–16.
235. Castelo-Soccio L, et al. Successful treatment of acyclovir-resistant herpes simplex virus with intralesional cidofovir. Arch Dermatol. 2010;146(2):124–6.
236. Andrei G, Snoeck R. Herpes simplex virus drug-resistance: new mutations and insights. Curr Opin Infect Dis. 2013;26(6):551–60.
237. Wald A, et al. Helicase-primase inhibitor pritelivir for HSV-2 infection. N Engl J Med. 2014;370(3):201–10.
238. Dropulic LK, Cohen JI. The challenge of developing a herpes simplex virus 2 vaccine. Expert Rev Vaccines. 2012;11(12):1429–40.
239. Belshe RB, et al. Efficacy results of a trial of a herpes simplex vaccine. N Engl J Med. 2012;366(1):34–43.

Viral Diseases: Molluscum Contagiosum Virus Infection of the Human Skin

240. Chen X, Anstey AV, Bugert JJ. Molluscum contagiosum virus infection. Lancet Infect Dis. 2013;13(10):877–88.
241. Schwartz JJ, Myskowski PL. Molluscum contagiosum in patients with human immunodeficiency virus infection: A review of twenty-seven patients. J Am Acad Dermatol. 1992;27(4):583–8.
242. Lynch PJ, Minkin W. Molluscum contagiosum of the adult: Probable venereal transmission. Arch Dermatol. 1968;98(2):141–3.
243. Dourmashkin R, Bernhard W. A study with the electron microscope of the skin tumour of molluscum contagiosum. J Ultrastruct Res. 1959;3(1):11–38.
244. Shelley WB, Burmeister V. Demonstration of a unique viral structure: the molluscum viral colony sac. Br J Dermatol. 1986;115(5):557–62.
245. Bugert JJ, Darai G. Stability of molluscum contagiosum virus DNA among 184 patient isolates: evidence for variability of sequences in the terminal inverted repeats. J Med Virol. 1991;33(3):211–7.
246. Senkevich TG, Bugert JJ, Sisler JR, Koonin EV, Darai G, Moss B. Genome sequence of a human tumorigenic poxvirus: prediction of specific host response-evasion genes. Science. 1996;273(5276):813–6.
247. Senkevich TG, Koonin EV, Bugert JJ, Darai G, Moss B. The genome of molluscum contagiosum virus: analysis and comparison with other poxviruses* 1. Virology. 1997;233(1):19–42.
248. Bugert JJ, Darai G. Recent advances in molluscum contagiosum virus research. Arch Virol Suppl. 1997;13:35–47.
249. Darai G, Reisner H, Scholz J, Schnitzler P, De Ruiz HL. Analysis of the genome of molluscum contagiosum virus by restriction endonuclease analysis and molecular cloning. J Med Virol. 1986;18(1):29–39.
250. Porter CD, Archard L. Characterisation by restriction mapping of three subtypes of molluscum contagiosum virus. J Med Virol. 1992;38(1):1–6.
251. Nakamura J, Muraki Y, Yamada M, Hatano Y, Nii S. Analysis of molluscum contagiosum virus genomes isolated in Japan. J Med Virol. 1995;46(4):339–48.
252. Scholz J, Rosen-Wolff A, Bugert J, Reisner H, White MI, Darai G, et al. Molecular epidemiology of molluscum contagiosum. J Infect Dis. 1988;158(4):898–900.
253. Scholz J, Rosen-Wolff A, Bugert J, Reisner H, White MI, Darai G, et al. Epidemiology of molluscum contagiosum using genetic analysis of the viral DNA. J Med Virol. 1989;27(2):87–90.
254. Thompson CH, De Zwart-Steffe RT, Biggs IM. Molecular epidemiology of Australian isolates of molluscum contagiosum. J Med Virol. 1990;32(1):1–9.
255. Saral Y, Kalkan A, Ozdarendeli A, Bulut Y, Doymaz MZ. Detection of Molluscum contagiosum Virus (MCV) subtype I as a single dominant virus subtype in Molluscum lesions from a Turkish population. Arch Med Res. 2006;37(3):388–91.
256. Konya J, Thompson CH. Molluscum contagiosum virus: antibody responses in persons with clinical lesions and seroepidemiology in a representative Australian population. J Infect Dis. 1999;179(3):701–4.
257. Sherwani S, Farleigh L, Agarwal N, Loveless S, Robertson N, Hadaschik E, et al. Seroprevalence of Molluscum contagiosum virus in German and UK populations. PLoS One [Research Support, Non-U.S. Gov't]. 2014;9(2):e88734.
258. Vreeswijk J, Leene W, Kalsbeek GL. Early interactions of the virus Molluscum contagiosum with its host cell virus-induced alterations in the basal and suprabasal layers of the epidermis. J Ultrastruct Res. 1976;54(1):37–52.
259. Viac J, Chardonnet Y. Immunocompetent cells and epithelial cell modifications in molluscum contagiosum. J Cutan Pathol. 1990;17(4):202–5.
260. Epstein WL, Fukuyama K. Maturation of molluscum contagiosum virus (MCV) in vivo: quantitative electron microscopic autoradiography. J Invest Dermatol. 1973;60(2):73–9.
261. Reed RJ, Parkinson RP. The histogenesis of molluscum contagiosum. Am J Surg Pathol. 1977;1(2):161–6.
262. Ku JK, Kwon HJ, Kim MY, Kang H, Song PI, Armstrong CA, et al. Expression of Toll-like receptors in verruca and molluscum contagiosum. J Korean Med Sci. 2008;23(2):307–14.
263. Minegishi Y, Saito M, Morio T, Watanabe K, Agematsu K, Tsuchiya S, et al. Human tyrosine kinase 2 deficiency reveals its requisite roles in multiple cytokine signals involved in innate and acquired immunity. Immunity. 2006;25(5):745–55.
264. Guitart J, Hurt MA. Pleomorphic T-cell infiltrate associated with molluscum contagiosum. Am J Dermatopathol. 1999;21(2):178–80.
265. Bhawan J, Dayal Y, Bhan AK. Langerhans cells in molluscum contagiosum, verruca vulgaris, plantar wart, and condyloma acuminatum. J Am Acad Dermatol. 1986;15(4):645–9.
266. Vermi W, Fisogni S, Scharer L, Kutzner H, Sozzani S, et al. Spontaneous regression of highly immunogenic molluscum contagiosum virus (MCV)-induced skin lesions is associated with plasmacytoid dendritic cells and IFN-DC infiltration. J Invest Dermatol. 2011;131:426–34.
267. Swiecki M, Colonna M. Disparate antiviral responses in Molluscum contagiosum virus-induced skin lesions. J Invest Dermatol. 2011;131(2):288–90.
268. Moss B, Shisler JL, Xiang Y, Senkevich TG. Immune-defense molecules of molluscum contagiosum virus, a human poxvirus. Trends Microbiol. 2000;8(10):473–7.
269. Xiang Y, Moss B. IL-18 binding and inhibition of interferon γ induction by human poxvirus-encoded proteins. Proc Natl Acad Sci. 1999;96(20):11537–42.
270. Xiang Y, Moss B. Correspondence of the functional epitopes of poxvirus and human interleukin-18-binding proteins. J Virol. 2001;75(20):9947–54.
271. Shisler JL, Senkevich TG, Berry MJ, Moss B. Ultraviolet-induced cell death blocked by a selenoprotein from a human dermatotropic poxvirus. Science. 1998;279(5347):102–5.
272. Bugert JJ, Lohmuller C, Damon I, Moss B, Darai G. Chemokine homolog of molluscum contagiosum virus: sequence conservation and expression. Virology. 1998;242(1):51–9.
273. Garvey TL, Bertin J, Siegel RM, Wang G, Lenardo MJ, Cohen JI. Binding of FADD and caspase-8 to molluscum contagiosum virus MC159 v-FLIP is not sufficient for its antiapoptotic function. J Virol. 2002;76(2):697–706.
274. Garvey TL, Bertin J, Siegel RM, Lenardo MJ, Cohen JI. The death effector domains (DEDs) of the molluscum contagiosum virus MC159 v-FLIP protein are not functionally interchangeable with each other or with the DEDs of caspase-8. Virology. 2002;300(2):217–25.
275. Thurau M, Everett H, Tapernoux M, Tschopp J, Thome M. The TRAF3-binding site of human molluscipox virus FLIP molecule MC159 is critical for its capacity to inhibit Fas-induced apoptosis. Cell Death Differ. 2006;13(9):1577–85.
276. Hawley TG. The natural history of molluscum contagiosum in Fijian children. J Hyg (Lond). 1970;68(04):631–2.
277. Gottlieb SL, Myskowski PL. Molluscum contagiosum. Int J Dermatol. 1994;33(7):453–61.
278. Simonart T, De Maertelaer V. Curettage treatment for molluscum contagiosum: a follow-up survey study. Br J Dermatol. 2008;159(5):1144–7.
279. All-Mutairi N, Al-Doukhi A, A-Farag S, Al-Haddad A. Comparative study on the efficacy, safety, and acceptability of

imiquimod 5% cream versus cryotherapy for molluscum contagiosum in children. Pediatr Dermatol. 2010;27(4):388–94.
280. Binder B, Weger W, Komericki P, Kopera D. Treatment of molluscum contagiosum with a pulsed dye laser: pilot study with 19 children. J Dtsch Dermatol Ges. 2008;6(2):121–5.
281. Weller R, O'Callaghan CJ, MacSween RM, White MI. Scarring in molluscum contagiosum: comparison of physical expression and phenol ablation. BMJ. 1999;319(7224):1540.
282. Coloe J, Morrell DS. Cantharidin use among pediatric dermatologists in the treatment of molluscum contagiosum. Pediatr Dermatol. 2009;26(4):405–8.
283. Syed TA, Lundin S, Ahmad M. Topical 0.3% and 0.5% podophyllotoxin cream for self-treatment of molluscum contagiosum in males. Dermatology. 1994;189(1):65–8.
284. Leslie KS, Dootson G, Sterling JC. Topical salicylic acid gel as a treatment for molluscum contagiosum in children. J Dermatolog Treat. 2005;16(5–6):336–40.
285. Saryazdi S. The comparative efficacy of benzoyl peroxide 10% cream and tretinoin 0.05% cream in the treatment of molluscum contagiosum. Abstract 10th World Congress on pediatric dermatology. Pediatr Dermatol. 2004;21(3).
286. Romiti R, Ribeiro AP, Grinblat BM, Rivitti EA, Romiti N. Treatment of molluscum contagiosum with potassium hydroxide: a clinical approach in 35 children. Pediatr Dermatol. 1999;16(3):228–31.
287. Romiti R, Ribeiro AP, Romiti N. Evaluation of the effectiveness of 5% potassium hydroxide for the treatment of molluscum contagiosum. Pediatr Dermatol. 2000;17(6):495.
288. Dohil M, Prendiville JS. Treatment of Molluseum contagiosum with oral cimetidine: clinical experience in 13 patients. Pediatr Dermatol. 1996;13(4):310–2.
289. Enns LL, Evans MS. Intralesional immunotherapy with Candida antigen for the treatment of Molluscum contagiosum in children. Pediatr Dermatol. 2011;28(3):254–8.
290. Na CH, Kim DJ, Kim MS, Kim JK, Shin BS. Successful treatment of molluscum contagiosum with intralesional immunotherapy by measles, mumps, and rubella vaccine: a report of two cases. Dermatol Ther. 2014;22.
291. van der Wouden JC, van der Sande R, van Suijlekom-Smit LW, Berger M, Butler CC, Koning S. Interventions for cutaneous molluscum contagiosum. Cochrane Database Syst Rev. 2009;4:CD004767.
292. Hanna D, Hatami A, Powell J, Marcoux D, Maari C, Savard P, et al. A prospective randomized trial comparing the efficacy and adverse effects of four recognized treatments of molluscum contagiosum in children. Pediatr Dermatol. 2006;23(6):574–9.
293. Monteagudo B, Cabanillas M, Acevedo A, de las Heras C, Suárez-Amor O, Ramírez-Santos A, et al. Curettage for the treatment of molluscum contagiosum: a descriptive study. Actas Dermosifiliogr. 2011;102(2):157–8.
294. Silverberg NB, Sidbury R, Mancini AJ. Childhood molluscum contagiosum: experience with cantharidin therapy in 300 patients. J Am Acad Dermatol. 2000;43(3):503–7.
295. Cathcart S, Coloe J, Morrell DS. Parental satisfaction, efficacy, and adverse events in 54 patients treated with cantharidin for molluscum contagiosum infection. Clin Pediatr (Phila). 2009;48(2):161–5.
296. Kose O, Ozmen I, Arca E. An open, comparative study of 10% potassium hydroxide solution versus salicylic and lactic acid combination in the treatment of molluscum contagiosum in children. J Dermatolog Treat. 2012;24(4):300-4.
297. Bayerl C, Feller G, Goerdt S. Experience in treating molluscum contagiosum in children with imiquimod 5% cream. Br J Dermatol. 2003;149:25–8.
298. Aldara (imiquimod) cream for topical use. DailyMed. http://dailymed.nlm.nih.gov/dailymed/lookup.cfm?setid=7fccca4e-8f-42b8-9555-8f78a5804ed3. Accessed 1 Apr 2014.
299. Gur I. The epidemiology of Molluscum contagiosum in HIV-seropositive patients: a unique entity or insignificant finding? Int J STD AIDS. 2008;19(8):503–6.
300. Koopman RJJ, Merrienboer FCJ, Vredden SGS, Dolmans WMV. Molluscum contagiosum: a marker for advanced HIV infection. Br J Dermatol. 1992;126(5):528–9.
301. Jung AC, Paauw DS. Diagnosing HIV-related disease: using the CD4 count as a guide. J Gen Intern Med. 1998;13(2):131–6.
302. Valentine CL, Diven D. Treatment modalities for molluscum contagiosum. Dermatol Ther. 2000;13(3):285–9.
303. Mc Cuaig C, Silverberg N, Santer M. Commentaries on 'interventions for cutaneous molluscum contagiosum'. Evid Based Child Health. 2011;6(5):1602–5.

Mosquito Bite Allergy

304. Garcia LS. Diagnostic medical parasitology. 5th ed. Washington D.C.: ASM Press; 2007. p. 682.
305. Brown AWA. The attraction of mosquitoes to hosts. JAMA. 1966;196:249–52.
306. Reunala T, Brummer-Korvenkontio H, Palosuo T. Are we really allergic to mosquito bites? Ann Med. 1994;26:301–6.
307. Peng Z, Simons FER. Mosquito allergy: immune mechanisms and recombinant salivary allergens. Int Arch Allergy Immunol. 2004;133:198–209.
308. James AA, Rossignol PA. Mosquito salivary glands: parasitological and molecular aspects. Parasitol Today. 1991;7:267–71.
309. Ribeiro JM. Vector salivation and parasite transmission. Mem Inst Oswaldo Cruz. 1987;82 Suppl 3:1–3.
310. Peng Z, Yang M, Simons FE. Immunologic mechanisms in mosquito allergy: correlation of skin reactions with specific IgE and IgG antibodies and lymphocyte proliferation response to mosquito antigens. Ann Allergy Asthma Immunol. 1996;77:238–44.
311. Oka K. Correlation of Aedes albopictus bite reaction with IgE antibody assay and lymphocyte transformation test to mosquito salivary antigens. J Dermatol. 1989;16:341–7.
312. Peng Z, Simons FE. A prospective study of naturally acquired sensitization and subsequent desensitization to mosquito bites and concurrent antibody responses. J Allergy Clin Immunol. 1998;101:284–6.
313. Mellanby K. Man's reaction to mosquito bites. Nature. 1946;158:554.
314. Oka K, Ohtaki N. Clinical observations of mosquito bite reactions in man: a survey of the relationship between age and bite reaction. J Dermatol. 1989;16:212–9.
315. Peng Z, Ho MK, Li C, et al. Evidence for natural desensitization to mosquito salivary allergens: mosquito saliva specific IgE and IgG levels in children. Ann Allergy Asthma Immunol. 2004;93:553–6.
316. Simons FE, Peng Z. Skeeter syndrome. J Allergy Clin Immunol. 1999;104:705–7.
317. Wongkamchai S, Techasintana P, Wisuthsarewong W, et al. Analysis of IgE-binding allergens in Culex quinquefasciatus saliva protein in mosquito bite allergic patients. Ann Allergy Asthma Immunol. 2007;98:200–1.
318. Robert AS, Christopher JS. Arthropod bites and stings. In: Fitzpatrick's dermatology in general medicine. 8th ed. New York: McGraw-Hill; 2012. p. 2599.
319. Asada H. Hypersensitivity to mosquito bites: a unique pathogenic mechanism linking Epstein-Barr virus infection, allergy and oncogenesis. J Dermatol Sci. 2007;45:153–60.
320. Pacheco SE, Gottschalk SM, Gresik MV, et al. Chronic active Epstein-Barr virus infection of natural killer cells presenting as severe skin reaction to mosquito bites. J Allergy Clin Immunol. 2005;116:470–2.

321. Tokura Y, Tamura Y, Takigawa M, et al. Severe hypersensitivity to mosquito bites associated with natural killer cell lymphocytosis. Arch Dermatol. 1990;126:362–8.
322. Chiu TM, Lin YM, Wang SC et al. Hypersensitivity to mosquito bites as the primary clinical manifestation of an EpsteineBarr virus infection. J Microbiol Immunol Infect. 2014; pii: S1684-1182(14)00011–5. doi: 10.1016/j.jmii.2014.01.008. [Epub ahead of print].
323. Brown A, Griffitts THD, Erwin S, et al. Arthus' phenomenon from mosquito bites: report of a case with experimental studies. South Med J. 1938;31:590–6.
324. Hidano A, Kawakami M, Yago A. Hypersensitivity to mosquito bite and malignant histiocytosis. Jpn J Exp Med. 1982;52:303–6.
325. Ishihara S, Ohshima K, Tokura Y, et al. Hypersensitivity to mosquito bites conceals clonal lymphoproliferation of Epstein-Barr viral DNA-positive natural killer cells. Jpn J Cancer Res. 1997;88:82–7.
326. Ishihara S, Okada S, Wakiguchi H, et al. Chronic active Epstein-Barr virus infection in children in Japan. Acta Paediatr. 1995;84:1271–5.
327. Mizuki M, Ueda S, Tagawa S, et al. Natural killer cell-derived large granular lymphocyte lymphoma of lung developed in a patient with hypersensitivity to mosquito bites and reactivated Epstein-Barr virus infection. Am J Hematol. 1998;59:309–15.
328. Ishihara S, Yabuta R, Tokura Y, et al. Hypersensitivity to mosquito bites is not an allergic disease, but an Epstein-Barr virus-associated lymphoproliferative disease. Int J Hematol. 2000;72:223–8.
329. Davis M, Perniciaro C, Dahl PR, et al. Exaggerated arthropod-bite lesions in patients with chronic lymphocytic leukemia: a clinical, histopatholoic, and immunopathologic study of eight patients. J Am Acad Dermatol. 1998;39:27–35.
330. Tsai WC, Luo SF, Liaw SJ, et al. Mosquito bite allergies terminating as hemophagocytic histiocytosis: report of a case. Taiwan Yi Xue Hui Za Zhi. 1989;88:639–42.
331. Fan PC, Chang HN. Hypersensitivity to mosquito bite: a case report. Gaoxiong Yi Xue Ke Xue Za Zhi. 1995;11:420–4.
332. Ruiz-Maldonado R, Parrilla FM, Orozco-Covarrubias ML. Edematous, scarring vasculitic panniculitis: a new multisystemic disease with malignant potential. J Am Acad Dermatol. 1995;32:37–44.
333. Tokura Y, Ishihara S, Tagawa S, et al. Hypersensitivity to mosquito bites as the primary clinical manifestation of a juvenile type of Epstein-Barr virus-associated natural killer cell leukemia/lymphoma. J Am Acad Dermatol. 2001;45:569–78.
334. Ohshima S, Ishii M, Asada H, et al. A possible mechanism of NK-cell lineage granular lymphocyte proliferative disorder (NK-GLDP) in a patient with chronic active Epstein-Barr virus infection (CAEBV) and severe hypersensitivity to mosquito bites (SHMB). Intern Med. 2002;41:651–6.
335. Schleupner CJ, Overall JC. Infectious mononucleosis and Epstein-Barr virus. Postgrad Med. 1979;65:83–105.
336. Kanai K, Kuwabara S, Mori M, et al. Leukocytoclastic-vasculitic neuropathy associated with chronic Epstein-Barr virus infection. Muscle Nerve. 2003;27:113e6.
337. Murakami K, Ohsawa M, Hu S, et al. Large-vessel arteritis associated with chronic active Epstein-Barr virus infection. Arthritis Rheum. 1998;41:369e73.
338. Asada H, Miyagawa S, Sumikawa Y, et al. CD4+ T-lymphocyte-induced Epstein-Barr virus reactivation in a patient with severe hypersensitivity to mosquito bites and Epstein-Barr virus-infected NK cell lymphocytosis. Arch Dermatol. 2003; 139:1601–7.
339. Kanno H, Onodera H, Endo M, et al. Vascular lesion in a patient of chronic active Epstein-Barr virus infection with hypersensitivity to mosquito bites: Vasculitis induced by mosquito bite with the infiltration of nonneoplastic Epstein-Barr virus-positive cells and subsequent development of natural killer/T-cell lymphoma with angiodestruction. Hum Pathol. 2005;36:212e8.
340. Penneys NS, Nayar JK, Berstein H, et al. Chronic pruritic eruption in patients with acquired immunodeficiency syndrome associated with increased antibody titers to mosquito salivary gland antigens. J Am Acad Dermatol. 1989;21:421–5.
341. Resneck JS, BeeK MV, Furmanski L, et al. Etiology of pruritic papular eruption with HIV infected in Uganda. JAMA. 2004;292:2614–21.
342. Fradin MS. Mosquitoes and mosquito repellents: a clinician's guide. Ann Intern Med. 1998;128:931–40.

Immunologically-Mediated Photodermatoses

343. Gruber-Wackermagel A, Byrne SN, Wolf P. Polymorphous light eruption: clinical aspects and pathogenesis. Dermatol Clin. 2014;32(3):315–34.
344. Nakamura M, Henderson M, Jacobsen G, et al. Comparison of photodermatoses in African-Americans and Caucasians: a follow-up study. Photodermatol Photoimmunol Photomed. 2014;30(5):231–8.
345. Chiam LY, Chong WS. Pinpoint popular polymorphous light eruption in Asian skin: a variant in darker-skinned individuals. Photodermatol Photoimmunol Photomed. 2009;25(2):71–4.
346. Straligos AJ, Antoniou C, Katsambas AD. Polymorphous light eruption. J Eur Acad Dermatol Venereol. 2002;16(3):193–206.
347. Gonzalez-Amaro R, Baranda L, Salazar-Gonzalez JF, et al. Immune sensitization against epidermal antigens in polymorphous light eruption. J Am Acad Dermatol. 1991;24(1):70–3.
348. McFadden JP, Norris PG, Cerio R, et al. Immunoreactivity in experimentally induced polymorphic light eruption. Acta Derm Venereol. 1994;74:283–5.
349. Norris PG, Morris J, McGibbon DM, et al. Polymorphic light eruption: an immunopathological study of evolving lesions. Br J Dermatol. 1989;120:173–80.
350. Kolgen W, Both H, Van Weelden H, et al. Epidermal Langerhans cell depletion after artificial ultraviolet B irradiation of human skin in vivo: apoptosis versus migration. J Invest Dermatol. 2002;118(5):812–7.
351. Kolgen W, Van Weelden H, Den Hengst S, et al. CD11b+cells and ultraviolet B-resistant CD1a+cells in skin of patients with polymorphous light eruption. J Invest Dermatol. 1999;113(1):4–10.
352. Hart PH, Grimbaldeston MA, Jaksic A, et al. Ultraviolet B-induced suppression of immune response in interleukin 4–/– mice: relationship to dermal mast cells. J Invest Dermatol. 2000;114(3):508–13.
353. Schornagel IJ, Sigurdsson V, Nijhuis EH, et al. Decreased neutrophil skin infiltration after UVB exposure in patients with polymorphous light eruption. J Invest Dermatol. 2004;123(1):202–6.
354. Byrne SN, Limon-Flores AY, Ullrich SE. Mast cell migration from the skin to the draining lymph nodes upon ultraviolet irradiation represents a key step in the induction of immune suppression. J Immunol. 2008;180(7):4648–55.
355. Lu LF, Lind EF, Gondek DC, et al. Mast cells are essential intermediaries in regulatory T-cell tolerance. Nature. 2006;442(7106):997–1002.
356. Roncarolo MG, Gregori S, Bacchetta R, et al. Tr1 cells and the counter-regulation of immunity: natural mechanisms and therapeutic applications. Curr Top Microbiol Immunol. 2014;380:39–68.
357. Wolf P, Gruber-Wackernagel A, Legat FJ, et al. Successful phototherapy of polymorphic light eruption patients is associated with a recruitment of mast cells in to the skin. J Invest Dermatol. 2010;130:50.

358. Gambichler T, Terras S, Kampilafkos P, et al. T regulatory cells and related immunoregulatory factors in polymorphic light eruption following ultraviolet A1 challenge. Br J Dermatol. 2013;169(6):1288–94.
359. Hiramoto K, Tanaka H, Yanagihara N, et al. Effect of 17beta-estradiol on immunosuppression induced by ultraviolet B irradiation. Arch Dermatol Res. 2004;295(8–9):307–11.
360. May E, Asadullah K, Zugel U. Immunoregulation through 1,25dihyroxyvitamin D3 and its analogs. Curr Drug Targets Inflamm Allergy. 2004;3(4):377–93.
361. Arnson Y, Amital H, Shoenfeld Y. Vitamin D and autoimmunity: new aetiological and therapeutic considerations. Ann Rheum Dis. 2007;66(9):1137–42.
362. Gruber-Wackernagel A, Obermayer-Pietsch B, Byrne SN, et al. Patient with polymorphic light eruption have decreased serum levels of 25-hydroxyvitamin-D3 that increase upon 311 nm UVB photohardening. Photochem Photobiol Sci. 2012;11(12):1831–6.
363. Diffey BI, Farr PM. The erythemal response to ultraviolet radiation in subjects with polymorphic light eruption. Br J Dermatol. 1986;114:103–8.
364. Bissonnette R, Nigen S, Bolduc C. Influence of the quantity of sunscreen applied on the ability to protect against ultraviolet-induced polymorphous light eruption. Photodermatol Photoimmunol Photomed. 2012;28(5):240–3.
365. Millard TP. Treatment of polymorphic light eruption. J Dermatol Treat. 2000;11:195–9.
366. Richards HL, Ling TC, Evangelou G, et al. Evidence of high levels of anxiety and depression in polymorphic light eruption and their association with clinical and demographic variants. Br J Dermatol. 2008;159(2):439–44.
367. Janssens AS, Pavel S, Out-Luiting JJ, et al. Normalized ultraviolet (UV) induction of Langerhans cell depletion and neutrophil infiltrates after artificial UVB hardening of patients with polymorphic light eruption. Br J Dermatol. 2005;152(6):1268–74.
368. Norris PG, Hawk JM. Successful treatment of severe polymorphous eruption with azathioprine. Arch Dermatol. 1989;125:1377–9.
369. Molin L, Volden G. Treatment of polymorphous light eruption with PUVA and prednisolone. Photodermatology. 1987;4:107–8.
370. Wiseman MC, Orr PH, Macdonald SM, et al. Actinic prurigo: clinical features and HLA associations in a Canadian Inuit population. J Am Acad Dermatol. 2001;44(6):952–6.
371. Duran de Rueda MM, Bernal JE, Ordonez CP. Actinic prurigo at sea level in Colombia. Int J Dermatol. 1989;28(4):228–9.
372. Ross G, Foley P, Baker C. Actinic prurigo. Photoderm Photoimmuno Photomed. 2008;24:272–5.
373. Hojyo-Tomoka M, Vega-Memije M, Cortes-Franco R, et al. Diagnosis and treatment of actinic prurigo. Dermatol Ther. 2003;16:40–4.
374. Valbuena MC, Muvdi S, Lim HW. Actinic prurigo. Dermatol Clin. 2014;32(3):335–44.
375. Grabczynska S, McGregor J, Kondeatis E, et al. Actinic prurigo and polymorphic light eruption: common pathogenesis and the importance of HLA-DR4/DRB1_0407. Br J Dermatol. 1999;140:232–6.
376. Crouch R, Foley P, Baker C. Actinic prurigo: a retrospective analysis of 21 cases referred to an Australian photobiology clinic. Aust J Dermatol. 2002;43:128–32.
377. Hojyo-Tomoka M, Vega-Memije M, Granados J, et al. Actinic prurigo: an update. Int J Dermatol. 1995;34:380–4.
378. Gomez A, Umana A, Trescalacios A. Immune responses to isolated human skin antigens in actinic prurigo. Med Sci Monit. 2006;12:106–13.
379. Gonzalez-Rodriguiz G, Ocadiz-Delgado R. T and B clonal populations in actinic prurigo, a photodermatosis. Gac Med Mex. 2001;137(1):15–20.
380. Torres-Alvarez B, Baranda L, Fuentes C, et al. An immunohistochemical study of UV-induced skin lesions in actinic prurigo. Resistance of Langerhans cells to UV light. Eur J Dermatol. 1998;8(1):24–8.
381. Arrese JE, Dominquez-Soto L, Hojyo-Tomoka MT, et al. Effectors of inflammation in actinic prurigo. J Am Acad Dermatol. 2001;44(6):958–61.
382. Ker KJ, Chong WS, Theng CS. Clinical characteristics of adult-onset actinic prurigo in Asians: a case series. Indian J Dermatol Venereol Leprol. 2013;39:783–8.
383. Collins P, Ferguson J. Narrow-band UVB (TLO1) phototherapy: an effective preventative treatment for the photodermatoses. Br J Dermatol. 1995;132:956–63.
384. McCoombes JA, Hirst LW, Green WR. Use of topical cyclosporin for conjunctival manifestations of actinic prurigo. Am J Opthalmol. 2000;130(6):830–1.
385. Estrada GI, Garibay-Escobar A, Nunez-Vazquez A, et al. Evidence that thalidomide modifies the immune response of patients suffering from actinic prurigo. Int J Dermatol. 2004;43:893–7.
386. Gupta G, Man I, Kemmett D. Hydroa vacciniforme: a clinical and follow-up study of 17 cases. J Am Acad Dermatol. 2000;42:208–13.
387. Wong SN, Tan SH, Khoo SW. Late-onset hydroa vacciniforme: two case reports. Br J Dermatol. 2001;144(4):874–7.
388. Wang T, Wang L, Xiong L, et al. A rare case of hydroa vacciniforme-like cutaneous T-cell lymphoma presenting mimicking herpes simples in an adult. Am J Dermatopathol. 2013;35(5):617–8.
389. Annamalai R. Hydroa vacciniforme in three alternate siblings. Arch Dermatol. 1971;103:224–5.
390. Huggins RH, Leithauser LA, Eide MJ, et al. Quality of life assessment and disease experience of patient members of a web-based hydroa vacciniforme support group. Photodermatol Photoimmunol Photomed. 2009;25(4):209–15.
391. Kim WS, Yeo UC, Chun HS, et al. A case of hydroa vacciniforme with unusual ear mutilation. Clin Exp Dermatol. 1998;23:70–2.
392. Hann SK, Im S, Park YK, et al. Hydroa vacciniforme with unusually severe scar formation: diagnosis by repetitive UVA phototesting. J Am Acad Dermatol. 1991;25:401–3.
393. Iwatsuki K, Satoh M, Yamamoto T, et al. Pathogenic link between hydroa vacciniforme and Epstein-Barr virus-associated hematologic disorders. Arch Dermatol. 2006;142(5):587–95.
394. Wang M, Wang S, Yang QP, et al. Hydroa vacciniforme-like lymphoma of an adult: a case report with review of the literature. Diagn Pathol. 2013,8.72.
395. Goldgeier MH, Nordlund JJ, Lucky AW. Reproduction of hydroa vacciniforme with UVA. J Am Acad Dermatol. 1983;9:279–80.
396. IwatsukiK XZ, Takata M, et al. The association of latent Epstein-Barr virus infection with hydroa vacciniforme. Br J Dermatol. 1999;140:715–21.
397. Sonnex TS, Hawk JM. Hydroa vacciniforme: a review of ten cases. Br J Dermatol. 1988;118:101–8.
398. Chantorn R, Lim HW, Shwayder TA. Photosensitivity disorders in children Part 1. J Am Acad Dermatol. 2012;67:1093e1–18.
399. Blackwell V, McGregor JM, Hawk JM. Hydroa vacciniforme presenting in an adult successfully treated with cyclosporin A. Clin Exp Dermatol. 1998;23:73–6.
400. Rhodes LE, White SI. Dietary fish oil as a photoprotective agent in hydroa vacciniforme. Br J Dermatol. 1998;138(1):173.
401. Chong WS, Khoo SW. Solar urticaria in Singapore: an uncommon photodermatoses seen in a tertiary dermatology center over a 10-year period. Photodermatol Photoimmunol Photomed. 2004;20:101–4.
402. Stratigos AJ, Antoniou C, Papathanakou E, et al. Spectrum of idiopathic photodermatoses in a Mediterranean country. Int J Dermatol. 2004;42:449–54.

403. Harris A, Burge SM, George SA. Solar urticaria in an infant. Br J Dermatol. 1997;136:105–7.
404. Williams-Arya P, Hogan MB, Wilson NW. Solar urticaria in a 6-year-old child. Ann Allergy Asthma Immunol. 1996;76(2):141–3.
405. Gardeazabal J, Gonzalez-Perez R, Bilbao I, et al. Solar urticaria enhanced through clothing. Photodermatol Photoimmunol Photomed. 1998;14:164–6.
406. Rose RF, Bhushan M, King CM. Solar angioedema: an uncommonly recognized condition? Photodermatol Photoimmunol Photomed. 2005;21:226–88.
407. Roelandts R, Ryckaert S. Solar urticaria: the annoying photodermatosis. Int J Dermatol. 1999;38:411–8.
408. Duschet P, Leyen P, Schwarz T, et al. Solar urticaria—effective treatment by plasmapheresis. Clin Exp Dermatol. 1987;12:185–8.
409. Sams Jr WM. Solar urticaria: studies of the active serum factor. J Allergy. 1970;45:295–301.
410. Rajka E. Passive transfer in light urticaria. J Allergy Clin Immunol. 1942;13:327–45.
411. Beal PL. Studies in solar urticaria. J Invest Dermatol. 1948;11:415–33.
412. Leenutaphong V, Holze E, Plewig G. Pathogenesis and classification of solar urticaria: a new concept. J Am Acad Dermatol. 1989;21(2):237–40.
413. Botto N, Warshaw E. Solar urticaria. J Am Acad Dermatol. 2008;59:909–20.
414. Murphy GM, Hawk JL. Broadening of action spectrum in a patient with solar urticaria. Clin Exp Dermatol. 1987;12:455–6.
415. Soter NA, Wasserman SI, Pathak MA, et al. Solar urticaria: release of mast cell mediators into the circulation after experimental challenge. J Invest Dermatol. 1979;72:282.
416. Plewig G, Wolff HH, Holzle E. Solar urticaria: immunoelectron microscopic study of leucocytoclastic vasculitis. Arch Dermatol Res. 1980;267:209.
417. Bernhard JD. Treatment of solar urticaria with terfenadine. J Am Acad Dermatol. 1993;28:668.
418. Roelandts R. Diagnosis and treatment of solar urticaria. Dermatol Ther. 2003;16:52–6.
419. Roelandts R. Pre-PUVA UVA desensitization for solar urticaria. Photodermatology. 1985;2:174–6.
420. Edström DW, Ros AM. Cyclosporin a therapy for severe solar urticaria. Photodermatol Photoimmunol Photomed. 1997;13:61–3.
421. Adamski H, Bedane C, Bonnevalle A. Solar urticaria treated with intravenous immunoglobulins. J Am Acad Dermatol. 2011;65(2):336–40.
422. Miyauchi H, Horio T. Detection of action, inhibition and augmentation spectra in solar urticaria. Dermatology. 1995;33:597–602.
423. Güzelbey O, Ardelean E, Magerl M, et al. Successful treatment of solar urticaria with anti-immunoglobulin E therapy. Allergy. 2008;63:1563–5.
424. Haylett AK, Nie Z, Brownrigg M, et al. Systemic photoprotection in solar urticaria with α-melanocyte stimulating hormone analogue [Nle4-D-Phe7]-α-MSH. Br J Dermatol. 2011;164(2):407–14.
425. Collins P, Ahamat R, Green C, et al. Plasma exchange therapy for solar urticaria. Br J Dermatol. 1996;134:1093–7.
426. Zak-Prelich M, Schwartz RA. Actinic reticuloid. Int J Dermatol. 1999;38:335–42.
427. Creamer D, McGregor JM, Hawk JL. Chronic actinic dermatitis occurring in young patients with atopic dermatitis. Br J Dermatol. 1998;139:1112–3.
428. Lim HW, Morison WL, Kamide R, et al. Chronic actinic dermatitis: an analysis of 51 patients evaluated in the United States and Japan. Arch Dermatol. 1994;130:1284–9.
429. Pappert A, Grossman M, DeLeo V. Photosensitivity as the presenting illness in four patients with human immunodeficiency viral infection. Arch Dermatol. 1994;130:618–23.
430. Chu AC, Robinson D, Hawk JL, et al. Immunologic differentiation of the Sezary syndrome due to cutaneous T-cell lymphoma and chronic actinic dermatitis. J Invest Dermatol. 1986;86(2):134.
431. Wolverton JE, Soter NA, Cohen DE. The natural history of chronic actinic dermatitis: an analysis at a single institution in the United States. Dermatitis. 2014;25(1):27–31.
432. Menage HP, Sattar NK, Haskard DO, et al. A study of the kinetics and pattern of E-selectin, VCAM-1, ICAM-1 expression in chronic actinic dermatitis. Br J Dermatol. 1996;134(2):262–8.
433. Willis I, Kligman AM. The mechanism of the persistent light reactor. J Invest Dermatol. 1968;51:385–94.
434. Baadsgaard O. In vivo ultraviolet irradiation of human skin results in profound perturbation of the immune system. Relevance to ultraviolet-induced skin cancer. Arch Dermatol. 1991;127:99–109.
435. Ross JS, Menage HP, Hawk JLM, et al. Sesquiterpene lactone contact sensitivity: clinical patterns of Compositae dermatitis and relationship to chronic actinic dermatitis. Contact Dermatitis. 1993;29:84–7.
436. Bilsland D, Ferguson J. Contact allergy to sunscreen chemicals in photosensitivity dermatitis/actinic reticuloid syndrome (PD/AR) and polymorphic light eruption (PLE). Contact Dermatitis. 1993;29:70–3.
437. Bakels V, van Oostveen JW, Preesman AH, et al. Differentiation between actinic reticuloid and cutaneous T cell lymphoma by T cell receptor gamma gene rearrangement analysis and immunophenotyping. J Clin Pathol. 1998;51:154–8.
438. Suga Y, Hashimoto Y, Matsuba S, et al. Topical tacrolimus for chronic actinic dermatitis. J Am Acad Dermatol. 2002;2002(46):321–3.
439. Murphy GM, Maurice PD, Norris PG, et al. Azathioprine treatment in chronic actinic dermatitis: a double-blind controlled trial with monitoring of exposure to ultraviolet radiation. Br J Dermatol. 1989;121(5):639.
440. Norris PG, Camp RD, Hawk JL. Actinic reticuloid response to cyclosporine. J Am Acad Dermatol. 1989;21(2):307–9.
441. Nousari HC, Anhalt GJ, Morison WL. Mycophenolate in psoralen-UV-A desensitization therapy for chronic actinic dermatitis. Arch Dermatol. 1999;135:1128–9.
442. Sinclair SE, Hindson C. PUVA therapy of chronic actinic dermatitis. Australas J Dermatol. 1988;29:117–9.
443. Toonstra J, Henquet CM, van Weelden H, et al. Actinic reticuloid. A clinical, photobiologic, histopathologic and follow-up study of 16 patients. J Am Acad Dermatol. 1989;21:205–14.

Contact Dermatitis

444. Bonamonte D, Foti C, Vestita M, Angelini G. Noneczematous contact dermatitis. ISRN Allergy. 2013;2013(361746):1–10. doi:10.1155/2013/361746.
445. Rietschel RL, Fowler JF, editors. Fisher's contact dermatitis. 5th ed. Philadelphia: Lippincott Williams & Wilkins; 2001. p. 75–76.
446. Burkhart CG. Pustular allergic contact dermatitis: a distinct clinical and pathological entity. Cutis. 1981;27(6):630–8.
447. Rodriguez-Martin M, Saez-Rodriguez M, Carnerero-Rodriguez A, et al. Pustular allergic contact dermatitis from topical minoxidil 5%. J Eur Acad Dermatol Venereol. 2007;21(5):701–2.
448. Sanchez-Motilla JM, Pont V, Nagore E, Rodriguez-Serna M, Sanchez JL, Aliaga A. Pustular allergic contact dermatitis from minoxidil. Contact Dermatitis. 1998;38(5):283–4.
449. Schoel J, Frosch PJ. Allergic contact eczema caused by rubber-containing substances simulating pustulosis palmaris. Derm Beruf Umwelt. 1990;38(6):178–80.
450. Tan CH, Rasool S, Johnston GA. Contact dermatitis: allergic and irritant. Clin Dermatol. 2014;32(1):116–24.

451. Davies RF, Johnston GA. New and emerging cosmetic allergens. Clin Dermatol. 2011;29(3):311–5.
452. Kulberg A, Schliemann S, Elsner P. Contact dermatitis as a systemic disease. Clin Dermatol. 2014;32(3):414–9.
453. Vocanson M, Hennino A, Rozieres A, Poyet G, Nicolas JF. Effector and regulatory mechanisms in allergic contact dermatitis. Allergy. 2009;64(12):1699–714.
454. Dhingra N, Shemer A, Correa da Rosa J, et al. Molecular profiling of contact dermatitis skin identifies allergen-dependent differences in immune response. J Allergy Clin Immunol. 2014;134(2):362–72.
455. Honda T, Egawa G, Grabbe S, Kabashima K. Update of immune events in the murine contact hypersensitivity model: toward the understanding of allergic contact dermatitis. J Invest Dermatol. 2013;133(2):303–15.
456. Saint-Mezard P, Berard F, Dubois B, Kaiserlian D, Nicolas JF. The role of CD4+ and CD8+ T cells in contact hypersensitivity and allergic contact dermatitis. Eur J Dermatol. 2004;14(3):131–8.
457. Fyhrquist N, Wolff H, Lauerma A, Alenius H. CD8+ T cell migration to the skin requires CD4+ help in a murine model of contact hypersensitivity. PLoS One. 2012;7(8):e41038.
458. Belsito DV. Patch testing: after 100 years, still the gold standard in diagnosing cutaneous delayed-type hypersensitivity. Arb Paul Ehrlich Inst Bundesamt Sera Impfstoffe Frankf A M. 1997;91:195–202.
459. Higgins E, Collins P. The relevance of 7-day patch test reading. Dermatitis. 2013;24(5):237–40.
460. Mitchell JC. Day 7 (D7) patch test reading – valuable or not. Contact Dermatitis. 1978;4(3):139–41.
461. Davis MD, Bhate K, Rohlinger AL, Farmer SA, Richardson DM, Weaver AL. Delayed patch test reading after 5 days: the mayo clinic experience. J Am Acad Dermatol. 2008;59(2):225–33.
462. Jonker MJ, Bruynzeel DP. The outcome of an additional patch-test reading on days 6 or 7. Contact Dermatitis. 2000;42(6):330–5.
463. Rietschel R, Fowler F, Fisher A. Practical aspects of patch testing. 16Y18. In: Rietschel R, Fowler F, Fisher A, editors. Fisher's contact dermatitis. 6th ed. Hamilton/Maidenhead: BC Decker/ McGraw-Hill Education; 2008. p. 6–18.
464. Wolf R, Orion E, Ruocco V, Baroni A, Ruocco E. Patch testing: facts and controversies. Clin Dermatol. 2013;31(4):479–86.
465. Medenica M, Rostenberg Jr A. A comparative light and electron microscopic study of primary irritant contact dermatitis and allergic contact dermatitis. J Invest Dermatol. 1971;56(4):259–71.
466. Astner S, Ulrich M. Spongiotic dermatitis. In: Hofmann-Wellenhof R, Pellacani G, Malvehy J, Soyer HP, editors. Reflectance confocal microscopy for skin diseases. 1st ed. Berlin/ Heidelberg: Springer-Verlag; 2012. p. 381–9.
467. Boone MA, Jemec GB, Del MV. Differentiating allergic and irritant contact dermatitis by high-definition optical coherence tomography: a pilot study. Arch Dermatol Res. 2014.
468. Wahlberg J, Lindberg M. Patch testing. In: Frosch P, Menne T, Lepoittevin J, editors. Contact dermatitis. London: Springer; 2006. p. 366–90.
469. Katta R, Schlichte M. Diet and dermatitis: food triggers. J Clin Aesthet Dermatol. 2014;7(3):30–6.
470. Krecisz B, Chomiczewska D, Kiec-Swierczynska M, Kaszuba A. Systemic contact dermatitis to nickel present in cocoa in 14-year-old boy. Pediatr Dermatol. 2011;28(3):335–6.
471. Pizzutelli S. Systemic nickel hypersensitivity and diet: myth or reality. Eur Ann Allergy Clin Immunol. 2011;43(1):5–18.
472. Dinkloh A, Worm M, Geier J, Schnuch A, Wollenberg A. Contact sensitization in patients with suspected cosmetic intolerance: results of the IVDK 2006–2011. J Eur Acad Dermatol Venereol. 2015;29:1071–81.
473. Wang WH, Li LF, Lu XY, Wang J. Cosmetic dermatitis in Chinese eczema patients patch tested with a modified European standard series of allergens. Contact Dermatitis. 2005;53(6):314–9.
474. Zhao J, Li LF. Contact sensitization to cosmetic series of allergens in a general population in Beijing. J Cosmet Dermatol. 2014;13(1):68–71.
475. Kumar P, Paulose R. Patch testing in suspected allergic contact dermatitis to cosmetics. Dermatol Res Pract. 2014;2014:695387.
476. Swinnen I, Goossens A. An update on airborne contact dermatitis: 2007–2011. Contact Dermatitis. 2013;68(4):232–8.
477. Thyssen JP, Johansen JD, Linneberg A, Menne T. The epidemiology of hand eczema in the general population – prevalence and main findings. Contact Dermatitis. 2010;62(2):75–87.
478. Clark SC, Zirwas MJ. Management of occupational dermatitis. Dermatol Clin. 2009;27(3):365–83, vii–viii.
479. Zhai H, Brachman F, Pelosi A, et al. A bioengineering study on the efficacy of a skin protectant lotion in preventing SLS-induced dermatitis. Skin Res Technol. 2000;6(2):77–80.
480. Schliemann-Willers S, Wigger-Alberti W, Elsner P. Efficacy of a new class of perfluoropolyethers in the prevention of irritant contact dermatitis. Acta Derm Venereol. 2001;81(6):392–4.
481. Ramsing DW, Agner T. Effect of glove occlusion on human skin (II). Long-term experimental exposure. Contact Dermatitis. 1996;34(4):258–62.
482. Pierard GE, Arrese JE, Rodriguez C, Daskaleros PA. Effects of softened and unsoftened fabrics on sensitive skin. Contact Dermatitis. 1994;30(5):286–91.
483. Loden M. Barrier recovery and influence of irritant stimuli in skin treated with a moisturizing cream. Contact Dermatitis. 1997;36(5):256–60.
484. Saary J, Qureshi R, Palda V, et al. A systematic review of contact dermatitis treatment and prevention. J Am Acad Dermatol. 2005;53(5):845.
485. Puviani M, Agostinis F, Milani M. Barrier repair therapy for facial atopic eczema with a non-steroidal emollient cream containing rhamnosoft, ceramides and iso-leucine. A six-case report series. Minerva Pediatr. 2014;66(4):307–11.
486. Sahle FF, Gebre-Mariam T, Dobner B, Wohlrab J, Neubert RH. Skin diseases associated with the depletion of stratum corneum lipids and stratum corneum lipid substitution therapy. Skin Pharmacol Physiol. 2014;28(1):42–55.
487. Perrenoud D, Gallezot D, van Melle G. The efficacy of a protective cream in a real-world apprentice hairdresser environment. Contact Dermatitis. 2001;45(3):134–8.
488. Vidmar DA, Iwane MK. Assessment of the ability of the topical skin protectant (TSP) to protect against contact dermatitis to urushiol (Rhus) antigen. Am J Contact Dermat. 1999;10(4):190–7.
489. Marks Jr JG, Fowler Jr JF, Sheretz EF, Rietschel RL. Prevention of poison ivy and poison oak allergic contact dermatitis by quaternium-18 bentonite. J Am Acad Dermatol. 1995;33(2 Pt 1):212–6.
490. Li Y, Li LF. Topical application of a Chinese medicine, Qingpeng ointment, ameliorates 2, 4-dinitrofluorobenzene-induced allergic contact dermatitis in BALB/c mice. Eur J Dermatol. 2013;23(6):803–6.
491. Taylor JS, Praditsuwan P, Handel D, Kuffner G. Allergic contact dermatitis from doxepin cream. One-year patch test clinic experience. Arch Dermatol. 1996;132(5):515–8.
492. Bonnel RA, La Grenade L, Karwoski CB, Beitz JG. Allergic contact dermatitis from topical doxepin: food and drug administration's postmarketing surveillance experience. J Am Acad Dermatol. 2003;48(2):294–6.
493. Brancaccio RR, Weinstein S. Systemic contact dermatitis to doxepin. J Drugs Dermatol. 2003;2(4):409–10.
494. Kaaber K, Menne T, Veien NK, Baadsgaard O. Some adverse effects of disulfiram in the treatment of nickel-allergic patients. Derm Beruf Umwelt. 1987;35(6):209–11.
495. Sharma AD. Disulfiram and low nickel diet in the management of hand eczema: a clinical study. Indian J Dermatol Venereol Leprol. 2006;72(2):113–8.

Drug Eruption

496. Roujeau JC, Stern RS. Severe adverse cutaneous reactions to drugs. N Engl J Med. 1994;332:959.
497. Naisbitt DJ, Pirmohamed M, Park BK. Immunological principles of T-cell-mediated adverse drug reactions in skin. Expert Opin Drug Saf. 2007;6:109–24.
498. Gell, P and Coombs, R. The classification of allergic reactions underlying disease. In Clinical Aspects of Immunology. Blackwell Science 1963:217–37.
499. Pichler WJ. Pharmacological interaction of drugs with antigen-specific immune receptors: the p-i concept. Curr Opin Allergy Clin Immunol. 2002;2:301–5.
500. Mallal S, Phillips E, Carosi G, et al. HLA-B* 5701 screening for hypersensitivity to abacavir. N Engl J Med. 2008;358:568–79.
501. Chen P, Lin J-J, Lu C-S, et al. Carbamazepine-induced toxic effects and HLA-B*1502 screening in Taiwan. N Engl J Med. 2011;364:1126–33.
502. McCormack M, Alfirevic A, Bourgeois S, et al. HLA-A*3101 and carbamazepine-induced hypersensitivity reactions in Europeans. N Engl J Med. 2011;364:1134–43.
503. Zhang FR, Liu H, Irwanto A, et al. HLA-B*13:01and the dapsone hypersensitivity syndrome. N Engl J Med. 2013;369:1620–8.
504. Breathnach SM. Mechanisms of drug eruptions: Part I. Austral J Dermatol 1995;36(3):121–7.
505. Anderson MW, deShazo RD. Studies of the mechanism of angiotensin-converting enzyme (ACE) inhibitor-associated angioedema: the effect of an ACE inhibitor on cutaneous responses to bradykinin, codeine, and histamine. J Allergy Clin Immunol. 1990;85:856–8.
506. Zuberbier T, Iffländer J, Semmler C, et al. Acute urticaria: clinical aspects and therapeutic responsiveness. Acta Derm Venereol. 1996;76:295–7.
507. Verma C, Vasudevan LC, Pragasam LC. Severe cutaneous adverse drug reactions. Med J Armed Forces India. 2013;69:375–83.
508. Roujeau JC, Bioulac-Sage P, Bourseau C, et al. Acute generalized exanthematous pustulosis. Analysis of 63 cases. Arch Dermatol. 1991;127:1333–8.
509. Sidoroff A, Halevy S, Bavinck JN, et al. Acute generalized exanthematous pustulosis (AGEP) – a clinical reaction pattern. J Cutan Pathol. 2001;28:113–9.

9 Diseases with Underlining Internal Conditions

Melissa Danesh, Jenny E. Murase, Zhirong Yao, Ruhong Cheng, Huaguo Li, Liangchun Wang, Jian-Zhong Zhang, and Jin Wei

Contents

M. Danesh, BS
Department of Dermatology, University of California San Francisco, San Francisco, CA, USA

J.E. Murase, MD (✉)
Department of Dermatology, University of California San Francisco, San Francisco, CA, USA

Department of Dermatology, Palo Alto Foundation Medical Group, 701 East El Camino Real (31-104), Mountain View, CA 94040, USA
e-mail: jemurase@gmail.com

Z. Yao (✉) • R. Cheng • H. Li
Department of Dermatology, Xinhua Hospital Affiliated to Shanghai Jiaotong University School of Medicine, Shenyang, China
e-mail: zryaosmu@sohu.com

L. Wang (✉)
Sun Yat-Sen Hospital, Guangzhou, China
e-mail: wliangch@mail.sysu.edu.cn

J.-Z. Zhang (✉) • J. Wei
Department of Dermatology, Peking University People's Hospital, Beijing 100044, China
e-mail: rmzjz@126.com

9.1 Dermatoses of Pregnancy

Melissa Danesh, BS and Jenny E. Murase, MD

9.1.1 Specific Dermatoses of Pregnancy

The specific dermatoses of pregnancy are defined as a group of pruritic inflammatory dermatoses associated exclusively with pregnancy and/or the immediate postpartum period [1]. Classification of this disease entity remains a topic of debate. The three generally accepted dermatoses include pemphigoid gestationis (PG), polymorphic eruption of pregnancy (PEP), and intrahepatic cholestasis of pregnancy (ICP) [2]. Apart from these three, a series of clinical entities in pregnancy have been previously documented including prurigo of pregnancy, pruritic folliculitis of pregnancy, and atopic dermatitis. However, recent literature has illustrated significant overlaps in clinical presentation and histopathology between these three presentations and, therefore, they will all be categorized together under the term "atopic eruption of pregnancy" (AEP) [3]. It is important to note that two of these four dermatoses (PG and ICP) may pose significant risk for the fetus, and that early recognition and appropriate diagnostic testing are imperative. This chapter will focus on diagnosis, pathogenesis, and management of the four aforementioned dermatoses of pregnancy.

X.-H. Gao, H.-D. Chen (eds.), *Practical Immunodermatology*, DOI 10.1007/978-94-024-0902-4_9

9.1.2 Pemphigoid Gestationis (PG)

Synonyms

Gestational pemphigoid
Herpes gestationis

Epidemiology
The incidence of pemphigoid gestationis in North America is estimated to be 1 in 50,000 pregnancies [4]. It most commonly appears in late pregnancy (mean onset 21 weeks) or immediately postpartum, but can appear in any of the three trimesters.

Pathogenesis
The dermoepidermal junction (DEJ) hemidesmosome contains a 180 kD protein (BP180) termed "bullous pemphigoid antigen 2 (BPAG2)." In PG, autoantibodies of the IgG1 class are generated against the NC16A domain of BPAG2 [5–8]. These serum antibodies activate the complement system via the classical pathway [9]. Complement activation leads to chemoattraction and degranulation of eosinophils [10]. Both the skin and the placenta are of ectodermal origin, sharing many of the same antigens. In PG, the serum IgG1 antibodies bind not only the basement membrane of the epidermis, but also to that of the major histocompatibility complex class II antigens within the chorionic villi (of paternal origin [11]) and to the basement membrane of the amnion [12, 13]. This is consistent with the hypothesis that the primary site of autoimmunity is in fact the placenta, which then cross-reacts with the skin.

Clinical Features and Risk to Fetus
PG is characterized by the sudden onset of intensely pruritic, urticarial erythema, papules, plaques, and tense blisters on the abdomen, often involving the periumbilical region [14] (Fig. 9.1a). The skin lesions may spread to the entire skin surface, though mucous membranes are usually not involved (Fig. 9.2a, b). While in the preblistering stage, differentiation of PG from PEP is difficult; a more advanced presentation of PG involves the development of tense blisters resulting in widespread erosions [1].

The potential negative impact on the pregnancy stems from the effects of these autoantibodies on the placenta. While the prognosis for the fetus is generally good, PG increases the tendency for small-for-gestational-age infants and prematurity [15, 16]. There is a risk of neonatal herpes gestationis in up to 10% of cases, though it is mild and self-limited [17]. There is no increase in fetal morbidity or mortality [18]. There is no maternal risk other than those involved with management of the dermatitis.

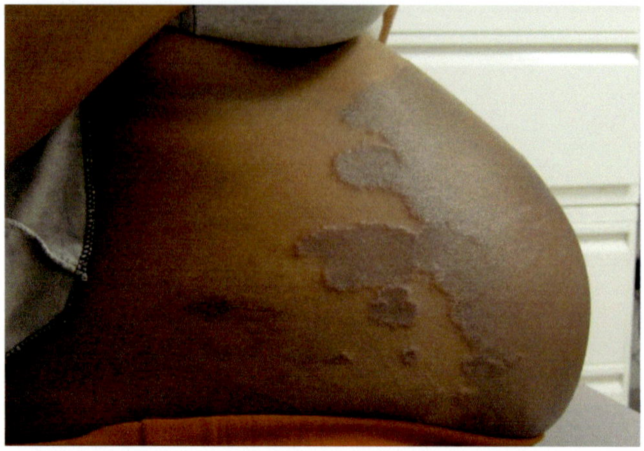

Fig. 9.1 Pemphigoid gestationis presenting in its classic form, involving the periumbilical area, in a large plaque with studded vesicles on the periphery. These vesicles are tested positive on direct immunofluorescence for linear deposition of C3 at the dermal-epidermal junction (Photo courtesy of Ronald O. Perelman Department of Dermatology)

Management
Diagnosis of PG involves direct immunofluorescence (DIF) of perilesional skin with the finding of linear deposition of C3, with or without IgG deposition, along the basement membrane.

Treatment of PG involves symptom management and prevention of blister formation. In milder disease, topical corticosteroids and oral antihistamines may suffice [19], but systemic corticosteroids [20, 21] have become the cornerstone of therapy (initially 0.5–1 mg/kg/day, slowly tapered as disease improves) [1, 22]. If the disease is refractory to the aforementioned treatments, intravenous immunoglobulin, cyclosporine, and immunophoresis have been suggested as alternatives [23–26].

9.1.3 Polymorphic Eruption of Pregnancy (PEP)

Synonyms

Pruritic urticarial papules and plaques of pregnancy (PUPPP)
Bourne's "toxemic rash of pregnancy"
Toxic erythema (or rash) of pregnancy
Nurse's "late-onset prurigo" of pregnancy

Epidemiology
Polymorphic eruption of pregnancy is estimated to affect between 1 in 130 and 1 in 300 pregnancies [27]. It is usually observed in primagravida women in the third trimester of pregnancy, and occasionally postpartum [28]. It has been correlated with multiple pregnancies and excess maternal weight gain [29].

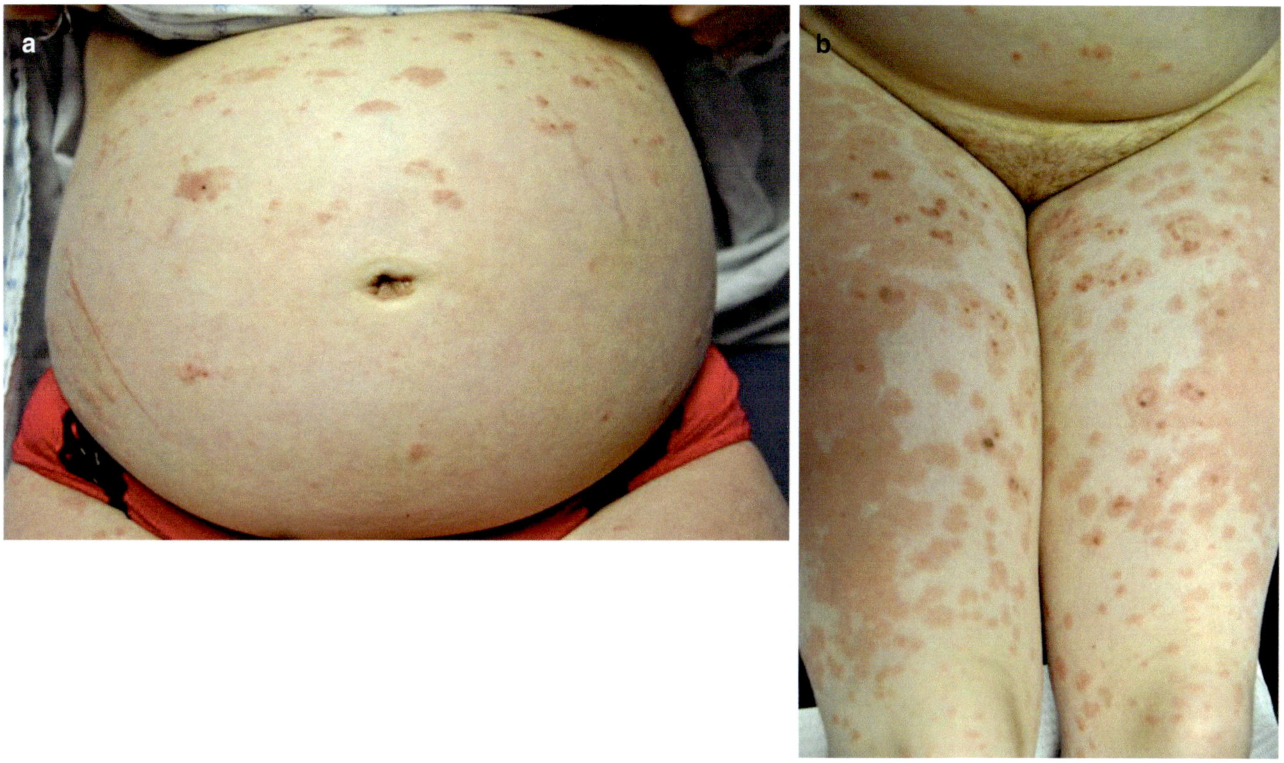

Fig. 9.2 (**a**) PG presenting on the abdomen. While PG usually involves the periumbilical area, this patient had umbilical sparing (Courtesy of George Kroumpouzos, MD, Norwell, MA). (**b**) The same patient with urticarial papules coalescent into plaques and small vesicles on the legs (Photos courtesy of George Kroumpouzos, MD, Norwell, MA)

Pathogenesis

The pathogenesis of PEP remains unknown. A negative DIF argues against an autoimmune mechanism [28]. The most current accepted hypothesis is that abdominal distention in pregnancy causes tissue damage that exposes previously unencountered antigen. This, in turn, could trigger an inflammatory response. This hypothesis is supported by the start of PEP within the striae of the skin and its association both with maternal weight gain and primigravida patients, particularly when the skin is distending at its fastest rate in the third trimester.

Clinical Features and Risk to Fetus

PEP is characterized by sudden onset of a pruritic eruption starting in the abdominal striae (Fig. 9.3). The periumbilical region is often spared. The eruption is polymorphous, presenting as erythematous urticarial papules and plaques, which spread from abdominal striae further to the abdomen, buttocks, proximal thighs (Fig. 9.4a, b), and arms. PEP may involve vesicles, purpura, or targetoid lesions as well, which is why the terms "polymorphous eruption of pregnancy" is now favored over the classic term "pruritic urticarial papules and plaques of pregnancy" [30, 31]. Palms, soles, and scalp are commonly spared [28].

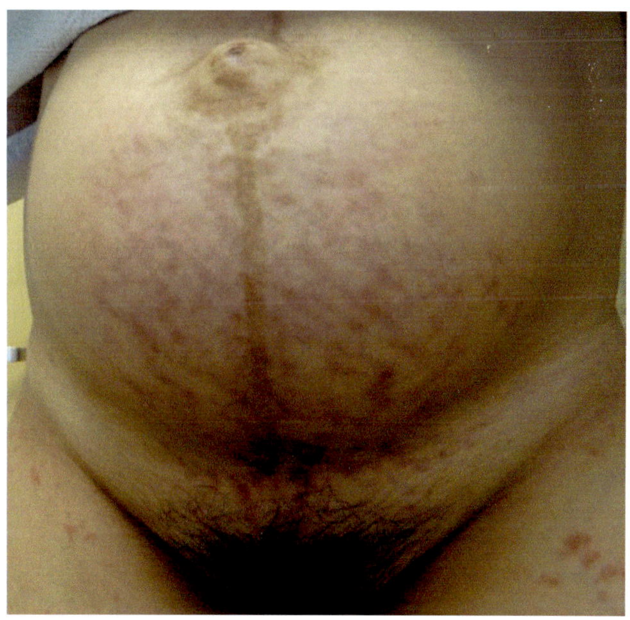

Fig. 9.3 Polymorphic eruption of pregnancy presenting as urticarial plaques in the lines of striae on the abdomen late in the third trimester

While PEP has the potential to be intensely pruritic, it portends no additional risk for the mother or the fetus.

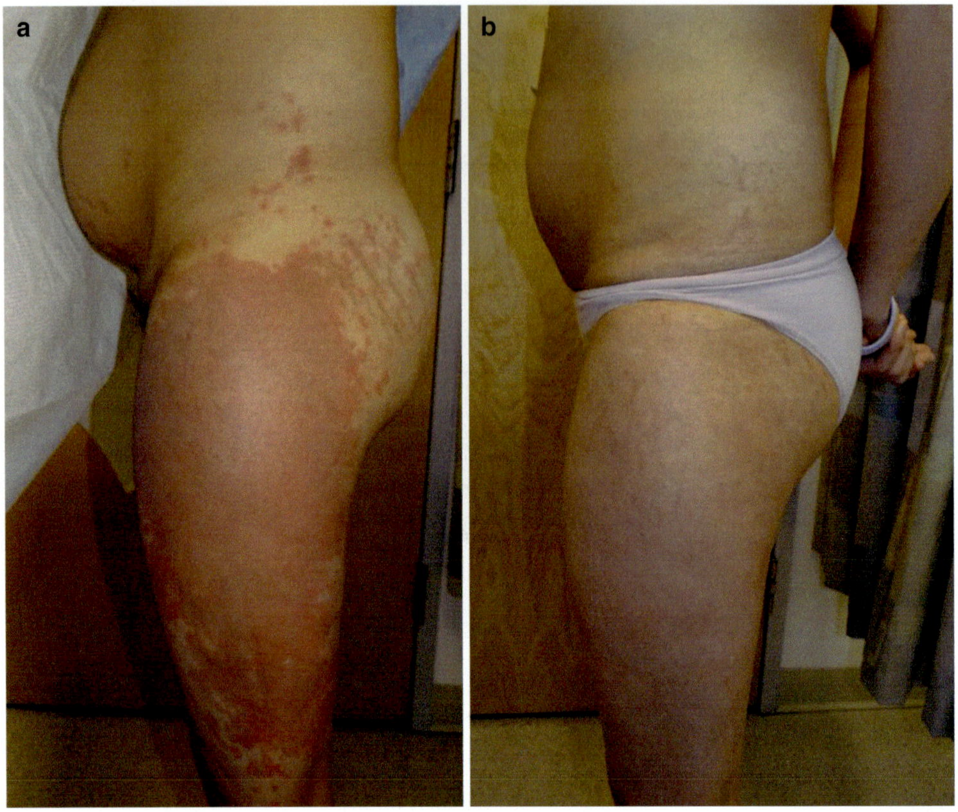

Fig. 9.4 (**a**) The same patient as pictured in Fig. 9.3 with prominent involvement on the lateral thighs and buttocks. (**b**) Three weeks postpartum. Following application of topical clobetasol, the dermatitis has almost completely resolved

Management
In the event that diagnosis is not clear from clinical presentations, a biopsy may be done to differentiate PEP from the prebullous stage of PG. The DIF in PG will be positive, while in PEP the histopathology will show nonspecific dermal lymphocytic infiltrate and the DIF will be negative.

Because this disease does not impact the prognosis of both the mother and fetus, symptomatic treatment is all that is usually required. Most patients will respond well to topical corticosteroids and oral antihistamines [28]. In refractory disease, short course of systemic cortisone can be used, and rarely early delivery of the fetus has been used for intractable pruritus [32, 33].

9.1.4 Atopic Eruption of Pregnancy (AEP)

Synonyms

Prurigo of pregnancy
Prurigo gestationis
Early-onset prurigo of pregnancy
Papular dermatitis of pregnancy
Pruritic folliculitis of pregnancy
Atopic dermatitis or eczema in pregnancy

Epidemiology
Atopic eruption of pregnancy is the most common specific dermatosis of pregnancy; however, incidence is unclear given its greatly contested diagnostic criteria [34]. Usually, AEP starts earlier in pregnancy, often before the third trimester, and tends to recur in subsequent pregnancies, and morbidity is higher than general population in subsequent pregnancies [3].

Pathogenesis
In pregnancy, a shift from T-helper 1 (Th1) to T-helper 2 (Th2) immunity has been described, likely secondary to the effects of estrogen. It has been found that Th1 cytokines (IL-2, interferon gamma, IL-12) are downregulated while Th2 cytokines (IL-4 and IL-10) are upregulated [35]. AEP is primarily a Th2regulated disease. As predicted, pregnancy will often induce a woman's first incidence or exacerbation of atopic cutaneous disease, classified under AEP. However, this is likely one of many heterogenous pathways contributing to this disease.

Clinical Features and Risk to Fetus
Some believe AEP is an extension of preexisting atopic dermatitis. However, in the majority of patients, pregnancy coincides with the patients' first ever incidence of atopic dermatitis or first flare since childhood [3]. Patients present with

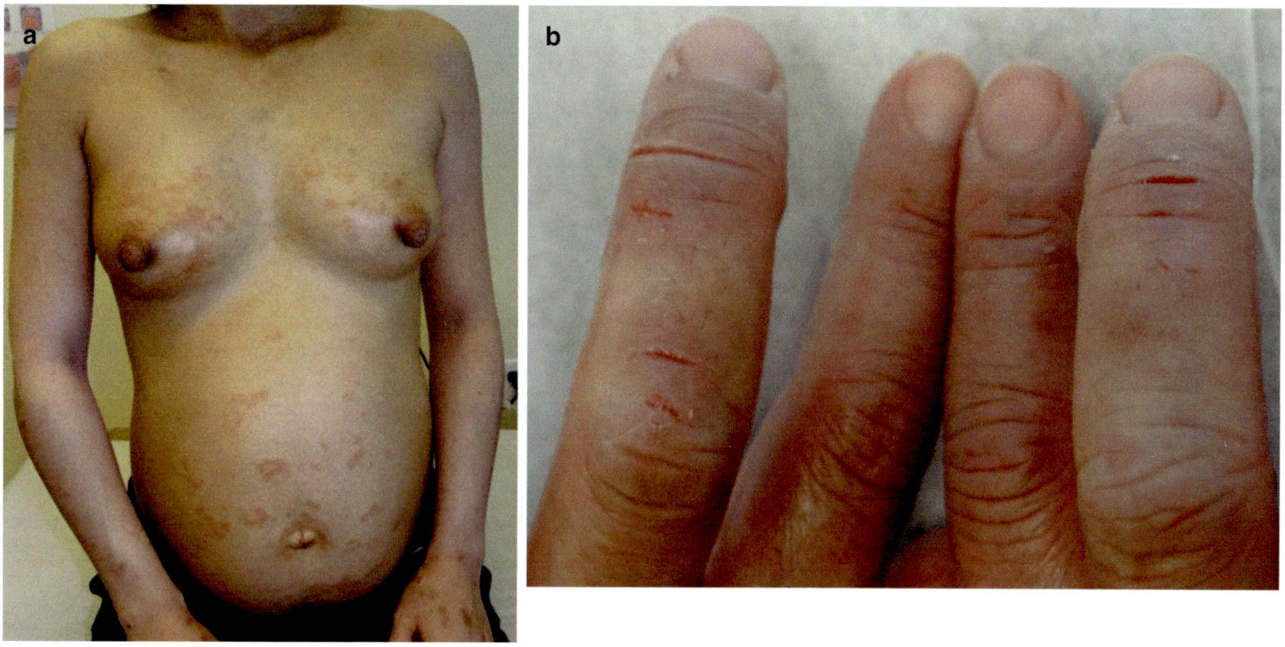

Fig. 9.5 (**a**) Atopic eruption of pregnancy, E-type (eczematous), in a patient with known atopic dermatitis. This patient is in her early second trimester. AEP often presents earlier in pregnancy than PEP. (**b**) Involvement of the hands is common in AEP, as well as other classic locations for atopic dermatitis such as the neck and antecubital fossa

severely dry skin and eczematous changes usually affecting the face, neck, and flexural surfaces (E-type for eczematous, Fig. 9.5a, b). Patients may also present with excoriated papules, predominantly on extensor surfaces (P-type for papular, Fig. 9.6a, b) [21].

AEP has no adverse risks to the mother or fetus' wellbeing.

Management

This is usually a diagnosis of exclusion. Cholestasis of pregnancy should be excluded in select cases with normal serum bile acids, and bacterial folliculitis may be ruled out with skin cultures. DIF will be negative.

Treatment of this dermatosis is mainly symptomatic, as neither maternal nor fetal wellbeing is endangered. This generally involves topical antipruritic agents and topical corticosteroids [36].

9.1.5 Intrahepatic Cholestasis of Pregnancy (ICP)

Synonyms

Obstetric cholestasis
Cholestasis of pregnancy
Prurigo (or pruritus) gravidarum
Jaundice of pregnancy

Epidemiology

The incidence of ICP varies widely based on geographic location suggesting a genetic predisposition, with a range from 0.2 to 2.4 % in Middle Europe to 15 % in parts of Chile and Bolivia. Positive family history of 27 % has been documented in those affected with ICP [37].

Pathophysiology

ICP is thought to be due to decreased excretion of bile salts, resulting in rise of serum bile salts and subsequent massive maternal pruritus. Importantly, the transfer of these toxic bile salts into fetal circulation can result in adverse fetal effects, such as cardiac depression and acute anoxia.

Clinical Features and Risk to Fetus

Classically ICP will present with sudden-onset pruritus in the late second or third trimester. Apart from excoriations or prurigo nodules that are self-induced secondary to scratching, ICP is not associated with any primary skin lesions. Pruritus can be severe, usually worse at night. Most commonly affected locations include the trunk (Fig. 9.7a), extensor extremities (Fig. 9.7b), palms, and soles. Apart from cutaneous symptoms, around 10–15 % [38] of patients develop jaundice within 2–4 weeks of initial pruritus; dark urine and light-colored stool may also be seen [39]. Symptoms usually resolve within 1–2 weeks of delivery.

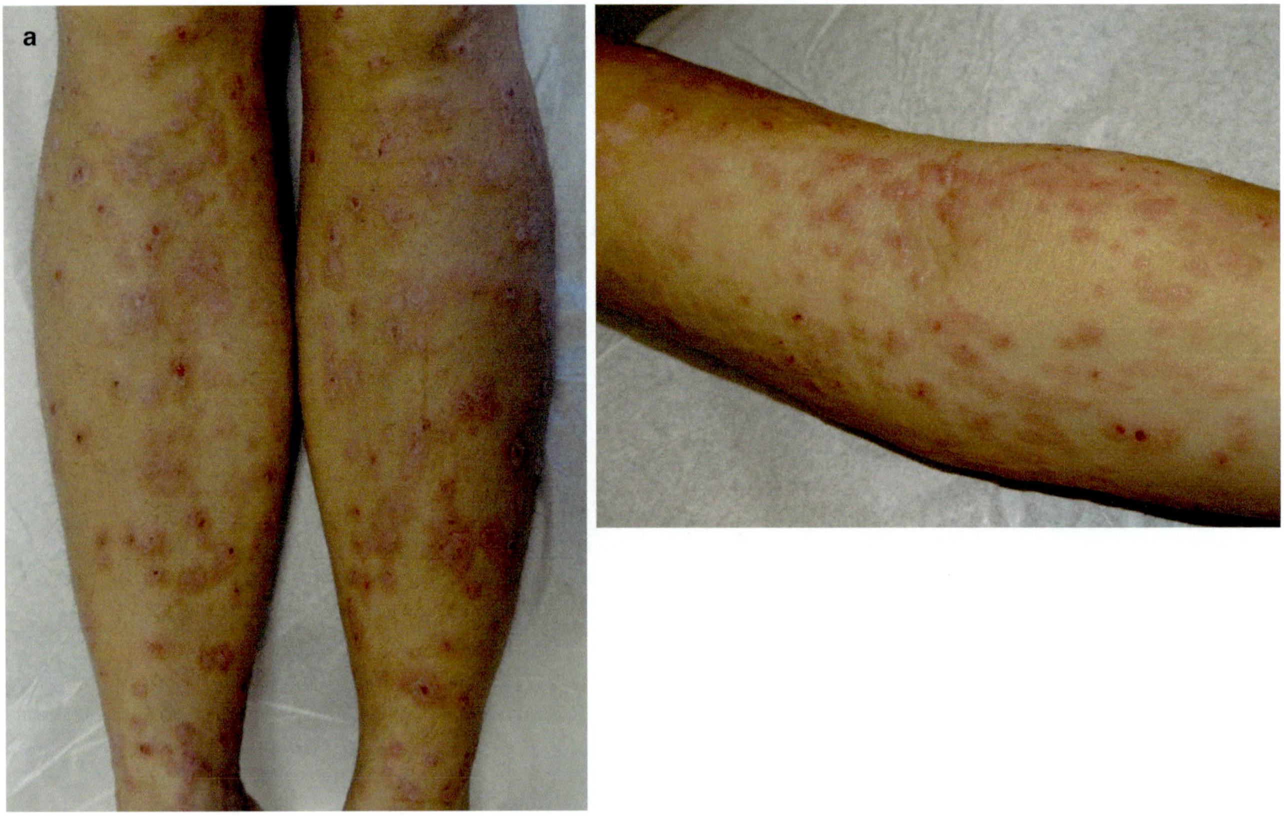

Fig. 9.6 (**a**) Atopic eruption of pregnancy, P-type (papular), involving the lower extremities. (**b**) AEP involving the upper extremities. This can be intensely pruritic

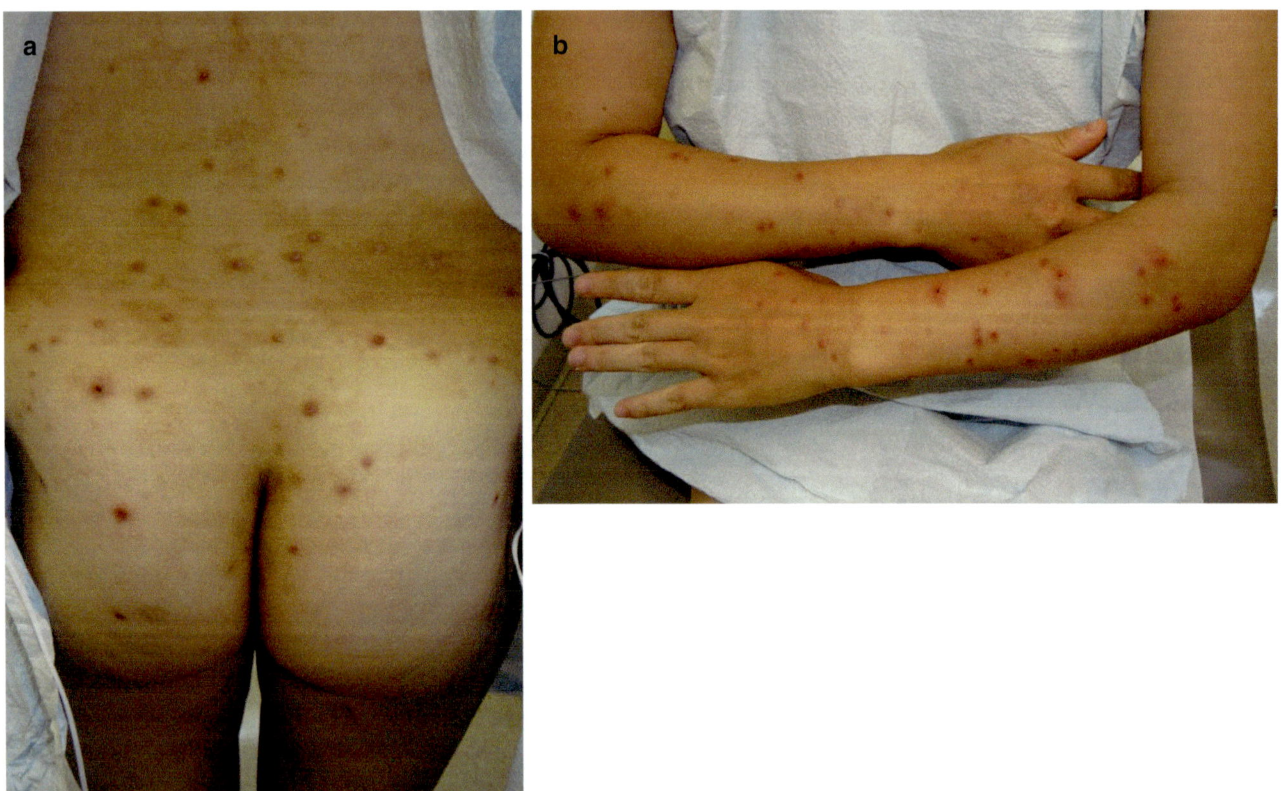

Fig. 9.7 (**a**) Intrahepatic cholestasis of pregnancy involves secondary skin lesions from scratching and no primary skin lesions. (**b**) Patients are often heavily excoriated in areas that they can reach to scratch such as the upper extremities. Interestingly the pruritus is also on the palms and soles

Risks in the pregnant patient include bleeding complications due to decreased vitamin K absorption and increased incidence of gallbladder disease. Risks to the fetus include preterm delivery (19–60 %) and intrauterine fetal death (0.75–1.6 %) [37].

Management

ICP is diagnosed in the setting of the absence of primary skin lesions, such as eczematous papules or vesicles, and elevated serum bile acids. In certain cases, elevation of liver function tests may also be seen.

Treatment goals in ICP include symptom reduction and decreasing risk of complications in the mother and fetus. Ursodeoxycholic acid is currently the first-line therapy for ICP (15 mg/kg per day until delivery). This medication provides relief from pruritus and decreases the rate of premature delivery [40].

Pregnancy and the Immune System

The human immune system aims to recognize and destroy non-self-antigens. Antigens of paternal origin can be detected in maternal serum, unrecognizable to the maternal immune system and targeted as non-self-antigens. However, the immune system has developed mechanisms to tolerate these non-self-antigens, through a shift away from cell-mediated immunity (Th1) to antibody-mediated immunity (Th2) during pregnancy and the expansion of T-regulatory cells [41]. This shift from Th1 to Th2 is thought to be due to the effect of increased estrogen [42]. As predicted, diseases that are primarily Th1 immune mediated (i.e., multiple sclerosis, rheumatoid arthritis, psoriasis, autoimmune thyroid disease, etc.) generally improve during pregnancy. However, due to an upregulation of Th2 cytokines, diseases that are primarily Th2 mediated, such as atopic dermatitis, lupus, and forms of pemphigus (i.e., pemphigus vulgaris or PG), are exacerbated. This is why intravenous immunoglobulin can be particularly effective for refractory autoinflammatory skin disease. Through our understanding of the effects of pregnancy on the immune system, we can develop strategies to better manage dermatologic conditions that have a tendency to flare during pregnancy.

9.2 Atopic Dermatitis

Zhirong Yao, Ruhong Cheng, and Huaguo Li

Atopic dermatitis (AD) is a chronic inflammatory disorder of skin characterized by an impaired immune response with the infiltration of inflammatory cells in skin, during which Th2 cytokines are prevalent at the acute stage while Th1 cytokines are prevalent at the chronic stage. Cells involved in the pathogenesis of AD include T lymphocytes, dendritic cells (Langerhans cells and inflammatory dendritic cells), keratinocytes, endothelial cells, eosinophils, and mast cells. During the course of the disease, chemokines and cytokines network is heavily involved [43]. Genetic factors, impaired skin barrier, and environmental factors (such as microbial organisms) contribute to the pathogenesis of AD together with immunological dysfunction.

T lymphocytes play a critical role in the atopic inflammation. Functionally, they secrete cytokines that are typical of Th2 cells (IL-3, 4, 5, 10, 13, and GM-CSF) and capable of inducing IgE produced by autologous B lymphocytes. Allergen-specific Th2 populations are prevalent in the initial phase of the immune response, while cytokines typical of Th1 response (IFN-gamma, IL-12) predominate in the late phase. Neutralizing Th2 cytokines in skin explants from AD patients [44] makes IL-17 functional, which could potentially restore antimicrobial peptides (AMP) expression and reduce microbial colonization. T cells could independently express IL-22 even with low expression of IL-17. Thus, Th17/22 helper cells and their cytokines (IL-17 and IL-22) are also involved and play an indispensable role in acute and chronic phases of AD [45]. Th17 cells are critical for the expression of AMP while Th22 cells could drive epidermal hyperplasia; $CD4^+$ Tcells, particularly activated Th2 cells, peripheral blood, and skin-homing $CD45RO^+CLA^+$T-cells, have been found to represent a major cellular source for IL-31 [46], which can induce pruritus. As a pruritic cytokine but not a Th2 cytokine in the classical sense, IL-31 can also promote Th2-driven inflammation [47]. IL-31 mRNA level strongly correlates with serum IL-31 protein level, disease severity as well as the subjective itch intensity. Moreover, IL-18-induced super Th1 cells, Th9 cells which produced IL-9 and IL-10, and regulatory T cells (Treg cells) are all considered to be involved in the inflammatory responses [48]. T lymphocytes activated by antigens express the skin-homing receptor CLA, which binds the E-selectin ELAM-1 expressed on endothelial cells of postcapillary venules, endowing T lymphocytes with a particular cutaneous tropism. IL-4, TNF-alpha, and IL-1 beta produced by multiple cells such as Th2 cells, Langerhans cells, and mast cells can further induce overexpression of adhesion molecules (ELAM-1, ICAM-1, and VCAM-1) on endothelial cells. These cytokines again increase the afflux of lymphocytes and eosinophils bearing skin-homing receptors [45].

Langerhans cells (LCs), a subpopulation of professional antigen-presenting cells present in normal epidermis, express on their membrane substantial amounts of high and low affinity receptors for IgE induced by IL-4 and IL-13 of Th2 lymphocytes. These LCs can therefore present the allergen efficiently, which has crossed the skin barrier and is bound to the specific IgE, to lymph node T lymphocytes such as Th1 and Th2 cells, and possibly also to Treg cells, initiating the immune reaction. Langerhans cells initiate epicutaneous sensitization with protein antigens and induce Th2-type immune responses via human thymic stromal lymphopoietin (TSLP, particularly expressed by keratinocytes of AD skin) signaling pathway [49]. Based on these data, AD can therefore be defined as an IgE-induced Th2 lymphocyte immune reaction. Inflammatory dendritic cells, appearing only in inflamed skin, are another form of dendritic cells involved in the pathogenesis of the disease. Contrary to Langerhans cells, inflammatory dendritic cells do not contain Birbeck granules. They present mainly in the dermis and express the high-affinity receptor for IgE in higher amounts than Langerhans cells. They can also be activated by TSLP. Inflammatory dendritic epidermal cells lead to Th1 polarization by producing IL-12 and IL-18 and by secreting proinflammatory cytokines [50]. Plasmacytoid dendritic cells, producing a large amount of IFN-alpha, are also present in the inflammatory infiltrate. Dendritic cells produce IL-25, which inhibits filaggrin synthesis and induces Th2 responses, thereby directly affecting skin barrier function [45].

Eosinophil skin infiltration is frequently observed in lesions of both AD patients and AD murine models [51]. Eosinophils are able to secrete a large amount of cytotoxic molecules, such as eosinophil cationic protein (ECP), major basic protein (MBP), and eosinophil peroxidase (EPO), into the skin, which are responsible for tissue damage. Total eosinophil counts, the expression level of ECP, along with serum IL-16 and total IgE, correlate with disease severity [45]. Kinetic studies of the cellular infiltration by atopy patch test showed that lymphocytes appear in the skin before the recruitment of eosinophils. Then, they induce activation, differentiation, and increase the survival of eosinophils by upregulation of IL-5 [45]. However, crossing STAT6 null mice, which have defects in Th2 differentiation and IgE class switching, with NC/Nga mice cannot prevent the development of AD-like skin lesions. The histological features of their skin lesions are similar to those of AD, even though these mice do not produce Th2 cytokines and IgE. Authors thereby indicate that a Th2 response is not absolutely necessary for the development of AD-like skin lesions; Instead, IFN-gamma and eosinophil skin infiltration may play an essential role [51]. Eosinophils, with expressing IL-31 receptor A (IL-31RA), are delayed to apoptosis with the presence of IL-31 [52].

Mast cells play a critical role in inflammatory responses, and they regulate eosinophil activation and recruitment, thus responding to challenge with an antigen and initiating an immune response [53]. Mast cells have FcεRI on their surface and generate the release of inflammatory mediators via the cross-linking of FcεRI by surface antigen and IgE. The number of IL-31-positive mast cells was upregulated in the lesion of AD patients, and human mast cell lines increased IL-31 in the presence of antimicrobial peptides which were highly expressed in the AD skin lesion [54]. A recent study identified that the population and maturation of mast cells were reduced in TSLP-deficient mice. Furthermore, TSLP induced the proliferation and differentiation of mast cells from bone marrow progenitors. The TSLP deficiency attenuated mast cell-mediated allergic reactions through the downregulation of STAT6 and MDM2 [55].

The biological mechanism described above was previously considered to exist almost exclusively in extrinsic AD patients (about 70 % of AD) with high levels of IgE and IgE antibodies. For intrinsic AD, a nonimmunological pathogenesis, at least in the atopic sense, was postulated more dependent on cutaneous hyperreactivity [45]. However, recent studies suggested a higher immune activation in patients with intrinsic AD compared with extrinsic AD, particularly of the Th17 and Th22 immune axes. Moreover, both extrinsic and intrinsic AD lesions showed marked Th2 activation (higher IL-4/IL-13 expression), suggesting that a Th2 bias is not the sole cause of high IgE levels in patients with extrinsic disease [56]. The immune pathogenesis for intrinsic AD requires further demonstration.

Genes associated with the structural abnormalities of the epidermis and immune dysregulation play a pivotal role in the etiology of AD. Genes involved in skin barrier include filaggrin gene and SPINK5 gene, encoding filaggrin and protease inhibitor lymphoepithelial Kazal-type-related inhibitor (LEKTI), respectively. Also, there are genes related to innate and adaptive immune systems. The linkage regions may vary among different populations, and there is no extensive overlap [57].

A primary structural abnormality of the stratum corneum (SC) exists in quite a few of AD, among which absence of filaggrin is the key factor in the pathogenesis of AD. Filaggrin deficiency resulted not only from the genotype [58–60] but also effected by inflammation and exogenous stressor [61]. Skin barrier dysfunction facilitates the penetration of environmental allergens. Atopic keratinocytes constitutively express mRNA and secrete proinflammatory cytokines (IL-1, TNF-alpha, and GM-CSF), which substantially increase after stimulation. These cytokines induce overexpression of adhesion molecules on endothelial cells, enhancing the recruitment of inflammatory cells. Keratinocytes in atopic skin also produce high levels of TSLP that initiates Th2 inflammatory responses. The particular keratinocyte reactivity can partly explain the persistent minimal inflammation in AD. Moreover, GM-CSF can activate Langerhans cells, increase their survival and allow, in association with IL-4, the differentiation of blood monocytes toward dendritic cells to present antigens [45].

There is a decreased production of antimicrobial peptides (cathelicidin LL-37; the human β-defensins HBD-1, HBD-2, and HBD-3; and dermcidin) in the skin of AD as a result of the high levels of IL-4, IL-13, and IL-10. This partly explains the high colonization of *S. aureus* or fungi, in normal and, especially, skin lesions of atopic patients. Deposits of fibronectin and fibrinogen further increase adhesiveness [45]. Scratching also increases the binding of *S. aureus* to the skin, and the increased amount of *S. aureus*-derived ceramidase can increase the permeability of the stratum corneum and aggravate skin barrier defect. *S. aureus* and its products again provide signals that induce sensitization and inflammation by multiple pathways [50].

Accumulating evidence links deficient signaling pathway to the mechanism of this multifactorial disease. The JAK–STAT pathway has been shown to play an important role in the dysregulation of immune responses in AD patients, including exaggeration of Th2 cell response, activation of eosinophils, maturation of B cells, suppression of regulatory T cells, upregulation of epidermal chemokines, proinflammatroy cytokines, and proangiogenic factors as well as downregulating antimicrobial peptides and factors which are responsible for skin barrier function [51]. In addition, deficient Notch signaling pathway is associated with key pathological features, both epidermal and immunological barrier dysfunctions, in AD. Molecular cross talk between Notch and epidermal inflammation, differentiation, barrier function, antimicrobial responses, and treatment regimens should be given more concentration [62].

The cutaneous hyperreactivity to itchy stimuli is clinically obvious. Itch is intense and leads to scratching, a further barrier deficit, and an increased risk of secondary bacterial colonization. The pathophysiology is too complex involving both neurophysiological and neuroimmunological aspects [63]. Pruritus results from the activation of small nerve endings in the skin by noxious mediators, such as neuropeptides, proinflammatory cytokines, and prostaglandins. Intradermal injection of substance P or histamine induces a different cutaneous response in the atopic subject, as compared to the healthy control, and the content of histamine and neuropeptides is altered in the atopic subjects. In the skin of AD individuals, an increased number of cutaneous nerve fibers and a strong representation of the histamine 4 receptor have been identified. Several new mediators, for example, IL-31 related above, serine proteases, and nerve growth factor, have been described associated with itch in AD [45]. Interestingly, TSLP can also activate cutaneous nerves to release neuropeptides [64]. More has to be studied about the mediators, receptors, and multidirectional pathways [63].

9.3 Paraneoplastic Dermatoses

Liangchun Wang

Paraneoplastic dermatoses are group of clinical mucocutaneous manifestations associated with a malignancy, but not directly related to the invasive tumor mass or to the metastatic tumor spread. Characteristically, they follow a course parallel to the tumor, resolving with successful treatment of the primary tumor, and tend to recur with its relapse or the onset of metastases. In this case, there is no presence of neoplastic cells in the skin [65–69].

The mechanism by which paraneoplastic dermatoses occur is not well understood, but may be related to the production of bioactive substances in response to the tumor, such as polypeptide hormones, hormone-like peptides, antibodies or immune complexes, cytokines, or growth factors [67, 70, 71].

The recognization of paraneoplastic dermatoses is very important. Mucocutaneous lesions may be the presenting sign of a previously unsuspected neoplasm, occurring late in the course of illness, or being the first sign of recurrence. The recognition of some typical skin manifestations may lead to the early diagnosis of a malignant process and result in a better prognosis. Besides, the only effective therapy for skin involvement is the treatment of the primary tumor [67, 68, 72, 73].

In this subject, we exclude the genodermatoses, which are part of a genetic syndrome. We discuss the paraneoplastic cutaneous manifestations closely associated with neoplasms, whose recognition implies a mandatory investigation of internal malignancy [65, 73, 74]. These include acanthosis nigricans, tripe palms, Leser–Trélat sign, erythema gyratum repens, necrolytic migratory erythema, acrokeratosis paraneoplastica of Bazex, paraneoplastic pemphigus, and dermatomyositis with or without polymyositis.

9.3.1 Acanthosis Nigricans

Acanthosis nigricans is characterized by hyperpigmented patches and/or plaques with a velvety texture, symmetrically distributed in intertriginous areas such as axillae, neck, groin, and popliteal and antecubital fossae. Histology reveals hyperkeratosis, papillomatosis, and some degree of acanthosis with elongated dermal projections. Melanin deposition is increased in epidermis. The dark color is mostly attributed to the hyperkeratosis [75, 76].

Most (80 %) cases of acanthosis nigricans are idiopathic or associated with obesity, insulin resistance, diabetes mellitus, and drug use [68, 76]. The malignant form generally occurs at a later age (more than 80 % of cases are over 40 years of age) and equally in both sexes without familial association [65, 72]. This form can be distinguished by its sudden onset, rapid and extensive development, and oral mucosal involvement. The most commonly associated malignancy are adenocarcinomas, of which, the majority are gastrointestinal origin. Other less reported tumors include uterus, breast, prostate, lung, bladder, ovary, and liver. Acanthosis nigricans can occur before, concomitantly, or after the diagnosis of tumor [65, 67, 77].

9.3.2 Tripe Palms

Tripe palms is also known as acanthosis palmaris, pachydermatoglyphy, palmar hyperkeratosis, palmar keratoderma, and acanthosis nigricans of the palms [78]. Some authors consider it as an entity of acanthosis nigricans only involved palms [71]. It presents velvety thickened palms with exaggerated skin ridges, roughly resembling to the bovine foregut, from which the term "tripe palms" is obtained. Tripe palms can present alone or in association with acanthosis nigricans. Histology shows hyperkeratosis, acanthosis, and papillomatosis [72].

This skin condition is strongly associated with solid malignancy. Lung carcinoma is the most frequent carcinoma, while gastric carcinoma is more common when patients present with tripe palms and acanthosis nigricans [79]. Breast and genitourinary tract cancers were also reported in certain cases. Tripe palms can precede, and occur simultaneously, or after the tumor [74, 80].

9.3.3 Leser–Trélat Sign

Leser–Trélat sign is a skin condition of numerous seborrheic keratoses in association with a possible internal malignancy. It occurs with acanthosis nigricans in some cases. Histology is nonspecific and shows the similarities between the two [77].

A sudden increase in the size and number of seborrheic keratoses with pruritus on the elderly strongly suggest an association of underlying tumors. All patients should be screened for neoplasms. Gastrointestinal adenocarcinoma is the most common tumor, which is followed by lymphoproliferative disorders [65, 81]. Other carcinomas including bladder, kidney, prostate, lung, and ovary were also reported [82]. Nonmalignant conditions such as pregnancy and benign tumors have been reported, but rarely. Leser–Trělat sign presents before or after the tumor, and the course is not always parallel with the tumor [83].

9.3.4 Erythema Gyratum Repens

Erythema gyratum repens is characterized by a widespread, serpiginous, polycyclic, and pruriginous erythema with fine scales around the edges, which is occasionally referred to as a "wood-grained" appearance [72]. It commonly involves the trunk and proximal portions of the extremities, and usually spares the face, hands, and feet. The most striking feature is the rapid progressing, about 1 cm/day [84]. Histology is nonspecific, demonstrating epidermal hyperkeratosis, parakeratosis, acanthosis, and spongiosis, with a superficial dermal perivascular mononuclear infiltrate [85].

About 80 % of patients with this skin condition are associated with malignancy. The most common malignancy is bronchial carcinoma (32 %), followed by esophageal cancer and breast cancer. Other cancers include those of uterus, bladder, cervix, prostate, and upper gastrointestinal tract. Other nonmalignant concurrent conditions include tuberculosis, pregnancy, and bullous dermatoses [85, 86].

The ratio of male to female is 2:1, and the average age of onset is 63 years [87]. About 80 % of cases have skin findings preceding the diagnosis of tumor. The average duration from the appearance of the rash to the diagnosis of tumor is 4–9 months. Skin manifestation is closely related to the tumor. Resolution of the rashes depends on the successful treatment of the neoplasia.

The differential diagnosis is erythema centrifugum annulare, which is not a paraneoplastic condition, only involves small area, and migrates slowly [88].

9.3.5 Necrolytic Migratory Erythema

The clinical appearance of necrolytic migratory erythema is polymorphous, but the most common manifestations are annular or arciform erythematous macules and papules, with the formation of superficial vesicles and blisters that rupture easily resulting in erosions and crusts, and hyperpigmentation after treatment [87, 89]. Lesions usually present in intertriginous areas such as groin, perineum, buttocks, as well as distal extremities, and central face. The involvement of perioral and perianal areas are most pronounced. Mucosal involvement frequently causes glossitis and cheilitis. The lesions are often complicated by infection with *Candida albicans* or *Staphylococcus aureus*. Histologically, changes are nonspecific and vary with the degree of involvement. It may present edema and irregular acanthosis with confluent parakeratosis, moderate perivascular inflammatory infiltrate with predominance of lymphocytes. There is pallor of the superficial epidermis, with dyskeratotic or nectotic keratinocytes. Multiple skin biopsies may be necessary to confirm the diagnosis. Candidal or bacterial superinfection commonly coexists [90].

Necrolytic migratory erythema is a characteristic of islet cell neoplasms, usually glucagonomas. The glucagonoma syndrome typically includes diabetes or glucose intolerance and hyperglucagonemia (typically greater than 1000 pg/mL), in addition to the rash [90]. Excess glucagon also causes weight loss, anemia, thromboembolic disease, hypoaminoacidemia, and psychiatric disturbances. This eruption may be easily recognized when presenting with weight loss, anemia, and diabetes. In rare cases, this condition can occur with chronic liver disease or malabsorption with villous atrophy. The differential diagnosis of dermatoses includes pemphigus foliaceus, acrodermatitis enteropathica, chronic mucocutaneous candidiasis, psoriasis, and severe seborrheic dermatitis [91, 92].

Necrolytic migratory erythema is more common in patients after 45 years of age. It can be an early or late manifestation of glucagonoma syndrome, and often resolves rapidly with surgical or chemotherapy treatment of glucagonoma [90, 92].

9.3.6 Acrokeratosis Paraneoplastica of Bazex

Violaceous erythematous papulosquamous plaques or patches initially arise on the acral sites of the body, such as the tip of the nose, helices of the ears, fingers, and toes, and progressively involve knees, elbows, trunk, and scalp later in the disease (Fig. 9.8) [93]. Nail dystrophy, characterized by horizontal or vertical ridging or onycholysis, and subungual hyperkeratosis may occur. Although the lesions clinically resemble psoriasis, their distribution is not typical of psoriasis, helping to distinguish the diagnosis. Histological examinations are nonspecific, showing hyperkeratosis, parakeratosis, acanthosis, dyskeratotic keratinocytes, and a perivascular lymphohistiocytic infiltrate [93–95].

The screening for an internal malignancy is strongly recommend when patients, especially male patients are older than 40 years present new onset of violaceous erythematous psoriasiform plaques on acral surfaces, especially the ears and nose. The most common associated tumors are squamous cell carcinoma that occur in the oropharynx, larynx, esophagus, and upper respiratory tract. Less frequently, tumors with or/and without metastases above the diaphragm include ductal breast cancer, cholangiocarcinoma, colon adenocarcinoma, and Hodgkin's disease [96, 97].

Skin manifestations may precede clinical manifestations of the underlying tumor over a few months to years and less often occur simultaneously or after tumor diagnosis. Skin eruptions closely follow the neoplastic course, with improvement after effective treatment of the neoplasia and reappearance with tumor recurrence, but nail changes may persist [93, 98].

9.3.7 Paraneoplastic Pemphigus

Paraneoplastic pemphigus (PNP) is an autoimmune disorder associated with benign and malignant lymphoproliferative processes [99, 100]. Intractable and painful hemorrhagic stomatitis is the most characteristic finding, which is often the first symptom in almost all PNP cases. The conjunctival and anorectal mucosa including penis are also frequently involved. The esophagus may be involved as well as the trachea and bronchi, with the potential risk of respiratory failure. Polymorphous eruptions are observed on the trunk and extremities, reminiscent of the features of pemphigus vulgaris, erythema multiforme, lichen planus, and/or graft-versus-host disease eruption. Involvement of the palms and plantars may often be severe, and paronychia may lead to nail shedding (Fig. 9.9) [101]. Histological findings include suprabasilar acantholysis, necrosis of keratinocytes, vacuolar interface dermatitis, and lichenoid inflammatory infiltrate. Multiple biopsies at different sites can reveal some of these features alone or in combination. In DIF, there is deposit of IgG (with or without C3) in the intercellular spaces of the epidermis and/or basement membrane. IIF shows positive cytoplasmic IgG staining of rat bladder epithelium [99, 102].

Most associated malignancies are derived from hematological origin. Non-Hodgkin lymphoma is the most common association followed by chronic lymphocytic leukemia, Castleman's disease, thymoma, and Waldenstrom's macroglobulinemia. All age groups may be affected. Solid tumors such as Castleman's disease are found in the younger group, mostly before the age of 35 years. PNP may appear prior to the diagnosis of solid tumors such as Castleman's disease and thymomas.

The exact etiology of the disease is unknown. Autoantibodies were detected from the supernatant of cultured lymphocytes of Castleman's disease, recognized cutaneous proteins with molecular weight equivalent to plakin family, and yielded positive staining on rat bladder sections as well, suggesting that autoantibodies produced by tumor

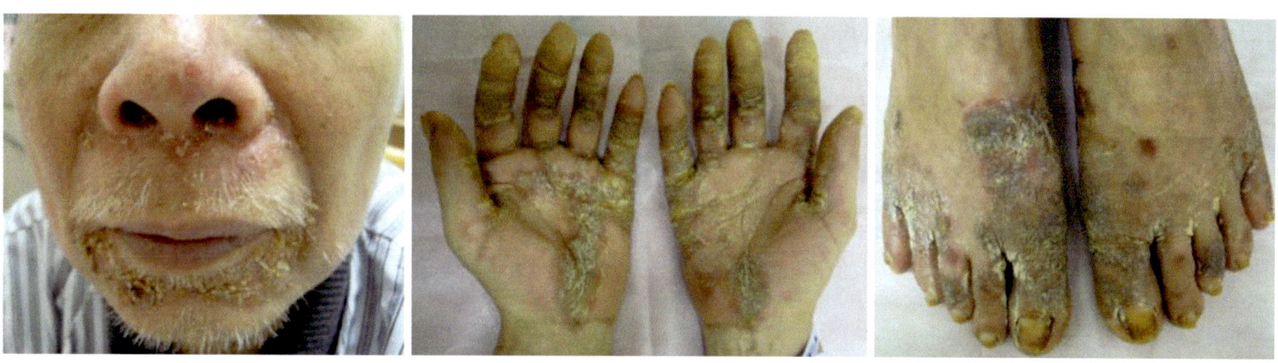

Fig. 9.8 Acrokeratosis paraneoplastica of Bazex

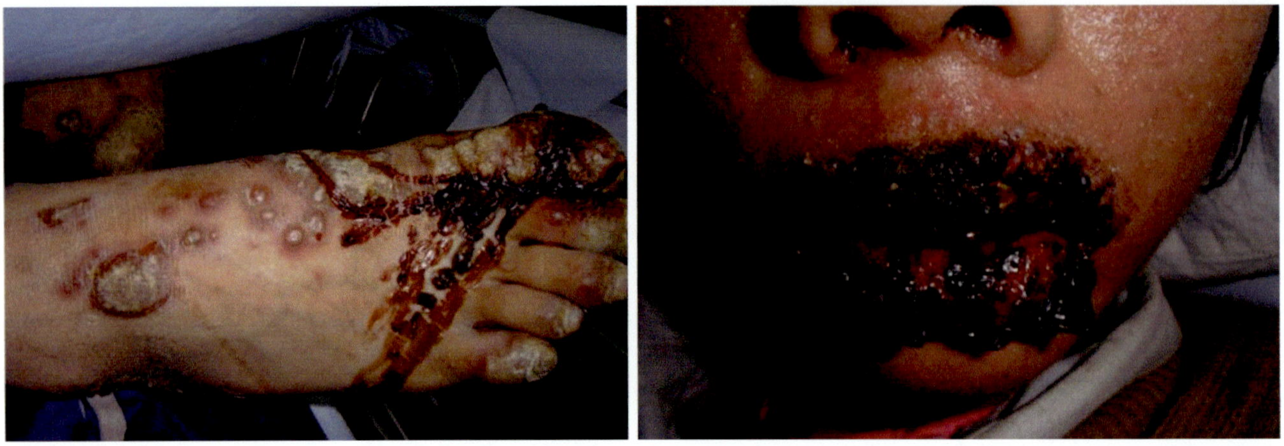

Fig. 9.9 Paraneoplastic pemphigus

cells play an important role in the pathogenesis of PNP associated with Castleman's disease [103, 104].

The diagnostic criteria (revised by Helm and Camissa) suggested for PNP can be divided into major criteria (polymorphous mucocutaneous eruption, concurrent internal neoplasia, antibodies with an immunoprecipitation specific standard) and minor criteria (histological evidence, DIF, and IIF). Three major criteria or two major and one minor are needed [99, 102, 105].

Disease activity and tumor burden do not usually correlate. Substantial or complete remissions have been observed in cases with benign tumors such as Castleman's disease or thymoma after tumor resection. Respiratory failure and infections are the major factors leading to death [105–108].

9.3.8 Dermatomyositis With or Without Polymyositis

Dermatomyositis (DM) is an idiopathic inflammatory disease that affects the skin and proximal muscles. Classic cutaneous findings include a purplish and edematous erythema of the upper eyelids (heliotrope rash), flat-topped erythematous or violaceous papules over the dorsal knuckles of the fingers, elbows, and knees (Gottron's papules), and photo-distributed poikiloderma on the V of the chest and back (hypo- and/or hyperpigmentation, telangectasia, and atrophy) [109]. Periungual telangiectasia, scalp pruritus, and erythema are other associated features [109, 110]. Skin biopsies are nonspecific and similar to findings seen in lupus erythematosus with epidermal atrophy, vacuolar interface dermatitis, and a perivascular lymphocytic infiltrate [110, 111]. Malaise, dysphagia, and weakness of proximal pectoral and pelvic muscles may be overt, subclinical, or absent. Magnetic resonance imaging (MRI) is highly sensitive to muscle disease. Muscle biopsies show perivascular and perifascicular inflammation, as well as ischemia and atrophy. Muscle enzymes such as creatine phosphokinase, aldolase, and transaminases are elevated. Most patients are antinuclear antibody positive. Antisynthetase antibodies can be an important predictor of pulmonary involvement [111–113].

Dermatomyositis with or without myositis has long been recognized as a potential paraneoplastic syndrome, with underlying malignancies in 30 % of adult patients. The rates of association with malignancy increase with age. Dermatomyositis in children is not associated with malignancies. Malignancies commonly associated with dermatomyositis include breast, lung, gastric, and genitourinary tumors, particularly ovarian cancer in women [72, 111, 114].

The musculocutaneous symptoms can precede, follow, or coincide with the detection of the cancer. Most tumors are diagnosed within 1 year following the development of dermatomyositis. Patients with newly diagnosed dermatomyositis should undergo a thorough physical examination, routine laboratory analysis, chest X-ray, and age-appropriate cancer screening. Patients should be closely monitored over several years, particularly if their findings are more prominent than myositis, and symptoms are poorly controlled [72, 111, 115].

Muscle symptoms usually improve with the treatment of the cancer, whereas cutaneous lesions may not response well. Corticosteroids, immunosuppressive medicine, IVIG, rituximab, and tumor necrosis factor (TNF)- inhibitors may help the resistant patients. Relapse of the rash can be a harbinger of tumor recurrence [111, 116].

9.4 Graft-Versus-Host Skin Disease

Jian-Zhong Zhang and Jin Wei

Graft-versus-host disease (GVHD) is a systemic disease which often occurs as the complication of allogeneic hematopoietic stem cell transplantation (HSCT), blood product transfusions, and solid organ transplantation [117]. It is induced by the reaction of donor T cells to recipient histoincompatible antigens [118]. The skin is the most commonly affected organ in GVHD, and dermatologists play a major role in both diagnosis and treatment.

9.4.1 Requirements for GVHD

Three classical requirements for GVHD were proposed by Billingham [119] in 1966. The first prerequisite is the transfer of viable immunocompetent cells to the host. Such transfer of foreign immune cells can occur by several kinds of medical therapies, such as bone marrow transplantation (BMT), solid organ transplantation, and blood product transfusions, which supply patients with a sufficient number of foreign immunocompetent cells to induce GVHD [120–122]. The second essential for GVHD is incompetence of the host to reject the foreign cells. The third requirement for GVHD is antigenic disparity between host and donor tissues [123]. Engrafted donor cells proliferate and attack in response to foreign antigens on host tissues [122].

9.4.2 Risk Factors for GVHD After Transplantation

Previous studies have identified a variety of factors associated with risks of GVHD, of which the main factors are as follows:

Donor–Recipient Factors

The major transplantation antigens in humans are the HLA products. The HLA gene complex is located on chromosome 6 and encodes for several products, including class I and II HLA antigens. Donor HLA mismatching is a dominant and characterized risk factor for GVHD in transplantation from related and unrelated donors and cord blood units [124–127]. In addition, graft failure, fatal infectious complications, and secondary lymphoproliferative disorders are common after HLA-disparate transplantation [128, 129].

Minor histocompatibility antigenic differences can also contribute to GVHD. Sex-mismatched H-Y Ags may be important minor histocompatibility Ags for GVH responses [130]. Clinical data suggest that 40–50 % of recipients of HLA-identical sibling transplants, as well as 50–90 % of recipients of unmodified marrow grafts from unrelated HLA-identical donors, developed GVHD because of unshared minor histocompatibility antigens [117, 129, 131].

Age

Older patient age is one of the most consistently reported factors significantly associated with an increased risk of GVHD [129, 132]. Patients younger than 20 years old have a 25 % incidence of GVHD, whereas patients older than 50 years may have three times as much [133, 134]. Other age-related variables, such as altered bacterial flora, latent viral infection, and less efficient repair mechanisms, may contribute to the increase of GVHD in older recipients. Advanced donor age is less well established as an independent risk factor for GVHD [134, 135].

Gender

Clinical data from MHC-matched BMT show that male recipients from female donors are at a greater risk of developing GVHD [136], particularly from a female donor who has been allosensitized to the putative H-Y male antigen through pregnancy or transfusion [137]. Male patients receiving marrow from an allosensitized sister have a higher incidence of GVHD than female patients receiving similar marrow (66 % vs. 39 %, respectively) [129, 134].

9.4.3 Classification of GVHD

GVHD has been traditionally divided into acute and chronic manifestations. Historically, the term "acute GVHD" has been defined temporally by the onset of GVHD signs and symptoms within the first 100 days of transplant, whereas chronic GVHD occurs after day 100 [138]. Greater appreciation that the 100-day mark is a somewhat artificial division between acute and chronic GVHD has led to a reclassification of acute and chronic disease definitions, based primarily on clinical manifestations and histological findings, known as a series of guidance papers of the National Institutes of Health (NIH) Consensus in 2004 and 2005 [139] (Table 9.1).

Table 9.1 Categories of acute and chronic graft-versus-host disease

Category	Time of symptoms after HCT or DLI	Presence of acute GVHD features	Presence of chronic GVHD features
Acute GVHD			
Classic	≤100 days	Yes	No
Persistent, recurrent, or late-onset	≥100 days	Yes	No
Chronic GVHD			
Classic	No time limit	No	Yes
Overlap syndrome	No time limit	Yes	Yes

Reprint from Filipovich et al. [139]

DLI donor lymphocyte infusion, *HCT* hematopoietic cell transplant

"Overlap syndrome": with features of both acute and chronic GVHD

"Late acute GVHD": acute manifestations after day 100

"Late acute": as "persistent" (continuation of an acute GVHD episode past day 100)

"Recurrent": a relapse of an earlier episode of acute GVHD, or "late-onset acute," which often occurs after withdrawal of immune suppression

9.4.4 Manifestations of Graft-Versus-Host Skin Disease

9.4.4.1 Acute Graft-Versus-Host Disease

Acute GVHD (aGVHD) occurs in approximately 40 % of patients who undergo allogeneic HSCT [140, 141]. The primary target organs of acute GVHD (aGVHD) are the skin, liver (cholestatic jaundice), and gastrointestinal (GI) tract (nausea, vomiting, and diarrhea). Frequently, skin involvement is the first sign of aGVHD, and most commonly presents as a rapid-onset, symmetric, morbilliform exanthem (Fig. 9.10), or folliculocentric erythematous papules [142], often beginning on the trunk, that become increasingly confluent over time [143]. The development of bullae or a positive Nikolsky sign heralds the onset of more severe disease characterized by epidermal denudation. Other epithelial surfaces, including the eye and mucous membranes, can also become extensively involved, resembling Stevens–Johnson syndrome/toxic epidermal necrolysis.

Histological confirmation is sometimes helpful, while it is often nonspecific [144]. Distinguishing between GVHD, drug reactions, or infectious exanthem is often difficult on clinical grounds alone. Initially, vacuolar changes are present at the basal cell layer, accompanied by a sparse lymphocytic infiltrate. The presence of scattered eosinophils, a hallmark feature of drug-induced and other hypersensitivity reactions, should not delay the diagnosis of acute GVHD if there is a strong clinical suspicion [144]. Pathological changes in the skin may confirm a clinical suspicion of GVHD but do not impact the grading or staging of the disease. Dyskeratotic epidermal cells, which may be contiguous to a "satellite lymphocyte," are characteristic of more advanced GVHD, but are also not specific to GVHD [145]. Disease progression results in clefts at the dermoepidermal junction followed by complete epidermal separation (Table 9.2) [146].

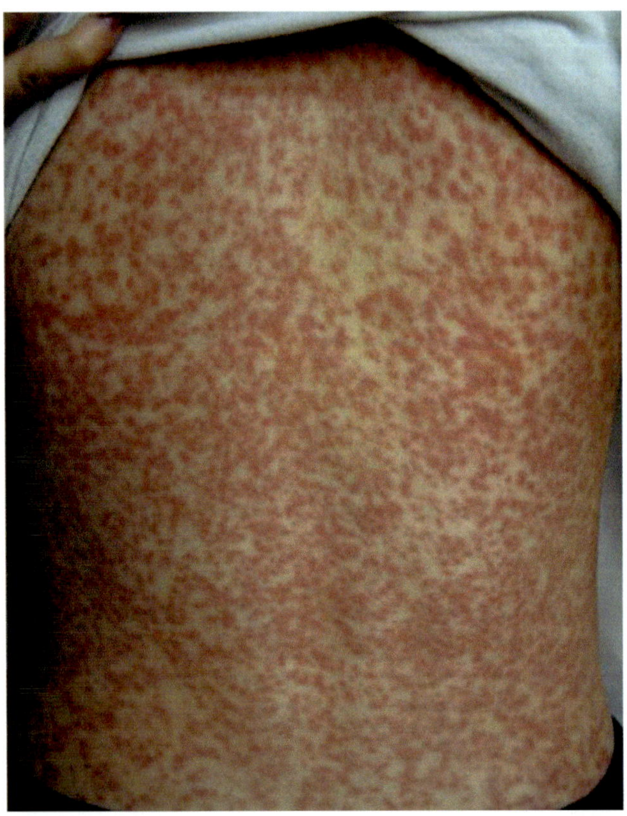

Fig. 9.10 Morbilliform exanthem in acute GVHD

9.4.4.2 Chronic Graft-Versus-Host Disease

Chronic GVHD (cGVHD) develops in approximately 30–70 % of patients who undergo allogeneic HSCT. The median onset is 4–6 months following HSCT, and symptoms usually present within 3 years of transplantation [139, 147]. The skin is the most common organ system involved at the time of initial cGVHD diagnosis; it is present in approximately 75 % of GVHD patients, followed by, in decreasing frequency, the oral mucosa, liver, and eye [148]. Less commonly, the GI tract, lung, esophagus, female genital tract, and joints are affected. Similar to aGVHD, chronic disease may result in significant morbidity and mortality [147].

9.4.4.3 Skin and Mucosal Manifestations

According to the NIH Consensus Development Project, the following skin manifestations are diagnostic of cGVHD which do not require a biopsy specimen to establish the diagnosis: poikiloderma, lichen planus-like eruptions, lichen sclerosus-like lesions, morphea-like sclerosis, and deep sclerosis/fasciitis [139]. Oral involvement with lichen planus-like features, leukoplakia/hyperkeratotic plaques, or restricted oral range of motion (in patients with sclerotic features) and vulvovaginal involvement with lichen planus-like features or scarring/stenosis, joint stiffness/fasciitis, and esophageal strictures are additional diagnostic manifestations sufficient to establish the diagnosis of cGVHD [139]. Various other clinical presentations are considered suggestive or distinctive, but are not sufficient to establish the diagnosis of cGVHD – at least for clinical trial purposes – in the absence of a confirmatory biopsy or other organ manifestation. Distinctive oral features of chronic GVHD include

Table 9.2 Histopathological staging of acute graft-versus-host disease

Grade	Histopathological features
0	Normal epidermis
1	Focal or diffuse vacuolar alteration of the basal cell layer
2	Grade 1 plus dyskeratotic squamous cells in the epidermis and/or hair follicle
3	Grade 2 plus subepidermal vesicle formation
4	Complete separation of the epidermis from dermis

Adapted from Lerner et al. [146]

mucoceles, xerostomia, mucosal atrophy, pseudomembrane formation, and noninfectious ulcers. Both acute and chronic GVHD may present with erythema, gingivitis, mucositis, and pain [139].

Lichen Planus-Like GVHD

The lichen planus-like lesion of cGVHD, well known as a kind of representative cutaneous manifestation of chronic GVHD, is indistinguishable clinically and histologically from classic lichen planus. The lesions can be focal, confluent, linear [149], folliculocentric, or even dermatomal. Lichen planus-like GVHD may have vesicles, and these must be distinguished from those of herpes simplex or varicella-zoster virus infection [150]. Disfiguring postinflammatory hyperpigmentation is a common problem with lichen planus-like GVHD, especially in darker skin individuals, and this may persist despite intervention [151]. The cutaneous manifestations of lichen planus-like GVHD are often polymorphic. If the epidermis is involved, it will have lichenoid features histologically; that is, there will be vacuolar degeneration of the basal layer, apoptotic cells within the epidermis, and a perivascular lymphohistiocytic infiltrate regardless of the clinical presentation.

Scleroderma-Like GVHD

Scleroderma-like skin changes are a prominent feature and a major source of morbidity in cGVHD. Sclerotic changes in the skin may occur at any level from the upper dermis to the muscle fascia. These can be divided by the extent of dermal, subcutaneous, and fascial involvement [152]. Involvement of the upper dermis results in well-circumscribed hyperpigmented plaques of superficial morphea (Fig. 9.11) or gray-white atrophic plaques of lichen sclerosus. Diffuse sclerotic involvement resembles scleroderma [153]. Fibrosis of the subcutaneous fat and/or fascia causes skin, particularly the medial arms or thighs to "ripple" and "dimple", resembling eosinophilic fasciitis. Fascial disease can also manifest as a "groove sign" – linear depressions between muscle groups or along the course of superficial blood vessels. New-onset limb edema may portend sclerotic skin involvement, or fascial involvement may occur insidiously, leading to a range of motion deficits and joint contractures without skin changes. If sclerotic changes are suspected, evaluation of joint range of motion in the affected area is recommended to follow progression of disease. Magnetic resonance imaging may aid in the diagnosis of fascial involvement [154]. Leopard-like changes, with hyperpigmented, scaly macules, may be localized or widespread and precede the sclerotic eruption [155]. Extensive deep sclerosis of the thorax may further contribute to the restrictive lung problems already associated with cGVHD. Alopecia and loss of skin appendages occur as the skin becomes more fibrotic, leading to decreased sweating and an often irreversible scarring alopecia [156] (Table 9.3).

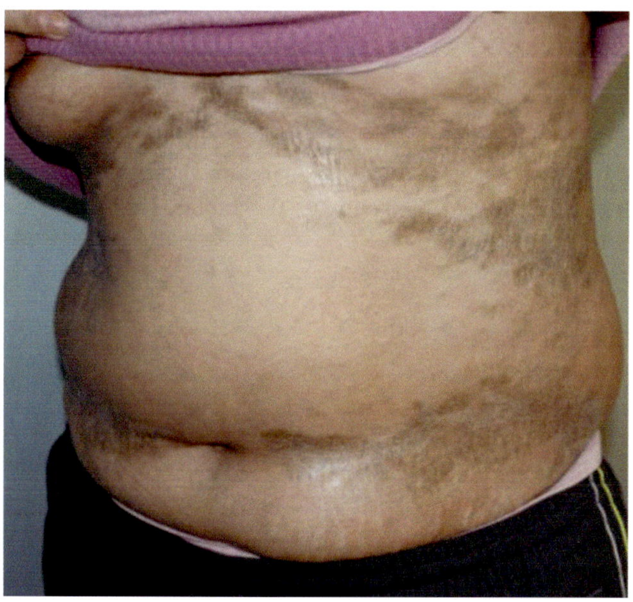

Fig. 9.11 Morphea-like lesions in chronic GVHD

Atopic Dermatitis (AD)-Like GVHD

The striking features of AD-like GVHD patients include pronounced itching, dry skin, dermatitis, and perifollicular accentuation. Also, high serum IgE level, peripheral eosinophilia, or both were common in the patient, often with good prognosis. The clinical and laboratory findings of which are quite similar to those of spontaneous AD [157].

Other Less Specific cGVHD Skin Changes

Other skin manifestations include pruritus, decreased sweating, erythema, and maculopapular rash. Nail changes include longitudinal ridging, splitting, brittle features, dystrophy, pterygium, and partial or complete nail loss. Periungual telangiectasias are occasionally present. These changes affect single or multiple nails, often correlate with the duration of the disease, and cause considerable morbidity for the patient [158]. Mucous membranes are affected in approximately 80% of patients with cGVHD [159]. Involvement of the oral cavity is also common in cGVHD and manifests as erythema, lichenoid changes, xerostomia, ulcers, and/or mucoceles [160]. Perioral sclerosis may result in a restricted ability to open the mouth. Candidiasis may result from salivary gland dysfunction. Genital involvement affects sexuality and overall quality of life [161]. Vulvovaginal involvement in female patients after transplant was reported [162], with the complaint of dryness, vulvodynia, pruritus, or dyspareunia. Diagnostic findings include vaginal scarring/stenosis and lichen planus-like features. Erosion, fissures, and ulcers are also common. Similarly, phimosis may occur in men. Mucosal strictures, like those of the esophagus, may require dilatation. In the setting of nondiagnostic cutaneous signs or symptoms after HSCT, alternative

Table 9.3 Cutaneous chronic GVHD

Clinical pattern	Description
Xerotic or asteatotic	Dry skin, frequently generalized; "dry dandruff" on scalp or fishlike scale as in ichthyosis
Keratosis pillaris-like	Perifollicular erythema or hyperpigmentation with papules or follicular keratotic, spiny protrusions
Lichen planus-like	Purplish to markedly hyperpigmented, polygonal papules with varying configurations: annular, reticulated or confluent; distribution may be follicular, linear, dermatomal or lupus-like; may be vesiculobullous at times
Lichen sclerosus-like	May be indistinguishable from the idiopathic variety with purple or gray-white smooth papules and plaques, plugged follicies and sclerosis of the papillary dermis; at times associated with fibrosis of deeper layers of the dermis or prominent atrophy
AD-like	Pronounced itching, dry skin, dermatitis, and perifollicular accentuation. Often with high serum IgE level, Peripheral eosinophilia
Papulosquamous/psoriasiform	Discrete guttate, annular or confluent erythematous scaly patches and plaques with micaceous scale that may involve any part of the body including scalp, face, hands, and feet
Poikiloderma	Variegated colors: erythema, hypo- and hyperpigmentation with cigarette-paper epidermis; suggestive of lupus when on the face
Dyspigmentation	May be punctuate or confetti-like; generally considered to be a postinflammatory phenomenon; may be associated with dermal fibrosis of varying depths and appear "leopard-like"; spontaneous depigmentation suggestive of vitiligo may be prominent
Reactive erythema	Urticarial or annular plaques with variable scale resembling erythema annulare centrifugum or lupus erythematosus
Erythroderma	Diffuse to generalized erythema over ≥80 % of the body accompanied by scaling, localized bullae or superficial erosions
Acral erythema	Diffuse or patchy erythema, edema and pain of distal fingers, toes, palms and soles; may appear targetoid or erythema multiforme-like with variable hyperkeratosis and erosions; early cases my resemble hand or foot eczema
Dermal fibrosis, superficial	Superficial and mid-dermal sclerosis resulting in indurated plaques with variable pigmentation; epidermis may be normal, atrophic, or bullous and skin can be moved over underlying structures; resembles morphea clinically
Rippled or cellulite-like fibrosis	Skin appears to be rippled in areas rich in adipose tissue-volar arms, abdomen and lateral thighs; caused by fibrosis of septae of subcutaneous fat
Dermal/subcutaneous fibrosis	Sclerosis involves all layers of the skin with loss of subcutaneous tissue, making it fixed to underlying bone; early on may be preceded by edema/lymphedema resulting in a peau d' orange appearance, associated with neuropathy and painful ulcers
Fasciitis	Superficial skin may have varying degrees of fibrosis or may not be fibrotic at all; prominent grooves are seen along the course of tendons; causes marked reduction of range of motion at joints; "prayer sign" is positive
Nails	Nails are generally thin with vertical ridging and vertical pigment bands; pterygia may be seen and entire nail may be lost; periungual telangiectasia is variable
Scalp	Patchy or moth-eaten scarring alopecia with variable epidermal and pigmentary changes and scarring

Reprint from Hymes et al. [156]

dermatologic diagnoses should be considered. Drug eruptions and viral exanthems may mimic cGVHD, or may also induce a flare of cutaneous cGVHD. Phototoxicity from voriconazole, an antifungal agent commonly employed in the HSCT setting, should also be considered in the differential diagnosis of a cGVHD flare [163].

9.4.5 Therapy

Treatment for cGVHD of the skin can be divided into skin-directed (including phototherapy) and systemic interventions. Systemic intervention may be chosen based on the severity of skin involvement, multiple organ involvement, or lack of response to skin-directed therapy. Other important considerations are risk of malignancy relapse, risk of infection, and rate of cGVHD disease progression [164].

9.4.5.1 Systemic Therapy

Corticosteroids

Corticosteroids are first-line therapy for both aGVHD and cGVHD. Prednisone 1 mg/kg/day is commonly used for aGVHD [165]. Higher-dose steroid regimens (e.g., 2 mg/kg/day) have no additional benefit in grade I–II aGVHD [166]. Doses less than 1 mg/kg/day are sometimes used in practice, but evidence is lacking in clinical trials [165]. Corticosteroids are effective for approximately 50 % of patients with aGVHD, particularly those with skin-limited disease [167]. For cGVHD, a common regimen is 1 mg/kg/day for 2 weeks, followed by reducing dosage over a period of 6–8 weeks [165]. Most patients who will respond to steroid therapy will do so within 3 months [168].

Tacrolimus and Cyclosporine (CSA)

The systemic calcineurin inhibitors tacrolimus and cyclosporine are used for GVHD prophylaxis as well as for active aGVHD [167]. CSA is a cyclic polypeptide that prevents T-cell activation by inhibiting interleukin-2 production and expression. While effective as GVHD prophylaxis, CSA has significant toxicities, including hypertension, nephrotoxicity, hypomagnesemia, tremors, seizures, anorexia, hypertrichosis, and gingival hyperplasia [169]. Tacrolimus is a macrolide lactone that closely resembles CSA in mechanism of action, spectrum of toxicities, and pharmacologic interactions. CSA and tacrolimus are generally viewed as equivalent when used for GVHD prophylaxis [170].

Other Systemic Therapy

Mycophenolate mofetil (MMF) is an inhibitor of purine synthesis via the inosine monophosphate dehydrogenase enzyme, and preferentially suppresses proliferation of B and T cells. It is associated with dose-dependent cytopenia and gastrointestinal adverse effects such as upper and lower enteritis [170].

Hydroxychloroquine (HCQ), a 4-aminoquinolone antimalarial drug, has also been employed in cGVHD with variable success. HCQ reduces proinflammatory cytokines such as IL-1, IL-6, and tumor necrosis factor-α, and has also been shown to interfere with antigen processing and presentation and to work synergistically with the calcineurin inhibitors to suppress proliferative T-cell responses in vitro [171, 172]. Responses were observed most commonly in skin, oral, and liver GVHD, and platelet count. Common side effects are gastrointestinal symptoms, neuropathy or myopathy, and retinopathy.

Rituximab is a chimeric mouse/human anti-CD20 antibody, which has been used for the treatment of B-cell malignancies and autoimmune disease. Recent studies have implicated B cells in the pathogenesis of cGVHD [173, 174], and rituximab is thought to modulate both the Th2 and humoral components of the disease. Responses have been reported most frequently for skin involvement, followed by oral mucosa, liver, and lung [175].

Imatinib mesylate is a multikinase inhibitor originally used for treatment of BCRABL-positive malignancies such as chronic myelogenous leukemia. Successful treatment of sclerotic-type cGVHD with imatinib 50–200 mg/day in the clinical setting has been reported [176, 177]. Side effects of imatinib include fluid retention, muscle cramps, diarrhea, and bone marrow toxicity.

Thalidomide has shown modest success in lichen planus-like cGVHD, but does not have efficacy in sclerotic disease [155, 178]. And use as cGVHD prophylaxis has been reported to increase risk of cGVHD [171]. Side effects of thalidomide include teratogenicity, sensory neuropathy, sedation, constipation, and granulocytopenia [167, 179].

Mesenchymal stem cells (MSCs) are multipotent progenitor cells found in the bone marrow and adipose tissue which have generated considerable interest for their immunomodulating effects [180, 181]. Interestingly, the immunomodulatory effects of MSCs are similar regardless of whether the cells are derived from HLA-identical, partially matched, or completely mismatched donors [182]. Some series showed that part of GVHD patients treated with MSC resulted in good response [183–185]. To date, significant adverse events related to MSC infusion have not been reported. However, additional clinical data are needed to characterize optimal dosage, number of infusions and time intervals, MSC growth medium, origin of MSC cells (adipose versus bone marrow), and the value of HLA matching.

9.4.5.2 Topical Therapy

Topical corticosteroids are first-line therapy for limited chronic cutaneous, oral and mucosal cGVHD, and may also be useful for symptomatic relief of mild cutaneous aGVHD. Medium-high potency topical corticosteroids provide relief for superficial skin changes such as a lichen planus-like rash or pruritus symptoms and avoid interference with graft-versus-malignancy effects. Unfortunately, topical corticosteroids may provide only short-term relief, and may lead to poor wound healing, skin atrophy, striae formation, and increased risk of local infection. Therefore, it is recommended that topical medications only be used for short periods and withdrawn or tapered following symptom relief [186].

The nonsteroidal topical immunomodulators, tacrolimus and pimecrolimus, are particularly beneficial for sites at risk of skin atrophy with topical steroids [187]. Topical tacrolimus and pimecrolimus have also been used to treat ocular and oral GVHD symptoms [188, 189]. Topical calcineurin inhibitor therapy is generally well tolerated; however, systemic absorption has been reported in GVHD patients following use on mucosal surfaces and in the pediatric setting [190].

9.4.5.3 Supportive Care Measures

Comprehensive management of the skin issues in the post-HSCT setting requires attention to other risks intrinsic to this population, including drug exposures, infection, and skin cancer. Ultraviolet radiation, drug eruptions, and systemic infections all may induce a flare of GVHD. Antifungal or antivirus drugs sometimes are necessary for good prevention of infection. Sun protection with chemical and/or physical blockers should be emphasized, particularly in patients taking photosensitizing antimicrobial agents, including voriconazole, which has also been associated with increased risk of squamous cell carcinoma in the immunocompromised setting [163, 191]. Patients should be educated regarding skin cancer risk and require regular surveillance for skin cancer. In addition, prompt evaluation of new areas of skin breakdown and other possible areas of skin infection are warranted.

In conclusion, the lack of a "criterion standard" diagnostic test 170, the psychological impact, the impaired body image, and functional performance due to the cutaneous involvement, as do threatens with infection and secondary tumors, all the above makes it imperative that dermatologists play an integral role in the multidisciplinary team needed to care for patients with graft-versus-host skin disease. All the above makes it imperative that dermatologists play an integral role in the multidisciplinary team needed to care for patients with graft-versus-host skin disease. It is important for dermatologists to be aware of its presentation in its many forms, the natural history of the disease, and the many variables that are factored into treatment decisions.

References

Dermatoses of Pregnancy

1. Ambros-Rudolph CM. Dermatoses of pregnancy. J Dtsch Dermatol Ges. 2006;4(9):748–59; quiz 760–1.
2. Lehrhoff S, Pomeranz MK. Specific dermatoses of pregnancy and their treatment. Dermatol Ther. 2013;26(4):274–84.
3. Ambros-Rudolph CM, et al. The specific dermatoses of pregnancy revisited and reclassified: results of a retrospective two-center study on 505 pregnant patients. J Am Acad Dermatol. 2006;54(3): 395–404.
4. Yancey KB. Herpes gestationis. Dermatol Clin. 1990;8(4): 727–35.
5. Morrison LH, et al. Herpes gestationis autoantibodies recognize a 180-kD human epidermal antigen. J Clin Invest. 1988;81(6):2023–6.
6. Diaz LA, et al. Isolation of a human epidermal cDNA corresponding to the 180-kD autoantigen recognized by bullous pemphigoid and herpes gestationis sera. Immunolocalization of this protein to the hemidesmosome. J Clin Invest. 1990;86(4):1088–94.
7. Karpati S, et al. Herpes gestationis: ultrastructural identification of the extracellular antigenic sites in diseased skin using immunogold techniques. Br J Dermatol. 1991;125(4):317–24.
8. Giudice GJ, et al. Bullous pemphigoid and herpes gestationis autoantibodies recognize a common non-collagenous site on the BP180 ectodomain. J Immunol. 1993;151(10):5742–50.
9. Carruthers JA, Ewins AR. Herpes gestationis: studies on the binding characteristics, activity and pathogenetic significance of the complement-fixing factor. Clin Exp Immunol. 1978;31(1):38–44.
10. Scheman AJ, et al. EVidence for eosinophil degranulation in the pathogenesis of herpes gestationis. Arch Dermatol. 1989;125(8): 1079–83.
11. Kelly SE, Black MM. Pemphigoid gestationis: placental interactions. Semin Dermatol. 1989;8(1):12–7.
12. Ortonne JP, et al. Herpes gestationis factor reacts with the amniotic epithelial basement membrane. Br J Dermatol. 1987;117(2): 147–54.
13. Borthwick GM, Holmes RC, Stirrat GM. Abnormal expression of class II MHC antigens in placentae from patients with pemphigoid gestationis: analysis of class II MHC subregion product expression. Placenta. 1988;9(1):81–94.
14. Holmes RC, et al. A comparative study of toxic erythema of pregnancy and herpes gestationis. Br J Dermatol. 1982;106(5): 499–510.
15. Lawley TJ, Stingl G, Katz SI. Fetal and maternal risk factors in herpes gestationis. Arch Dermatol. 1978;114(4):552–5.
16. Shornick JK, Black MM. Fetal risks in herpes gestationis. J Am Acad Dermatol. 1992;26(1):63–8.
17. Karna P, Broecker AH. Neonatal herpes gestationis. J Pediatr. 1991;119(2):299–301.
18. Holmes RC, Black MM. The fetal prognosis in pemphigoid gestationis (herpes gestationis). Br J Dermatol. 1984;110(1):67–72.
19. Al-Fares SI, Jones SV, Black MM. The specific dermatoses of pregnancy: a re-appraisal. J Eur Acad Dermatol Venereol. 2001;15(3):197–206.
20. Ponnighaus JM, Ziegler H, Kowalzick L. Herpes gestationis – oral corticosteroids cannot be avoided. Zentralbl Gynakol. 1998; 120(11):548–50.
21. Kroumpouzos G, Cohen LM. Specific dermatoses of pregnancy: an evidence-based systematic review. Am J Obstet Gynecol. 2003;188(4):1083–92.
22. Semkova K, Black M. Pemphigoid gestationis: current insights into pathogenesis and treatment. Eur J Obstet Gynecol Reprod Biol. 2009;145(2):138–44.
23. Kreuter A, et al. Intravenous immune globulin in the treatment of persistent pemphigoid gestationis. J Am Acad Dermatol. 2004;51(6):1027–8.
24. Hern S, et al. A severe persistent case of pemphigoid gestationis treated with intravenous immunoglobulins and cyclosporin. Clin Exp Dermatol. 1998;23(4):185–8.
25. Doiron P, Pratt M. Antepartum intravenous immunoglobulin therapy in refractory pemphigoid gestationis: case report and literature review. J Cutan Med Surg. 2010;14(4):189–92.
26. Sereno CFP, Marques-Gomes M, Cirne-Castro J. Refractory herpes gestationis responsive to intravenous immunoglobulin: a case report. J Am Acad Dermatol. 2005;52(3 Supplement):P116.
27. Roger D, et al. Specific pruritic diseases of pregnancy. A prospective study of 3192 pregnant women. Arch Dermatol. 1994;130(6):734–9.
28. Ghazeeri G, Kibbi AG, Abbas O. Pruritic urticarial papules and plaques of pregnancy: epidemiological, clinical, and histopathological study of 18 cases from Lebanon. Int J Dermatol. 2012;51(9):1047–53.
29. Cohen LM, et al. Pruritic urticarial papules and plaques of pregnancy and its relationship to maternal-fetal weight gain and twin pregnancy. Arch Dermatol. 1989;125(11):1534–6.
30. Alcalay J, et al. Pruritic urticarial papules and plaques of pregnancy. A review of 21 cases. J Reprod Med. 1987;32(4):315–6.
31. Aronson IK, et al. Pruritic urticarial papules and plaques of pregnancy: clinical and immunopathologic observations in 57 patients. J Am Acad Dermatol. 1998;39(6):933–9.
32. Petropoulou H, Georgala S, Katsambas AD. Polymorphic eruption of pregnancy. Int J Dermatol. 2006;45(6):642–8.
33. Beltrani VP, Beltrani VS. Pruritic urticarial papules and plaques of pregnancy: a severe case requiring early delivery for relief of symptoms. J Am Acad Dermatol. 1992;26(2):266–7.
34. Vaughan J, et al. A prospective study of 200 women with dermatoses of pregnancy correlating clinical findings with hormonal and immunopathological profiles. Br J Dermatol. 1999;141(1):71–81.
35. Garcia-Gonzalez E, et al. Immunology of the cutaneous disorders of pregnancy. Int J Dermatol. 1999;38(10):721–9.
36. Dermatology, B., volume set/Jean L Bolognia [et al.]. editors: Jean L Bolognia, Joseph L Jorizzo, Ronald P Rapini. 2008, Elsevier Limited.
37. Glantz A, Marschall H-U, Mattsson L-Å. Intrahepatic cholestasis of pregnancy: relationships between bile acid levels and fetal complication rates. Hepatology. 2004;40(2):467–74.
38. Lunzer MR. Jaundice in pregnancy. Baillieres Clin Gastroenterol. 1989;3(2):467–83.
39. Reyes H, et al. Steatorrhea in patients with intrahepatic cholestasis of pregnancy. Gastroenterology. 1987;93(3):584–90.

40. Bacq Y, et al. Efficacy of ursodeoxycholic acid in treating intrahepatic cholestasis of pregnancy: a meta-analysis. Gastroenterology. 2012;143(6):1492–501.
41. Aluvihare VR, Kallikourdis M, Betz AG. Regulatory T cells mediate maternal tolerance to the fetus. Nat Immunol. 2004;5(3): 266–71.
42. Doria A, et al. Th2 immune deviation induced by pregnancy: the two faces of autoimmune rheumatic diseases. Reprod Toxicol. 2006;22(2):234–41.

Atopic Dermatitis

43. Nedoszytko B, Sokołowska-Wojdyło M, Ruckemann-Dziurdzińska K, et al. Chemokines and cytokines network in the pathogenesis of the infammatory skin diseases: atopic dermatitis, psoriasis and skin mastocytosis. Postepy Dermatol Alergol. 2014;2:84–91.
44. Howell MD, et al. Cytokine milieu of atopic dermatitis skin subverts the innate immune response to vaccinia virus. Immunity. 2006;24:341–8.
45. Giannetti A, Scarabello A, Miglietta S, Bassoli S. Atopic eczema or atopic dermatitis. Dermatol Sex Transm Dis. 2013;Chapter 51:969–71.
46. Rabenhorst A, Hartmann K. Interleukin-31: a novel diagnostic marker of allergic diseases. Curr Allergy Asthma Rep. 2014;14:423.
47. Stott B, Lavender P, Lehmann S, et al. Human IL-31 is induced by IL-4 and promotes TH2-driven inflammation. J Allergy Clin Immunol. 2013;132:446–54.
48. Auriemma M, Vianale G, Amerio P, et al. Cytokines and T cells in atopic dermatitis. Eur Cytokine Netw. 2013;24:37–44.
49. Novak N. An update on the role of human dendritic cells in patients with atopic dermatitis. J Allergy Clin Immunol. 2012;129: 879–86.
50. Bieber T. Atopic dermatitis. N Engl J Med. 2008;358:1483–94.
51. Bao L, Zhang H, Chan LS. The involvement of the JAK-STAT signaling pathway in chronic inflammatory skin disease atopic dermatitis. JAKSTAT. 2013;2:e24137.
52. Cheung PF, Wong CK, Ho AW, et al. Activation of human eosinophils and epidermal keratinocytes by Th2 cytokine IL-31: implication for the immunopathogenesis of atopic dermatitis. Int Immunol. 2010;22:453–67.
53. Angel CE, George E, Brooks AE, Ostrovsky LL, Brown TL, Dunbar PR. Cuttingedge: CD1a1 antigen-presenting cells in human dermis respond rapidly to CCR7 ligands. J Immunol. 2006;176:5730–4.
54. Kopfnagel V, Harder J, Werfel T. Expression of antimicrobial peptides in atopic dermatitis and possible immunoregulatory functions. Curr Opin Allergy Clin Immunol. 2013;13:531–6.
55. Han NR, Oh HA, Nam SY, Moon PD, Kim DW, Kim HM, Jeong HJ. TSLP induces mast cell development and aggravates allergic reactions through the activation of MDM2 and STAT6. J Invest Dermatol. 2014;134(10):2521–30.
56. Suárez-Fariñas M, Dhingra N, Gittler J, et al. Intrinsic atopic dermatitis shows similar TH2 and higher TH17 immune activation compared with extrinsic atopic dermatitis. J Allergy Clin Immunol. 2013;132:361–70.
57. Mu Z, Zhao Y, Liu X, et al. Molecular biology of atopic dermatitis. Clin Rev Allerg Immunol. 2014;47:193–218.
58. Zhang H, Guo YF, Wang WZ, et al. Mutations in the filaggrin gene in Han Chinese patients with atopic dermatitis. Allergy. 2011;66:420–7.
59. Li M, Liu Q, Liu JB, et al. Mutations analysis in filaggrin gene in northern China patients with atopic dermatitis. J Eur Acad Dermatol Venereol. 2013;27(2):169–74.
60. Cheng R, Li M, Zhang H, et al. Common FLG mutation K4671X not associated with atopic dermatitis in Han Chinese in a family association study. PLoS One. 2012;7(11):e49158.
61. Thyssen JP, Kezic S. Causes of epidermal filaggrin reduction and their role in the pathogenesis of atopic dermatitis. J Allergy Clin Immunol. 2014;134:792–9.
62. Melnik BC. The potential role of impaired notch signalling in atopic dermatitis. Acta Derm Venereol. 2015;95:5–11.
63. Buddenkotte J, Steinhoff M. Pathophysiology and therapy of pruritus in allergic and atopic diseases. Allergy. 2010;65:805–21.
64. Wilson SR, The L, Batia LM, et al. The epithelial cell-derived atopic dermatitis cytokine TSLP activates neurons to induce itch. Cell. 2013;155:285–95.

Paraneoplastic Dermatoses

65. Silva JA, Mesquita Kde C, Igreja AC, et al. Paraneoplastic cutaneous manifestations: concepts and updates. An Bras Dermatol. 2013;88:9–22.
66. Outerbridge CA. Cutaneous manifestations of internal diseases. Vet Clin North Am. 2013;43:135–52.
67. Ehst BD, Minzer-Conzetti K, Swerdlin A, Devere TS. Cutaneous manifestations of internal malignancy. Curr Probl Surg. 2010;47: 384–445.
68. Pipkin CA, Lio PA. Cutaneous manifestations of internal malignancies: an overview. Dermatol Clin. 2008;26:1–15, vii.
69. Brenner S, Tamir E, Maharshak N, Shapira J. Cutaneous manifestations of internal malignancies. Clin Dermatol. 2001;19: 290–7.
70. Maverakis E, Goodarzi H, Wehrli LN, Ono Y, Garcia MS. The etiology of paraneoplastic autoimmunity. Clin Rev Allergy Immunol. 2012;42:135–44.
71. Braverman IM. Skin manifestations of internal malignancy. Clin Geriatr Med. 2002;18:1–19, v.
72. Chung VQ, Moschella SL, Zembowicz A, Liu V. Clinical and pathologic findings of paraneoplastic dermatoses. J Am Acad Dermatol. 2006;54:745–62; quiz 63–6.
73. Thomas I, Schwartz RA. Cutaneous paraneoplastic syndromes: uncommon presentations. Clin Dermatol. 2005;23:593–600.
74. Ramos ESM, Carvalho JC, Carneiro SC. Cutaneous paraneoplasia. Clin Dermatol. 2011;29:541–7.
75. Higgins SP, Freemark M, Prose NS. Acanthosis nigricans: a practical approach to evaluation and management. Dermatol Online J. 2008;14:2.
76. Krawczyk M, Mykala-Ciesla J, Kolodziej-Jaskula A. Acanthosis nigricans as a paraneoplastic syndrome. Case reports and review of literature. Pol Arch Med Wewn. 2009;119:180–3.
77. Thiers BH, Sahn RE, Callen JP. Cutaneous manifestations of internal malignancy. CA Cancer J Clin. 2009;59:73–98.
78. Cohen PR, Grossman ME, Almeida L, Kurzrock R. Tripe palms and malignancy. J Clin Oncol. 1989;7:669–78.
79. Cohen PR, Grossman ME, Silvers DN, Kurzrock R. Tripe palms and cancer. Clin Dermatol. 1993;11:165–73.
80. Moore RL, Devere TS. Epidermal manifestations of internal malignancy. Dermatol Clin. 2008;26:17–29, vii.
81. Shah KR, Boland CR, Patel M, Thrash B, Menter A. Cutaneous manifestations of gastrointestinal disease: part I. J Am Acad Dermatol. 2013;68:189 e1-21; quiz 210.
82. Yeh JS, Munn SE, Plunkett TA, Harper PG, Hopster DJ, du Vivier AW. Coexistence of acanthosis nigricans and the sign of Leser-Trelat in a patient with gastric adenocarcinoma: a case report and literature review. J Am Acad Dermatol. 2000;42:357–62.
83. Schwartz RA. Sign of Leser-Trelat. J Am Acad Dermatol. 1996;35:88–95.

84. Joseph JV, Turner KJ, Bramwell SP. Dermatomyositis: a rare initial presentation of adenocarcinoma of the prostate. J Urol. 2002;168:637.
85. Stone SP, Buescher LS. Life-threatening paraneoplastic cutaneous syndromes. Clin Dermatol. 2005;23:301–6.
86. Boyd AS, Neldner KH, Menter A. Erythema gyratum repens: a paraneoplastic eruption. J Am Acad Dermatol. 1992;26:757–62.
87. Eubanks LE, McBurney E, Reed R. Erythema gyratum repens. Am J Med Sci. 2001;321:302–5.
88. Tyring SK. Reactive erythemas: erythema annulare centrifugum and erythema gyratum repens. Clin Dermatol. 1993;11:135–9.
89. Adam DN, Cohen PD, Ghazarian D. Necrolytic migratory erythema: case report and clinical review. J Cutan Med Surg. 2003;7:333–8.
90. Geria AN, Holcomb KZ, Scheinfeld NS. Necrolytic acral erythema: a review of the literature. Cutis. 2009;83:309–14.
91. van Beek AP, de Haas ER, van Vloten WA, Lips CJ, Roijers JF, Canninga-van Dijk MR. The glucagonoma syndrome and necrolytic migratory erythema: a clinical review. Eur J Endocrinol. 2004;151:531–7.
92. Tierney EP, Badger J. Etiology and pathogenesis of necrolytic migratory erythema: review of the literature. MedGenMed. 2004;6:4.
93. Valdivielso M, Longo I, Suarez R, Huerta M, Lazaro P. Acrokeratosis paraneoplastica: Bazex syndrome. J Eur Acad Dermatol Venereol. 2005;19:340–4.
94. Bolognia JL, Brewer YP, Cooper DL. Bazex syndrome (acrokeratosis paraneoplastica). An analytic review. Medicine (Baltimore). 1991;70:269–80.
95. Rao R, Shenoi SD. Acrokeratosis paraneoplastica (Bazex syndrome): an atypical presentation. Dermatol Online J. 2004;10:21.
96. Sharma V, Sharma NL, Ranjan N, Tegta GR, Sarin S. Acrokeratosis paraneoplastica (Bazex syndrome): case report and review of literature. Dermatol Online J. 2006;12:11.
97. Zarzour JG, Singh S, Andea A, Cafardi JA. Acrokeratosis paraneoplastica (Bazex syndrome): report of a case associated with small cell lung carcinoma and review of the literature. J Radiol Case Rep. 2011;5:1–6.
98. Abreu Velez AM, Howard MS. Diagnosis and treatment of cutaneous paraneoplastic disorders. Dermatol Ther. 2010;23:662–75.
99. Anhalt GJ, Kim SC, Stanley JR, et al. Paraneoplastic pemphigus. An autoimmune mucocutaneous disease associated with neoplasia. N Engl J Med. 1990;323:1729–35.
100. Yong AA, Tey HL. Paraneoplastic pemphigus. Australas J Dermatol. 2013;54:241–50.
101. Nousari HC, Deterding R, Wojtczack H, et al. The mechanism of respiratory failure in paraneoplastic pemphigus. N Engl J Med. 1999;340:1406–10.
102. Camisa C, Helm TN. Paraneoplastic pemphigus is a distinct neoplasia-induced autoimmune disease. Arch Dermatol. 1993; 129:883–6.
103. Frew JW, Murrell DF. Paraneoplastic pemphigus (paraneoplastic autoimmune multiorgan syndrome): clinical presentations and pathogenesis. Dermatol Clin. 2011;29:419–25, viii.
104. Wang L, Bu D, Yang Y, Chen X, Zhu X. Castleman's tumours and production of autoantibody in paraneoplastic pemphigus. Lancet. 2004;363:525–31.
105. Zimmermann J, Bahmer F, Rose C, Zillikens D, Schmidt E. Clinical and immunopathological spectrum of paraneoplastic pemphigus. J Dtsch Dermatol Ges. 2010;8:598–606.
106. Frew JW, Murrell DF. Current management strategies in paraneoplastic pemphigus (paraneoplastic autoimmune multiorgan syndrome). Dermatol Clin. 2011;29:607–12.
107. Sehgal VN, Srivastava G. Paraneoplastic pemphigus/paraneoplastic autoimmune multiorgan syndrome. Int J Dermatol. 2009;48: 162–9.
108. Wang J, Zhu X, Li R, et al. Paraneoplastic pemphigus associated with Castleman tumor: a commonly reported subtype of paraneoplastic pemphigus in China. Arch Dermatol. 2005;141:1285–93.
109. Iorizzo 3rd LJ, Jorizzo JL. The treatment and prognosis of dermatomyositis: an updated review. J Am Acad Dermatol. 2008;59: 99–112.
110. Smith ES, Hallman JR, DeLuca AM, Goldenberg G, Jorizzo JL, Sangueza OP. Dermatomyositis: a clinicopathological study of 40 patients. Am J Dermatopathol. 2009;31:61–7.
111. Iaccarino L, Ghirardello A, Bettio S, et al. The clinical features, diagnosis and classification of dermatomyositis. J Autoimmun. 2014;48–49:122–7.
112. Zaba LC, Fiorentino DF. Skin disease in dermatomyositis. Curr Opin Rheumatol. 2012;24:597–601.
113. Strowd LC, Jorizzo JL. Review of dermatomyositis: establishing the diagnosis and treatment algorithm. J Dermatolog Treat. 2013;24:418–21.
114. Femia AN, Vleugels RA, Callen JP. Cutaneous dermatomyositis: an updated review of treatment options and internal associations. Am J Clin Dermatol. 2013;14:291–313.
115. Ungprasert P, Bethina NK, Jones CH. Malignancy and idiopathic inflammatory myopathies. N Am J Med Sci. 2013;5:569–72.
116. Gordon PA, Winer JB, Hoogendijk JE, Choy EH. Immunosuppressant and immunomodulatory treatment for dermatomyositis and polymyositis. Cochrane Database Syst Rev. 2012;8:CD003643.

Graft-Versus-Host Skin Disease

117. Johnson ML, et al. Graft-versus-host reactions in dermatology. J Am Acad Dermatol. 1998;38(3):369–92.
118. Yasunori I, et al. T cell immunity and graft-versus-host disease (GVHD). Autoimmun Rev. 2006;5:1–9.
119. Billingham RE. The biology of graft-versus-host reactions. Harvey Lect. 1966;62:21–78.
120. Leitman SF, Holland PV. Irradiation of blood products: indications and guidelines. Transfusion. 1985;25:293–300.
121. Alexander G, Portman B. Graft-versus-host disease after liver transplantation. Hepatology. 1990;11:144–5.
122. Joysey VC, Wood H, Ramsbottom S, Morgan H, Ford C, Horsford J, et al. Lymphocyte chimerism after organ transplantation. Transplant Proc. 1992;24:2519–22.
123. Hymes SR, Alousi AM, Cowen EW. Graft-versus-host disease: part I. Pathogenesis and clinical manifestations of graft-versus-host disease. J Am Acad Dermatol. 2012;66(4):515.e1-18; quiz 533–4.
124. Petersdorf EW. Genetics of graft-versus-host disease: the major histocompatibility complex. Blood Rev. 2013;27(1):1–12.
125. Ash RC, Casper JT, Chitambar CR, Hansen R, Bunin N, Truitt RL, et al. Successful allogeneic transplantation of T-cell-depleted bone marrow from closely HLAmatched unrelated donors. N Engl J Med. 1990;322:485–94.
126. Elkins WL. Cellular immunology and the pathogenesis of graft-versus-host reactions. Prog Allergy. 1971;15:78–187.
127. Beatty PG, Clift RA, Mickelson EM, Nisperos BB, Flournoy N, Martin PJ, et al. Marrow transplantation from related donors other than HLA-identical siblings. N Engl J Med. 1985;313:765–71.
128. Beatty PG, Hansen JA, Anasetti C, Sanders J, Buckner CD, Storb R, et al. Marrow transplantation from unrelated HLA-matched volunteer donors. Transplant Proc. 1989;21:2993–4.
129. Witherspoon RP, Deeg HJ, Storb R. Secondary malignancies after marrow transplantation for leukemia or aplastic anemia. Transplant Sci. 1994;4:33–41.
130. Toubai T, Tawara I, Sun YP, et al. Induction of acute GVHD by sex-mismatched H-Y antigens in the absence of functional

radiosensitive host hematopoietic-derived antigen-presenting cells. Blood. 2012;119(16):3844–53.
131. Martin PJ. Increased disparity for minor histocompatibility antigens as a potential cause of increased GVHD risk in marrow transplantation from unrelated donors compared with related donors. Bone Marrow Transplant. 1991;8:217–23.
132. Hahn T, McCarthy Jr PL, Zhang MJ, et al. Risk factors for acute graft-versus-host disease after human leukocyte antigen-identical sibling transplants for adults with leukemia. J Clin Oncol. 2008;26(35):5728–34.
133. Storb R, Thomas ED. Graft-versus-host disease in dog and man: the Seattle experience. Immunol Rev. 1985;88:215–38.
134. Klingeman HG, Storb R, Fefer A, Deeg HG, Appelbaum FR, Buckner CD, et al. Bone marrow transplantation in patients aged 45 years and older. Blood. 1986;67:770–6.
135. Weisdorf D, Hakke R, Blazar B, Miller W, McGlave P, Ramsey N, et al. Risk factors for acute graft-versus-host disease in histocompatible donor bone marrow transplantation. Transplantation. 1991;51:1197–203.
136. Randolph SS, Gooley TA, Warren EH, et al. Female donors contribute to a seslective graft-versus-leukemia effect in male recipients of HLA-matched, related hematopoietic stem cell transplants. Blood. 2004;103(1):347–52.
137. Michallet M, Corront B, Bosson JL, Reiffers J, Marit G, Maraninchi D, et al. Risk factors for GVHD: study of 157 patients from Bordeaux, Grenoble, Marseille. Bone Marrow Transplant. 1988;3 Suppl 1:226.
138. Gale RP, Bortin MM, van Bekkum DW, Biggs JC, Dicke KA, Gluckman E, et al. Risk factors for acute graft-versus-host disease. Br J Haematol. 1987;67:397–406.
139. Filipovich AH, Weisdorf D, Pavletic S, Socie G, Wingard JR, Lee SJ, et al. National Institutes of Health consensus development project on criteria for clinical trials in chronic graft-versus-host disease: I. Diagnosis and staging working group report. Biol Blood Marrow Transplant. 2005;11:945–56.
140. Hari P, Carreras J, Zhang MJ, Gale RP, Bolwell BJ, Bredeson CN, et al. Allogeneic transplants in follicular lymphoma: higher risk of disease progression after reduced-intensity compared to myeloablative conditioning. Biol Blood Marrow Transplant. 2008;14:236–45.
141. Ferrara JL, Levine JE, Reddy P, Holler E. Graftversus-host disease. Lancet. 2009;373:1550–61.
142. Hausermann P, Walter RB, Halter J, Biedermann BC, Tichelli A, Itin P, et al. Cutaneous graft-versushost disease: a guide for the dermatologist. Dermatology. 2008;216:287–304.
143. Friedman KJ, LeBoit PE, Farmer ER. Acute follicular graft-vs-host reaction. A distinct clinicopathologic presentation. Arch Dermatol. 1988;124:688–91.
144. Marra DE, McKee PH, Nghiem P. Tissue eosinophils and the perils of using skin biopsy specimens to distinguish between drug hypersensitivity and cutaneous graft-versus-host disease. J Am Acad Dermatol. 2004;51:543–6.
145. Hymes SR, Farmer ER, Lewis PG, Tutschka PJ, Santos GW. Cutaneous graft-versus-host reaction: prognostic features seen by light microscopy. J Am Acad Dermatol. 1985;12:468–74.
146. Lerner KG, Kao GF, Storb R, Buckner CD, Clift RA, Thomas ED. Histopathology of graft-vs.-host reaction (GvHR) in human recipients of marrow from HL-A-matched sibling donors. Transplant Proc. 1974;6:367–71.
147. Lee SJ. Have we made progress in the management of chronic graft-vs-host disease? Best Pract Res Clin Haematol. 2010;23: 529–35.
148. Lee SJ, Flowers ME. Recognizing and managing chronic graft-versus-host disease. Hematology Am Soc Hematol Educ Program. 2008;2008:134–41.
149. Beers B, Kalish RS, Kaye VN, Dahl MV. Unilateral linear lichenoid eruption after bone marrow transplantation: an unmasking of tolerance to an abnormal keratinocyte clone? J Am Acad Dermatol. 1993;28:888–92.
150. Schauder CS, Hymes SR, Rapini RP, Zipf TF. Vesicular graftversus-host disease. Int J Dermatol. 1992;31:509–10.
151. Aractingi S, Janin A, Devergie A, Bourges M, Socie G, Gluckman E. Histochemical and ultrastructural study of diffuse melanoderma after bone marrow transplantation. Br J Dermatol. 1996;134:325–31.
152. Pavletic SZ, Martin P, Lee SJ, et al. Measuring therapeutic response in chronic graft-versus-host disease: National Institutes of Health Consensus Development Project on Criteria for Clinical Trials in Chronic Graft-versus-Host Disease: IV. Response Criteria Working Group Report. Biol Blood Marrow Transplant. 2006;12:252–66.
153. Kroft EB, Berkhof NJ, van de Kerkhof PC, Gerritsen RM, de Jong EM. Ultraviolet A phototherapy for sclerotic skin diseases: a systematic review. J Am Acad Dermatol. 2008;59:1017–30.
154. Clark J, Yao L, Pavletic SZ, Krumlauf M, Mitchell S, Turner ML, et al. Magnetic resonance imaging in sclerotic-type chronic graft-vs-host disease. Arch Dermatol. 2009;145:918–22.
155. Penas PF, Jones-Caballero M, Aragues M, Fernandez-Herrera J, Fraga J, Garcia-Diez A. Sclerodermatous graft-vs-host disease: clinical and pathological study of 17 patients. Arch Dermatol. 2002;138:924–34.
156. Hymes SR, Turner ML, Champlin RE, Couriel DR. Cutaneous manifestations of chronic graft-versus-host disease. Biol Blood Marrow Transplant. 2006;12(11):1101–13.
157. Wei J, Zhang Y, Xu HJ, Jin J, Zhang JZ. Atopic dermatitiselike presentation of graft-versus-host disease: a novel form of chronic cutaneous graft-versus-host disease. J Am Acad Dermatol. 2013;69:34–9.
158. Sanli H, Arat M, Oskay T, Gurman G. Evaluation of nail involvement in patients with chronic cutaneous graft versus host disease: a single-center study from Turkey. Int J Dermatol. 2004; 43:176–80.
159. Sullivan KM, Shulman HM, Storb R, et al. Chronic graftversus-host disease in 52 patients: adverse natural course and successful treatment with combination immunosuppression. Blood. 1981;57:267–76.
160. Carpenter PA. How I conduct a comprehensive chronic graft-versus host disease assessment. Blood. 2011;118:2679–87.
161. Spinelli S, Chiodi S, Costantini S, et al. Female genital tract graft-versus-host disease following allogeneic bone marrow transplantation. Haematologica. 2003;88:1163–8.
162. Hymes SR, Farmer ER, Burns WH, et al. Bullous sclerodermalike changes in chronic graft-vs-host disease. Arch Dermatol. 1985;121:1189–92.
163. Patel AR, Turner ML, Baird K, Gea-Banacloche J, Mitchell S, Pavletic SZ, et al. Voriconazole-induced phototoxicity masquerading as chronic graft-versus-host disease of the skin in allogeneic hematopoietic cell transplant recipients. Biol Blood Marrow Transplant. 2009;15:370–6.
164. Wu PA, Cowen EW. Cutaneous graft-versus-host disease-clinical considerations and management. Curr Probl Dermatol. 2012;43:101–15.
165. Wolff D, Gerbitz A, Ayuk F, Kiani A, Hildebrandt GC, Vogelsang GB, et al. Consensus conference on clinical practice in chronic graft-versus-host disease (GVHD): first-line and topical treatment of chronic GVHD. Biol Blood Marrow Transplant. 2010;16:1611–28.
166. Mielcarek M, Storer BE, Boeckh M, Carpenter PA, McDonald GB, Deeg HJ, et al. Initial therapy of acute graft-versus-host disease with low-dose prednisone does not compromise patient outcomes. Blood. 2009;113:2888–94.
167. Penas PF, Fernandez-Herrera J, Garcia-Diez A. Dermatologic treatment of cutaneous graft versus host disease. Am J Clin Dermatol. 2004;5:403–16.

168. Vogelsang GB. How I treat chronic graft-versushost disease. Blood. 2001;97:1196–201.
169. Rossi SJ, Schroeder TJ, Hariharan S, First MR. Prevention and management of the adverse effects associated with immunosuppressive therapy. Drug Saf. 1993;9:104–31.
170. Hymes SR, Alousi AM, Cowen EW. Graft-versus-host disease: part II. Management of cutaneous graft-versus-host disease. J Am Acad Dermatol. 2012;66(4):535.e1-16.
171. Gilman AL, Chan KW, Mogul A, Morris C, Goldman FD, Boyer M, et al. Hydroxychloroquine for the treatment of chronic graft-versus-host disease. Biol Blood Marrow Transplant. 2000;6:327–34.
172. Ziegler HK, Unanue ER. Decrease in macrophage antigen catabolism caused by ammonia and chloroquine is associated with inhibition of antigen presentation to T cells. Proc Natl Acad Sci U S A. 1982;79:175–8.
173. Miklos DB, Kim HT, Miller KH, Guo L, Zorn E, Lee SJ, et al. Antibody responses to H-Y minor histocompatibility antigens correlate with chronic graftversus-host disease and disease remission. Blood. 2005;105:2973–8.
174. Miklos DB, Kim HT, Zorn E, Hochberg EP, Guo L, Mattes-Ritz A, et al. Antibody response to DBY minor histocompatibility antigen is induced after allogeneic stem cell transplantation and in healthy female donors. Blood. 2004;103:353–9.
175. Kharfan-Dabaja MA, Mhaskar AR, Djulbegovic B, Cutler C, Mohty M, Kumar A. Efficacy of rituximab in the setting of steroid-refractory chronic graftversus-host disease: a systematic review and metaanalysis. Biol Blood Marrow Transplant. 2009;15:1005–13.
176. Moreno-Romero JA, Fernandez-Aviles F, Carreras E, Rovira M, Martinez C, Mascaro Jr JM. Imatinib as a potential treatment for sclerodermatous chronic graft-vs-host disease. Arch Dermatol. 2008;144:1106–9.
177. Olivieri A, Locatelli F, Zecca M, Sanna A, Cimminiello M, Raimondi R, et al. Imatinib for refractory chronic graft-versus-host disease with fibrotic features. Blood. 2009;114:709–18.
178. Parker PM, Chao N, Nademanee A, O'Donnell MR, Schmidt GM, Snyder DS, et al. Thalidomide as salvage therapy for chronic graft-versus-host disease. Blood. 1995;86:3604–9.
179. Koc S, Leisenring W, Flowers ME, Anasetti C, Deeg HJ, Nash RA, et al. Thalidomide for treatment of patients with chronic graft-versus-host disease. Blood. 2000;96:3995–6.
180. Le Blanc K, Tammik L, Sundberg B, Haynesworth SE, Ringden O. Mesenchymal stem cells inhibit and stimulate mixed lymphocyte cultures and mitogenic responses independently of the major histocompatibility complex. Scand J Immunol. 2003;57:11–20.
181. Tse WT, Pendleton JD, Beyer WM, Egalka MC, Guinan EC. Suppression of allogeneic T-cell proliferation by human marrow stromal cells: implications in transplantation. Transplantation. 2003;75:389–97.
182. Ringden O, Le Blanc K. Mesenchymal stem cells for treatment of acute and chronic graft-versus-host disease, tissue toxicity and hemorrhages. Best Pract Res Clin Haematol. 2011;24: 65–72.
183. Le Blanc K, Frassoni F, Ball L, Locatelli F, Roelofs H, Lewis I, et al. Mesenchymal stem cells for treatment of steroid-resistant, severe, acute graft-versus-host disease: a phase II study. Lancet. 2008;371:1579–86.
184. Weng JY, Du X, Geng SX, Peng YW, Wang Z, Lu ZS, et al. Mesenchymal stem cell as salvage treatment for refractory chronic GVHD. Bone Marrow Transplant. 2010;45:1732–40.
185. Zhou H, Guo M, Bian C, Sun Z, Yang Z, Zeng Y, et al. Efficacy of bone marrow-derived mesenchymal stem cells in the treatment of sclerodermatous chronic graft-versus-host disease: clinical report. Biol Blood Marrow Transplant. 2010;16:403–12.
186. Wolff D, Schleuning M, von Harsdorf S, Bacher U, Gerbitz A, Stadler M, et al. Consensus conference on clinical practice in chronic GVHD: second-line treatment of chronic graft-versus-host disease. Biol Blood Marrow Transplant. 2011;17:1–17.
187. Choi CJ, Nghiem P. Tacrolimus ointment in the treatment of chronic cutaneous graft-vs-host disease: a case series of 18 patients. Arch Dermatol. 2001;137:1202–6.
188. Riemens A, te Boome L, Imhof S, Kuball J, Rothova A. Current insights into ocular graft-versus-host disease. Curr Opin Ophthalmol. 2010;21:485–94.
189. Ziemer M, Gruhn B, Thiele JJ, Elsner P. Treatment of extensive chronic cutaneous graft-versus-host disease in an infant with topical pimecrolimus. J Am Acad Dermatol. 2004;50:946–8.
190. Prot-Labarthe S, Therrien R, Champagne MA, Duval M, Joubert C. Toxic serum levels of tacrolimus after topical administration in an infant with severe cutaneous graft-versus-host disease. Bone Marrow Transplant. 2007;40:295–6.
191. Cowen EW, Nguyen JC, Miller DD, McShane D, Arron ST, Prose NS, et al. Chronic phototoxicity and aggressive squamous cell carcinoma of the skin in children and adults during treatment with voriconazole. J Am Acad Dermatol. 2010;62:31–7.

Multifactorial Diseases with Immunological Involvement

10

Ting Xiao, Hong-Duo Chen, Jixin Gao, Gang Wang, Jeffrey D. Cizenski, Darlene Gou, Alan Menter, Li-Ping Zhao, Ru Yan, Yan Wu, Jinping Yuan, Hong-Hui Xu, Xing-Hua Gao, and Hong-Duo Chen

Contents

10.1 Urticaria

Ting Xiao and Hong-Duo Chen

Urticaria is a disease with transient itching wheals/hives and/or angioedema. Urticaria is divided into acute urticaria (AU) or chronic urticaria (CU, duration more than 6 weeks) [1]. Urticaria may be the skin manifestation of food allergy, drug allergy, anaphylaxis, autoimmune disorders, or infections.

10.1.1 Etiology and Pathogenesis

Urticaria can be caused by different stimuli. The pathogenesis include autoreactive/autoimmune, infectious, allergic, or nonallergic. Causative infections include common viral infections, EB virus, herpes simplex virus, *Helicobacter pylori*, hepatitis B and C, bacterial infections, and parasitic infections [2–5]. IgE-mediated reactions may are causes of some cases of AU. The reactions may result from foods, medications, or other allergens including ingested allergens, injected allergens, and rarely inhaled allergens [2–5]. However, IgE-mediated reactions are rare in CU [6, 7]. Quite many cases of chronic urticaria have no identifiable cause and are called chronic idiopathic urticaria (CIU) [5]. Mast cells play a key role in all types of urticaria. Upon stimulation, the mast cells are activated to release inflammatory mediators (including histamine, prostaglandins, leukotrienes)

T. Xiao (✉) • H.-D. Chen • R. Yan • Y. Wu (✉) • J. Yuan
H.-H. Xu (✉) • X.-H. Gao • H.-D. Chen
Department of Dermatology, No.1 Hospital of China Medical University, Shenyang 110001, China
e-mail: cmuxt@126.com; jlwuyan@126.com; xuhonghui@hotmail.com

J. Gao, MD, PhD • G. Wang, MD, PhD (✉)
Department of Dermatology, Xijing Hospital, Fourth Military Medical University, Xi'an, China
e-mail: xjwgang@fmmu.edu.cn

J.D. Cizenski, MD • D. Gou, BS • A. Menter, MD (✉)
Division of Dermatology, Baylor University Medical Center, Dallas, TX, USA
e-mail: amderm@gmail.com

L.-P. Zhao (✉)
Department of Dermatology, General Hospital of Shenyang Military Command, Shenyang, China
e-mail: zhaolp1@163.com

X.-H. Gao, H.-D. Chen (eds.), *Practical Immunodermatology*, DOI 10.1007/978-94-024-0902-4_10

that induce dermal or deeper edema [2–4]. Non-IgE-mediated release of mast cell mediators can be caused by aspirin or the NSAIDs [5]. Thyroid autoantibodies are positive in approximately 20 % of CU patients [8, 9]. Specific IgG antibodies against the FcεR1α subunit component of the high-affinity IgE receptor can be detected in 30–50 % of CU patients [5, 10–12]. Though the autologous serum skin test (ASST) and autologous plasma skin test (APST) have been suggested by some authors as screening test for autoantibody-associated CU [13], there is no evidence demonstrating the tests identify a distinct subgroup of CU. In vitro/ex vivo studies indicate that memory T cells, sCD154, and basophil histamine responsiveness play roles in the pathogenesis of autoantibody-associated CU [5, 14–16].

10.1.2 Diagnosis and Types

The diagnosis is made on typical case history, symptoms, and signs. Diagnostic testing should depend on patient history and likely causes [1, 5]. Chronic urticaria is divided into chronic spontaneous urticaria (CSU) and chronic inducible urticaria [1, 17, 18]. The latter includes special types of CU: symptomatic dermographism, cold urticaria, delayed pressure urticaria, solar urticaria, heat urticaria, vibratory angioedema, cholinergic urticaria, contact urticaria, and aquagenic urticaria, which may be triggered by scratch, cold, pressure, sunlight, heat, vibrations, sweating, contact, or water [1, 19, 20].

10.1.3 Differential Diagnosis

If the individual lesions persist for more than 24 h, accompanied by pain and hyperpigmentation, urticarial vasculitis should be suspected. Skin biopsy should be considered [1, 5]. The European Academy of Allergy and Clinical Immunology (EAACI)/the Global Allergy and Asthma European Network (GA2LEN)/the European Dermatology Forum (EDF)/the World Allergy Organization (WAO) guideline (2013 revision) lists the following diseases and syndromes that present with hives and/or angioedema or are related to urticaria for historical reasons, as differential diagnoses of urticaria: maculopapular cutaneous mastocytosis (urticaria pigmentosa), bradykinin-mediated angioedema (e.g., hereditary angioedema), cryopyrin-associated periodic syndrome (CAPS; urticarial rash, recurrent fever attacks, arthralgia or arthritis, eye inflammation, fatigue, and headaches), Schnitzler's syndrome (recurrent urticarial rash and monoclonal gammopathy, recurrent fever attacks, bone and muscle pain, arthralgia or arthritis, and lymphadenopathy), Gleich's syndrome (episodic angioedema with eosinophilia), and Well's syndrome (granulomatous dermatitis with eosinophilia) [1]. In addition, the American Academy of Allergy, Asthma and Immunology (AAAAI)/American College of Allergy, Asthma and Immunology (ACAAI) guideline (2014) listed gestational pemphigoid, autoimmune progesterone-induced dermatitis, hypereosinophilic syndrome, erythema multiforme, bullous pemphigoid, and polymorphous light eruption as differential diagnoses of urticaria, and raised cheilitis granulomatosa (Melkersson–Rosenthal syndrome) as a differential diagnosis of angioedema [5].

10.1.4 Treatment

Acute urticaria should be treated with nonsedating antihistamines. Short course steroids should be used in severe cases [1, 5]. Adrenaline is indicated in cases with anaphylaxis [5].

Both the EAACI/GA2LEN/EDF/WAO guideline (2013 revision) and the AAAAI/ACAAI guideline (2014) recommend nonsedating H1-antihistamines at standard or licensed doses as the first-line treatment of CSU or CIU. Second-generation H1-antihistamines up to four times the standard or licensed dose are recommended as second-line treatment for patients with CSU who do not respond to the standard dose. Omalizumab, leukotriene antagonists, and cyclosporine are suggested as third-line therapies for refractory cases [21–23]. For cases with exacerbations, short courses of steroids (up to 10 days) may be administered [1]. The AAAAI/ACAAI guideline (2014) recommends dose advancement of second-generation H1-antihistamines, combining first- and second-generation H1-antihistamines, adding H2-antihistamines and/or an antileukotriene agent as second-line therapies of CU. Moreover, potent antihistamines including hydroxyzine and doxepin are recommended as third-line therapies. Finally, omalizumab and immunosuppressants are recommended for refractory cases [5].

10.2 Psoriasis

Jixin Gao, MD, PhD and Gang Wang, MD, PhD

Psoriasis is one of the most common skin diseases characterized by raised, well-demarcated, erythematous oval plaques with adherent scales. A classical process may begin an episode as a relatively self-limiting guttate type which usually follows a streptococcal pharyngitis, but with consequences majorly same as the most common chronic plaque type, the lesions of which could persist for years and with high relapsing tendency. The recurrences may be induced by streptococcal infection, season change, mental pressure, or without any certain incentives. Typical pathological manifestation includes hyperkeratosis, parakeratosis, acanthosis, and inflammatory infiltration of neutrophils in the epidermis and mainly lymphocytes in the dermis.

Until now, psoriasis has already been known as a chronic inflammatory disease closely induced by T cell mediated immune response, with the participation of abundant related cytokines, especially Th1/Th17 related cytokines [24–27]. To maneuver biologics better and further develop new biologics, dermatologists should be familiar with the immunopathogenesis of psoriasis.

A commonly accepted process of psoriasis related to immune response is started by the CD8$^+$ T cells recognizing the streptococcal M protein determinant in the palatine tonsils and homologous keratin determinant (Keratin 17) in the skin, and the amplifying and sustaining processes are maneuvered by CD4$^+$ T cells (Th1/Th17/Th22) and γδT cells in some kind of self-maintaining vicious circles with the participation of various cytokines [28–30]. The complicated pathogenesis network of psoriasis is crossing multilevels, from keratinocytes' biological behavior to the innate immune and adaptive immune response, and then the underlying susceptibility gene loci [31], which heavily troubled researchers but also offered multiple therapeutic targets especially for biologics aiming at immunopathogenesis of psoriasis.

10.2.1 Cytokines Storm in the Pathogenesis of Psoriasis

Nowadays, people use the term *cytokine storm* to describe the significant change and vital effects of various cytokines in the process of psoriasis. This cytokines network nearly involves all the ones participating in the skin-related immune system, such as TNF-α, IFN-γ, IL-17 family, IL-10 family (including IL-22), IL-10 family (including IL-23), IL-1 family, IL-36 subfamily, IL-37, and others [26].

1. TNF-α: TNF-α is mostly from macrophages and monocytes. In psoriatic skin, it comes from activated T cells and APCs, and gene variants susceptible to psoriasis were also found in TNF-α pathway, like *TNIP1* and *TNFAIP3* [32]. TNF-α exacerbates psoriasis by initiating Langerhans cell migration [33], induction of VEGF, inhibiting apoptosis of keratinocytes, promoting proliferation of keratinocytes, etc. [34]. Its downstream mediators like IL-1β, iNOS, and chemokines like IL-8, etc., further contribute to the migration and activation of DCs, recruiting T cells and neutrophils, and microabscess formation [35, 36]. What worth more concern is its synergy with other cytokines, especially the IL-17 family. TNF-α alone can only induce little reaction of keratinocytes unless cooperating with IL-17A [37], IL-17C [38], and other cytokines. Furthermore, TNF-α could stabilize IL-17A mRNA [39] and increase IL-17R expression on keratinocyte [40], while IL-17A also induces TNFR expression in turn [26]. Now, TNF-α is taken as a central enigmatic cytokine in the development of many autoimmune diseases in addition to psoriasis.
2. Interferons: Both type I IFNs (IFN-α and IFN-β) and type II IFN (IFN-γ) are believed to be important in the process of psoriasis. IFN-α and IFN-β are mostly from plasmacytoid dendritic cells (pDCs) [41], and seem to contribute to triggering psoriasis, but absent in chronic lesions [42]. IFN-γ secreted by T cells could induce the expression of HLA-DR in keratinocytes, and further contribute to the epidermal and vascular alteration [43]. It may cooperate with IL-17A to prime APCs and augment Th17 response [44]. However, despite their rising serum level, skin level, and highly respected role in the triggering effect of psoriasis-related T cells, all attempts that targeted either type I IFN (IFN-α) [45], or type II IFN (IFN-γ) [46] failed to show efficacy on psoriasis. Thus, IFNs' role in the process of psoriasis sounds important from the pathophysiological view, but not irreplaceable, or only of key importance in a small group of patients.
3. IL-17 family: Consisting of six ligands and five receptors [47], IL-17 family's physical function predominantly contributes to antifungal infection, especially to *Candida* species, by stimulating local cells (both immune cells and keratinocytes) to produce antimicrobial peptides and pro-inflammatory cytokines and chemokines [44]. T cells, especially Th17 cells, thought to be the major source of IL-17s and IL-17A subtype, are the major culprits to exacerbate psoriasis [44, 48], whereas IL-17C was newly found and expressed more strongly in skin than IL-17A and mainly produced by keratinocytes [49]. However, IL-17A is from various immune cells besides Th17 cells, including other acquired immunocytes like Tc17 cells [44, 50, 51], and innate immunocytes like NK cells, γδ T cells, mast cells, neutrophils [52], innate lymphoid cells (ILCs) [53], and mucosa-associated invariant T cells (MAIT) [54], with wide functions, and contribute to more various diseases. Thus, biologics under clinical trials targeting this cytokine family are still focusing on IL-17A now, with two against IL-17A [55–57] and one inhibiting its receptor [58]. As these clinical trials all delivered good news, agents targeting IL-17C may be worth further exploring in future, especially for psoriasis.

   Further targets in the IL-17 related signal pathway are also coming into concern [59], and a RORγT inverse agonist (TMP778) has already been produced to block IL-17 gene expression [60], although it has not entered clinical trial yet.
4. IL-12 family: Within IL-12 family, IL-12 and IL-23 are in special relationship to each other. They are with similar structure, effect, and source, but with clear lines on those aspects mentioned above at the same time. For example, they are both of great importance to psoriasis as the upstream of Th1/Th17 arm, but they facilitate Th1 and

Th17 cells, respectively [61, 62]. They share the same p40 subunit and belong to the same family together with IL-27 and IL-35 [27]. They are both produced mostly by APCs, but of different kinds, as IL-12 is majorly from skin macrophages [63] and IL-23 is majorly from keratinocytes [64] and dendritic cells [62, 65]. As several polymorphisms associated with psoriasis were found in both *IL12B and IL23R* genes [66–68], some polymorphisms in their shared subunit devote to different results, as one may increase the expression of IL-12 p40 and increase IL-12 level to promote Th1 reaction, but at the same time decrease IL-23 level [67]. Biologics targeting their shared subunit p40 or IL-23 specific p19 subunits are all under clinical trials with promising results [69, 70].

5. IL-10 family: With traditional member like IL-10 along with IL-28, IL-29, and recent densely concerned IL-22 (belonging to its IL-20 subfamily, together with IL-19, IL-20, IL-24, and IL-26) [71], and their biologics' ambiguous clinical efficacy, the IL-10 family's role in psoriasis is always full of controversies. As the parental member, IL-10 could be produced by regulatory T cells (although majorly from macrophage and monocytes in vivo), and a phase II clinical trial showed promising results [72], but required long-term administration of overwhelming dose with unbearable side effects, which exhaust people's interest. IL-20 subfamily is secreted majorly by myeloid and epithelial cells; except IL-22, their receptors are on epithelial cells with the downstream connection to transcription factor STAT3, to promote tissue repairing, wound healing, and antimicrobial expression [73]. Unlike other members, IL-22 is mostly from T cells [74] and ILCs [75] in psoriatic lesions, and elevated in serum and skin of psoriasis patients [73]. Along with IL-1 and IL-17, or alone, IL-22 inhibits epidermal differentiation and causes hyperplasia [73] but not proliferation [76]. One variant on its promoter was shown to be related to childhood-onset psoriasis [77]. Putting all these together made IL-22 an attractive therapeutic target, but only one product is under clinical trial (fezakinumab (ILV-094)) without any published results yet, while biologics targeting other members of IL-20 subfamily like anti-IL-20 brought some disappointing results [26]. Beside these undesirable situations, there are still suggestions that IL-19 and anti-IL-20R biologics should be further attempted [26] for their abundant expression in psoriasis and direct action on epidermis [73].
6. IL-1 family: IL-1 family (including 11 ligands and 9 receptors), as the first cytokine family detected in skin, which receptors have a vast distribution on keratinocytes, fibroblasts, vascular endothelium, and lymphocytes, plays key roles in antigen presentation and development of skin Th17 response in psoriasis [44, 78]. At the same time, as a subfamily of the IL-1 family, IL-36 subfamily is more specifically important to psoriasis. IL-36 receptor could not be found on T cells or neutrophils [79], but exclusively distributed on the skin and other epithelia directly contacting with the environment [80–82]. What is more important, loss of function in IL-36R antagonist gene *IL-36RN* was found to be tightly related to psoriasis pustulosa, especially the generalized variant (GPP) [83, 84]. Both make IL-36 subfamily an interested therapeutic target.
7. Other psoriasis-related cytokines: Among the cytokine storm, there are much more cytokines with unclear or relatively clear function but proven to be unusable as a therapeutic target. IL-6 is one of the latest ones, secreted by Th0 cells as a proinflammatory cytokine that could stimulate both Th17 and Th22 cells, but its inhibition has proven to be unbeneficial [26]. IL-13 serves as a typical Th2 cytokine in central immunity [26] in psoriatic skin; it is co-secreted and synergized with IFN-γ, IL-17A, and IL-22 by T cells [85, 86]. A polymorphism serving as a risk allele for psoriasis was also found on *IL13* gene [87], but with unclear function and still far from possible application on clinic. Another cytokine worth noticing is IL-37. In contrary to most cytokines' change in psoriasis, level of IL-37 decreased apparently in lesions [88]. Both in vitro studies on cell lines [89] and in vivo studies on murine models [90] indicated IL-37 inflammation inhibition due to external stimuli, which makes it a potential target in future.

10.2.2 Anticytokine Therapies

1. TNF-α: TNF-α antagonist now is no doubt the mainstream biologics in treating psoriasis, with three agents including infliximab, adalimumab, and etanercept. (a) Of these, infliximab is the first biologic applied in treating psoriasis and psoriasis arthritis. As a chimeric antibody with mainly human origin Fc portion and murine Fab portion, it targets both soluble and membrane-bound TNF-α [91]. It is used intravenously per 8 weeks after an initiating stage and could reach PASI score of 75 in 80% of patients, with fast enough onsets [92]. (b) Adalimumab is a fully humanized monoclonal antibody, also binding both soluble and membrane-bound forms of TNF-α [91], which had been approved by FDA in treating psoriasis and psoriasis arthritis. It is used in the same frequency with infliximab but subcutaneously, which may bring better compliance [93, 94]. Its efficacy could reach PASI score of 75 within 16 weeks in 80% of patients [95]. (c) Etanercept is a dimeric protein fused with the IgG1 Fc portion and TNF-α receptor p75 protein; it is not a monoclonal antibody, and could bind soluble TNF only, but not membrane-bound form [91]. Its efficacy was reported to be reaching PASI score of 75 in 49% of patients [96].

Despite the more or less effective rates of TNF-α targeting biologics, decreased efficacy in certain cases is the most common problem [97, 98], and it may be due to the development of anti-idiotype antibodies (even with fully humanized adalimumab) [97] or shift of set points in the cytokines network. The major risk which should be concerned is infection, especially the reactivation of tuberculosis. Other risks include congestive heart failure, central demyelinating disease, and drug-induced lupus (especially in humanized antibodies). Interestingly, TNF-α may also bring additional benefits like reducing risks of cardiovascular disease and diabetes [98–101].

2. IL-12/23: This group of biologics is getting prevailing attention secondary to the TNF-α group. Ustekinumab and apilimod are targeting both IL-12 and IL-23, and several IL-23-specific antagonists are still under development, while another anti-IL-12/23 antibody, briakinumab has been withdrawn for safety concerns [102]. Ustekinumab, a fully-human mAb targeting the p40 subunit shared by both IL-12 and IL-23, have showed more than 60 % of PASI 75 in 12 weeks when administered subcutaneously [103], which also works on psoriatic arthritis [104] and still effective on anti-TNFα-experienced patients [105]. Apilimod is not an antibody but a small molecule targeting PIKfyve (a class III PI kinase) which could block and inhibit IL-12/IL-23 through TLR pathway [106], and was reported to help 50 % of patients to reach a medium or higher improvement [107]. Two IL-23 specific antagonists (guselkumab and tildrakizumab), which are specifically targeting p19 subunit, have passed phase 1 and phase 2 studies, respectively [102]. Guselkumab, a human mAb, has brought a 100 % PASI 75 using the highest dose [108]. Tildrakizumab, a humanized IgG1/x antibody, also reached a PASI 75 improvement in about 74 % of patients using the highest dose. Both were considered to be with a low rate of adverse effects [109, 110]. In addition, APG2305 is another IL-23 inhibitor, short peptide, which could be administered orally and still under study [111].

   Cardiovascular risks are the main problem with this group of biologics, which lead directly to withdraw the development of briakinumab [112], although related statistical significance was not reached in meta-analysis over 20 studies on briakinumab and ustekinumab [113]. Another theoretical risk is still the infections, but with no clinical cases reported yet [103].

3. IL-17: Three under-study biologics targeting IL-17 are all fully humanized monoclonal IgG antibodies. Secukinumab, a IgG1k subtype anti-IL-17A antibody, could bring PASI 75 in over 80 % of patients in a large scale of phase 3 clinical trials, together with PASI 90 on over 50 % of patients, by subcutaneous injection [114]; it can also greatly improve ACR response, enthesitis, dactylitis, skin function, and quality-of-life measurement on psoriatic arthritis patients [104, 115, 116]. The IgG4 subtype ixekizumab is also against IL-17A with outstanding and early efficacy; the overall PASI 75 is over 80 % in phase 2 study, and what is more brilliant is reaching PASI 100 on nearly 40 % of patients in a highest two doses, efficacy was recorded early in the first week [56]. Its phase 3 clinical trials are still ongoing [102]. Brodalumab is an IgG2 subtype antibody against IL-17RA which broadly blocks IL-17 signal transduction pathway from IL-17A to IL-17 F which shares the same receptor. This antibody also managed PASI 75 in over 80 % of patients in a phase 2 study [58]; another phase 2 study that focuses on psoriatic arthritis also showed promising results [117].

   As IL-17 family is naturally involved in antifungal immunity, Candida infections were reported to be of 4.7 % in Secukinumab study [114]. Grade 2 or 3 of neutropenia is occasionally found in both Secukinumab and Brodalumab clinical trials [114, 117].

4. IL-22: As mentioned above, there is one anti-IL-22 monoclonal antibody called fezakinumab under phase 1 study with no result released until now [118].
5. IL-1 family and IL-36 subfamily: As an IL-1R antagonist, anakinra has to be administrated frequently for its short half-life compared with TNF antibodies; it has moderate efficacy in treating psoriasis valgaris, but remarkable for the pustular type, especially those carrying *IL36RN* mutations [119, 120]. Though IL-36 targeting is much more attractive than IL-1, there is still no product with accomplished clinical trial yet [121].
6. Nonbiological therapies: Tofacinitnib is a JAK1/3 inhibitor and could block IL-4, IL-17, IL-22, and IFN-γ in vitro. Tofacitinib has already been written into the guideline of RA treatment; its phase 3 clinical trial on treating psoriasis also has made over 60 % of patients reach the PASI 75 [122]. Apremilast could inhibit phosphodiesterase 4 to decrease cytokines like TNF-α, IL-2, IL-12, and IL-23. Its efficacies on psoriasis and psoriatic arthritis are also promising [123]. BMS-582949 is an orally taken p38 MAP kinase inhibitor which could block TNF-α and IL-1β; its phase 2a clinical trial to psoriasis is still under process [124].

Anticytokine therapies are the mainstream development in the future. Anti-TNF-α biologics are popular already. IL-17/23 antagonists have been developed recently, but need better evaluation in clinical trials and preliminary application. Biologics targeting other related cytokines and underlying signaling pathways worth further exploration.

Although simple therapies should be persistent as far as possible, alternative applications of different biologics might help coping with and even avoiding the production of anti-idiotype antibodies. Furthermore, the combination of biologics targeting different targets could be taken into consideration in order to cope with the shifting of set points in the cytokines network. These might all bring much more complicated problems on expected cross talk among different signaling pathways and side effects.

10.3 Drug Eruptions: Erythema Multiforme and SJS/TEN

Jeffrey D. Cizenski, MD Darlene Gou, BS and Alan Menter, MD

10.3.1 Introduction Paragraph About Spectrum of EM Major/Minor->SJS->TEN

Erythema multiforme (EM) was historically considered to be part of a spectrum of diseases with Stevens-Johnson syndrome (SJS) and toxic epidermal necrolysis (TEN). Currently, based on inciting factors and clinical presentation, EM should be considered a separate diagnostic entity from SJS and TEN. We will be discussing the aforementioned conditions in this chapter with evidence that delineates EM from SJS and TEN.

10.3.1.1 EM Introduction

EM is an acute skin eruption consisting of symmetric red papules that often progress to "targetoid" lesions. These typical lesions, classically associated with EM, can occasionally present as papular atypical targets [125]. EM most commonly appears on the face and extremities, predominantly on the hands and wrists. The most well-documented inciting event for EM is infection with herpes simplex virus (HSV) [126]. EM is further delineated into two subsets, EM minor and EM major. Mucosal involvement and systemic symptoms can also occur in EM which constitutes EM major. EM major can also have the atypical papular lesions as described above. This is in contrast to EM minor which lacks mucosal involvement and systemic symptoms.

EM can be differentiated from SJS and TEN based on the morphology of the lesions as well as the inciting factors for the eruption [127]. Clinically in SJS/TEN, the lesions appear as dusky macules, indicative of impending necrosis. SJS/TEN can also have macular atypical targets and progress to larger bullous lesions. The causative factor for SJS/TEN also differs from EM, with drugs being the most common culprit as opposed to HSV induction of EM. The clinical course of disease in EM is usually self-limiting as opposed to SJS/TEN which are associated with significant morbidity and mortality.

10.3.1.2 Epidemiology

The incidence of EM is not well defined, but has been estimated to be <1 % [128]. EM tends to occur mostly in younger adults, between the ages of 20 and 40. There also appears to be a slight male predominance.

10.3.1.3 Etiology (See Table 10.1)

As mentioned briefly above, the development of EM is most closely linked with a preceding infection [128]. Viruses, namely HSV, as well as bacteria and fungi have been recognized as common precipitants. *Mycoplasma pneumoniae* has also been identified as a causative agent, especially in children [130]. Less commonly, medications have been found to trigger EM. Antibiotics, antiepileptics, NSAIDS, and sulfonamides have all been documented as the most common drugs to cause EM (French [131]). These drugs only account for around 10 % of cases of EM, whereas upwards of 90 % of cases are attributed to infections. Other less commonly reported cases of EM have been induced by parapoxvirus and histoplasmosis.

10.3.1.4 Pathogenesis

Understanding that HSV infection is the main inciting event in the development of EM allows further investigation into the pathogenesis of the eruption. However, it is important to note that the majority of people afflicted with HSV do not develop EM. In HSV patients, current thinking points to EM being a cutaneous immune reaction to viral antigen in certain genetically susceptible individuals, as HSV DNA has been detected in EM skin biopsies [132]. However, HSV has not been cultured from EM lesions indicating that the DNA replication may be at a low level.

Table 10.1 Common etiologies of erythema multiforme (Bolognia [129])

Infectious causes of EM *Viral* Herpes simplex virus (most common viral) Parapoxvirus (orf) Varicella zoster virus Adenovirus Epstein Barr virus Cytomegalovirus Parvovirus B19 Human immunodeficiency virus *Bacterial* *Mycoplasma pneumoniae* (most common bacterial) *Salmonella* *Mycobacterium tuberculosis* *Fungal* *Histoplasma capsulatum*	*Drug-induced causes of EM* Nonsteroidal anti-inflammatories Sulfonamides Antiepileptics Antibiotics
Exposures causing EM Poison Ivy	*Systemic disease causes of EM* Lupus (Rowell's syndrome) Inflammatory bowel disease Behcet's disease

Herpes labialis is the most common HSV infection preceding the development of EM [133], often presenting up to 2 weeks prior to the initial cutaneous manifestations of EM. Both HSV-1 and HSV-2 can cause EM, with cases of HSV-associated EM in children/young adults predominantly related to HSV-1. No defined genetic associations for patients who develop EM have been found.

One mechanism for how EM is induced by HSV involves phagocytosis of viral particles by Langerhans cells. Once the virus has been engulfed, the Langerhans cells travel to the epidermis and viral DNA is then transmitted to keratinocytes. This process is facilitated by E-cadherin expression and the presence of adhesion molecules on endothelial cells. CD4+ Th1 cells that are specific for HSV produce interferon gamma in response to viral antigens thus inducing inflammation and lysis of keratinocytes consistent with the lesions in EM [134, 135]. Patients with HSV who develop EM appear to have a normal host immune response to the virus, but may have difficulty with clearance. HSV DNA has been detected up to 3 months in previously healed lesions.

10.3.1.5 Clinical Presentation

EM lesions are typically pruritic and may be associated with a burning sensation. The onset of the eruption is quite abrupt as most lesions are fully developed morphologically within 72 h [132] (Fig. 10.1). The lesions remain fixed at the same site for at least 7 days [136]. Lesions often resolve within 14 days and generally heal without issue. Patients with HSV-associated EM frequently have recurrence of the eruption. In patients who are immunosuppressed this is more frequent. Postinflammatory hypo-/hyperpigmentation may occur in areas where EM lesions were present, but generally lesions fade over time.

As mentioned previously, EM and SJS/TEN are now considered to be distinct clinical and pathological entities. The eruptions also present with different cutaneous features. When describing the morphology of the lesions in EM, the characteristic presentation is that of the typical target lesion. These targets tend to have a well-defined border and have a regular round shape. Three distinct zones typify the target lesions: two rings of color change consisting of dark red central zone surrounded by a pale ring of edema along with a red-pink halo at the periphery of the lesion. The central zone often displays bulla formation or crust (Fig. 10.2). The initial presentation of EM often consists of round erythematous papules that evolve into classic target lesions [137].

Atypical targets can also be present; these lesions are round, edematous, and palpable. Usually these lesions have a rather poorly defined border and do not have three full distinct zones of color change. These atypical targets can be present in both EM minor and major. These differ from the macular lesions that exemplify SJS and TEN, which may have a poorly defined border and only two zones of change but are by and large not palpable.

The upper half of the body tends to be the classical area affected by EM. The lesions predominate on the face and extremities, specifically the dorsal hands and the forearms [138]. Lesions can be grouped together with the lower extremities less frequently involved. Koebnerization has been reported to occur in EM with typical target lesions appearing within areas of sunburn or other cutaneous injury [137]. The Koebner phenomenon must occur prior to the onset of EM, as lesions do not develop in traumatized areas once the eruption has already occurred.

Mucosal lesions can also be a component of EM, specifically EM major. Very rarely does EM minor have mucosal involvement and when it does it tends to be very mild. Vesicles and bullae are the primary mucosal lesions in EM major, and they can develop into painful erosions within the oral cavity. The external lip surface can also be involved painful erosions and crusts. Systemic symptoms are largely reserved to EM major, with predominant symptoms being asthenia, fever, and arthralgias.

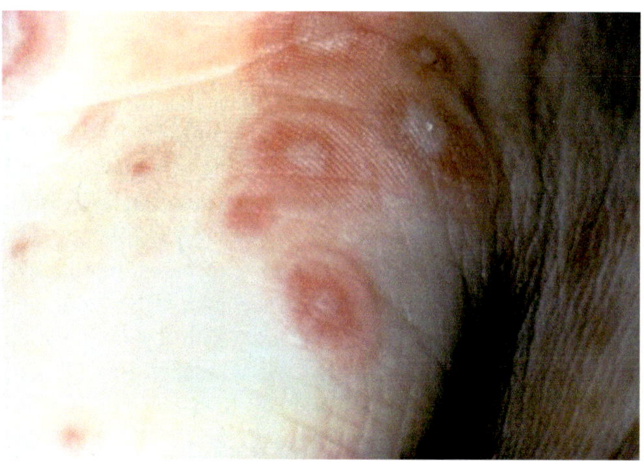

Fig. 10.1 Classic targetoid lesions of erythema multiforme

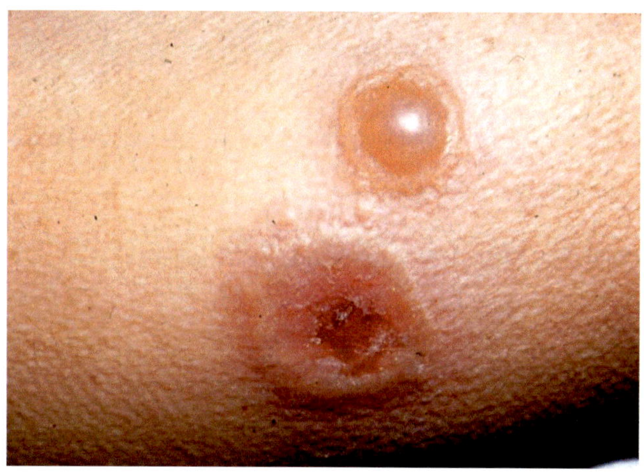

Fig. 10.2 Atypical bullous lesion of erythema mutiforme

10.3.1.6 Histopathology

EM does have characteristic, but not specific findings. The site of biopsy within the EM lesion influences the histology. While the diagnosis of EM can be aided by pathology, in the majority of cases, clinical findings and history are confirmatory. As described above, inflammation causes lysis of keratinocytes and as a result apoptotic keratinocytes are seen microscopically [139] (Fig. 10.3). A superficial perivascular infiltrate of lymphocytes is seen with migration into the epidermis, in addition to spongiosis as well as vacuolar change of the basal keratinocytes with extravasation of erythrocytes [140]. Direct immunofluorescence is nonspecific, with granular deposits of IgM and C3 reported at the dermoepidermal junction.

10.3.1.7 Differential Diagnosis (See Table 10.2)

The differential diagnosis for EM is broad and often confusing for the nondermatologist. Diffuse urticaria and EM are frequently confused. However, there are definitive criteria in place to distinguish between these two entities [138]. The best way to distinguish between these two entities is by observing the central zone. In urticaria, there is normal uninvolved skin located centrally in the lesion. In contrast, EM is characterized by a central bullous, necrotic, or dusky zone.

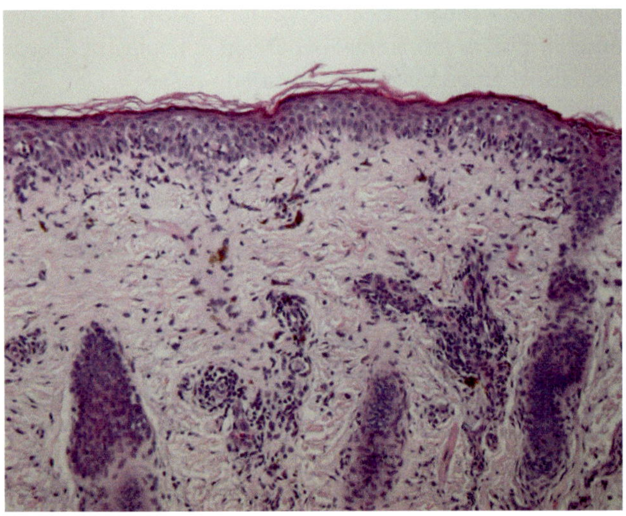

Fig. 10.3 Apoptotic keratinocytes are seen microscopically along with a superficial perivascular infiltrate of lymphocytes. In addition there is spongiosis as well as vacuolar change of the basalkeratinocytes with extravisation of erythrocytes

Table 10.2 Differential diagnosis of erythema multiforme

Diffuse urticaria
Fixed drug eruption
Rowell syndrome
Kawasaki disease
Erythema annulare centrifugum
Paraneoplastic pemphigus
Polymorphous light eruption

In urticaria, the lesions are transient, predominantly fading within 24 h. As mentioned above, EM lesions are fixed for at least 7 days after appearance. Urticarial eruptions also differ from EM with new lesions appearing daily, whereas in EM all of the lesions appear within 72 h of initial onset. Symptoms of angioedema (e.g., lips and eyelids) are commonly seen in conjunction with urticaria, but are normally not observed in EM (Schofield [141]).

The characteristic target lesion that is seen in EM can often be mistaken by other targetoid lesions seen in entities such as fixed drug eruptions, cutaneous lupus/Rowell syndrome, Kawasaki disease, and erythema annulare centrifugum (Weston [142]). Distinguishing between fixed drug eruption and EM relies on clinical features as the histology of the two can overlap. In fixed drug eruption, there are generally fewer lesions at the time of presentation when compared to EM. Rowell syndrome has been described as the presence of targetoid lesions resembling EM in the presence of a positive ANA with cutaneous lupus (Zeitouni [143]). While clinically these lesions may resemble EM, they differ histopathologically and in serology.

EM may also mimic polymorphous light eruption, especially in children with recurrent episodes of EM secondary to HSV infection. Lesions of EM can appear in photodistributed areas, and if the eruption of EM occurs following sun exposure in the springtime, this may confound the true diagnosis (Wolf [144]). A recent history of herpetic lesions will aid in the identification of EM.

10.3.1.8 Treatment

Overall, EM is a self-limited disease, but as described above the recurrence of the eruption is not infrequent. Therapeutic options are available to treat the acute eruption as well as to decrease the incidence of recurrence. If bullous lesions become eroded, topical antibacterial preparations help to prevention superinfection. Topical corticosteroids and systemic antihistamines may also be used if patients report itching and burning. Patients with ocular involvement should be immediately referred to an ophthalmologist. Painful oral lesions require treatment with topical anesthetic mouthwashes and potent topical steroid gels. Treatment of severe oral lesions with prednisone has been reported to be effective [146]. However, other authors argue that this may increase the chronicity of the disease and prolong duration [147, 148].

With respect to EM induced by HSV, antiviral therapy is of no value, once cutaneous lesions have appeared. In contrast, individuals with recurrent episodes secondary HSV should be maintained on chronic antiviral therapy with acyclovir, which is highly effective in preventing HSV-induced EM (Tatnall [145]). A 6-month course of oral acyclovir twice daily demonstrated benefit when compared to placebo. If EM is induced by other causes (e.g., *Mycoplasma pneumoniae*), treatment of the inciting event should be implemented.

10.3.2 SJS/TEN Section

10.3.2.1 Introduction

Stevens-Johnson syndrome (SJS) and toxic epidermal necrolysis (TEN) are severe mucocutaneous reactions characterized by extensive sloughing of the epidermis. SJS and TEN are now considered to be two parts of a disease continuum. As discussed earlier, this continuum has previously included erythema multiforme (EM). The current prevailing view is that while EM and SJS/TEN may have similar mucosal erosions they have very different cutaneous lesions [127]. Inflammatory infiltrates found in EM and SJS/TEN are markedly distinct with EM having dense T-lymphocyte infiltrates and SJS/TEN having cell-poor infiltrates with macrophages and dendrocytes [149]. Additionally, while EM is a cell-mediated immune process against infections such as herpes simplex virus or mycoplasma antigens deposited in skin, SJS/TEN is predominantly triggered by a response to drugs or their metabolites. SJS and TEN are serious conditions and potentially fatal with patients ideally to be treated in a burn intensive care unit.

Classification of SJS and TEN is still controversial because it is based on the percent of body surface area affected, and does not take into account the causative factor. The most widely accepted categorization system comes from Bastuji-Garin et al., who proposed SJS, SJS/TEN overlap, and TEN with and without "spots" [125] (Table 10.3).

10.3.2.2 Etiology

The vast majority of SJS/TEN cases are caused by medications or their metabolites. A summary of causative agents is presented in Table 10.4. Hundreds of drugs have been purported to cause SJS/TEN, with a number of them classified as high risk. These include sulfonamides, NSAIDS, antiepileptic drugs, and antibiotics. These drugs have been extensively reviewed by the RegiSCAR group, formerly known as the EuroSCAR group [150]. Schwartz et al. found that TEN occurs between 7 days and 8 weeks after drug administration, with a mean time of onset ranging between 6 days and 2 weeks [151]. Readministration of the offending drug will precipitate TEN within hours [152]. Patients with SJS/TEN induced by antibiotics were found to have a shorter incubation period and a higher morbidity and mortality than in SJS/TEN induced by antiepileptic drugs [153]. Recently several chemotherapeutic agents have been found to cause SJS/TEN, including antimetabolites such as cladribine, gemcitabine, and permetrexed as well as more targeted chemotherapeutics such as imatinib, nilotinib, dasatinib, and ipilimumab [154, 155].

Infections can cause up to 15 % of SJS, whereas it is less commonly a cause of TEN [156]. There are reports of SJS/TEN arising from *Mycoplasma pneumoniae*, herpes simplex virus, cytomegalovirus reactivation, and dengue virus. Rare reports have associated SJS/TEN with herbal medicines, vaccination, and systemic diseases [156–163].

Table 10.3 Classification of SJS/TEN based on clinical features

SJS	Detachment below 10 % BSA plus widespread erythematous or purpuric macules or flat atypical targets
SJS/TEN overlap	Detachment between 10 and 30 % BSA plus widespread purpuric macules or flat atypical targets
TEN with spots	Detachment above 30 % BSA plus widespread purpuric macules or flat atypical targets
TEN without spots	Detachment above 10 % BSA with large epidermal sheets and without any purpuric macule or targets

10.3.2.3 Epidemiology

SJS and TEN are rare diseases, with an incidence of 1–7.1 and 0.4–1.4 cases per million per year worldwide, respectively [164]. The combined incidences of SJS and SJS/TEN do overlap. Women account for over 60 % of cases [165]. The average age is typically found to be higher in TEN than SJS [166]. There have been multiple studies showing an association between SJS/TEN and HIV, with one study showing a thousandfold increase in incidence of SJS/TEN in

Table 10.4 Etiologies of SJS/TEN [150–163]

A. High-risk drugs
Nevirapine
Lamotrigine
Carbamazepine
Phenytoin
Phenobarbital
Anti-infective sulfonamides, particularly cotrimoxazole
Sulfasalazine
Allopurinol
Nonsteroidal anti-inflammatory drugs, particularly oxicam
B. Low-risk drugs
Setraline
Acetic acid NSAIDS
Macrolides
Quinolones
Cephalosporins
Tetracyclines
Aminopenicillins
C. Infectious agents
Mycoplasma pneumoniae
Herpes simplex virus
Cytomegalovirus
Varicella virus
Dengue virus
D. Other etiologies
Herbal medications
Ophiopogonis tuber
Vaccinations, including varicella vaccination, influenza vaccination, hepatitis B vaccination, BCG vaccine
Contrast medium
Graft-versus-host disease
Systemic lupus erythromatosus

HIV positive patients. Eight out of the 167 patients (4.8 %) with SJS, TEN, and SJS/TEN overlap in a 2-year period in Germany were found to have AIDS [167]. Certain antiretroviral therapies may also play a role; the non-nucleoside reverse transcriptase inhibitor nevirapine is well known as a high-risk medication, with SJS/TEN occurring in 0.3 % of patients on nevirapine therapy [168].

Genetic Associations

Human leukocyte antigens (HLAs) are a strong marker for SJS/TEN in specific ethnic groups. The finding that HLA-B*5701 was strongly associated with hypersensitivity to abacavir sparked growing interest in the role of HLA in severe drug reactions [169, 170]. Carbamazapine-induced SJS/TEN was subsequently found to have a 100 % association with HLA-B*1502 in 44 Han Chinese patients [171]. In a study on SJS/TEN related to cold medicines including NSAIDS and multi-ingredient cold medications, HLA-B*44:03 was associated with SJS/TEN in an Indian and Brazilian population, but not a Korean population. In addition, researchers found that HLA-A*02:06 may be weakly associated with SJS/TEN in Koreans, but not the Indian and Brazilian population [172]. HLA-B*5801 was strongly associated with allopurinol-related SJS/TEN in Japanese patients [173]. Other HLA haplotypes have been associated with specific drug-induced SJS/TEN cases in various ethnic groups (see Table 10.5). While these haplotypes are risk factors, they have not been found to be sufficient nor necessary to explain all disease cases. However as more SJS/TEN-HLA associations emerge, genetic databases will hopefully allow prescriptions to be tailored to an individual's genetic risk [174, 175].

10.3.2.4 Pathogenesis

The complete pathophysiology of SJS/TEN has yet to be fully elucidated. Fas and granulysin-mediated apoptotic pathways, reactive oxygen species, and cytokine-induced amplification of apoptosis are all implicated.

Table 10.5 Genetic associations in SJS/TEN [169–180]

HLA haplotype	Ethnic group	Associated drug
HLA-B*1502	Han Chinese, Malay, Indian, Thai	Carbamazepine
HLA-B*1502	Thai	Phenytoin
HLA-B*1511	Japanese	Carbamazepine
HLA-A*3101	Northern Europeans	Carbamazepine
HLA-B*44:03	Indian, Brazilian	NSAIDS, multi-ingredient cold medications
HLA-B*5901	Korean, Japanese	Methazolamide
HLA-B*5701	Caucasians	Abacavir
HLA-A*02:06	Korean	NSAIDS, multi-ingredient cold medications
HLA-B*5801	Japanese, Thai	Allopurinol

FAS

TEN patients have long been shown to have high levels of Fas ligand (FasL), with dense keratinocyte localization of FasL in affected skin. In addition, the lytic activity of keratinocyte-bound FasL could be blocked by addition of FasL-binding monoclonal antibody. Further investigations did not demonstrate the expression of FasL on keratinocytes; however, soluble Fas ligand (sFasL) was found to be secreted by peripheral blood mononuclear cells obtained from TEN/SJS patients when exposed to the causal drug. In vitro analyses of cultured keratinocytes showed the sera of TEN/SJS-induced keratinocyte apoptosis [175, 181, 182]. The serum levels of sFasL do not correlate with SJS/TEN severity [183], and FasL has been shown to be increased in drug-induced hypersensitivity reactions. This suggest that sFasL may not be specific for SJS/TEN, and higher levels of sFasL may be more of an indicator for hepatic damage [184].

Granulysin

Granulysin is a pro-apoptotic protein secreted in two forms by cytotoxic T-lymphocytes (CTLs) and natural killer (NK) cells. It is made as a 15 kD molecule and portions from the amino and carboxy termini are cleaved into a 9kD form. The 9kD form is released in granules along with granzyme B and perforin via receptor-mediated exocytosis, while the 15kD form is constitutively secreted. Chung et al. detected granulysin in TEN blisters, and found that the predominant cells in SJS/TEN blister fluid were CTL, NK, and natural killer T cells. The severity of the lesions correlated with granulysin levels, and granulysin demonstrated a dose-dependent cytotoxicity in vitro. Intradermal injection of granulysin in nude mice produced lesions resembling SJS/TEN [185]. Subsequently, serum levels of granulysin were found to be increased in 4 of 5 patients with SJS/TEN before skin detachment or the development of mucosal lesions, whereas granulysin levels were increased in only 1 of 24 patients with ordinary drug-induced skin reactions [186].

Granzyme B and Perforin

Granzyme B and perforin also play important roles in keratinocyte apoptosis. After being exocytosed in granules by cytolytic T cells, these proteins create channels in the cell membrane and activate caspases thus causing cell apoptosis. Mononuclear cells from TEN blister fluid were shown to induce apoptosis in the pretense of anti-Fas antibodies, but not in the presence of EGTA and $MgCl_2$, inhibitors of calcium-dependent perforin/granzyme B-mediated cell lysis [187]. Granzyme B and perforin were present in higher levels in SJS/TEN patients in comparison to control subjects [188].

Oxidative Stress

Oxidative stress is also implicated in SJS/TEN. Glutathione-S-transferase-pi, a marker of oxidative stress in keratinocytes, is expressed in greater abundance in TEN compared with other cutaneous drug reactions [189]. By interfering with intracellular processes and damaging membranes, reactive oxygen species trigger pro-apoptotic pathways including FasL and tumor necrosis factor alpha (TNF-α). TNF-α activates TNFA-R1, causing caspase activation, Fas and FasL expression, and cell death. TNF-α is elevated in blister fluid, skin, and sera of TEN patients [190–192]. TNF-α also stimulates nitric oxide production. Nitric oxide is also involved in FasL expression, activating caspases via p53 inhibition, and interfering with the electron transport chain thus worsening oxidative stress [193, 194]. Inducible NO synthase (iNOS) has been shown to be increased in the prebullous skin samples of patients with SJS/TEN [195].

Other Pathways

Other apoptotic pathways implicated in SJS/TEN include the activation of CTL and NK via recognition of keratinocyte-bound HLA-E. Keratinocytes in affected skin express HLA-E, which sensitizes keratinocytes to killing by CD94/NKG2C-positive CTL. Flow cytometry showed increased CD94/NKG2C-positive CTL and NK cells in patients with SJS/TEN [196]. Takahashi et al. found Treg cells were present in normal frequency but have impaired function during the acute stage of TEN. After disease resolution, Treg cells regain function, suggesting that a transient impairment in function is related to severe epidermal damage, whereas in drug-induced hypersensitivity syndrome there is a gradual loss of Treg function which may increase the risk of subsequent autoimmunity [197].

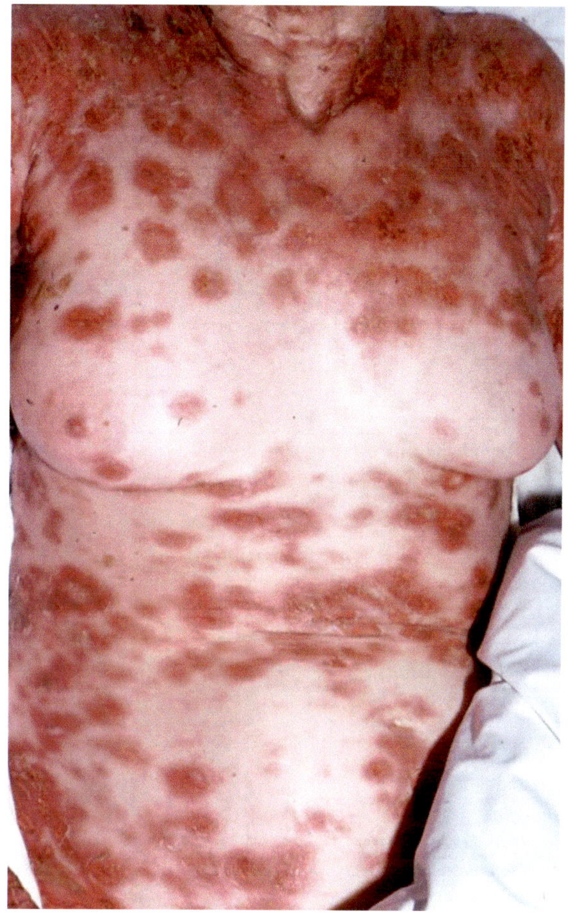

Fig. 10.4 Erosions and full thickness ulcerations with sloughing of skin in a patient with TEN

10.3.2.5 Clinical Manifestations (See Fig. 10.4)

SJS and TEN typically have a prodrome of fever, malaise, cough, rhinorrhea, conjunctivitis, and anorexia. Subsequently, a painful, symmetric, macular rash appears initially on the face and trunk with subsequent spread to the extremities [175]. This rash may be morbiliform or consist of atypical targetoid macules [151, 198, 199]. The Nikolsky sign is present in TEN, i.e., gentle lateral pressure induces large sheets of epidermal sloughing. Flaccid bullae, skin erosions, and ulceration of mucosal surfaces develop over 1 day to 2 weeks [199]. Mucosal sites affected in order of frequency include the oral cavity, conjunctiva, urogenital epithelium, trachea, bronchi, esophageal membranes, and rarely, intestines [199–203]. A variable period of re-epithelialization begins within several days and occurs over the ensuing 1–3 weeks. Mucosal sites and areas of pressure, maceration, or infection are slower to heal.

Complications (See Table 10.6)

Complications in SJS/TEN are frequently seen, and include massive fluid loss through denuded skin, electrolyte imbalance, acute renal failure, hypovolemic shock, insulin resistance, and hypercatabolic state. Cytokines involved in the pathogenesis of TEN may have a direct effect on destruction of tubular cells, the glomerular filtration barrier, and mesangial cells [204]. Involvement of pulmonary mucosa in addition to severe systemic disease may lead to respiratory failure; patients who develop adult respiratory distress syndrome require prolonged mechanical ventilation. Other pulmonary complications include pulmonary edema, bacterial pneumonitis, and bronchiolitis obliterans. Long-term pulmonary abnormalities have been observed, showing a persistent reduction in carbon monoxide diffusing capacity of 35–40% of normal [203, 205–207]. Hematologic abnormalities, in particular anemia and leukopenia, are common [208]. Persistent neutropenia heralds a poor prognosis, whereas recovery of the granulocyte count portends a favorable outcome [209]. Lee et al. found SJS/TEN patients to have mild hepatocellular-type liver injury of relatively brief duration, whereas those with drug reaction with eosinophilia and drug-induced hypersensitivity syndrome had severe and prolonged hepatocellular injury in addition to cholestatic liver injury [210].

Due to loss of the epidermal barrier, patients are at high risk of bacterial infection and death from sepsis. In one study, bacteremia was detected in 48 out of 179 patients with

Table 10.6 Complications of SJS/TEN [203–207, 209–216]

A. Fluid and electrolyte loss/imbalance
B. Metabolic
Hypercatabolic state
Insulin resistance
C. Pulmonary
Acute respiratory distress syndrome
Pulmonary edema
Bacterial pneumonitis
Bronchiolitis obliterans
Bronchiectasis
D. Hematologic
Anemia
Neutropenia
Leukopenia
Disseminated intravascular coagulation
E. Gastrointestinal
Diarrhea
Ulceration
Perforation
Intussuception
Gastrointestinal bleeding
F. Hepatic
Hepatocellular damage
Hypoalbuminemia
G. Renal
Acute renal failure
Microalbuminuria
H. Infections
Staphylococcus aureus
Pseudomonas aeruginosa
Enterobactereiaceae
Candida species
Polymicrobial gram-negative bacteria

SJS/TEN, with *Staphylococcus aureus*, *Pseudomonas aeruginosa*, and Enterobacteriaceae being the most commonly found pathogens, although polymicrobial gram negative and candidal infections can also occur. The percent of body surface area involved was the main predictor of systemic infection with more than 50 % of deaths in patients with SJS/TEN attributable to sepsis [211, 212].

10.3.2.6 Histopathologic Findings (Fig. 10.5)

Massive keratinocyte apoptosis in SJS and TEN leads to subepidermal bullae with separation of the epidermis from the dermis at the dermoepidermal junction. There is occasional edema in the papillary dermis. The dermal infiltrate is sparse in SJS/TEN and consists mainly of macrophages and dendrocytes [159]. The paucicellular nature of SJS/TEN is consistent with the theory that widespread keratinocyte death is mediated by cytokines rather than by cell-mediated death [182, 217]. While TEN is described as having a paucicellular infiltrate, 22 % of patients in one series had biopsies showing intermediate or extensive dermal infiltrates [159]. In a subsequent study, the extent of inflammation correlated with poorer outcomes [217].

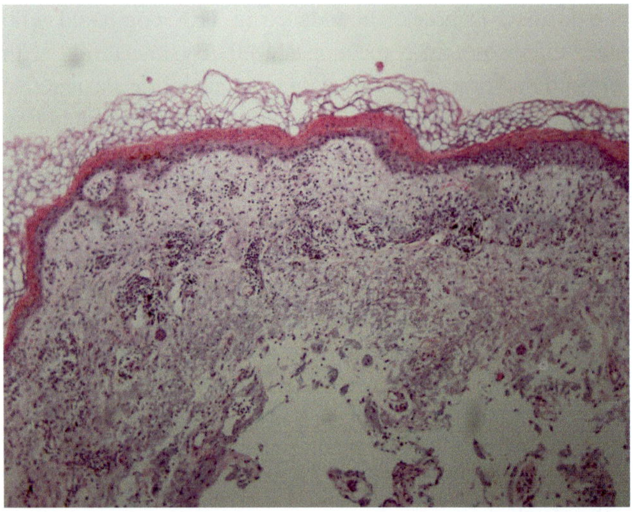

Fig. 10.5 Massive keratinocyte apoptosis in SJS and TEN leads to subepidermal bullae with separation of the epidermis from the dermis at the dermoepidermal junction. There is also papillary dermal edema with a sparse inflammatory infiltrate

10.3.2.7 Differential Diagnosis

The differential diagnosis of SJS/TEN is broad, and includes erythema multiforme, acute generalized exanthematous pustulosis, staphylococcal scalded skin syndrome, drug eruption with eosinophilia and systemic symptoms, drug-induced linear IgA bullous dermatosis, and graft-versus-host disease. The clinical and histological features of these conditions, outlined by Schwartz et al., are shown in Table 10.7.

1. Erythema multiforme. This is typically induced by infection with herpes simplex or *Mycoplasma pneumoniae* infection, and less often by medications.
2. Acute generalized exanthematous pustulosis (AGEP). This is a rare eruption typically caused by drugs characterized by nonfollicular sterile pustules on a background of edematous erythema. AGEP may have nonerosive mucosal lesions along with blisters and targetoid lesions. Histopathologically, subcorneal or intraepidermal pustules with papillary dermal edema and focal necrotic keratinocytes are seen [218].
3. Staphylococcal scalded skin syndrome (SSSS). This is caused by epidermolytic toxins produced by staphylococci and is typically seen in young children. Detachment of the epidermal layer is seen; however, there is no mucous membrane involvement as there is in TEN. In addition, histology of SSSS shows sloughing of the superficial epidermis, whereas in TEN there is full-thickness epidermal necrosis and sloughing [219, 220].
4. Drug eruption with eosinophilia and systemic symptoms (DRESS) syndrome. This can similarly present with atypical targetoid plaques, bullae and lip erosions, but full-thickness epidermal denudation is not present, and the

Table 10.7 Differential diagnosis of SJS/TEN [151]

	Type of differentiation from TEN	
Disease	Clinical	Histological
Erythema multiforme minor	Typical or atypical target lesions; symmetric acral predominance; lack of mucosal involvement; most commonly caused by infections	Clinical features facilitate distinction; epidermal cell death far less extensive
Erythema multiforme major	Typical or atypical target lesions; symmetric acral predominance; most commonly caused by infections; minimal epidermal exfoliation and bullae	Clinical features facilitate distinction; epidermal cell death far less extensive; scattered necrotic keratinocytes
Staphylococcal scalded skin syndrome	No mucositis and superficial epidermal peeling	Intraepidermal blistering
Drug-induced linear IgA	Rare mucositis and annular distribution of bullae	Direct immunofluorescence studies reveal linear deposits of IgA along the basement membrane
Drug reaction with eosinophilia and systemic symptoms	Atypical targetoid plaques, bullae, and lip erosions	Lack of full-thickness epidermal denudation; prominent cellular infiltrate
Severe acute graft-versus-host disease	Foliculocentric distribution of eruption and acral to proximal spread of bullae	Indistinguishable from TEN
Acute generalized exanthematous pustulosis	Rare, nonerosive mucous membrane involvement	Intraepidermal pustules and focal necrotic keratinocytes

infiltrate in DRESS syndrome is prominent rather than paucicellular [221].

5. Drug-induced linear IgA bullous dermatosis. This presents with the sudden onset of tense bullae in annular or herpetiform configuration. Vancomycin is the most commonly implicated medication. Mucosal erosions or ulcers may also be present. Immunofluoresecence shows typical linear deposition of IgA along the basement membrane zone [222, 223].
6. GVHD. While mild acute graft-versus-host disease (GVHD) is easily distinguished from SJS/TEN, severe acute GVHD is characterized by generalized erythroderma with bullae formation and desquamation. Histologically, there is full thickness epidermal necrosis and can be indistinguishable from TEN. GVHD typically has a folliculocentric eruption early in the course, and the rash spreads from limbs to the trunk in contrast to that of SJS/TEN [224, 225].

10.3.2.8 Treatment

A multidisciplinary management team is necessary for the treatment of SJS/TEN, with three areas of focus: withdrawal of the offending agent, supportive care, and active intervention [226]. Patients with SJS/TEN should ideally be diagnosed early and transferred expeditiously to a burn intensive care unit. This correlates with decreased rates of bacteremia, septicemia, and mortality [227–229]. Burn units are ideal for providing contact isolation, temperature regulation, fluid balance, and monitoring for infection.

The offending agent must be discontinued immediately. Supportive therapy must be initiated early with fluid and electrolyte replacement, acid–base equilibrium regulation, serum protein and glucose control, and wound management. The traditional approach to wound management is aggressive debridement, or using whirlpool therapy to remove necrotic epidermis. Others are more conservative, evacuating blister exudate and leaving the detached epidermis in place as a biologic dressing, so-called antishear wound care. In an observational study at a center which used both traditional and the antishear approaches there were equivalent mortality figures [230, 231].

Denuded or debrided skin should be covered. A variety of products including paraffin gauze, biologic allografts or xenografts, and newer products including Biobrane™, Aquacel® Ag, and Veloderm® should be considered [232]. Biobrane™ is a temporary biosynthetic bilaminar membrane which has shown to have less serum protein loss, diminished pain, and decreased time to mobilization when compared to antiseptic solution and daily dressing changes. No difference in mortality between the two groups has been shown [233–235]. Severe or widespread denudation unresponsive to traditional methods of coverage can be successfully treated with umbilical cord mesenchymal stem cells (UC-MSCs). Three patients treated with UC-MSC showed an interruption of cutaneous blistering and wound healing. This innovative treatment modality has yet to be further explored [236, 237].

Appropriate measures for contact isolation and infection prevention should be undertaken, and include sterile handling and antiseptic solutions. Initial blood, skin, and urine cultures should be taken; skin cultures should be repeated at 48-h intervals [238, 239]. Prophylactic antibiotics are not recommended. If antibiotics are indicated, culture and sensitivity data should drive antibiotic selection when possible [227].

Ophthalmic Care

Immediate attention and continued observation of ocular involvement should be undertaken early to establish a baseline of ocular health and to avoid permanent ocular sequelae. Cleaning of eyelids with continual lubrication with drops or ointments is recommended for all patients. Topical steroid treatment and steroid pulse therapy starting from disease onset are important for improvement of visual prognosis as well as the prevention of corneal epithelial stem cell loss [240, 241]. Amniotic membrane transplantation applied to eyelid margins, palpebral conjunctiva, and ocular surface has shown promising results in treating ocular and eyelid inflammation [242, 243]. Gas-permeable scleral contact lens therapy is also a component of visual rehabilitation, and has found to be useful for refractory ocular surface disease [244]. The "Triple-TEN" is a novel combination treatment strategy proposed by Tomlins et al. [245]. It is comprised of subconjunctival triamcinolone administered into each fornices, placement of amniotic membrane tissue mounted on a polycarbonate skirt over the corneal and limbal regions, and insertion of a steepy curved acrylic scleral shell spacer to vault the lids away from the globe. A trial of 2 patients produced resolution of ocular surface inflammation and at 1-year follow-up, no progression of conjunctival cicatrization or evidence of limbal epithelial stem cell failure.

Systemic Steroids

Systemic steroids have been the traditional agent utilized for treating SJS/TEN for decades. However, there is little evidence that corticosteroids confer a benefit, and in face studies have shown an increased morbidity and mortality when steroids are used. In addition, corticosteroids are associated with increased risk of infection and duration of hospital stay. However, other studies have shown improvement in mortality rates when corticosteroids are used [246–248].

IVIG

Human intravenous immunoglobulin (IVIG) was proposed as therapy for TEN by Viard et al., based on the finding that IVIG inhibited Fas-FasL binding in vitro [249]. In the protocol used by Viard et al., IVIG was infused at a dose of 0.7 g/kg daily for 4 days leading to a total dose of 2.8 g/kg. Methylprednisolone at a dose of 250 mg every 6 h was given for the first 48 h. Subsequent studies have modified the dosing with conflicting results [246, 250, 251]. In 2012, Huang et al. reported a meta-analysis of IVIG efficacy against TEN. Adults treated with high-dose IVIG exhibited significantly lower mortality than those treated with low-dose IVIG, and pediatric patients treated with IVIG had significantly lower mortality than adults. While IVIG is now considered the standard of care, future randomized controlled trials will allow for a better understanding of the exact role of IVIG in treating SJS/TEN [252].

Plasmapheresis

Plasmapheresis has been shown to dramatically halt TEN progression and produce re-epithelialization in patients refractory to systemic corticosteroids and IVIG. However, it is unclear if the benefits of plasmapheresis are due to removal of the culprit drug or the inflammatory and pro-apoptotic mediators. There have been case series of non-responsive patients, and there are no randomized controlled trials of plasmapheresis in SJS/TEN [253–257].

Cyclosporine

The calcineurin inhibitor cyclosporine has been used to treat TEN for over 25 years [258, 259]. In 2000, Arévalo et al. published a case series of 11 patients treated with cyclosporine 3 mg/kg daily for 12 days. Cyclosporine was well tolerated and there were no patient deaths in this trial [260]. This was followed by a more recent trial of 29 patients with SJS/TEN treated with cyclosporine for at least 10 days which showed a lower death rate than predicted and decreased progression of epidermal detachment [261]. In 2014, cyclosporine was found to have a greater mortality benefit over IVIG in treating SJS/TEN in a retrospective review of 71 patients [262].

Thalidomide and TNF-Alpha Inhibitory Drugs

In 1998, Wolkenstein et al. conducted a randomized controlled trial of thalidomide versus placebo in TEN; however, due to excess mortality in the thalidomide group the study was discounted. Thalidomide lowers release of TNF-α from monocytes; however, in the thalidomide group plasma levels of TNF-α were higher than in the placebo group suggesting a paradoxical enhancement of TNF-α production [263]. Other TNF-α inhibitors have also been reported to have successful outcomes in patients with TEN. Cessation of further progression of TEN has been shown even with a single dose of infliximab [264, 265]. Etanercept has also been used successfully as treatment for TEN, though no randomized controlled trials exist for these biologic agents [266, 267].

10.4 Vasculitis

Li-Ping Zhao

Vasculitis represents a specific pattern of inflammation of the blood vessel wall, affecting both arteries and veins; it can occur in any organ system of the body. Vasculitis may be idiopathic or secondary to a medication, infection, neoplasm, or systemic inflammatory disease. It is primarily due to leukocyte migration and resultant damage. Children and adults, males and females, and individuals of any ethnic background can be affected. Vasculitis may be idiopathic or secondary to established extravascular diseases, such as trauma, systemic inflammatory conditions, infection, connective tissue disease, malignancy, and drug hypersensitivity, and has similar clinicopathological features with other conditions, which had characteristic features of prevailing vessel inflammation such as atherosclerosis, systemic sclerosis (SSc), and thrombotic microangiopathies. Inflammation of the vasculature results in vessel wall destruction and increased permeability, leading to extravasation of blood cells, aneurysm formation, and stenosis. Clinically, these processes present as infarction of the affected organ, tissue ischemia, or hemorrhage. Ascribable to different organs and caliber of vessels involved, vasculitis can manifest with a wide spectrum of clinical findings from a self-limiting course, benign, or to death.

Small blood vessels are ubiquitous in the skin. They include capillaries, postcapillary venules, and arterioles. Small blood vessels are typically 50 μm or less in diameter and may not have a fully developed muscular layer, which are found in the superficial and mid-dermis of the skin. Medium-sized blood vessels, with fully developed muscular layers, are larger than 50 μm, usually including the small arteries and veins that reside within the deep dermis or subcutis. Large vessels include the aorta and are named arteries. Cutaneous involvement occurs almost exclusively with vasculitis of small- and medium-sized vessels; Large-vessel vasculitides rarely have cutaneous manifestations, but a key concept is that vasculitis of all three major categories can affect any size artery. It is very important to realize that medium-vessel vasculitis and even large-vessel vasculitis can affect small arteries. Therefore, the large vessel vasculitides (e.g., giant cell arteritis) are mentioned only briefly. In addition, some vasculitic disorders are accompanied by a skin eruption that is not the result of cutaneous vasculitis, as exampled by Kawasaki disease, in which there is a vasculitis of the coronary arteries but not the skin.

Erythema and purpuric macules would be present when small, superficial vessels are involved, whereas severe lesions including palpable purpura, livedo, vesicles, urticaria, ulcers, subcutaneous nodules, necrosis, and distal gangrene would be present increasingly when larger vessels in deeper dermis are involved. Multiple lesion types often occur, as a range of blood vessel sizes may be involved. Inflammation of blood vessels produce the chemical mediators, resulting in a variety of systemic findings, such as fever, malaise, weight loss, arthritis, arthralgias, night sweats, myalgia, and laboratory abnormalities [268–270]. Because different disease processes can result in similiar lesions, and because many diseases can have similar lesions, prognosis cannot only be determined from physical examination [270–272]. In order to further classify suspected vasculitis and identify extracutaneous involvement, a complete history, physical exam, systemic review, and laboratory workup are essential. Biopsy and clinical histological correlation provide the gold standard for diagnosis and determination of both the degree of systemic involvement and uncovering underlying causes for the vasculitic process (Table 10.8).

Table 10.8 Suggested laboratory workup for suspected vasculitis

Standard workup
Complete blood count w/differential
Complete metabolic panel (including creatinine)
Urinalysis with microscopic evaluation
Biopsy for hematoxylin and eosin staining
Biopsy for direct immunofluorescence
Infectious serologies (blood, urine, swabs)
Rheumatoid factor
C-reactive protein
Antinuclear antibody
Antineutrophil cytoplasmic antibody
Cryoglobulins
Complement (C3, C4, and CH50)
Hepatitis panel
Stool guaiac
Chest X-ray
HIV
Serum protein electrophoresis/urine protein electrophoresis
Other tests to consider based on the individual case
Renal biopsy
Nerve conduction studies
Hypercoagulability panel
Echocardiogram

Adapted from [273]

Data obtained from lab investigations are essential to make decisions regarding prognosis and treatment modalities. For example, low levels of serum complement, a known mediator of vascular inflammation, indicate excessive consumption, suggesting more extensive or systemic involvement [274]. Elevation of erythrocyte sedimentation rate (ESR) can present in up to 50 % of patients with limited cutaneous vasculitis; however, significant elevations (up to 60 mm/h) of ESR have been associated with higher rates of systemic involvement [275].

Histopathology of skin biopsies stained by both routine hematoxylin and eosin (H&E) as well as direct immunofluorescence (DIF) is essential for determining whether physical findings represent true vasculitis or other conditions that can clinically mimic vasculitis. Lesions between 24 and 48 h after their appearance should be obtained, as sampling before or after this time range may result in false-negative results on DIF. Biopsies with perivascular lymphocytic inflammation or thrombosis are characteristic of older lesions. When suspicion of vasculitis is high but histology is not associated with clinical findings, biopsy should be repeated. Similarly, biopsy must reach to sufficient depth to include the afflicted vessels. Ulcerated lesions should not be avoided [268]. The diagnosis of vasculitis is confirmed explicitly by the presence of an inflammatory infiltrate within and around the walls of vessel with fibrin deposition. These areas of fibrinoid necrosis are accompanied by swelling and necrosis of endothelial cells of vessel, as well as secondary changes such as necrosis leading to purpura and infarction and erythrocyte extravasation [268, 270]. Apoptotic cells may be seen frequently as well as overlying ulceration. Determination of vessel size, depth, type of cellular infiltrate, and degree of involvement on H&E stains helps in diagnosis, classification, and generation of differential diagnoses.

The pathogenesis of vasculitis is related to vessel wall injury resulting in fibrinoid necrosis in the vessel walls, which can be immune-mediated, toxin-mediated, or from direct infection. The pathogenesis caused by immune-mediated is more likely to result in extracutaneous involvement [273]. (1) Deposition of immune complexes result in complement activation, further recruitment of cytokines and inflammatory cells, and expression of adhesion molecules such as P-selectin, E-selectin, and intercellular adhesion molecule 1 (ICAM-1). Endothelial cell retraction results in vascular deposition of immune complexes, edema, neutrophil infiltration, thrombosis, and hemorrhage. (2) Immunofluorescence is an extremely necessary diagnostic tool in the assessment of cutaneous vasculitis, especially in the small-vessel vasculitis. Deposition of IgG, IgA, IgM, and C3 in or around vessel wall detected by DIF characterizes antibody and immune complex-mediated vasculitis, and the patterns of Ig and C3 deposition further classify vasculitis. Lesion age is essential to evaluation, as up to 30 % of immune-mediated vasculitides are negative on DIF by 72 h, and only C3 is detected on DIF after this point [276].

Serological testing is routine in the assessment of vasculitis. In antineutrophil cytoplasmic antibodies (ANCA)-associated vasculitides [277], antibodies against cytoplasmic (c-ANCA) neutrophil-derived products are directed against proteinase 3 (PR3) and antibodies against perinuclear (p-ANCA) neutrophil-derived products are directed against myeloperoxidase (MPO) and elastase. Many inflammatory cytokines can induce the translocation of these targets to the surface of neutrophils, and binding of ANCAs and adherence to endothelial cells, finally causing damage to vessel walls [278]. Titers may predict disease activity or clinical relapse [279]. Acute infections can be accompanied with transient elevations in ANCAs; so, serial testing is recommended [280]. Enzyme-linked immunosorbent assay (ELISA) is a more sensitive and specific assay for c-ANCA, and immunofluorescence is preferred for p-ANCA.

It is difficult to make a satisfactory classification of systemic vasculitis, as the pathogenesis of vasculitis is not very clear and there is incomplete insight underlying pathogenetic events [281]. Classification of vasculitis in the skin is typically based on the type of inflammatory response and the size of predominantly affected blood vessels, combined with DIF examination and laboratory workup. Classification of vasculitis correlates with disease etiology and affect the treatment decisions [273]. Classification schemes outlined by the Chapel Hill Consensus Criteria or the American College of Rheumatology are mentioned in most texts [282–284].

The Chapel Hill Consensus Conference has released an updated classification of primary systemic vasculitides, and seven main vasculitis groups have been proposed: large-vessel vasculitides, small-vessel vasculitides, medium-vessel vasculitides, variable-vessel vasculitides, single-organ vasculitides, vasculitides associated with systemic disease, and vasculitides associated with probable etiology (Table 10.9) [285].

Table 10.9 2012 Chapel Hill Consensus Conference on the nomenclature of vasculitides

Large vessel vasculitides
Takayasu arteritis (TA)
Giant cell arteritis (GCA)
Medium vessel vasculitides
Polyarteritis nodosa (PAN)
Kawasaki disease (KD)
Small vessel vasculitides
Antineutrophil cytoplasmic antibody (ANCA)-associated vasculitides (AAV)
Microscopic polyangiitis (MPA)
Granulomatosis with polyangiitis (Wegener's) (GPA)
Eosinophilic granulomatosis with polyangiitis (Churg–Strauss, EGPA)
Immune complex small-vessel vasculitides
Antiglomerular basement membrane disease
Cryoglobulinemic vasculitis (CV)
IgA vasculitis (Henoch–Schönlein) (IgAV)
Hypocomplementemic urticarial vasculitis (anti-C1q vasculitis)
Variable vessel vasculitides
Behçet's disease
Cogan's syndrome
Single-organ vasculitides
Cutaneous leucocytoclastic angiitis
Cutaneous arteritis
Primary central nervous system vasculitis
Isolated aortitis
Others
Vasculitides associated with systemic disease
Lupus vasculitis
Rheumatoid vasculitis
Sarcoid vasculitis
Others
Vasculitides associated with probable etiology
Hepatitis C virus-associated cryoglobulinemic vasculitis
Hepatitis B virus-associated vasculitis
Syphilis-associated aortitis
Drug-associated immune complex vasculitis
Drug-associated ANCA-associated vasculitis
Cancer-associated vasculitis
Others

Adapted from [285]

10.4.1 Large-Vessel Vasculitides (LVV)

CHCC 2012 [285] defines LVV as vasculitis affecting the aorta and its major branches more often than other vasculitides; however, any size artery may be affected. The group of large-vessel vasculitides is comprised of Takayasu's arteritis (TA) and giant cell arteritis (GCA). The major discriminator between TA and GCA is the age of the patient. Large-vessel vasculitides rarely have cutaneous manifestations and will be mentioned only briefly.

10.4.1.1 Takayasu's Arteritis (TA)

TA is arteritis, often granulomatous, predominantly affecting the aorta and its major branches [285]. Onset usually is in patients younger than 50 years, in particular women of child-bearing age. TA has a higher incidence in Asia and Latin America [286]. It usually involves the whole subdiaphragmatic arterial tree and pulmonary artery. TA has a lower rate of progression of vessel wall remodeling and enhanced formation of collateral vessels than GCA [287]. TA has a lower rate of aneurysm formation than GCA, [288]. Involvement of large vessels can occasionally manifest as lesions of the scalp and tongue [289]. Cutaneous large-vessel vasculitis (CLVV) is rare, as there are simply no large vessels found in the skin.

10.4.1.2 Giant Cell Arteritis (GCA)

GCA is arteritis, often granulomatous, usually affecting the aorta and its major branches, with a predilection for the branches of the carotid and vertebral arteries, often involving the temporal artery. It involves mainly supradiaphragmatic space and segmental. GCA often affects patients older than 50 years of age and has a significant epidemiological impact in the elderly Caucasian population. Common symptoms are jaw claudication, new-onset headache, and scalp tenderness. GCA is usually accompanied with systemic inflammation (fever, fatigue, elevated erythrocyte sedimentation rate (ESR)) and polymyalgia rheumatica (PMR) in which pathogenesis is unknown, and is an inflammatory disease characterized by pain of the shoulders, neck, and hips. Typical and frequent complications of GCA are aortic aneurysm formation, vision loss, and ischemic stroke [273].

10.4.1.3 Treatment

High-dose glucocorticosteroids are the most effective drugs in the treatment of GCA and should be initiated immediately after the diagnosis is suspected [290]. The initial dose of oral prednisolone is 40–60 mg per day and is maintained until inflammatory mediators have normalized and symptoms have resolved. Most patients have stopped treatment by 2 years. Glucocorticosteroids are usually ordered in TA in association with immunosuppressive drugs such as azathioprine or methotrexate [291]. Antitumor necrosis factor (TNF) agents are effective in TA, whereas biological agents are ambiguously effective in GCA [292].

10.4.2 Medium-Vessel Vasculitides (MVV)

MVV is vasculitis predominantly affecting medium arteries defined as the main visceral arteries and their branches. However, any size artery may be affected [285]. Cutaneous MVV is clinically present with livedo, nodules, ulcerations, or digital infarcts. Wedge biopsy without necrotic or ulcerated areas is typically needed for sufficient diagnostic yield. Vasculitis of these vessels is often referred to as necrotizing vasculitis, reflecting the coagulative necrosis, hyalinization, and degeneration of muscular layers, where it is more readily visible. Occasionally, nerve or muscle biopsy can provide additional diagnostic information if histology is inconclusive. The group of medium-vessel vasculitides comprises Kawasaki's disease (KD) and polyarteritis nodosa (PAN).

10.4.2.1 Kawasaki's Disease (KD)

KD is arteritis associated with the mucocutaneous lymph node syndrome, predominantly affecting medium and small arteries. Coronary arteries are often involved. KD usually occurs in infants and young children. KD is virtually known in patients aged under 5 years, more common in Afro-Caribbean and Japanese ethnic cohorts. KD is severe and potentially life threatening, because it usually involves coronary arteries, despite its self-limiting course. Common clinical signs include cervical (often unilateral) lymphadenopathy, fever, nonexudative conjunctivitis, reddening and fixation of lips and tongue, polymorphic diffused exanthema, nonpitting edema of the dorsa of hands and desquamating exanthema of soles and palms. After an early phase of predominant perivasculitis, inflammation of medium-sized artery in KD progresses toward the involvement of the medial and intimal layers [293]. There are predominant infiltrating CD8+T cells, macrophages, and IgA-secreting plasma cells, as well as frequent vessel wall damage and formation of aneurysms. Centripetal activation of the endothelium is related to frequent thrombosis and resultant end-organ ischemia. KD late stages present stenoses and aneurysms. KD is, virtually, the primary cause of heart disease in children.

Current treatment in KD consist of intravenous immunoglobulins (IVIG) and antiplatelet agents, such as aspirin, abiciximab [294], and anti-TNF agents [295]. Despite treatment, children with KD still have a 5–10 % risk of developing coronary artery lesions and need for more effective therapies [296]. TNF blockade does not markedly make dendritic cells endowed with a tolerogenic function expanding and the resultant a somewhat complex remodeling of the immune network that occurs in KD patients during subacute phases of KD responding to therapy [297].

10.4.2.2 Polyarteritis Nodosa (PAN)

PAN is an extremely rare necrotizing arteritis of medium or small arteries without glomerulonephritis or vasculitis in arterioles, capillaries, or venules, and not associated with ANCA [285]. It is a multisystem vasculitis characterized by segmental necrotizing vasculitis that involves predominantly medium-sized blood vessels. Cutaneous PAN is a "skin-limited" variant which follows a benign but chronic course. It is characterized by stenosing and micro-aneurysmatic lesions [298]. Fibrinoid necrosis and lymphocyte infiltrate and dense neutrophil are usual findings [299]. DIF may show deposits of C3, IgM, and fibrin within vessel walls or perivascularly. The absence of ANCA is a valuable clinical feature in distinguishing PAN from microscopic polyangiitis [300].

The pathogenesis is virtually under investigation: most cases are still under investigation because of difficulty in differentiating it from other vasculitides, especially microscopic polyangiitis (MPA) and the epidemiological shift toward nonhepatitis B virus (HBV)-associated PAN [301, 302]. HBV infection is thought to be an etiological trigger in approximately 7% of patients with classic PAN [303]. Cutaneous PAN has been associated with other infections, including streptococcal (especially in children), parvovirus B19, and HIV. Inflammatory conditions associated with both classic and cutaneous PAN include inflammatory bowel disease, SLE, and familial Mediterranean fever. Hairy cell leukemia has also been observed in association with classic PAN.

Current treatments are as those employed in small-vessel vasculitides [290, 303, 304].

Patients with idiopathic classic PAN should be treated with systemic corticosteroids or cyclophosphamide. Antiviral interferon-2a and, more recently, lamivudine are commonly used for the treatment of HBV-associated PAN [305]. Combination therapy with short-term corticosteroids, plasma exchange, and antiviral agents has been effective in several open-label trials [306].

For cutaneous PAN, topical or intralesional corticosteroids may benefit localized areas of cutaneous involvement, but oral corticosteroids may be warranted for progressive or extensive disease. Successful therapies, based upon anecdotal reports, include IVIg, sulfapyridine (especially in patients with associated Crohn's disease), low-dose methotrexate (7.5–15 mg/week), and pentoxifylline (400 mg orally, three times daily) [307]. Patients with evidence of a streptococcal infection should be treated with penicillin. Digital necrosis has been reported to improve with intravenous prostaglandins or calcium channel blockers.

10.4.3 Small-Vessel Vasculitides (SVV)

SVV [285] include immune complex and antineutrophil cytoplasmic antibodies (ANCA)-associated vasculitides (AAV). They include Wegener's granulomatosis, Churg–Strauss syndrome, microscopic polyangiitis, Henoch–Schönlein purpura, essential cryoglobulinemic vasculitis, and cutaneous leukocytoclastic angiitis.

10.4.3.1 Immune Complex SVV

Immune complex SVV is vasculitis with moderate to marked vessel wall deposits of complement components and immunoglobulin predominantly affecting small vessels [285]. Immune complex SVV include antiglomerular basement membrane (anti-GBM) disease, cryoglobulinemic vasculitis (CV), IgA vasculitis (Henoch–Schönlein) (IgAV), and hypocomplementemic urticarial vasculitis (HUV) (anti-C1q vasculitis).

Anti-GBM disease is vasculitis which affects pulmonary capillaries, glomerular capillaries, or both, and has basement membrane deposition of antibasement membrane autoantibodies [285]. The pathogenesis of this involves formation of immune complexes in situ between GBM antigens and anti-GBM antibodies, resulting in the activation of inflammatory mediators.

Hypocomplementemic urticarial vasculitis (HUV) was the least common immune complex vasculitis affecting small vessels and associated with anti-C1q antibodies [285]. Glomerulonephritis, arthritis, obstructive pulmonary disease, and ocular inflammation are common.

10.4.3.2 IgA Vasculitis (IgAV) (Henoch–Schönlein Purpura, HSP)

HSP, synonyms of which are anaphylactoid purpura, purpura rheumatica, cutaneous small-vessel vasculitis secondary to circulating IgA immune complexes, is with IgA1-dominant immune deposits, affecting small vessels [285]. Classically, it is a specific form of CSVV that typically affects children following a respiratory tract infection. HSP is the most common form of vasculitis in children and can also occur in adults. It follows a seasonal pattern, with a peak in incidence during the winter. In children, HSP affects boys and girls equally, while in adults, there is a slight male predominance. It is presenting with palpable purpura mainly at lower extremities, arthritis, gastrointestinal involvement (ischemia, enteric hemorrhage, intussusception), mainly with abdominal pain and renal disease (commonly hematuria), with features undistinguishable from isolated IgA nephropathy (Berger's disease) being relatively common [285, 298, 308]. Urticaria, vesicles, bullae, and foci of necrosis can also be seen. Ulcerative lesions have been reported in HIV-positive patients [309]. Individual lesions usually regress within 10–14 days, with resolution of skin involvement over a period of several weeks to months, although recurrences are observed in 5–10 % of patients [307].

Although several studies have reported that a substantial minority of HSP patients have positive antistreptolysin O (ASLO) titers, no causal role for group Ab-hemolytic streptococci has been demonstrated [310]. As with other forms of CSVV, immune complexes are presumed to play a role in the pathogenesis of HSP. The role of complement is suggested in HSP patients with inherited C2 or C4 deficiency, as it is likely that these molecules play a role in the clearance of immune complexes and/or antigens from apoptotic cells [311]. It is also likely that immunoglobulin deposition in the vessel wall results in complement activation and vascular damage [312]. Approximately 50 % of patients develop systemic involvement such as neuropathy, nephritis, and gastrointestinal involvement (GI) [313]. GI can develop hemorrhage and necrosis of the bowel from mesenteric vasculitis and pulmonary hemorrhages [314].

There are no specific serology associations with IgA vasculitis. Urinalysis is a necessary laboratory workup for the patient with suspected IgAV, as hematuria is the most sensitive measurement for renal involvement.

Histopathology shows a neutrophil-rich SSV of the superficial dermis with leukocytoclasia and few eosinophils. DIFs reveal IgA deposits being the most prominent in small, superficial vessels, providing the gold standard for diagnosis, and C3 and fibrin deposits are seen. Although IgA deposition in the vessel wall supports the diagnosis of HSP, this histological finding is not entirely specific, and can be seen in patients with autoimmune connective tissue diseases, acute hemorrhagic edema of infancy, Wegener's granulomatosis, and drug hypersensitivity reactions [315]. A study showed that 82 % of all adults with CSVV demonstrated some vascular IgA deposition [316], and thus a diagnosis of HSP is supported by an IgA predominance in the correct clinical setting.

Skin lesions usually have an initial response to glucocorticosteroids, followed by rapid relapse upon completion of treatment. Glomerulonephritis responds well to alkylating agents. Severe renal manifestations are usually treated with high-dose corticosteroids, either alone or in combination with immunosuppressive agents, plasmapheresis, or IVIG [294, 317], whereas other manifestations are usually self-limiting or controlled by nonsteroid anti-inflammatory drugs or moderate doses of oral corticosteroids.

10.4.3.3 Cryoglobulinemic Vasculitis (CV)

CV is vasculitis with cryoglobulin immune deposits affecting small vessels and associated with cryoglobulins in serum [285]. The incidence of CV peaks in middle age and in regions with a high incidence of hepatitis C virus (HCV) infection. Monoclonal or oligoclonal immunoglobulins combining with rheumatoid factor cryoglobulins form cryoglobulins underlying humoral responses related to autoimmunity (e. g. Sjögren's syndrome), chronic infection (mainly HCV), or B cell malignancies. Common features of CV are purpura, mainly in the lower limbs, and skin ulcers, possibly with arthralgia or arthritis. Glomerulonephritis is less common, and peripheral nerve involvement is often mild [318].

Treatments for HCV-related CV depend on antiviral agents such as peginterferon (IFN) plus ribavirin [319], whereas in nonviral CV, AAV-like regimens are considered [290]. Antiviral agents include anti-B cell agents such as rituximab as the standard-of-care treatment for CV, given their obvious safety and efficacy [320].

10.4.3.4 Antineutrophil Cytoplasmic Antibodies (ANCA)-associated Vasculitides (AAV)

AAV is a necrotizing vasculitis, with few or no immune deposits, predominantly affecting small vessels and is characterized by the presence of circulating ANCA (MPO-ANCA or PR3-ANCA) [285]. Mounting evidence indicates that the ANCA specificity identifies distinct categories of disease [321, 322]. In contrast to immune complex deposition, specific antibodies, known as antineutrophil cytoplasmic antibodies (ANCA), are directed against intracellular neutrophilic ANCA targets which are known to translocate to the neutrophil's cell surface following primary activation by cytokines such as TNF-alpha. Upon binding, ANCA activate neutrophils, resulting in a respiratory burst and the release of enzymes from granules as well as cytokines that lead to endothelial damage and recruitment of additional inflammatory cells. Two major ANCA targets are proteinase 3 (PR3-ANCA), giving rise to cytosplasmic (C)-ANCA pattern, and myeloperoxidase (MPO-ANCA), giving rise to perinuclear (P)-ANCA pattern on ethanol-fixed neutrophils. These antigens are found within the cytoplasm of neutrophils, but can also be found on the cell surface of a subset of neutrophils [323, 324].

Occasionally, other autoantigens can be targeted by ANCA, such as cathepsin G, lactoferrin, lysozyme, bacterial permeability increasing factor, hLAMP-2, and elastase. ANCA can even coexist with ANA, as reported in cases of drug-induced vasculitis associated with chronic hydralazine or minocycline use [325].

It has been established that incidence of venous thromboembolism in all AAV increases (but not in patients with PAN) [326, 327]. AAV patients also are at a higher risk of arterial thrombosis, and 14 % of patients develop GPA or MPA within 5 years [328]. Arterial and venous thrombosis often occur during the active phases of vasculitis and are not obviously related to conventional prothrombotic risk factors, rather suggesting a potential link with inflammation and defective regulation of the thrombogenic action of leukocytes [329, 330].

A combination of intravenous or oral glucocorticoids with cyclophosphamide is often used for induction of remission in patients with severe or generalized AAV or with a 5-factor score ≥1 [290, 331, 332]. Encouraging results from the Rituximab in Vasculitis (RITUXVAS) trials and Rituximab for ANCA-associated Vasculitis (RAVE) [333, 334] indicate that rituximab might be an alternative to cyclophosphamide, as it might be ordered in the standard-of-care treatment [335, 336]. Methotrexate plus high-dose glucocorticoids could be used for remission induction in nonorgan or nonlife-threatening AAV. Standard treatment plus plasma exchange are usually recommended to patients with severe renal involvement, although it does not notably effect the overall survival [290]. Various agents, such as azathioprine, methotrexate, and rituximab, are used to maintain remission [337].

10.4.3.5 Granulomatosis with Polyangiitis (GPA)

GPA (formerly named Wegener's granulomatosis) is necrotizing granulomatous inflammation and necrotizing vasculitis affecting predominantly small to medium vessels and is a complex rare multisystemic disease usually involving the upper and lower respiratory tract [286, 338]. Clinical features of classic GPA include respiratory tract and renal disease in up to 95 % and 75 % of patients, respectively, although various limited clinical phenotypes can occur and present to clinicians in various subspecialties. GPA is characterized by antiproteinase 3 antibodies (cANCA), destructive granulomatous lesions of the upper and lower respiratory tract, of the eye and of the ear, necrotizing crescentic glomerulonephritis, leading to end-stage renal disease in 20–25 % of patients within 5 years and systemic vasculitis [339]. Over the same time period, clinical relapses are seen in up to 50 % of patients [324]. Systemic features such as arthromyalgias and fever are common, while involvement of nervous system and skin is less common. The natural history of the disease might involve persistent exposure to respiratory infections and irritant agents [339]. There are currently no reliable disease biomarkers that can sensitively predict flares of GPA in an individual patient.

Management of GPA varies greatly from one case to another based on the extent of systemic involvement (localized/limited vs multisystemic disease) and relapsing nature of the disease.

10.4.3.6 Microscopic Polyangiitis (MPA)

MPA is necrotizing vasculitis, with few or no immune deposits, predominantly affecting small vessels [285]. Necrotizing glomerulonephritis is very common.

In contrast to GPA, MPA is characterized by systemic small vasculitis, including a very common pauci-immune glomerulonephritis, but without evidence of systemic granulomatous disease. Serologically, MPA presents with antimyeloperoxidase (MPO) antibodies (pANCA). Chronic lung damage in MPA, while common, tends to assume a more restrictive fibrosing pattern different from that seen in GPA and EGPA. Another distinctive feature is that MPA has a significantly lower relapse rate compared to GPA [324]. Peripheral nerve, skin, lung, and gastrointestinal involvements are, in fact, exquisitely vasculitic in MPA. Renal involvement in MPA is frequent and often severe.

An increased incidence of venous thromboembolism in all AAV (but not to patients with PAN) has been established [326, 327]. AAV patients also are at higher risk of arterial thrombosis, with 14 % of patients experiencing a cardiovascular event within 5 years of GPA or MPA diagnosis [328]. Venous and arterial thrombosis often occur during the active phases of vasculitis and are not apparently associated with conventional prothrombotic risk factors, rather suggesting a potential link with inflammation and defective regulation of the thrombogenic action of leukocytes [329, 330].

10.4.3.7 Eosinophilic Granulomatosis with Polyangiitis (EGPAn)

EGPA (formerly Churg–Strauss' syndrome) is a rare eosinophil-rich and systemic necrotizing granulomatous inflammation often involving the respiratory tract associated with asthma and eosinophilia and predominantly affecting small to medium vessels [285]. ANCA is more frequent in EGPA when glomerulonephritis is present [340]. P-ANCA, or MPO, is detectable in 40–50 % of patients. Clinical features include allergy, palpable purpura, hypereosinophilia, nasal polyposis, peripheral neuropathy, and a history of allergic asthma, usually improving just before the onset of vasculitis. The EGPA prevalence is highest at a mean age of 48, with an equal gender distribution, although the syndrome can occur at any age [341]. Although the annual incidence is low in the general population, 2.4–13 per million persons, it is relatively high in asthma patients, 34.6–64.6 per million persons [342, 343]. Gastrointestinal, pulmonary, and cardiac involvement with either eosinophilic and granulomatous infiltration or vasculitic lesions are also common [344]. Renal involvement is less common than in other AAV. It is not easy to diagnose EGPA because of its low incidence and the variety of clinical features at each of its stages. Additionally, the definite causes and pathophysiology of EGPA remain not well understood [345].

Treatment approaches depend on disease severity refractoriness to therapies or extension to vital organs [290, 346]. Before steroid treatment was used routinely in EGPA, the mortality rate in the 3 months after diagnosis was as high as 50 % [347]. However in a study of treatment with steroid and immunosuppressants in 2005, it was reported that the 5-year survival rate was up to 98 % [348, 349].

10.4.4 Variable-Vessel Vasculitides

VVV is vasculitis with no predominant type of vessel involvement, that is, VVV can affect vessels of any size (small, medium, and large) and type (arteries, veins, and capillaries) [285]. Vasculitides that are included in this category are Behcet's disease (BD) and Cogan's syndrome (CS), neither of which frequently affects the kidneys.

10.4.5 Single-Organ Vasculitides (SOV)

SOV is vasculitis in a single organ with no features indicating a limited expression of a systemic vasculitis [285]. The vessel type and involved organ should be included in the name (e.g., cutaneous small vessel vasculitis, testicular arteritis, central nervous system vasculitis).

10.4.5.1 Cutaneous Small-Vessel Vasculitis (CSVV)

CSVV is a general term applied to any patient with small-vessel vasculitis of the skin, irrespective of clinical severity or etiology. It is the synonym of cutaneous leukocytoclastic angiitis, cutaneous leukocytoclastic vasculitis, hypersensitivity angiitis, and cutaneous necrotizing venulitis. Infectious agents, cytokines, exogenous chemicals, and circulating immune entities not strong enough to activate complement can cause CSVV by inducing an inflammatory cascade in the endothelium of small vessel. Most usually triggered by drugs or infections, the onset of a single crop of lesions is acute with both nonpalpable and palpable erythematous, purpuric papules and vesicles or urticarial lesions dependent on areas such as the lower extremities, as well as areas affected by trauma (pathergy) or under tight-fitting clothing. Lesions appear about 5–20 days after initial exposure and 2–4 days after repeat exposures [350]. Of note, the diameter can range from 1 mm to several centimeters. Although they are usually asymptomatic, the lesions can be associated with burning, pain, or pruritus. Residual postinflammatory hyperpigmentation may persist for months. Constitutional and/or musculoskeletal symptoms, such as fevers, weight loss, arthralgias, and myalgias, may accompany flares of CSVV. Gastrointestinal, genitourinary, or neurological symptoms should raise the suspicion of a systemic vasculitis. These cases tend to be single episodes, and infection, systemic inflammatory conditions, and malignancy can result in relapsing cycles. Although constitutional symptoms caused by mediators of inflammation released locally are common, extracutaneous involvement is rare [307].

Approximately 90 % of patients will have spontaneous resolution of cutaneous lesions within several weeks or a few months, while another 10 % will have chronic or recurrent disease at intervals of months to years [307]. If there is an underlying cause for CSVV, such as an autoimmune connective tissue disease or neoplasm, this will also impact on the patient's prognosis. The ESR increases in up to 50 % of cases, while urinalysis and complement levels are normal. There are no specific serological markers for CLA, resulting in an exclusive diagnosis of exclusion, and normal complementemic urticarial vasculitis is likely to be a clinical variant of this condition [351].

On histology, there is a neutrophil-predominant vasculitis of superficial vessels with varying numbers of surrounding eosinophils. DIF is positive in about half of these biopsies, indicating mild to moderately intense granular IgM deposits with weak or absent C3. The lack of complement involvement may be associated with the relatively benign course of this condition and low level of systemic involvement.

Treatment includes resolution of underlying systemic condition or removal of the offending agent in cases with a known trigger. Immunosuppressive treatment is necessary in CLA, in the most severe cases, aiming at reducing constitutional symptoms and synovitis. Moderately dosed glucocorticosteroids (0.5 mg/kg/day) are used until symptoms resolve. Recalcitrant cases warrant more extensive treatment.

10.4.6 Vasculitis Associated with Systemic Conditions or Probable Etiology

This vasculitis may be secondary to and is related to a systemic disease [285], such as a number of inflammatory, infectious, malignant diseases, autoimmune, and as well as pregnancy [352–358]. Hematological cancers are most common among correlative malignant diseases. The diagnosis should have a prefix specifying the associated systemic disease (e.g., rheumatoid vasculitis, lupus vasculitis, etc.) [285]. Likewise, vasculitis related to a probable etiology should have a prefix specifying the association (e.g., hepatitis B virus-associated vasculitis, hydralazine-associated MPA, hepatitis C virus-associated cryoglobulinemic vasculitis, etc.). These categories emphasize that a patient with vasculitis should always search primary cause.

10.5 Eosinophilic Dermatoses

Ru Yan and Yan Wu

10.5.1 Wells' Syndrome (Eosinophilic Cellulitis)

Wells' syndrome (WS) was first described by Wells in 1971 [359]. Wells' syndrome (WS) is a rare inflammatory skin disease of uncertain pathogenesis, and is histologically characterized by eosinophilic infiltration and flame figures. Wells reported four cases with characteristically cutaneous lesions, similar to bacterial cellulitis and histopathologically showing dermal eosinophilia with distinctive "flame figures". In 1979, Wells and Smith introduced the term "eosinophilic cellulitis" [360–362].

10.5.1.1 Immunopathogenesis of WS

The etiology and pathogenesis of Wells' syndrome are unclear; the cause may be idiopathic, or represent a nonspecific reaction to infection, surgery, drug reactions, or underlying hematological disorders [363, 364]. Other possible causative factors are inheritance, cancer, Raynaud's phenomenon, and urticaria.

10.5.1.2 Clinical Spectrum of WS

The literature has been in confusion for describing this manifestation: recurrent granulomatous dermatitis with eosinophilia and eosinophilic cellulitis are other names that have been used. The appearance of Wells' syndrome (WS) is variable and may be confused with cellulitis, urticaria, urticarial vasculitis, persistent insect bites, and contact dermatitis [364].

Wells' syndrome (WS) always has a benign course; systemic manifestations like fever, lymphaden anomaly, and arthralgias can occur [361]. After several weeks, without any residual scarring, the lesions resolve spontaneously. Recurrences over many years are common [364]. The classical feature is a tender or mild pruritus, which has typical histology characterized by tissue eosinophilia, edema, and "flame" figures [360]. Other reported clinical symptoms include papular and nodular eruptions. It may be recurrent and proceed at a variable time by a pruritic papular eruption [365].

10.5.1.3 Histological Features of WS

Mitchell et al. divided the histological features of Wells' syndrome into three stages [366]. The appearance of the skin in the first stage is spreading rapidly, poorly demarcated, edematous macules or patches. In the second stage, the skin appears indurated and grayish, with less inflammation. In the third stage, the skin is atrophic and grayish, without residual scarring.

Depending on the stage of the process, the histopathological findings vary. However, intense dermal edema with diffuse eosinophilic infiltration can appear in the acute and subacute stages [367–369].

10.5.1.4 Laboratory Examination of WS

The frequent accompanying feature is that of eosinophilia of the peripheral blood film or bone marrow; other serum investigations are often normal [370].

10.5.1.5 Diagnostic Approach of WS

The diagnosis of Wells' syndrome should be based on the typical clinical symptoms and the process of the disease with its recurrences and distinct histopathology [364].

The differentiation between Wells' syndrome and hypereosinophilic syndrome (HES) is important, as HES is a fatal multisystem disease if left untreated [371]. Further differential diagnosis includes urticaria, especially cold-induced and cholinergic types.

10.5.1.6 Management of WS

Treatment is often unnecessary as lesions typically develop rapidly and resolve spontaneously. Systemic and topical steroids, such as dapsone, are effective treatments [365]. Systemic steroids are the most effective treatment. In order to limit steroid side effects, Coldiron and Robinson suggest to give low-dose, alternate-day treatments [372]. Then, the dose is tapered [373].

10.5.2 Hypereosinophilic Syndrome

Jinping Yuan and Yan Wu

The hypereosinophilic syndrome (HES) is characterized by the presence of marked unexplained blood and tissue eosinophilia associated with a variety of clinical manifestations [374]. HES is a chronic disorder with significant morbidity and mortality [375]. In recent years, the concept of HESs has expanded beyond the previously defined "idiopathic HESs" to include a diversity of disorders in which eosinophils and eosinophils activation are believed to play a primary role in disease pathogenesis [376].

10.5.2.1 Pathophysiology of HES

The pathophysiology of HES is not well understood. Several mechanisms have been proposed as the causes of dysregulated overproduction and proliferation due to a primary defect in hematopoietic stem cells, overproduction of eosinophilopoietic cytokines such as IL-5, and functional abnormalities of the eosinophilopoietic cytokines. However, how and why these overproduced eosinophils infiltrate the target organs and cause symptoms are unknown [374]. Hypereosinophilic syndromes include various phenotypes defined based on the immunogenetic abnormality, which results in abnormal bone marrow and organ eosinophil proliferation [377].

10.5.2.2 Clinical Spectrum of HES

Ninety percent of patients reported are male, mostly between the ages of 20 and 50. Children cases are rare. Presenting symptoms include fever, cough, fatigue, malaise, muscle pains, and skin eruptions [378]. In HES, skin, heart, neurological, and lung involvement were commonly reported, in addition to cardiac manifestations, which have the highest lethal potential [377]. The most frequent clinical manifestations include skin abnormalities, cardiac failure, and neurological deficits, but the disease's presence differs between patients, and every organ can be affected [379].

10.5.2.3 Diagnostic Approach of HES

Four criteria have been used to define HES: (1) blood eosinophilia $\geq$1500/mm^3 for longer than 6 months; (2) eosinophils' increase in bone marrow; (3) lack of evidence for parasitic, allergic, or other known causes of eosinophilia; and (4) evidences for skin and organ involvement [376, 379]. Recently, the following new criteria have been proposed: blood eosinophilia of $\geq$1,500/mm^3 present on at least two occasions with no other apparent etiologies for the degree of eosinophilia, such as viral infections, hypoadrenalism, and neoplasms [374]. Other diseases characterized by eosinophilia include eosinophilic esophagitis (EE) and eosinophilic gastroenteritis (EG), referring to excess eosinophil infiltration of the esophagus and the stomach or intestines, respectively [380].

10.5.2.4 Management of HES

Conventional therapies include corticosteroids, cytotoxic agents, interferon-α or bone marrow transplantation. Some of these options, such as corticosteroids and cytotoxic agents, were previously more widely used in HES in general [376]. All patients, even asymptomatic, should be treated; the goal of therapy is cytogenetic and molecular remission. Such patients are often unresponsive to corticosteroid therapy. However, if there is evidence of cardiac involvement in diagnosis, corticosteroids should be given concomitantly with initiation of imatinib to prevent acute myocarditis. Mepolizumab, an anti-IL-5 antibody, has recently been shown to be an extremely well tolerated and effective corticosteroid-sparing agent in patients with FIP1L1-PDGFRA-negative HES; this promising agent may or may not be currently available in the setting of compassionate use programs. Appropriate treatment is dependent in part on the ability to make an accurate etiological diagnosis and to judge the clinical urgency for introducing an eosinophil-lowering agent [381, 382].

10.6 Neutrophilic Dermatoses

Hong-Hui Xu, Xing-Hua Gao, and Hong-Duo Chen

Neutrophilic dermatoses are a heterogeneous group of diseases characterized by the accumulation of polymorphonuclear neutrophil infiltration in the skin without infectious cause. The cutaneous manifestations include vesicles, pustules, plaques, nodules, and ulcers. The same patient can present with several different types of lesions. The pathophysiology of the disease remains to be elucidated. The neutrophilic infiltrates of other organs including lungs, enterogastric, and kidneys result in extracutaneous manifestations. The assessment of neutrophilic dermatosis includes identification of the type of cutaneous lesion, and a search for possible extracutaneous involvement and associated disease. The management strategies for these conditions are similar.

Some patients have overlapping features of Sweet's syndrome (SS) and pyoderma gangrenosum (PG), and some patients with Behçet's disease (BD) can develop SS lesions. So, it is proposed that neutrophilic dermatosis is a continuous spectrum [383]. We will discuss SS, PG, and BD, respectively.

10.6.1 Sweet's Syndrome

10.6.1.1 Introduction

Sweet's syndrome (SS), also termed as acute febrile neutrophilic dermatosis, was first described by Robert Douglas Sweet in 1964. It is characterized by acute onset of tender erythematous plaques, nodules, papules, fever, arthralgia, peripheral neutrophilia, increased erythrocyte sedimentation rate, and a diffuse infiltrate of mature neutrophils with a typical band-like pattern in the upper dermis.

SS is categorized into five groups based upon associated medical conditions: (1) classic or idiopathic, (2) inflammatory conditions associated with either infectious or immune system disorders, (3) malignancy-associated, (4) pregnancy, and (5) drugs-associated.

10.6.1.2 Pathogenesis

The pathogenesis of SS is not fully understood. Some patients develop SS after infection, inflammation, vaccination, or drug exposure, suggesting that SS is a result of hypersensitivity reaction [384]. The neutrophils may play a role in the process of SS, which is supported by the histopathological changes, peripheral neutrophilia, and the response to drugs that disturb neutrophil activity.

Cytokines appear to play an etiological role in the pathogenesis of SS. Alterations of granulocyte colony-stimulating factor (G-CSF), macrophage colony-stimulating factor (GM-CSF), interferon-gamma, interleukin-1 (IL-1), IL-3, IL-6, and IL-8 have been detected in SS patients [385–387]. Refractory idiopathic SS patients' response to TNF-α inhibitors and IL-1 receptor antagonists indicated a significant role of TNF-alpha in the pathogenesis of SS [388, 389].

10.6.1.3 Clinical Features

SS most often occurs between 30 and 50 years of age, with a female predominance. Patients develop single or multiple, painful erythematous to violaceous papules or nodules, which progress into edematous plaques. The lesions often present with a pseudovesicular appearance secondary to the pronounced edema in the papillary dermis. The lesions develop central clearing, giving annular or arcuate appearance with time. The lesions ultimately resolve without scarring. These lesions may be tender, pruritic, or asymptomatic. SS occurs anywhere, most frequently on the head, neck, and upper and lower extremities. The trunk, hands, and mucosal surfaces can also be affected.

Patients also suffer from pathergy, a phenomenon of new lesions developing after trauma. Other uncommon skin features include bullous, ulcerative, erythema nodosum-like, pustular, or hemorrhagic lesions. Lesions may recur in about 50 % patients.

Subcutaneous SS is a rare subtype of SS, characterized by erythematous, tender dermal nodules mimicking erythema nodosum when they are located on the legs. Tissue evaluation may be necessary to differentiate subcutaneous SS from erythema nodosum.

SS is idiopathic in up to 50 % patients, while underlying malignancy (10–20 %), autoimmune conditions, or pregnancy can be seen. The malignancy-associated SS affects men and women equally. When associated with malignancy, vesiculobullous variant is common, with ulcerative lesions mimicking pyoderma gangrenosum (PG) [390].

Extracutaneous manifestations most commonly are the ocular and mucosal involvement. Ocular involvement may cause a sore and red eye and can lead to ulceration and loss of vision due to conjunctivitis, dacryoadenitis, keratitis, and episcleritis. Oral ulcers are uncommon in patients with classical SS, however, more frequent in hematological disorder-associated SS. SS patients often have systemic symptoms of fever, arthralgias, or myalgias when the disease is active.

10.6.1.4 Associated Diseases

Up to 20 % of SS cases occur with an underlying malignancy, most commonly hematological disease. An association with solid tumors is rare, but carcinomas of the genitourinary tract, breast, and gastrointestinal tract have been reported. SS may follow, precede, or appear concurrently with the diagnosis of malignancy. SS may occur as a sign of malignancy undiagnosed or recurrence of established malignancy.

SS is rarely associated with inflammatory bowel disease (IBD, including Crohn's disease and ulcerative colitis), BD, rheumatoid arthritis, and autoimmune thyroid disease. The skin manifestations of SS may precede or parallel the activity of the bowel disease. Some may appear during the remission period of the bowel disease. Interstitial lung disease (ILD) has been reported in SS patients, which indicate a poor prognosis [390].

10.6.1.5 Histopathology

The characteristic histopathological presentation is papillary edema and a diffuse nodular and perivascular neutrophilic infiltrate in the upper reticular dermis without evidence of vasculitis.

A histiocytoid variant of SS, characterized by a dermal, and sometimes subcutaneous, infiltrate of immature myeloid cells, has been described. This pattern of infiltrate can be mistaken for leukemia cutis [391].

In subcutaneous SS, the neutrophilic infiltrate may involve the septa, lobules, or both, with the dermis spared. The most common pattern is neutrophilic lobular panniculitis, and sometimes is admixed with scattered eosinophils.

10.6.1.6 Workup

Laboratory testing should include a complete blood count with differential. Evaluation of acute erythrocyte sedimentation rate (ESR), C-reactive protein (CRP), antinuclear antibodies, rheumatoid factor, antistreptolysin O antibody, urinalysis, and serum biochemistries (hepatic and renal function) should also be made.

Initial malignancy evaluation in newly diagnosed SS patients include stool guaiac slide test, carcinoembryonic antigen level, and chest roentgenograms, and complete blood cell count and differential to assess for a leukocytosis or an underlying leukemia should be done.

10.6.1.7 Diagnosis

The diagnostic criteria was originally proposed in Su and Liu in 1986 and modified by von den Driesch in 1994. Establishment of the diagnosis of SS required both major and at least two minor criteria (Table 10.10).

Since neoplasms may occur concurrently in SS patients without a prior cancer, Cohen and Kurzrock proposed the malignancy evaluation including: (1) a detailed medical history; (2) a thorough physical examination; and (3) laboratory tests including blood cell count, urinalysis, stool occult blood test, serum chemistries, and pap test. SS may precede the malignancy by years; so, it is reasonable to repeat the blood cell count every 6–12 months and to examine for a solid tumor [393].

Table 10.10 Criteria for diagnosis of SS [392]. Two major and two minor criteria are needed

Major criteria
1. Abrupt onset of painful erythematous plaques or nodules
2. Predominantly neutrophilic infiltration in the dermis without leukocytoclatic vasculitis
Minor criteria
1. Preceding infection or vaccinations; association with malignancies, inflammatory disorders, or pregnacy; exposure to drug
2. Accompanying fever, arthralgia, or malaise
3. Leukocytosis
4. Excellent response to systemic corticosteroids
5. ESR > 20 mm; increased C-reactive protein

10.6.1.8 Treatment

The first approach to treating SS is identifying the underlying cause and treating it if there is one. Systemic corticosteroid is first-line treatment for SS. Once the diagnosis is established, prednisone should be initiated. A dose of 0.5–1 mg/kg/day usually achieves a rapid response in days to weeks and can be tapered.

Antineutrophil therapies, including colchicine, dapsone, and potassium iodide are helpful. Potassium iodide and dapsone have a similar steroid-sparing effect.

For refractory SS patients, cyclosporine or cyclophosphamide can be administered in either monotherapy or in combination with steroids.

TNF blockers, like infliximab, may be considered for patients with arthritis of IBD. These agents have been reported to be successful in refractory SS cases [394].

10.6.1.9 Prognosis

SS may recur or relapse over years. Although SS typically has a good prognosis, the accompanied disorders may alter the prognosis. Since SS may be associated with infectious or inflammatory disorders, or malignancy, it is necessary to investigate the underlying diseases. Furthermore, SS may precede the malignancy; it is important to monitor the later development of such a condition, especially the hematological malignancy.

10.6.2 Pyoderma Gangrenosum

10.6.2.1 Introduction

Pyoderma gangrenosum (PG) is a rare noninfectious inflammatory neutrophilic dermatosis of unknown etiology. It is characterized by painful cutaneous ulcer associated with underlying systemic disease in the majority of cases. PG affects patients of all ages, but more commonly those at ages between 20 and 55 years, without a clear gender predilection. Diagnosis of PG requires exclusion of other causes of skin ulceration such as infection, malignant neoplasms, and vasculitic syndromes.

10.6.2.2 PG and Immunity

PG is thought to be related to autoinflammatory and autoimmune [395]. It can be associated with IBD, haematological malignancies, and rheumatological disorders. The etiopathophysiology is not fully understood. It is considered that PG is mediated by T lymphocytes and subsequent macrophages, which produce IL-8 attracting neutrophils which play the central pathogenetic role in PG. Besides IL-8, elevations of a variety of cytokines, including IL-1β, IL-6, IFN-γ, G-CSF, TNF-α in the serum as well as in the lesional skin, have been reported [396–398]. IL-1β plays a key role in triggering the neutrophilic inflammation of the skin [399]. IL-1 promotes the production and release of cytokines, such as TNF-α, IFN-γ, and IL-8. The biological medications targeting these cytokines (TNF-α and IL-1) are effective in treating PG [400, 401]. IL-17, together with IL-1 and TNF-α, induces the production of metalloproteinases (MMPs) resulting in the damage of the tissue. The overexpression of MMP-9 and MMP-10 were found in the skin lesions [402]. IL-17 antagonist may be a potential for refractory PG.

10.6.2.3 Clinical Manifestations

The lesions begin as papules or pustules, the centers of which break down becoming necrotic ulcers in serpiginous pattern with violacious, undermined borders. The ulcers are often covered with purulent exudates, blood, and necrotic tissue, and are painful. The ulcerations heal with cribriform scars, which is a hallmark of the disease. PG can affect any body site including breast, hand, trunk, head and neck, and peristomal skin, with a predilection for the pretibial area. PG usually occurs at the site of trauma, and pathergy is common in PG; therefore, surgical debridement should be avoided.

Clinically, PG is classified into four types: ulcerative, pustular, bullous, and vegetative. The variants may overlap.

Ulcerative PG, also known as classic PG, is the most common type of PG. The characteristic feature is a necrotic and mucopurulent tender ulcer with an edematous, violaceous, and undermined border. This type is usually associated with inflammatory diseases including IBD, arthritis, or monoclonal gammopathies. Most patients suddenly develop tender ulcers, which enlarge rapidly. It can also present less aggressively as one or two slow-growing ulcers, and the pain is relatively mild.

Pustular PG manifests as painful pustules on the extensor aspects of the extremities and upper trunk. It is considered a superficial form of ulcerative PG in which the pustules remain in the pustular stage. Pustular PG is often associated with active IBD.

Bullous PG is another superficial variant, characterized by rapidly evolving vesicles or bullae with central necrosis and an areola of erythema. The lesions occur more commonly on the arms and face. This type of PG is usually associated with myeloproliferative diseases like leukemia.

Vegetative PG is a localized, nonaggressive form of PG, with verrucous and ulcerative lesions. It is usually not associated with systemic conditions, and generally responds to milder therapies.

PG patients are often accompanied with fever, myalgia, arthralgia, and malaise. Extracutaneous involvements include oropharynx, upper airway, eye, genitalia, and lung.

10.6.2.4 Associations

PG is frequently associated with a systemic disease such as IBD, rheumatoid arthritis, seronegative arthritis, hematological disorders. These diseases may precede, follow, or occur simultaneously with PG. Up to 7 % of PG patients are associated with hematological malignancy, most commonly myelodysplastic syndrome and acute myeloid leukemia.

10.6.2.5 Histopathology

Histopathological features of PG are nonspecific, including dermal edema, suppurative inflammation with dense neutrophilic infiltrates in the dermis and subcutaneous fat, which can also be seen in skin infections. Leukocytoclastic vasculitis is often present.

The changes are diverse depending on the type and the evolution stage of the lesion, and even the site of a given lesion.

A biopsy from early lesions shows neutrophil infiltration (with or without lymphocyte), which often occurs diffusely in the deeper dermis and involves follicular structures. Later, a mixed inflammatory infiltrate, more prominent hemorrhage, necrosis, and fibrosis in the reticular dermis and subcutaneous tissue can be observed. As lesions regress, macrophages and plasma cells invade the dermis showing granulomatous reactions. In the end stage, fibrosis results in scar formation. The vascular changes in early lesions appear as endothelial edema, perivascular neutrophil infiltrate without fibrinoid necrosis. Focal vasculitis in fully developed lesions can be seen, which may be a secondary phenomenon.

10.6.2.6 Workup

A thorough approach to the workup of the patient is paramount to work through the other entities that may imitate PG. Although the histopathological changes are nonspecific, they are valuable in ruling out other causes of ulceration. An incisional biopsy from the edge of the ulcer and the surrounding skin is very important. Negative cultures and special stains are needed to exclude infectious diseases.

For up to 50 % of PG patients are associated with systemic disorders, workup for PG includes searching for extracutaneous involvement and underlying coexisting conditions. Helpful laboratories include a blood cell count, erythrocyte sedimentation rate (ESR), liver and renal function tests, protein electrophoresis, antineutrophilic cytoplasmic antibodies, antiphospholipid antibodies, and cryoglobulins. Chest X-ray or computed tomography and colonoscopy should be considered when respiratory or intestinal symptoms are present.

10.6.2.7 Diagnosis

Diagnosis of PG depends on clinical features and histopathology. PG should be considered in patients with painful, rapidly expanding, serpiginous ulcers. No criteria have been generally adopted. A proposed criteria requires two major criteria: (i) rapid progression of a painful, necrolytic, cutaneous ulcer with an irregular, violaceous, and undermined border; and (ii) exclusion of other causes of cutaneous ulceration; and at least two minor criteria, including (a) a history suggestive of pathergy or a clinical finding of cribiform scarring, (b) systemic diseases associated with PG, (c) histopathological findings (sterile dermal neutrophilia, mixed inflammation, lymphocytic vasculitis), and (d) rapid response to systemic corticosteroid treatment [403].

PG is a diagnosis of exclusion. Histopathological and cultures must be performed to rule out other differentials such as vasculitis, cutaneous malignancies, and infections (bacterial, fungal, amoebic).

10.6.2.8 Treatment

The goal of management is to control inflammation, optimize wound healing, and relieve pain. PG patients usually require aggressive immunosuppressive therapy (prednisone and/or cyclosporine) to induce disease remission and long-term maintenance therapy with another less toxic agent for months to years to prevent relapses. Associated disease must be treated promptly.

Corticosteroid (prednisone 1 mg/kg/day) is considered first-line treatment, and cyclosporine (3–5 mg/kg/day) can be used as a second-line treatment in chronic and steroid-resistant cases. Alternative treatments include thalidomide, minocycline, colchicine, dapsone, mycophenolate mofetil, azathioprine, and high-dose intravenous immunoglobulin.

Anti-TNF agents, etanercept, infliximab, and adalimumab, have been found effective in the treatment of recalcitrant PG. Case reports have demonstrated the effectiveness of ustekinumab (anti-IL-12/23), ixekizumab (anti-IL-17), and brodalumab (anti-IL-17R). IL-1 antagonists (i.e., anakinra and gevokizumab) have produced a very good response in patients with PAPA syndrome.

Systemic therapy combined with topical tacrolimus or steroids, and gentle wound care is ideal. Hyperbaric oxygen therapy has been found to be an effective adjunct in wound healing. The outcomes of surgery usually are not optimistic.

The management strategy is individualized and based on evaluation of each case.

10.6.2.9 Prognosis

Poor prognostic factors include older age at onset and associations with systemic diseases. Death can occur in patients with severe associated diseases, particularly with an underlying hematological malignancy. Sepsis is the leading cause of death.

10.6.3 Behçet's Disease

10.6.3.1 Introduction

Behçet's disease (BD) is a chronic, relapsing, inflammatory vasculitis involving vessels of all sizes. It is clinically characterized by multisystemic manifestations including cutaneous lesions such as aphthous stomatitis, genital ulcers, erythema nodosum-like lesions, and papulopustular lesions, as well as uveitis, epididymitis, arthritis (swollen, painful, stiff joints), and neurological and gastrointestinal symptoms. BD is thought to be an autoimmune and autoinflammatory response in a genetically predisposed individual triggered by an infectious or environmental agent.

Onset of BD is usually in the third or fourth decades. Men and women are equally affected in the West, but the course of the disease is more severe in men. A male predominance in Middle Eastern countries is seen. Familial cases have been reported.

BD usually begins with recurrent aphthous ulcers. Usually, there is a delay in diagnosis after the presence of the first sign.

10.6.3.2 Pathogenesis

The exact cause is still unknown, but it is believed that a complex genetic predisposition, environmental factors, and immunological abnormalities cause the disease. People carrying the human leukocyte antigen (HLA)-B51 are more prone to develop BD. Herpes simplex virus and *Streptococcus sanguis*, which activate the immune system, contribute to the development of BD.

10.6.3.3 BD and Immunity

It is likely that hypersensitivity of T cells to an infectious agent plays a key role in the pathogenesis. Complex interactions among antigen-presenting cells (APCs), Th1 lymphocytes, and neutrophils are the basis of the immune aberrations observed in patients with BD. APCs either primary or secondary to their stimulation with Th1 cytokines including IFN-γ and TNF-α cause overproduction of IL-12 and IL-18, which eventually drive an immune response toward Th1. Additionally, enhanced production of IFN-γ, TNF-a, IL-8, IL-17, and IL-18 might lead to a state which is characterized by neutrophil hyperactivity. Serum/plasma levels of several cytokines, including TNF-α, IFN-γ, IL-1, IL-8, IL-12, soluble IL-2R (IL-2R), and TNF receptor, have been reported to be correlated with the clinical activity of BD [404].

Treatments targeting TNF have successfully been used in BD patients who are refractory to standard of care [405]. IL-1 and IL-6 have also been reported to be promising targets in patients resistant to other regimens [406]. Favorable responses to IL-1 blockade have been described for BD mucocutaneous lesions and uveitis [407, 408].

10.6.3.4 Clinical Features

Mucocutaneous Manifestations

Recurrent and painful oral ulcers are seen in approximately 97–100 % of all BD patients. They usually present as the initial sign, and most often occur on the gingiva, tongue, and buccal or labial mucosae. Aphthous lesions mostly recur more than three times a year. It begins as a painful papule, which rapidly becomes ulcerated with white to yellowish pseudomembrane on the surface of the ulcer and an erythematous halo surrounding the ulcer. Three types of aphthae can develop: (1) minor aphthae, the most common type with a diameter of less than 10 mm, usually heal spontaneously within 7–10 days without scarring; (2) major aphthae, characterized by deep and painful ulcers with a diameter of more than 10 mm, may cause scarring after the wound healing; (3) herpetiform aphthae appear as multiple ulcers.

50–85 % of BD patients develop genital ulcers, which start as a painful papule or papulopustule. The lesions tend to occur on the scrotum, inguinal region and penis in men, and on the vulva in women. They usually resolve in 2–4 weeks with scarring.

Cutaneous lesions of BD include papulopustular lesions, erythema nodosum-like lesions, PG-like lesions, SS-like lesions, acneiform lesions, acral purpuric papulonodules, and superficial and/or deep thrombophlebitis. Skin lesions can occur in combinations.

Small, recurrent, disseminated papulopustules of proximal extremity are the most common findings in BD. They are seen in 30–96 % of patients. Erythema nodosum-like lesions are localized symmetrically on the lower extremities, as well as on the thighs and sacral region. Women are more prone to develop erythema nodosum-like lesions. They usually heal in 1–6 weeks. Acneiform lesions include inflammatory papules, pustules, and cysts, which mostly locate on the back, chest, shoulder area, and less commonly on the face. SS-like lesions can be seen in approximately 4 % of BD patients.

Superficial thrombophlebitis migrans are more frequent in men presenting with dusky, red nodules on the medial side of the legs. Superficial thrombosis can present as palpable masses along the veins. Pathergy tests are more likely to be positive when the disease is active.

10.6.3.5 Eye Involvement

About half of the BD patients have eye involvement, which may be the initial manifestation of the disease. Behçet's uveitis (BU) is characterized by chronic panuveitis or posterior uveitis with necrotizing retinal vasculitis and tends to be more recurrent and sight threatening than other endogenous uveitides. The disease usually presents with acute inflammatory episodes that resolve within days or weeks. Recurrent episodes may result in permanent vision loss.

10.6.3.6 Joints

Up to 50 % of BD patients have either arthritis or arthralgia affecting knee, ankle, wrist, and elbow joints. Symptoms usually heal within a few weeks, without causing deformities.

10.6.3.7 Gastrointestinal Symptoms

Patients with gastrointestinal involvement usually have abdominal pain, diarrhea, nausea, or vomiting. Gastrointestinal bleeding is rarely seen.

10.6.3.8 Neurological Symptoms

Neuro-BD, accounting for 5–10 % of BD patients, is recognized approximately 5 years after the diagnosis. Patients are usually young. The symptoms include cognitive changes, sphincter dysfunction, severe headaches, papilledema, and motor or ocular nerve paralysis.

10.6.3.9 Histopathology

Histopathologically, BD typically displays as a pattern of leukocytoclastic vasculitis (LCV), a neutrophilic vascular reaction, septal panniculitis, and lobular panniculitis with vasculitis. Vascular thrombosis may also be present. Acneiform lesions show changes of suppurative or granulomatous folliculitis. EN-like lesions display deep dermal and septal perivascular lymphocytic infiltrates, with lymphocytic infiltration of vessel walls, but without granulomatous changes. Direct immunofluorescence studies reveal IgM and C3 in a diffuse distribution of aphthous lesions, but less likely in EN-like lesions or other lesions of BD.

10.6.3.10 Workup

There are currently no specific laboratory tests for BD. Abnormal laboratory results include leukocytosis, increased erythrocyte sedimentation rate and C-reactive protein, as well as elevations in immunoglobulins IgG, IgA, and IgM.

10.6.3.11 Diagnosis

In 1990, the ISG published its diagnostic criteria, which includes the presence of recurrent oral ulceration, as well as at least two other features, such as recurrent genital ulceration, ocular lesions, cutaneous lesions, and a positive pathergy test.

10.6.3.12 Treatment

There is no cure for BD. The goal of the treatment is to relieve the symptoms when the disease is active, prevent complications, and maintain the remission. The treatment strategy depends on the severity of symptoms, disease duration, and the age and the associations. The medications including corticosteroids, dapsone, colchicine, immunosuppressants, interferon-alpha, and biologics have been used for BD. Colchicine, dapsone, and thalidomide are effective for mild-to-moderate mucocutaneous lesions. If the therapy fails, oral corticosteroids may be added.

10.6.3.13 Corticosteroids

Corticosteroids are the most commonly used drug for rapid suppression of inflammatory process during acute exacerbations, to reduce severe joint pain, skin sores, eye disease, or CNS symptoms. For mild disease, topical or intralesional corticosteroids are recommended.

10.6.3.14 Cyclosporine

Cyclosporine shows effectiveness for oral and genital ulcers, erythema nodosum-like lesion, and thrombophlebitis. Due to its rapid action, cyclosporine is the first-line drug besides corticosteroids. Because of its side effects such as hypertension, renal impairment, and neurotoxicity, cyclosporine is generally reserved for ocular diseases or arthritis. Close monitoring of liver and kidney functions and blood pressure is required.

10.6.3.15 Azathioprine (AZA)

Oral AZA may decrease eye involvement, reduce the frequency and severity of oral and skin lesions, thus improving the long-term prognosis of BD. If patients do not respond to corticosteroids, cyclosporine of AZA should be considered.

10.6.3.16 TNF-α Antagonist

Anti-TNF agents, etanercept and infliximab, show remarkable effect for uveitis, orogenital ulcers, and skin lesions which are refractory to conventional drugs.

10.6.3.17 Interferon-Alpha (IFN-α)

IFN-α (3 million units every other day) shows a significant effect on decreasing pain, oral and genital ulcers, and skin lesions. Long-lasting remissions in patients with severe ocular disease have been reported after cessation of the drug. Side effects include alopecia, influenza-like symptoms, leukopenia, and depression. IFN-α should not be combined with AZA for causing severe leukopenia.

10.6.3.18 Prognosis

Poor prognostic factors include male sex, arterial involvement, and the frequent flares. Uveitis has a potential for visual loss.

References

Urticaria

1. Zuberbier T, Aberer W, Asero R, et al. The EAACI/GA2LEN/EDF/WAO guideline for the definition, classification, diagnosis, and management of urticaria: the 2013 revision and update. Allergy. 2014;69(7):868–87.
2. Burmester GR, Pezzutto A. Color atlas of immunology. 1st ed. Stuttgart: Georg Thieme Verlag; 2006. p. 200–1.
3. Roecken M, Grevers G, Burgdorf W. Color atlas of allergic diseases. 1st ed. Stuttgart: Georg Thieme Verlag; 2006. p. 116–7.
4. Spickett G. Oxford handbook of clinical immunology and allergy. 3rd ed. UK: Oxford University Press; 2013. p. 129–32.
5. Bernstein JA, Lang DM, Khan DA, et al. The diagnosis and management of acute and chronic urticaria: 2014 update. J Allergy Clin Immunol. 2014;133(5):1270–7.

6. Kaplan AP. What the first 10,000 patients with chronic urticaria have taught me:a personal journey. J Allergy Clin Immunol. 2009;123:713–7.
7. Di Lorenzo G, Pacor ML, Mansueto P, Martinelli N, Esposito-Pellitteri M, Lo Bianco C, et al. Food-additive-induced urticaria: a survey of 838 patients with recurrent chronic idiopathic urticaria. Int Arch Allergy Immunol. 2005;138:235–42.
8. Leznoff A, Josse RG, Denburg J, Dolovich J. Association of chronic urticaria and angioedema with thyroid autoimmunity. Arch Dermatol. 1983;119:636–40.
9. Leznoff A, Sussman GL. Syndrome of idiopathic chronic urticaria and angioe- dema with thyroid autoimmunity: a study of 90 patients. J Allergy Clin Immunol. 1989;84:66–71.
10. Ferrer M, Kinet JP, Kaplan AP. Comparative studies of functional and binding assays for IgG anti-Fc(epsilon)RIalpha (alpha-subunit) in chronic urticaria. J Allergy Clin Immunol. 1998;101:672–6.
11. Tong LJ, Balakrishnan G, Kochan JP, Kinet JP, Kaplan AP. Assessment of auto- immunity in patients with chronic urticaria. J Allergy Clin Immunol. 1997;99:461–5.
12. Puccetti A, Bason C, Simeoni S, Millo E, Tinazzi E, Beri R, et al. In chronic idiopathic urticaria autoantibodies against Fc epsilon-RII/CD23 induce histamine release via eosinophil activation. Clin Exp Allergy. 2005;35:1599–607.
13. Niimi N, Francis DM, Kermani F, O'Donnell BF, Hide M, Kobza-Black A, et al. Dermal mast cell activation by autoantibodies against the high affinity IgE receptor in chronic urticaria. J Invest Dermatol. 1996;106:1001–6.
14. Garmendia JV, Zabaleta M, Aldrey O, Rivera H, De Sanctis JB, Bianco NE, et al. Immunophenotype characteristics of peripheral blood mononuclear leukocytes of chronic idiopathic urticaria patients. Invest Clin. 2006;47:361–9.
15. Garmendia JV, Zabaleta M, Blanca I, Bianco NE, De Sanctis JB. Total and biologically active serum-soluble CD154 in patients with chronic idiopathic urticaria. Allergy Asthma Proc. 2004;25:121–5.
16. Eckman JA, Hamilton RG, Gober LM, Sterba PM, Saini SS. Basophil phenotypes in chronic idiopathic urticaria in relation to disease activity and autoantibodies. J Invest Dermatol. 2008;128: 1956–63.
17. Zuberbier T, Maurer M. Urticaria: current opinions about etiology, diagnosis and therapy. Acta Derm Venereol. 2007;87:196–205.
18. Magerl MA, Altrichter S, Boodstein N, Gu€zelbey O, Keßler B, Krause K, et al. Urticaria – classification and strategies for diagnosis and treatment. CME Dermatol. 2008;3:2 18.
19. Ventura MT, Napolitano S, Menga R, Cecere R, Asero R. Anisakis simplex hyper sensitivity is associated with chronic urticaria in endemic areas. Int Arch Allergy Immunol. 2013;160:297–300.
20. Daschner A, Pascual CY. Anisakis simplex: sensitization and clinical allergy. Curr Opin Allergy Clin Immunol. 2005;5:281–5.
21. Kaplan AP. Treatment of chronic spontaneous urticaria. Allergy Asthma Immunol Res. 2012;4:326–31.
22. Metz M, Maurer M. Omalizumab in chronic urticaria. Curr Opin Allergy Clin Immunol. 2012;12:406–11.
23. Ivyanskiy I, Sand C, Francis ST. Omalizumab for chronic urticaria: a case series and overview of the literature. Case Rep Dermatol. 2012;4:19–26.

Psoriasis

24. Di Cesare A, Di Meglio P, Nestle FO. The IL-23/Th17 axis in the immunopathogenesis of psoriasis. J Invest Dermatol. 2009;129(6): 1339–50.
25. Zaba LC, et al. Effective treatment of psoriasis with etanercept is linked to suppression of IL-17 signaling, not immediate response TNF genes. J Allergy Clin Immunol. 2009;124(5):1022–10. e1–395.
26. Baliwag J, Barnes DH, Johnston A. Cytokines in psoriasis. Cytokine. 2015;73(2):342–50.
27. Hijnen D, et al. CD8(+) T cells in the lesional skin of atopic dermatitis and psoriasis patients are an important source of IFN-gamma, IL-13, IL-17, and IL-22. J Invest Dermatol. 2013; 133(4):973–9.
28. Jin L, Wang G. Keratin 17: a critical player in the pathogenesis of psoriasis. Med Res Rev. 2014;34(2):438–54.
29. Fu M, Wang G. Keratin 17 as a therapeutic target for the treatment of psoriasis. J Dermatol Sci. 2012;67(3):161–5.
30. Grine L, et al. An inflammatory triangle in psoriasis: TNF, type I IFNs and IL-17. Cytokine Growth Factor Rev. 2014;26(1):25–33.
31. Puig L, Julia A, Marsal S. The pathogenesis and genetics of psoriasis. Actas Dermosifiliogr. 2014;105(6):535–45.
32. Nair RP, et al. Genome-wide scan reveals association of psoriasis with IL-23 and NF-kappaB pathways. Nat Genet. 2009;41(2): 199–204.
33. Villablanca EJ, Mora JR. A two-step model for Langerhans cell migration to skin-draining LN. Eur J Immunol. 2008;38(11): 2975–80.
34. Avramidis G, et al. The role of endothelial cell apoptosis in the effect of etanercept in psoriasis. Br J Dermatol. 2010;163(5): 928–34.
35. Gottlieb AB, et al. TNF inhibition rapidly down-regulates multiple proinflammatory pathways in psoriasis plaques. J Immunol. 2005;175(4):2721–9.
36. Schmuth M, et al. Expression of the C-C chemokine MIP-3 alpha/CCL20 in human epidermis with impaired permeability barrier function. Exp Dermatol. 2002;11(2):135–42.
37. Chiricozzi A, et al. Integrative responses to IL-17 and TNF-alpha in human keratinocytes account for key inflammatory pathogenic circuits in psoriasis. J Invest Dermatol. 2011;131(3):677–87.
38. Johnston A, et al. Keratinocyte overexpression of IL-17C promotes psoriasiform skin inflammation. J Immunol. 2013;190(5): 2252–62.
39. Hartupee J, et al. IL-17 enhances chemokine gene expression through mRNA stabilization. J Immunol. 2007;179(6):4135–41.
40. Johnston A, et al. Early tissue responses in psoriasis to the antitumour necrosis factor-alpha biologic etanercept suggest reduced interleukin-17 receptor expression and signalling. Br J Dermatol. 2014;171(1):97–107.
41. Nestle FO, et al. Plasmacytoid predendritic cells initiate psoriasis through interferon-alpha production. J Exp Med. 2005;202(1): 135–43.
42. Albanesi C, et al. Chemerin expression marks early psoriatic skin lesions and correlates with plasmacytoid dendritic cell recruitment. J Exp Med. 2009;206(1):249–58.
43. Das RP, Jain AK, Ramesh V. Current concepts in the pathogenesis of psoriasis. Indian J Dermatol. 2009;54(1):7–12.
44. Kryczek I, et al. Induction of IL-17+ T cell trafficking and development by IFN-gamma: mechanism and pathological relevance in psoriasis. J Immunol. 2008;181(7):4733–41.
45. Bissonnette R, et al. A randomized, double-blind, placebo-controlled, phase I study of MEDI-545, an anti-interferon-alfa monoclonal antibody, in subjects with chronic psoriasis. J Am Acad Dermatol. 2010;62(3):427–36.
46. Johnson-Huang LM, et al. A single intradermal injection of IFN-gamma induces an inflammatory state in both non-lesional psoriatic and healthy skin. J Invest Dermatol. 2012;132(4):1177–87.
47. Gaffen SL. Structure and signalling in the IL-17 receptor family. Nat Rev Immunol. 2009;9(8):556–67.
48. Lowes MA, et al. Psoriasis vulgaris lesions contain discrete populations of Th1 and Th17 T cells. J Invest Dermatol. 2008; 128(5):1207–11.

49. Johnston A, et al. Keratinocyte overexpression of IL-17C promotes psoriasiform skin inflammation. J Immunol. 2013;190(5):2252–62.
50. Ortega C, et al. IL-17-producing CD8+ T lymphocytes from psoriasis skin plaques are cytotoxic effector cells that secrete Th17-related cytokines. J Leukoc Biol. 2009;86(2):435–43.
51. Res PC, et al. Overrepresentation of IL-17A and IL-22 producing CD8 T cells in lesional skin suggests their involvement in the pathogenesis of psoriasis. PLoS One. 2010;5(11):e14108.
52. Lin AM, et al. Mast cells and neutrophils release IL-17 through extracellular trap formation in psoriasis. J Immunol. 2011; 187(1):490–500.
53. Villanova F, et al. Characterization of innate lymphoid cells in human skin and blood demonstrates increase of NKp44+ ILC3 in psoriasis. J Invest Dermatol. 2014;134(4):984–91.
54. Teunissen MB, et al. The IL-17A-producing CD8+ T-cell population in psoriatic lesional skin comprises mucosa-associated invariant T cells and conventional T cells. J Invest Dermatol. 2014;134(12):2898–907.
55. Papp KA, et al. Efficacy and safety of secukinumab in the treatment of moderate-to-severe plaque psoriasis: a randomized, double-blind, placebo-controlled phase II dose-ranging study. Br J Dermatol. 2013;168(2):412–21.
56. Leonardi C, et al. Anti-interleukin-17 monoclonal antibody ixekizumab in chronic plaque psoriasis. N Engl J Med. 2012;366(13): 1190–9.
57. Rich P, et al. Secukinumab induction and maintenance therapy in moderate-to-severe plaque psoriasis: a randomized, double-blind, placebo-controlled, phase II regimen-finding study. Br J Dermatol. 2013;168(2):402–11.
58. Papp KA, et al. Brodalumab, an anti-interleukin-17-receptor antibody for psoriasis. N Engl J Med. 2012;366(13):1181–9.
59. Gaffen SL, et al. The IL-23-IL-17 immune axis: from mechanisms to therapeutic testing. Nat Rev Immunol. 2014;14(9):585–600.
60. Skepner J, et al. Pharmacologic inhibition of RORgammat regulates Th17 signature gene expression and suppresses cutaneous inflammation in vivo. J Immunol. 2014;192(6):2564–75.
61. Sigmundsdottir H, et al. Differential effects of interleukin 12 and interleukin 10 on superantigen-induced expression of cutaneous lymphocyte-associated antigen (CLA) and alphaEbeta7 integrin (CD103) by CD8+ T cells. Clin Immunol. 2004;111(1):119–25.
62. Wilson NJ, et al. Development, cytokine profile and function of human interleukin 17-producing helper T cells. Nat Immunol. 2007;8(9):950–7.
63. Yawalkar N, et al. Expression of interleukin-12 is increased in psoriatic skin. J Invest Dermatol. 1998;111(6):1053–7.
64. Piskin G, et al. In vitro and in situ expression of IL-23 by keratinocytes in healthy skin and psoriasis lesions: enhanced expression in psoriatic skin. J Immunol. 2006;176(3):1908–15.
65. Lee E, et al. Increased expression of interleukin 23 p19 and p40 in lesional skin of patients with psoriasis vulgaris. J Exp Med. 2004;199(1):125–30.
66. Cargill M, et al. A large-scale genetic association study confirms IL12B and leads to the identification of IL23R as psoriasis-risk genes. Am J Hum Genet. 2007;80(2):273–90.
67. Johnston A, et al. Susceptibility-associated genetic variation at IL12B enhances Th1 polarization in psoriasis. Hum Mol Genet. 2013;22(9):1807–15.
68. Nair RP, et al. Polymorphisms of the IL12B and IL23R genes are associated with psoriasis. J Invest Dermatol. 2008;128(7): 1653–61.
69. Desmet J, et al. Structural basis of IL-23 antagonism by an Alphabody protein scaffold. Nat Commun. 2014;5:5237.
70. Quiniou C, et al. Specific targeting of the IL-23 receptor, using a novel small peptide noncompetitive antagonist, decreases the inflammatory response. Am J Physiol Regul Integr Comp Physiol. 2014;307(10):R1216–30.
71. Commins S, Steinke JW, Borish L. The extended IL-10 superfamily: IL-10, IL-19, IL-20, IL-22, IL-24, IL-26, IL-28, and IL-29. J Allergy Clin Immunol. 2008;121(5):1108–11.
72. Asadullah K, et al. IL-10 is a key cytokine in psoriasis. Proof of principle by IL-10 therapy: a new therapeutic approach. J Clin Invest. 1998;101(4):783–94.
73. Sa SM, et al. The effects of IL-20 subfamily cytokines on reconstituted human epidermis suggest potential roles in cutaneous innate defense and pathogenic adaptive immunity in psoriasis. J Immunol. 2007;178(4):2229–40.
74. Sabat R, Ouyang W, Wolk K. Therapeutic opportunities of the IL-22-IL-22R1 system. Nat Rev Drug Discov. 2014;13(1):21–38.
75. Ward NL, Umetsu DT. A new player on the psoriasis block: IL-17A- and IL-22-producing innate lymphoid cells. J Invest Dermatol. 2014;134(9):2305–7.
76. Boniface K, et al. IL-22 inhibits epidermal differentiation and induces proinflammatory gene expression and migration of human keratinocytes. J Immunol. 2005;174(6):3695–702.
77. Nikamo P, et al. Genetic variants of the IL22 promoter associate to onset of psoriasis before puberty and increased IL-22 production in T cells. J Invest Dermatol. 2014;134(6):1535–41.
78. Natsuaki Y, et al. Perivascular leukocyte clusters are essential for efficient activation of effector T cells in the skin. Nat Immunol. 2014;15(11):1064–9.
79. Foster AM, et al. IL-36 promotes myeloid cell infiltration, activation, and inflammatory activity in skin. J Immunol. 2014;192(12): 6053–61.
80. Johnston A, et al. IL-1F5, –F6, –F8, and -F9: a novel IL-1 family signaling system that is active in psoriasis and promotes keratinocyte antimicrobial peptide expression. J Immunol. 2011;186(4): 2613–22.
81. Kumar S, et al. Identification and initial characterization of four novel members of the interleukin-1 family. J Biol Chem. 2000;275(14):10308–14.
82. Smith DE, et al. Four new members expand the interleukin-1 superfamily. J Biol Chem. 2000;275(2):1169–75.
83. Onoufriadis A, et al. Mutations in IL36RN/IL1F5 are associated with the severe episodic inflammatory skin disease known as generalized pustular psoriasis. Am J Hum Genet. 2011;89(3):432–7.
84. Marrakchi S, et al. Interleukin-36-receptor antagonist deficiency and generalized pustular psoriasis. N Engl J Med. 2011; 365(7):620–8.
85. Hijnen D, et al. CD8(+) T cells in the lesional skin of atopic dermatitis and psoriasis patients are an important source of IFN-gamma, IL-13, IL-17, and IL-22. J Invest Dermatol. 2013;133(4):973–9.
86. Koga C, et al. Possible pathogenic role of Th17 cells for atopic dermatitis. J Invest Dermatol. 2008;128(11):2625–30.
87. Nair RP, et al. Genome-wide scan reveals association of psoriasis with IL-23 and NF-kappaB pathways. Nat Genet. 2009;41(2): 199–204.
88. Li B, et al. Transcriptome analysis of psoriasis in a large case–control sample: RNA-seq provides insights into disease mechanisms. J Invest Dermatol. 2014;134(7):1828–38.
89. Sharma S, et al. The IL-1 family member 7b translocates to the nucleus and down-regulates proinflammatory cytokines. J Immunol. 2008;180(8):5477–82.
90. Nold MF, et al. IL-37 is a fundamental inhibitor of innate immunity. Nat Immunol. 2010;11(11):1014–22.
91. Garcia-Valladares I, Cuchacovich R, Espinoza LR. Comparative assessment of biologics in treatment of psoriasis: drug design and clinical effectiveness of ustekinumab. Drug Des Devel Ther. 2011;5:41–9.
92. Menter A, et al. A randomized comparison of continuous vs. intermittent infliximab maintenance regimens over 1 year in the treatment of moderate-to-severe plaque psoriasis. J Am Acad Dermatol. 2007;56(1):31.e1–15.

93. Thaci D, et al. Adalimumab for the treatment of moderate to severe psoriasis: subanalysis of effects on scalp and nails in the BELIEVE study. J Eur Acad Dermatol Venereol. 2015;29(2):353–60.
94. Turner D, et al. Adalimumab for the treatment of psoriasis. Health Technol Assess. 2009;13 Suppl 2:49–54.
95. Mrowietz U, et al. An assessment of adalimumab efficacy in three Phase III clinical trials using the European Consensus Programme criteria for psoriasis treatment goals. Br J Dermatol. 2013; 168(2):374–80.
96. Strober BE, et al. Efficacy and safety results from a phase III, randomized controlled trial comparing the safety and efficacy of briakinumab with etanercept and placebo in patients with moderate to severe chronic plaque psoriasis. Br J Dermatol. 2011; 165(3):661–8.
97. Bartelds GM, et al. Anti-infliximab and anti-adalimumab antibodies in relation to response to adalimumab in infliximab switchers and anti-tumour necrosis factor naive patients: a cohort study. Ann Rheum Dis. 2010;69(5):817–21.
98. Wolbink GJ, et al. Development of antiinfliximab antibodies and relationship to clinical response in patients with rheumatoid arthritis. Arthritis Rheum. 2006;54(3):711–5.
99. Solomon DH, et al. Association between disease-modifying antirheumatic drugs and diabetes risk in patients with rheumatoid arthritis and psoriasis. JAMA. 2011;305(24):2525–31.
100. Wu JJ, Poon KY. Tumor necrosis factor inhibitor therapy and myocardial infarction risk in patients with psoriasis, psoriatic arthritis, or both. J Drugs Dermatol. 2014;13(8):932–4.
101. Wu JJ, et al. Association between tumor necrosis factor inhibitor therapy and myocardial infarction risk in patients with psoriasis. Arch Dermatol. 2012;148(11):1244–50.
102. Mease PJ. Inhibition of interleukin-17, interleukin-23 and the TH17 cell pathway in the treatment of psoriatic arthritis and psoriasis. Curr Opin Rheumatol. 2015;27(2):127–33.
103. Papp KA, et al. Efficacy and safety of ustekinumab, a human interleukin-12/23 monoclonal antibody, in patients with psoriasis: 52-week results from a randomised, double-blind, placebo-controlled trial (PHOENIX 2). Lancet. 2008;371(9625):1675–84.
104. McInnes IB, et al. Efficacy and safety of ustekinumab in patients with active psoriatic arthritis: 1 year results of the phase 3, multicentre, double-blind, placebo-controlled PSUMMIT 1 trial. Lancet. 2013;382(9894):780–9.
105. Ritchlin C, et al. Efficacy and safety of the anti-IL-12/23 p40 monoclonal antibody, ustekinumab, in patients with active psoriatic arthritis despite conventional non-biological and biological anti-tumour necrosis factor therapy: 6-month and 1 year results of the phase 3, multicentre, double-blind, placebo-controlled, randomised PSUMMIT 2 trial. Ann Rheum Dis. 2014;73(6):990–9.
106. Cai X, et al. PIKfyve, a class III PI kinase, is the target of the small molecular IL-12/IL-23 inhibitor apilimod and a player in Toll-like receptor signaling. Chem Biol. 2013;20(7):912–21.
107. Wada Y, et al. Apilimod inhibits the production of IL-12 and IL-23 and reduces dendritic cell infiltration in psoriasis. PLoS One. 2012;7(4):e35069.
108. Sofen H, et al. Guselkumab (an IL-23-specific mAb) demonstrates clinical and molecular response in patients with moderate-to-severe psoriasis. J Allergy Clin Immunol. 2014;133(4):1032–40.
109. Zandvliet A, et al. Tildrakizumab, a novel anti-IL-23 monoclonal antibody, is unaffected by ethnic variability in Caucasian, Chinese, and Japanese subjects. Int J Clin Pharmacol Ther. 2015; 53(2):139–46.
110. Tausend W, Downing C, Tyring S. Systematic review of interleukin-12, interleukin-17, and interleukin-23 pathway inhibitors for the treatment of moderate-to-severe chronic plaque psoriasis: ustekinumab, briakinumab, tildrakizumab, guselkumab, secukinumab, ixekizumab, and brodalumab. J Cutan Med Surg. 2014;18(3):156–69.
111. Gudjonsson JE, Johnston A, Ellis CN. Novel systemic drugs under investigation for the treatment of psoriasis. J Am Acad Dermatol. 2012;67(1):139–47.
112. Mitra A, Fallen RS, Lima HC. Cytokine-based therapy in psoriasis. Clin Rev Allergy Immunol. 2013;44(2):173–82.
113. Ryan C, et al. Association between biologic therapies for chronic plaque psoriasis and cardiovascular events: a meta-analysis of randomized controlled trials. JAMA. 2011;306(8):864–71.
114. Langley RG, et al. Secukinumab in plaque psoriasis – results of two phase 3 trials. N Engl J Med. 2014;371(4):326–38.
115. McInnes IB, et al. Efficacy and safety of secukinumab, a fully human anti-interleukin-17A monoclonal antibody, in patients with moderate-to-severe psoriatic arthritis: a 24-week, randomised, double-blind, placebo-controlled, phase II proof-of-concept trial. Ann Rheum Dis. 2014;73(2):349–56.
116. McInnes IB, et al. Efficacy and safety of secukinumab, a fully human anti-interleukin-17A monoclonal antibody, in patients with moderate-to-severe psoriatic arthritis: a 24-week, randomised, double-blind, placebo-controlled, phase II proof-of-concept trial. Ann Rheum Dis. 2014;73(2):349–56.
117. Mease PJ, et al. Brodalumab, an anti-IL17RA monoclonal antibody, in psoriatic arthritis. N Engl J Med. 2014;370(24):2295–306.
118. Study evaluating the safety and tolerability of ILV-094 in subjects with psoriasis. 2012. Clinical trial.gov.
119. Huffmeier U, et al. Successful therapy with anakinra in a patient with generalized pustular psoriasis carrying IL36RN mutations. Br J Dermatol. 2014;170(1):202–4.
120. Huffmeier U, et al. Successful therapy with anakinra in a patient with generalized pustular psoriasis carrying IL36RN mutations. Br J Dermatol. 2014;170(1):202–4.
121. Wolf J, Ferris LK. Anti-IL-36R antibodies, potentially useful for the treatment of psoriasis: a patent evaluation of WO2013074569. Expert Opin Ther Pat. 2014;24(4):477–9.
122. Papp KA, et al. Efficacy and safety of tofacitinib, an oral Janus kinase inhibitor, in the treatment of psoriasis: a Phase 2b randomized placebo-controlled dose-ranging study. Br J Dermatol. 2012;167(3):668–77.
123. Papp K, et al. Efficacy of apremilast in the treatment of moderate to severe psoriasis: a randomised controlled trial. Lancet. 2012;380(9843):738–46.
124. Kupetsky EA, Mathers AR, Ferris LK. Anti-cytokine therapy in the treatment of psoriasis. Cytokine. 2013;61(3):704–12.

Drug Eruptions: Erythema Multiforme and SJS/TEN

125. Bastuji-Garin S, Rzany B, Stern RS, Shear NH, Naldi L, Roujeau J. Clinical classification of cases of toxic epidermal necrolysis, stevens-johnson syndrome, and erythema multiforme. Arch Dermatol. 1993;129(1):92–6.
126. Auquier-Dunant A, Mockenhaupt M, Naldi L, Correia O, Schröder W, Roujeau J-C. Correlations between clinical patterns and causes of erythema multiforme majus, Stevens-Johnson syndrome, and toxic epidermal necrolysis: results of an international prospective study. Arch Dermatol. 2002;138(8):1019–24.
127. Assier H, Bastuji-Garin S, Revuz J, Roujeau JC. Erythema multiforme with mucous membrane involvement and Stevens-Johnson syndrome are clinically different disorders with distinct causes. Arch Dermatol. 1995;131(5):539–43.
128. Huff JC, Weston WL, Tonnesen MG. Erythema multiforme: a critical review of characteristics, diagnostic criteria, and causes. J Am Acad Dermatol. 1983;8(6):763–75.
129. Bolognia JL, Cooper DL, Glusac EJ. Toxic erythema of chemotherapy: a useful clinical term. J Am Acad Dermatol. 2008;59(3):524–9.

130. Schalock PC, Dinulos JGH, Pace N, Schwarzenberger K, Wenger JK. Erythema multiforme due to Mycoplasma pneumoniae infection in two children. Pediatr Dermatol. 2006;23(6):546–55.
131. French S. Manipulative therapy or NSAIDS do not provide additional benefit to quality baseline care for acute back pain. Aust J Physiother. 2008;54(1):75.
132. Brice SL, Krzemien D, Weston WL, Huff JC. Detection of herpes simplex virus DNA in cutaneous lesions of erythema multiforme. J Invest Dermatol. 1989;93(1):183–7.
133. Schofield JK, Tatnall FM, Leigh IM. Recurrent erythema multiforme: clinical features and treatment in a large series of patients. Br J Dermatol. 1993;128(5):542–5.
134. Aurelian L, Ono F, Burnett J. Herpes simplex virus (HSV)-associated erythema multiforme (HAEM): a viral disease with an autoimmune component. Dermatol Online J. 2003;9(1):1.
135. Ono F, Sharma B, Smith CC, Burnett JW, Aurelian L. CD34+ cells in the peripheral blood transport herpes simplex virus DNA fragments to the skin of patients with erythema multiforme (HAEM). J Invest Dermatol. 2005;124(6):1215–24.
136. Hebra F, Fagge CH. On diseases of the skin, including the exanthemata: translated and edited by CH Fagge, vol. 1. London: The New Sydenham Society; 1866.
137. Huff JC, Weston WL. Recurrent erythema multiforme. Medicine. 1989;68(3):133–40.
138. Brice SL, Huff JC, Weston WL. Erythema multiforme. Curr Probl Dermatol. 1990;2(1):5–25.
139. Howland WW, Golttz LE, Weston WL, Huff JC. Erythema multiforme: clinical, histopathologic, and immunologic study. J Am Acad Dermatol. 1984;10(3):438–46.
140. Ackerman AB, Penneys NS, Clark WH. Erythema multiforme exudativum: distinctive pathological process. Br J Dermatol. 1971;84(6):554–66.
141. Schofield JK, Tatnall FM, Leigh IM. Recurrent erythema multiforme: clinical features and treatment in a large series of patients. Br J Dermatol. 1993;128(5):542–5.
142. Weston WL, Brice SL. Atypical forms of herpes simplex-associated erythema multiforme. J Am Acad Dermatol. 1998;39(1): 124–6.
143. Zeitouni NC, Funaro D, Cloutier RA, Gagne E, Claveau J. Redefining Rowell's syndrome. Br J Dermatol. 2000;142(2):343–6.
144. Wolf P, Soyer HP, Fink-Puches R, Huff JC, Kerl H. Recurrent post-herpetic erythema multiforme mimicking polymorphic light and juvenile spring eruption: report of two cases in young boys. Br J Dermatol. 1994;131(3):364–7.
145. Tatnall FM, Schofield JK, Leigh IM. A double-blind, placebo-controlled trial of continuous acyclovir therapy in recurrent erythema multiforme. Br J Dermatol. 1995;132(2):267–70.
146. Bean SF, Quezada RK. Recurrent oral erythema multiforme: clinical experience with 11 patients. JAMA. 1983;249(20):2810–2.
147. Farthing PM, Maragou P, Coates M, Tatnall F, Leigh IM, Williams DM. Characteristics of the oral lesions in patients with cutaneous recurrent erythema multiforme. J Oral Pathol Med. 1995;24(1):9–13.
148. Tatnall FM, Schofield JK, Leigh IM. A double-blind, placebo-controlled trial of continuous acyclovir therapy in recurrent erythema multiforme. Br J Dermatol. 1995;132(2):267–70.
149. Paquet P, Pierard GE. Erythema multiforme and toxic epidermal necrolysis: a comparative study. Am J Dermatopathol. 1997;19(2):127–32.
150. Roujeau J-C, Allanore L, Liss Y, Mockenhaupt M. Severe cutaneous adverse reactions to drugs (SCAR): definitions, diagnostic criteria, genetic predisposition. Dermatol Sinica. 2009;27(2):203–9.
151. Schwartz RA, McDonough PH, Lee BW. Toxic epidermal necrolysis: part I. Introduction, history, classification, clinical features, systemic manifestations, etiology, and immunopathogenesis. J Am Acad Dermatol. 2013;69(2):173.e1–113; quiz 185–176.
152. Guillaume J, Roujeau J, Revuz J, Penso D, Touraine R. THe culprit drugs in 87 cases of toxic epidermal necrolysis (lyell's syndrome). Arch Dermatol. 1987;123(9):1166–70.
153. Dayal S, Monga B, JainVk A. Anuradha. Comparative evaluation of antimicrobial and anticonvulsant induced cases of Steven Johnson syndrome and toxic epidermal necrolysis. Int J Pharma Col Clin Sci. 2014;3:1–6.
154. Reyes-Habito CM, Roh EK. Cutaneous reactions to chemotherapeutic drugs and targeted therapies for cancer: part I. Conventional chemotherapeutic drugs. J Am Acad Dermatol. 2014;71(2):203.e201–12. quiz 215–206.
155. Reyes-Habito CM, Roh EK. Cutaneous reactions to chemotherapeutic drugs and targeted therapy for cancer: part II. Targeted therapy. J Am Acad Dermatol. 2014;71(2):217.e1–211; quiz 227–218.
156. Strom BL, Carson JL, Halpern AC, et al. Using a claims database to investigate drug-induced Stevens-Johnson syndrome. Stat Med. 1991;10(4):565–76.
157. Chowdhury AD, Oda M, Markus AF, Kirita T, Choudhury CR. Herbal medicine induced Stevens-Johnson syndrome: a case report. Int J Paediatrc Dent/Br Paedod Soc Inter Assoc Dent Children. 2004;14(3):204–7.
158. Ball R, Ball LK, Wise RP, Braun MM, Beeler JA, Salive ME. Stevens-Johnson syndrome and toxic epidermal necrolysis after vaccination: reports to the vaccine adverse event reporting system. Pediatr Infect Dis J. 2001;20(2):219–23.
159. Rzany B, Hering O, Mockenhaupt M, et al. Histopathological and epidemiological characteristics of patients with erythema exudativum multiforme major, Stevens-Johnson syndrome and toxic epidermal necrolysis. Br J Dermatol. 1996;135(1):6–11.
160. Tay Y-K, Huff JC, Weston WL. Mycoplasma pneumoniae infection is associated with Stevens-Johnson syndrome, not erythema multiforme (von Hebra). J Am Acad Dermatol. 1996;35(5):757–60.
161. Grieb G, Alazemi M, Das R, Dunda SE, Fuchs PC, Pallua N. A rare case of toxic epidermal necrolysis with unexpected fever resulting from dengue virus. Case Rep Dermatol. 2010;2(3):189–94.
162. Fournier S, Bastuji-Garin S, Mentec H, Revuz J, Roujeau JC. Toxic epidermal necrolysis associated with Mycoplasma pneumoniae infection. Eur J Clin Microbiol Infect Dis. 1995;14(6):558–9.
163. Mandelcorn R, Shear NH. Lupus-associated toxic epidermal necrolysis: a novel manifestation of lupus? J Am Acad Dermatol. 2003;48(4):525–9.
164. Lissia M, Mulas P, Bulla A, Rubino C. Toxic epidermal necrolysis (Lyell's disease). Burns: J Inter Soc Burn Inj. 2010;36(2): 152–63.
165. Levi N, Bastuji-Garin S, Mockenhaupt M, et al. Medications as risk factors of Stevens-Johnson syndrome and toxic epidermal necrolysis in children: a pooled analysis. Pediatrics. 2009;123(2): e297–304.
166. Schöpf E, Stühmer A, Rzany B, Victor N, Zentgraf R, Kapp J. Toxic epidermal necrolysis and stevens-johnson syndrome: an epidemiologic study from west Germany. Arch Dermatol. 1991;127(6):839–42.
167. Rzany B, Mockenhaupt M, Stocker U, Hamouda O, Schöpf E. INcidence of stevens-johnson syndrome and toxic epidermal necrolysis in patients with the acquired immunodeficiency syndrome in Germany. Arch Dermatol. 1993;129(8):1059.
168. Metry DW, Lahart CJ, Farmer KL, Hebert AA. Stevens-Johnson syndrome caused by the antiretroviral drug nevirapine. J Am Acad Dermatol. 2001;44(2 Suppl):354–7.
169. Hetherington S, Hughes AR, Mosteller M, et al. Genetic variations in HLA-B region and hypersensitivity reactions to abacavir. Lancet. 2002;359(9312):1121–2.
170. Mallal S, Nolan D, Witt C, et al. Association between presence of HLA-B*5701, HLA-DR7, and HLA-DQ3 and hypersensitivity to HIV-1 reverse-transcriptase inhibitor abacavir. Lancet. 2002; 359(9308):727–32.

171. Chung WH, Hung SI, Hong HS, et al. Medical genetics: a marker for Stevens-Johnson syndrome. Nature. 2004;428(6982):486.
172. Ueta M, Kannabiran C, Wakamatsu TH, et al. Trans-ethnic study confirmed independent associations of HLA-A*02:06 and HLA-B*44:03 with cold medicine-related Stevens-Johnson syndrome with severe ocular surface complications. Sci Rep. 2014;4:5981.
173. Kaniwa N, Saito Y, Aihara M, et al. HLA-B locus in Japanese patients with anti-epileptics and allopurinol-related Stevens-Johnson syndrome and toxic epidermal necrolysis. Pharmacogenomics. 2008;9(11):1617–22.
174. Lonjou C, Borot N, Sekula P, et al. A European study of HLA-B in Stevens-Johnson syndrome and toxic epidermal necrolysis related to five high-risk drugs. Pharmacogenet Genomics. 2008;18(2):99–107.
175. Downey A, Jackson C, Harun N, Cooper A. Toxic epidermal necrolysis: review of pathogenesis and management. J Am Acad Dermatol. 2012;66(6):995–1003.
176. Locharernkul C, Loplumlert J, Limotai C, et al. Carbamazepine and phenytoin induced Stevens-Johnson syndrome is associated with HLA-B* 1502 allele in Thai population. Epilepsia. 2008;49(12):2087–91.
177. Kim S-H, Kim M, Lee KW, et al. HLA-B* 5901 is strongly associated with methazolamide-induced Stevens-Johnson syndrome/toxic epidermal necrolysis. Pharmacogenomics. 2010;11(6):879–84.
178. Chang CC, Too CL, Murad S, Hussein SH. Association of HLA-B* 1502 allele with carbamazepine-induced toxic epidermal necrolysis and Stevens–Johnson syndrome in the multi-ethnic Malaysian population. Int J Dermatol. 2011;50(2):221–4.
179. Tassaneeyakul W, Jantararoungtong T, Chen P, et al. Strong association between HLA-B* 5801 and allopurinol-induced Stevens–Johnson syndrome and toxic epidermal necrolysis in a Thai population. Pharmacogenet Genomics. 2009;19(9):704–9.
180. Kaniwa N, Saito Y, Aihara M, et al. HLA-B* 1511 is a risk factor for carbamazepine-induced Stevens-Johnson syndrome and toxic epidermal necrolysis in Japanese patients. Epilepsia. 2010;51(12): 2461–5.
181. Viard I, Wehrli P, Bullani R, et al. Inhibition of toxic epidermal necrolysis by blockade of CD95 with human intravenous immunoglobulin. Science. 1998;282(5388):490–3.
182. Abe R, Shimizu T, Shibaki A, Nakamura H, Watanabe H, Shimizu H. Toxic epidermal necrolysis and Stevens-Johnson syndrome are induced by soluble Fas ligand. Am J Pathol. 2003;162(5):1515–20.
183. Stur K, Karlhofer FM, Stingl G. Soluble FAS ligand: a discriminating feature between drug-induced skin eruptions and viral exanthemas. J Invest Dermatol. 2007;127(4):802–7.
184. Tohyama M, Shirakata Y, Sayama K, Hashimoto K. The influence of hepatic damage on serum soluble Fas ligand levels of patients with drug rashes. J Allergy Clin Immunol. 2009;123(4):971–2; author reply 972.
185. Chung W-H, Hung S-I, Yang J-Y, et al. Granulysin is a key mediator for disseminated keratinocyte death in Stevens-Johnson syndrome and toxic epidermal necrolysis. Nat Med. 2008; 14(12):1343–50.
186. Abe R, Yoshioka N, Murata J, Fujita Y, Shimizu H. Granulysin as a marker for early diagnosis of the Stevens–Johnson syndrome. Ann Intern Med. 2009;151(7):514–5.
187. Nassif A, Bensussan A, Boumsell L, et al. Toxic epidermal necrolysis: effector cells are drug-specific cytotoxic T cells. J Allergy Clin Immunol. 2004;114(5):1209–15.
188. Posadas SJ, Padial A, Torres MJ, et al. Delayed reactions to drugs show levels of perforin, granzyme B, and Fas-L to be related to disease severity. J Allergy Clin Immunol. 2002;109(1):155–61.
189. Paquet P, Pierard GE. Glutathione-S-transferase pi expression in toxic epidermal necrolysis: a marker of putative oxidative stress in keratinocytes. Skin Pharmacol Physiol. 2007;20(2):66–70.
190. Nagata S. Apoptosis by death factor. Cell. 1997;88(3):355–65.
191. Abe R. Toxic epidermal necrolysis and Stevens–Johnson syndrome: soluble Fas ligand involvement in the pathomechanisms of these diseases. J Dermatol Sci. 2008;52(3):151–9.
192. Nassif A, Moslehi H, Le Gouvello S, et al. Evaluation of the potential role of cytokines in toxic epidermal necrolysis. J Invest Dermatol. 2004;123(5):850–5.
193. Kroncke KD, Fehsel K, Kolb-Bachofen V. Nitric oxide: cytotoxicity versus cytoprotection – how, why, when, and where? Nitric Oxide: Biol Chem/off J Nitric Oxide Soc. 1997;1(2): 107–20.
194. Brüne B, von Knethen A, Sandau KB. Nitric oxide and its role in apoptosis. Eur J Pharmacol. 1998;351(3):261–72.
195. Lerner LH, Qureshi AA, Reddy BV, Lerner EA. Nitric oxide synthase in toxic epidermal necrolysis and Stevens-Johnson syndrome. J Invest Dermatol. 2000;114(1):196–9.
196. Morel E, Escamochero S, Cabanas R, Diaz R, Fiandor A, Bellon T. CD94/NKG2C is a killer effector molecule in patients with Stevens-Johnson syndrome and toxic epidermal necrolysis. J Allergy Clin Immunol. 2010;125(3):703–10, 710.e701–710. e708.
197. Takahashi R, Kano Y, Yamazaki Y, Kimishima M, Mizukawa Y, Shiohara T. Defective regulatory T cells in patients with severe drug eruptions: timing of the dysfunction is associated with the pathological phenotype and outcome. J Immunol. 2009; 182(12):8071–9.
198. Schwartz RA. Toxic epidermal necrolysis. Cutis. 1997;59(3): 123–8.
199. Revuz J, Penso D, Roujeau J, et al. Toxic epidermal necrolysis: clinical findings and prognosis factors in 87 patients. Arch Dermatol. 1987;123(9):1160–5.
200. Emberger M, Lanschuetzer CM, Laimer M, Hawranek T, Staudach A, Hintner H. Vaginal adenosis induced by Stevens-Johnson syndrome. J Eur Acad Dermatol Venereol: JEADV. 2006;20(7): 896–8.
201. Jha AK, Goenka MK. Colonic involvement in Stevens-Johnson syndrome: a rare entity. Dig Endosc: Off J Japan Gastroenterol Endosc Soc. 2012;24(5):382.
202. Lebargy F, Wolkenstein P, Gisselbrecht M, et al. Pulmonary complications in toxic epidermal necrolysis: a prospective clinical study. Intensive Care Med. 1997;23(12):1237–44.
203. de Prost N, Mekontso-Dessap A, Valeyrie-Allanore L, et al. Acute respiratory failure in patients with toxic epidermal necrolysis: clinical features and factors associated with mechanical ventilation. Crit Care Med. 2014;42(1):118–28.
204. Blum L, Chosidow O, Rostoker G, Philippon C, Revuz J, Roujeau J-C. Renal involvement in toxic epidermal necrolysis. J Am Acad Dermatol. 1996;34(6):1088–90.
205. Lebargy F, Wolkenstein P, Gisselbrecht M, et al. Pulmonary complications in toxic epidermal necrolysis: a prospective clinical study. Intensive Care Med. 1997;23(12):1237–44.
206. Wallis C, McClymont W. Case reports Toxic epidermal necrolysis with adult respiratory distress syndrome. Anaesthesia. 1995; 50(9):801–3.
207. McIvor RA, Zaidi J, Peters WJ, Hyland RH. Acute and chronic respiratory complications of toxic epidermal necrolysis. J Burn Care Rehabil. 1996;17(3):237–40.
208. Roujeau JC, Chosidow O, Saiag P, Guillaume JC. Toxic epidermal necrolysis (Lyell syndrome). J Am Acad Dermatol. 1990;23(6 Pt 1): 1039–58.
209. Westly E, Wechsler HL. Toxic epidermal necrolysis: granulocytic leukopenia as a prognostic indicator. Arch Dermatol. 1984; 120(6):721–6.
210. Lee T, Lee YS, Yoon S-Y, et al. Characteristics of liver injury in drug-induced systemic hypersensitivity reactions. J Am Acad Dermatol. 2013;69(3):407–15.

211. de Prost N, Ingen-Housz-Oro S, Duong T, et al. Bacteremia in Stevens-Johnson syndrome and toxic epidermal necrolysis: epidemiology, risk factors, and predictive value of skin cultures. Medicine. 2010;89(1):28–36.
212. Avakian R, Flowers FP, Araujo OE, Ramos-Caro FA. Toxic epidermal necrolysis: a review. J Am Acad Dermatol. 1991;25(1, Part 1):69–79.
213. Carter FM, Mitchell CK. Toxic epidermal necrolysis – an unusual cause of colonic perforation. Report of a case. Dis Colon Rectum. 1993;36(8):773–7.
214. Sakai N, Yoshizawa Y, Amano A, et al. Toxic epidermal necrolysis complicated by multiple intestinal ulcers. Int J Dermatol. 2008;47(2):180–2.
215. Chosidow O, Delchier JC, Chaumette MT, et al. Intestinal involvement in drug-induced toxic epidermal necrolysis. Lancet. 1991;337(8746):928.
216. Bouziri A, Khaldi A, Hamdi A, et al. Toxic epidermal necrolysis complicated by small bowel intussusception: a case report. J Pediatr Surg. 2011;46(2):e9–11.
217. Quinn AM, Brown K, Bonish BK, et al. UNcovering histologic criteria with prognostic significance in toxic epidermal necrolysis. Arch Dermatol. 2005;141(6):683–7.
218. Sidoroff A, Halevy S, Bavinck JNB, Vaillant L, Roujeau J-C. Acute generalized exanthematous pustulosis (AGEP) – A clinical reaction pattern. J Cutan Pathol. 2001;28(3):113–9.
219. Ladhani S, Joannou CL, Lochrie DP, Evans RW, Poston SM. Clinical, microbial, and biochemical aspects of the exfoliative toxins causing staphylococcal scalded-skin syndrome. Clin Microbiol Rev. 1999;12(2):224–42.
220. Gentilhomme E, Faure M, Piemont Y, Binder P, Thivolet J. Action of staphylococcal exfoliative toxins on epidermal cell cultures and organotypic skin. J Dermatol. 1990;17(9):526–32.
221. Husain Z, Reddy BY, Schwartz RA. DRESS syndrome: part I. Clinical perspectives. J Am Acad Dermatol. 2013;68(5):693.e691–14.
222. Khan I, Hughes R, Curran S, Marren P. Drug-associated linear IgA disease mimicking toxic epidermal necrolysis. Clin Exp Dermatol. 2009;34(6):715–7.
223. Wojnarowska F, Marsden RA, Bhogal B, Black MM. Chronic bullous disease of childhood, childhood cicatricial pemphigoid, and linear IgA disease of adults. A comparative study demonstrating clinical and immunopathologic overlap. J Am Acad Dermatol. 1988;19(5 Pt 1):792–805.
224. Stone N, Sheerin S, Burge S. Toxic epidermal necrolysis and graft vs. host disease: a clinical spectrum but a diagnostic dilemma. Clin Exp Dermatol. 1999;24(4):260–2.
225. Jeanmonod P, Hubbuch M, Grunhage F, et al. Graft-versus-host disease or toxic epidermal necrolysis: diagnostic dilemma after liver transplantation. Trans Infect Dis: Off J Transpl Soc. 2012;14(4):422–6.
226. Borchers AT, Lee JL, Naguwa SM, Cheema GS, Gershwin ME. Stevens–Johnson syndrome and toxic epidermal necrolysis. Autoimmun Rev. 2008;7(8):598–605.
227. Palmieri TL, Greenhalgh DG, Saffle JR, et al. A multicenter review of toxic epidermal necrolysis treated in U.S. burn centers at the end of the twentieth century. J Burn Care Rehabil. 2002;23(2):87–96.
228. Chave TA, Mortimer NJ, Sladden MJ, Hall AP, Hutchinson PE. Toxic epidermal necrolysis: current evidence, practical management and future directions. Br J Dermatol. 2005;153(2):241–53.
229. McGee T, Munster A. Toxic epidermal necrolysis syndrome: mortality rate reduced with early referral to regional burn center. Plast Reconstr Surg. 1998;102(4):1018–22.
230. Dorafshar AH, Dickie SR, Cohn AB, et al. Antishear therapy for toxic epidermal necrolysis: an alternative treatment approach. Plast Reconstr Surg. 2008;122(1):154–60.
231. Spies M, Sanford AP, Aili Low JF, Wolf SE, Herndon DN. Treatment of extensive toxic epidermal necrolysis in children. Pediatrics. 2001;108(5):1162–8.
232. Melandri D. Lyell's syndrome skin lesions treated by Veloderm. J Eur Acad Dermatol Venereol: JEADV. 2007;21(3):426–7.
233. Bradley T, Brown RE, Kucan JO, Smoot III EC, Hussmann J. Toxic Epidermal necrolysis: a review and report of the successful use of biobrane for early wound coverage. Ann Plast Surg. 1995;35(2):124–32.
234. Arévalo JM, Lorente JA. Skin coverage with biobrane biomaterial for the treatment of patients with toxic epidermal necrolysis. J Burn Care Res. 1999;20(5):406–10.
235. Boorboor P, Vogt PM, Bechara FG, et al. Toxic epidermal necrolysis: use of Biobrane® for skin coverage reduces pain, improves mobilisation and decreases infection in elderly patients. Burns: J Inter Soc Burn Inj. 2008;34(4):487–92.
236. Li X, Wang D, Lu Z, Chen J, Zhang H, Sun L. Answer to 'Toxic epidermal necrolysis with failure of re-epithelialization. Could umbilical cord mesenchymal stem cell transplantation have a role?'. J Eur Acad Dermatol Venereol. 2013;27(7):925.
237. Li X, Wang D, Lu Z, Chen J, Zhang H, Sun L. Umbilical cord mesenchymal stem cell transplantation in drug-induced Stevens-Johnson syndrome. J Eur Acad Dermatol Venereol. 2013; 27(5):659–61.
238. Schwartz RA, McDonough PH, Lee BW. Toxic epidermal necrolysis: part II. Prognosis, sequelae, diagnosis, differential diagnosis, prevention, and treatment. J Am Acad Dermatol. 2013;69(2):187.e181–116; quiz 203–184.
239. Letko E, Papaliodis DN, Papaliodis GN, Daoud YJ, Ahmed AR, Foster CS. Stevens-Johnson syndrome and toxic epidermal necrolysis: a review of the literature. Ann Aallergy Asthma Immunol: Off Publ Am Coll Allergy Asthma Immunol. 2005;94(4):419–36; quiz 436–418, 456.
240. Araki Y, Sotozono C, Inatomi T, et al. Successful treatment of Stevens-Johnson syndrome with steroid pulse therapy at disease onset. Am J Ophthalmol. 2009;147(6):1004–11, 1011.e1001.
241. Sotozono C, Ueta M, Koizumi N, et al. Diagnosis and treatment of Stevens-Johnson syndrome and toxic epidermal necrolysis with ocular complications. Ophthalmology. 2009;116(4):685–90.
242. Gregory DG. Treatment of acute Stevens-Johnson syndrome and toxic epidermal necrolysis using amniotic membrane: a review of 10 consecutive cases. Ophthalmology. 2011;118(5):908–14.
243. Ciralsky JB, Sippel KC, Gregory DG. Current ophthalmologic treatment strategies for acute and chronic Stevens-Johnson syndrome and toxic epidermal necrolysis. Curr Opin Ophthalmol. 2013;24(4):321–8.
244. Segal O, Barkana Y, Hourovitz D, et al. Scleral contact lenses may help where other modalities fail. Cornea. 2003;22(4):308–10.
245. Tomlins PJ, Parulekar MV, Rauz S. "Triple-TEN" in the treatment of acute ocular complications from toxic epidermal necrolysis. Cornea. 2013;32(3):365–9.
246. Schneck J, Fagot JP, Sekula P, Sassolas B, Roujeau JC, Mockenhaupt M. Effects of treatments on the mortality of Stevens-Johnson syndrome and toxic epidermal necrolysis: a retrospective study on patients included in the prospective EuroSCAR study. J Am Acad Dermatol. 2008;58(1):33–40.
247. Halebian PH, Corder VJ, Madden MR, Finklestein JL, Shires GT. Improved burn center survival of patients with toxic epidermal necrolysis managed without corticosteroids. Ann Surg. 1986;204(5):503.
248. Worswick S, Cotliar J. Stevens-Johnson syndrome and toxic epidermal necrolysis: a review of treatment options. Dermatol Ther. 2011;24(2):207–18.
249. Viard I, Wehrli P, Bullani R, et al. Inhibition of toxic epidermal necrolysis by blockade of CD95 with human intravenous immunoglobulin. Science. 1998;282(5388):490–3.

250. Faye O, Roujeau JC. Treatment of epidermal necrolysis with high-dose intravenous immunoglobulins (IV Ig): clinical experience to date. Drugs. 2005;65(15):2085–90.
251. Roujeau JC, Bastuji-Garin S. Systematic review of treatments for Stevens-Johnson syndrome and toxic epidermal necrolysis using the SCORTEN score as a tool for evaluating mortality. Ther Adv Drug Safety. 2011;2(3):87–94.
252. Huang YC, Li YC, Chen TJ. The efficacy of intravenous immunoglobulin for the treatment of toxic epidermal necrolysis: a systematic review and meta-analysis. Br J Dermatol. 2012;167(2):424–32.
253. Sakellariou G, Koukoudis P, Karpouzas J, et al. Plasma exchange (PE) treatment in drug-induced toxic epidermal necrolysis (TEN). Int J Artif Organs. 1991;14(10):634–8.
254. Egan CA, Grant WJ, Morris SE, Saffle JR, Zone JJ. Plasmapheresis as an adjunct treatment in toxic epidermal necrolysis. J Am Acad Dermatol. 1999;40(3):458–61.
255. Chaidemenos GC, Chrysomallis F, Sombolos K, Mourellou O, Ioannides D, Papakonstantinou M. Plasmapheresis in toxic epidermal necrolysis. Int J Dermatol. 1997;36(3):218–21.
256. Furubacke A, Berlin G, Anderson C, Sjöberg F. Lack of significant treatment effect of plasma exchange in the treatment of drug-induced toxic epidermal necrolysis? Intensive Care Med. 1999;25(11):1307–10.
257. Koštál M, Bláha M, Lánská M, et al. Beneficial effect of plasma exchange in the treatment of toxic epidermal necrolysis: a series of four cases. J Clin Apher. 2012;27(4):215–20.
258. Hewitt J, Ormerod AD. Toxic epidermal necrolysis treated with cyclosporin. Clin Exp Dermatol. 1992;17(4):264–5.
259. Renfro L, Grant-Kels JM, Daman LA. Drug-induced toxic epidermal necrolysis treated with cyclosporin. Int J Dermatol. 1989;28(7):441–4.
260. Arévalo JM, Lorente JA, González-Herrada C, Jiménez-Reyes J. Treatment of toxic epidermal necrolysis with cyclosporin A. J Trauma Acute Care Surg. 2000;48(3):473–8.
261. Valeyrie-Allanore L, Wolkenstein P, Brochard L, et al. Open trial of ciclosporin treatment for Stevens-Johnson syndrome and toxic epidermal necrolysis. Br J Dermatol. 2010;163(4):847–53.
262. Kirchhof MG, Miliszewski MA, Sikora S, Papp A, Dutz JP. Retrospective review of Stevens-Johnson syndrome/toxic epidermal necrolysis treatment comparing intravenous immunoglobulin with cyclosporine. J Am Acad Dermatol. 2014;71(5):941–7.
263. Wolkenstein P, Latarjet J, Roujeau JC, et al. Randomised comparison of thalidomide versus placebo in toxic epidermal necrolysis. Lancet. 1998;352(9140):1586–9.
264. Kreft B, Wohlrab J, Bramsiepe I, Eismann R, Winkler M, Marsch WC. Etoricoxib-induced toxic epidermal necrolysis: Successful treatment with infliximab. J Dermatol. 2010;37(10):904–6.
265. Fischer M, Fiedler E, Marsch WC, Wohlrab J. Antitumour necrosis factor-α antibodies (infliximab) in the treatment of a patient with toxic epidermal necrolysis. Br J Dermatol. 2002;146(4):707–9.
266. Famularo G, Di Dona B, Canzona F, Girardelli CR, Cruciani G. Etanercept for toxic epidermal necrolysis. Ann Pharmacother. 2007;41(6):1083–4.
267. Gubinelli E, Canzona F, Tonanzi T, Raskovic D, Didona B. Toxic epidermal necrolysis successfully treated with etanercept. J Dermatol. 2009;36(3):150–3.

Vasculitis

268. Rencic A, Rivadeneira A, Cummins D, Nousari CH. Cutaneous vasculitides. In: Kerdel F, editors. Dermatology: just the facts. New York: McGraw-Hill. 2003, p. 45–57.
269. Suresh E. Diagnostic approach to patients with suspected vasculitis. Postgrad Med J. 2006;82(970):483–8.
270. Carlson JA, Chen KR. Cutaneous vasculitis update: neutrophilic muscular vessel and eosinophilic, granulomatous, and lymphocytic vasculitis syndromes. Am J Dermatopathol. 2007;29(1):32–43.
271. Kao NL, Broy S, Tillawi I. Malignant angioendotheliomatosis mimicking systemic necrotizing vasculitis. J Rheumatol. 1992; 19(7):11–5.
272. Thomas R, Vuitch F, Lakhanpal S. Angiocentric T cell lymphoma masquerading as cutaneous vasculitis. J Rheumatol. 1994; 21(4):760–2.
273. Ibrahim SF, Nousari CH. Clinical and basic immunodermatology. London: Springer; 2008.
274. Blanco R, Martinez-Taboada VM, Rodriguez Valverde V, Garcia-Fuentes M. Cutaneous vasculitis in children and adults. Associated diseases and etiologic factors in 303 patients. Medicine (Baltimore). 1998;77(6):403–18.
275. Sais G, Vidaller A, Jucgla A, et al. Prognostic factors in leukocytoclastic vasculitis: a clinicopathologic study of 160 patients. Arch Dermatol. 1998;134(3):309–15.
276. Kulthanan K, Pinkaew S, Jiamton S, Mahaisavariya P, Suthipinittharm P. Cutaneous leukocytoclastic vasculitis: the yield of direct immunofluorescence study. J Med Assoc Thai. 2004;87(5):531–5.
277. Grzeszkiewicz TM, Fiorentino DF. Update on cutaneous vasculitis. Semin Cutan Med Surg. 2006;25(4):221–5.
278. Heeringa P, Huugen D, Tervaert JW. Anti-neutrophil cytoplasmic autoantibodies and leukocyte-endothelial interactions: a sticky connection? Trends Immunol. 2005;26(11):561–4.
279. Birck R, Schmitt WH, Kaelsch IA, van der Woude FJ. Serial ANCA determinations for monitoring disease activity in patients with ANCA-associated vasculitis: systematic review. Am J Kidney Dis. 2006;47(1):15–23.
280. Hermann J, Demel U, Stunzner D, Daghofer E, Tilz G, Graninger W. Clinical interpretation of antineutrophil cytoplasmic antibodies: parvovirus B19 infection as a pitfall. Ann Rheum Dis. 2005;64(4):641–3, Epub 2004 Oct 14.
281. Luqmani RA, Suppiah R, Grayson PC, Merkel PA, Watts R. Nomenclature and classification of vasculitis – update on the ACR/EULAR diagnosis and classification of vasculitis study (DCVAS). Clin Exp Immunol. 2011;164 Suppl 1:11–3.
282. Jennette JC, Falk RJ, Andrassy K, et al. Nomenclature of systemic vasculitides. Proposal of an international consensus conference. Arthritis Rheum. 1994;37(2):187–92.
283. Rao JK, Allen NB, Pincus T. Limitations of the 1990 American College of Rheumatology classification criteria in the diagnosis of vasculitis. Ann Intern Med. 1998;129(5):345–52.
284. Sorensen SF, Slot O, Tvede N, Petersen J. A prospective study of vasculitis patients collected in a five year period: evaluation of the Chapel Hill nomencla ture. Ann Rheum Dis. 2000;59(6):478–82.
285. Jennette JC, Falk RJ, Bacon PA, et al. 2012 revised International Chapel Hill Consensus Conference nomenclature of vasculitides. Arthritis Rheum. 2013;65:1–11.
286. Langford C. Takayasu's arteritis. In: Hochberg MC, Silman AJ, Smolen JS, Weinblatt ME, editors. Rheumatology. Oxford: Elsevier; 2010. p. 1567–73.
287. Weyand CM, Goronzy JJ. Medium- and large-vessel vasculitis. N Engl J Med. 2003;349:160–9.
288. Chauhan SK, Singh M, Nityanand S. Reactivity of gamma/delta T cells to human 60-kd heat-shock protein and their cytotoxicity to aortic endothelial cells in Takayasu arteritis. Arthritis Rheum. 2007;56:2798–802.
289. Dourmishev AL, Erafimova DK, Vassileva SG, et al. Segmental ulcerative vasculitis: a cutaneous manifestation of Takayasu's arteritis. Int Wound J. 2005;2(4):340–5.
290. Mukhtyar C, Guillevin L, Cid MC, et al. EULAR recommendations for the management of large vessel vasculitis. Ann Rheum Dis. 2009;68:318–23.

291. Tombetti E, Franchini S, Papa M, Sabbadini MG, Baldissera E. Treatment of refractory Takayasu arteritis with tocilizumab: seven Italian patients from a single referral center. J Rheumatol. 2013;40(12):2047–51.
292. Mekinian A, Neel A, Sibilia J, et al. Efficacy and tolerance of infliximab in refractory Takayasu arteritis: French multicentre study. Rheumatology (Oxford). 2012;51:882–6.
293. Burns JC. Kawasaki disease. In: Hochberg MC, Silman AJ, Smolen JS, Weinblatt ME, editors. Rheumatology. Oxford: Elsevier; 2010. p. 1583–6.
294. Chan M, Luqmani R. Pharmacotherapy of vasculitis. Expert Opin Pharmacother. 2009;10:1273–89.
295. Burns JC, Best BM, Mejias A, et al. Infliximab treatment of intravenous immunoglobulin-resistant Kawasaki disease. J Pediatr. 2008;153:833–8.
296. Breunis WB, Davila S, Shimizu C, et al. Disruption of vascular homeostasis in patients with Kawasaki disease: involvement of vascular endothelial growth factor and angiopoietins. Arthritis Rheum. 2012;64:306–15.
297. Burns JC, Song Y, Bujold M, et al. Immune-monitoring in Kawasaki disease patients treated with infliximab and intravenous immunoglobulin. Clin Exp Immunol. 2013;174:337–44.
298. Langford CA. Vasculitis. J Allergy Clin Immunol. 2010;125: S216–25.
299. Ishiguro N, Kawashima M. Cutaneous polyarteritis nodosa: a report of 16 cases with clinical and histopathological analysis and a review of the published work. J Dermatol. 2010;37:85–93.
300. Guillevin L, Lhote F, Amouroux J, Gherardi R, Callard P, Casassus P. Antineutrophil cytoplasmic antibodies, abnormal angiograms and pathological findings in polyarteritis nodosa and Churg-Strauss syndrome: indications for the classification of vasculitides of the polyarteritis Nodosa Group. Br J Rheumatol. 1996;35:958–64. [PubMed: 8883433].
301. Lidar M, Lipschitz N, Langevitz P, Shoenfeld Y. The infectious etiology of vasculitis. Autoimmunity. 2009;42:432–8.
302. de Menthon M, Mahr A. Treating polyarteritis nodosa: current state of the art. Clin Exp Rheumatol. 2011;29:S110–6.
303. Gayraud M, Guillevin L, le Toumelin P, et al. Long-term followup of polyarteritis nodosa, microscopic polyangiitis, and Churg-Strauss syndrome: analysis of four prospective trials including 278 patients. Arthritis Rheum. 2001;44:666–75.
304. Chan M, Luqmani R. Pharmacotherapy of vasculitis. Expert Opin Pharmacother. 2009;10:1273–89.
305. Gayraud M, Guillevin L, le Toumelin P, et al. Long-term followup of polyarteritis nodosa, microscopic polyangiitis, and Churg-Strauss syndrome: analysis of four prospective trials including 278 patients. Arthritis Rheum. 2001;44:666–75.
306. Guillevin L, Mahr A, Cohen P, et al. Short-term corticosteroids then lamivudine and plasma exchanges to treat hepatitis B virus-related polyarteritis nodosa. Arthritis Rheum. 2004;51:482–7.
307. Fiorentino DF. Cutaneous vasculitis. J Am Acad Dermatol. 2003;48:311–40.
308. Suzuki H, Kiryluk K, Novak J, Moldoveanu Z, Herr AB, Renfrow MB, et al. The pathophysiology of IgA nephropathy. J Am Soc Nephrol. 2011;22:1795–803. [PubMed: 21949093].
309. Birchmore D, Sweeney C, Choudhury D, et al. IgA multiple myeloma presenting as Henoch-Schonlein purpura/polyarteritis nodosa overlap syndrome. Arthritis Rheum. 1999;39(4):698–703.
310. Gonzalez-Gay MA, Garcia-Porrua C. Systemic vasculitides. Best Pract Res Clin Rheumatol. 2002;16:833–45.
311. Stefansson Thors V, Kolka R, Sigurdardottir SL, et al. Increased frequency of C4B*Q0 alleles in patients with Henoch- Schonlein purpura. Scand J Immunol. 2005;61:274–8.
312. Kawana S, Shen GH, Kobayashi Y, Nishiyama S. Membrane attack complex of complement in Henoch- Schonlein purpura skin and nephritis. Arch Dermatol Res. 1990;282:183–7.
313. Garcia-Porrua C, Gonzalez-Louzao C, Llorca J, et al. Predictive factors for renal sequelae in adults with Henoch-Schonlein purpura. J Rheumatol. 2001;28(5):1019–24.
314. Besbas N, Duzova A, Topaloglu R, et al. Pulmonary haemorrhage in a 6-year-old boy with Henoch-Schonlein purpura. Clin Rheumatol. 2001;20(4):293–6.
315. Magro CM, Crowson AN. The cutaneous neutrophilic vascular injury syndromes: a review. Semin Diagn Pathol. 2001;18:47–58.
316. Barnadas MA, Perez E, Gich I, et al. Diagnostic, prognostic and pathogenic value of the direct immunofluorescence test in cutaneous leukocytoclastic vasculitis. Int J Dermatol. 2004;43:19–26.
317. Pillebout E, Alberti C, Guillevin L, et al. Addi-tion of cyclophosphamide to steroids provides no benefit compared with steroids alone in treating adult patients with severe Henoch Schonlein purpura. Kidney Int. 2010;78:495–502.
318. Quartuccio L, Isola M, Corazza L, et al. Performance of the preliminary classification criteria for cryoglobulinaemic vasculitis and clinical manifestations in hepatitis C virus-unrelated cryoglobulinaemic vasculitis. Clin Exp Rheumatol. 2012;30:S48–52.
319. Fabrizi F, Dixit V, Messa P. Antiviral therapy of symptomatic HCV-associated mixed cryoglobulinemia: meta-analysis of clinical studies. J Med Virol. 2013;85:1019–27.
320. Saadoun D, Rosenzwajg M, Landau D, Piette JC, Klatzmann D, Cacoub P. Restoration of peripheral immune homeostasis after rituximab in mixed cryoglobulinemia vasculitis. Blood. 2008;111:5334–41.
321. Lyons PA, Rayner TF, Trivedi S, et al. Genetically distinct subsets within ANCA-associated vasculitis. N Engl J Med. 2012;367: 214–23.
322. Lionaki S, Blyth ER, Hogan SL, et al. Classification of antineutrophil cytoplasmic autoantibody vasculitides: the role of antineutrophil cytoplasmic autoantibody specificity for myeloperoxidase or proteinase 3 in disease recognition and prognosis. Arthritis Rheum. 2012;64:3452–62.
323. Kallenberg CGM. Advances in pathogenesis and treatment of ANCA-associated vasculitis. Discov Med. 2014;18(99):195–201.
324. Tarzi RM, Pusey CD. Current and future prospects in the management of granulomatosis with polyangiitis (Wegener's granulomatosis). Ther Clin Risk Manag. 2014;10:279–93.
325. Lenert P, Icardi M, Dahmoush L. ANA (+) ANCA (+) systemic vasculitis associated with the use of minocycline: case-based review. Clin Rheumatol. 2013;32(7):1099–106.
326. Merkel PA, Lo GH, Holbrook JT, et al. Brief communication: high incidence of venous thrombotic events among patients with Wegener granulomatosis: the Wegener's Clinical Occurrence of Thrombosis (WeCLOT) Study. Ann Intern Med. 2005;142:620–6.
327. Allenbach Y, Seror R, Pagnoux C, Teixeira L, Guilpain P, Guillevin L. High frequency of venous thromboembolic events in Churg-Strauss syndrome, Wegener's granulomatosis and microscopic polyangiitis but not polyarteritis nodosa: a systematic retrospective study on 1130 patients. Ann Rheum Dis. 2009;68:564–7.
328. Suppiah R, Judge A, Batra R, et al. A model to predict cardiovascular events in patients with newly diagnosed Wegener's granulomatosis and microscopic polyangiitis. Arthritis Care Res (Hoboken). 2011;63:588–96.
329. Springer J, Villa-Forte A. Thrombosis in vasculitis. Curr Opin Rheumatol. 2013;25:19–25.
330. Gaffo AL. Thrombosis in vasculitis. Best Pract Res Clin Rheumatol. 2013;27:57–67.
331. Cohen P, Pagnoux C, Mahr A, et al. Churg-Strauss syndrome with poor-prognosis factors: a prospective multicenter trial comparing glucocorticoids and six or twelve cyclophosphamide pulses in forty-eight patients. Arthritis Rheum. 2007;57:686–93.
332. Langford CA. Cyclophosphamide as induction therapy for Wegener's granulomatosis and microscopic polyangiitis. Clin Exp Immunol. 2011;164 Suppl 1:31–4.

333. Jones RB, Tervaert JW, Hauser T, et al. Rituximab versus cyclophosphamide in ANCA-associated renal vasculitis. N Engl J Med. 2010;363:211–20.
334. Stone JH, Merkel PA, Spiera R, et al. Rituximab versus cyclophosphamide for ANCA-associated vasculitis. N Engl J Med. 2010;363:221–32 (Specks U, Merkel PA, Seo P et al. Efficacy of remission-induction regimens for ANCA-associated vasculitis. N Engl J Med 2013; 369: 417–27).
335. Niles J. Rituximab in induction therapy for anti-neutrophil cytoplasmic antibody (ANCA) vasculitis. Clin Exp Immunol. 2011; 164 Suppl 1:27–30.
336. Guerry MJ, Brogan P, Bruce IN, et al. Recommendations for the use of rituximab in anti-neutrophil cytoplasm antibodyassociated vasculitis. Rheumatology (Oxford). 2012;51:634–43.
337. Luqmani R. Maintenance of clinical remission in ANCAassociated vasculitis. Nat Rev Rheumatol. 2013;9:127–32.
338. Falk RJ, Gross WL, Guillevin L, et al; American College of Rheumatology, the American Society of Nephrology, and the European League Against Rheumatism. Granulomatosis with polyangiitis (Wegener's): an alternative name for Wegener's granulomatosis. Arthritis Rheum. 2011;63:863–4.
339. Jennette JC. Nomenclature and classification of vasculitis: lessons learned from granulomatosis with polyangiitis (Wegener's granulomatosis). Clin Exp Immunol. 2011;164 Suppl 1:7–10.
340. Sinico RA, Di Toma L, Maggiore U, Tosoni C, Bottero P, Sabadini E, et al. Renal involvement in Churg-Strauss syndrome. Am J Kidney Dis. 2006;47:770–9. [PubMed: 16632015].
341. Guillevin L, Cohen P, Gayraud M, Lhote F, Jarrousse B, Casassus P. Churg-Strauss syndrome: clinical study and long-term follow-up of 96 patients. Medicine (Baltimore). 1999;78:26–37.
342. Dunogue B, Pagnoux C, Guillevin L. Churg-strauss syndrome: clinical symptoms, complementary investigations, prognosis and outcome, and treatment. Semin Respir Crit Care Med. 2011; 32:298–309.
343. Szczeklik W, Jakiela B, Adamek D, Musial J. Cutting edge issues in the Churg-Strauss syndrome. Clin Rev Allergy Immunol. 2013;44:39–50.
344. Sinico RA, Bottero P, Guillevin L. Antineutrophil cytoplasmic autoantibodies and clinical phenotype in patients with Churg-Strauss syndrome. J Allergy Clin Immunol. 2012;130:1440. Author reply, 1.
345. Szczeklik W, Jakiela B, Adamek D, Musial J. Cutting edge issues in the Churg-Strauss syndrome. Clin Rev Allergy Immunol. 2013;44:39–50.
346. Guillevin L, Pagnoux C, Seror R, Mahr A, Mouthon L, Le Toumelin P. The Five-Factor Score revisited: assessment of prognoses of systemic necrotizing vasculitides based on the French Vasculitis Study Group (FVSG) cohort. Medicine (Baltimore). 2011;90:19–27.
347. Baldini C, Talarico R, Della Rossa A, Bombardieri S. Clinical manifestations and treatment of Churg-Strauss syndrome. Rheum Dis Clin North Am. 2010;36:527–43.
348. Bourgarit A, Le Toumelin P, Pagnoux C, et al. Deaths occurring during the f irst year after treatment onset for polyarteritis nodosa, microscopic polyangiitis, and Churg-Strauss syndrome: a retrospective analysis of causes and factors predictive of mortality based on 595 patients. Medicine (Baltimore). 2005;84:323–30.
349. Phillip R, Luqmani R. Mortality in systemic vasculitis: a systematic review. Clin Exp Rheumatol. 2008;26(5 Suppl 51):S94–104.
350. Koutkia P, Mylonakis E, Rounds S, Erickson A. Leucocytoclastic vasculitis: an update for the clinician. Scand J Rheumatol. 2001;30(6):315–22.
351. Davis MD, Daoud MS, Kirby B, et al. Clinicopathologic correlation of hypocomplementemic and normocomplementemic urticarial vasculitis. J Am Acad Dermatol. 1998;38(6 pt 1): 899–905.
352. Jaing TH, Hsueh C, Chiu CH, et al. Cutaneous lymphocytic vasculitis as the presenting feature of acute lymphoblastic leukemia. J Pediatr Hematol Oncol. 2002;24(7):555–7.
353. Kembre PS, Mahajan S, Kharkar V, Khopkar U. Cutaneous vasculitis as a presenting feature of multiple myeloma: a report of 2 cases. Indian J Dermatol Venereol Leprol. 2006;72(6):437–9.
354. Koulaouzidis A, Campbell S, Bharati A, et al. Primary biliary cirrhosis associated pustular vasculitis. Ann Hepatol. 2006;5(3): 177–8.
355. Ferrero P, Orzan F, Marchisio F, Trevi G. Vasculitis mimicking bacterial endocarditis. Ital Heart J. 2003;4(11):816–8.
356. Golden MP, Hammer SM, Wanke CA, et al. Cytomegalovirus vasculitis. Case reports and review of the literature. Medicine (Baltimore). 1994;73(5):246–55.
357. Lee YS, Lee SW, Lee JR, Lee SC. Erythema induratum with pulmonary tuberculosis: histopathologic features resembling true vasculitis. Int J Dermatol. 2001;40(3):193–6.
358. Feldmann R, Rieger W, Sator PG, Gschnait F, Breier F. Schonlein-Henoch purpura during pregnancy with successful outcome for mother and newborn. BMC Dermatol. 2002;2:1.

Eosinophilic Dermatoses: Wells' Syndrome (Eosinophilic Cellulitis)

359. Wells GC. Recurrent granulomatous dermatitis with eosinophilia. Trans St Johns Hosp Dermatol Soc. 1971;57:46–56.
360. Fujimoto N, Wakabayashi M, Kato T, Nishio C, Tanaka T. Wells syndrome associated with Churg–Strauss syndrome. Clin Exp Dermatol. 2011;36(1):46–8.
361. Barreiros H, Matos D, Furtado C, Cunha H, Bártolo E. Wells syndrome in a child triggered by parvovirus B19 infection? J Am Acad Dermatol. 2012;67(4):1667.
362. Gilliam AE, Bruckner AL, Howard RM, Lee BP, Wu S, Frieden IJ. Bullous "cellulitis" with eosinophilia:case report and review of Wells' syndrome in childhood. Pediatrics. 2005;116: 149–55.
363. Van den Hoogenband HM. Eosinophilic cellulitis as a result of onchocerciasis. Clin Exp Dermatol. 1983;8:405–8.
364. Weiss G, Shemer A, Confino Y, Kaplan B, Trau H. Wells' syndrome: report of a case and review of the literature. Int J Dermatol. 2001;40(2):148–52.
365. Holme SA, McHenry P. Nodular presentation of eosinophilic cellulitis (Wells' syndrome). Clin Exp Dermatol. 2001;26(8): 677–9.
366. Mitchell AJ, Anderson TF, Headington JT, Rasmussen JE. Recurrent granulomatous dermatitis with eosinophilia. Int J Dermatol. 1984;3: 198–202.
367. Wells CG. Recurrent granulomatous dermatitis with eosinophilia. Trans St Johns Hosp Dermatol Soc. 1971;57:46–56.
368. Wells CG, Smith NP. Eosinophilic cellulitis. Br J Dermatol. 1979;100:101–9.
369. McKee PH. Pathology of the skin. 2nd ed. London: Mosby-Wolfe; 1996. p. 29–30.
370. Fisher GB, Greer KE, Cooper PH. Eosinophilic cellulitis (Wells' Syndrome). Int J Dermatol. 1985;24:101–7.
371. Bogenrieder T, Griese DP, Schiffner R, et al. Wells' syndrome associated with idiopathic hypereosinophilic syndrome. Br J Dermatol. 1997;137:978–82.
372. Coldiron BM, Robinson JK. Low-dose alternate-day prednisone for persistent Wells' syndrome. Arch Dermatol. 1989;125: 1625–6.
373. Anderson CR, Jenkins D, Tron V, Prendiville JS. Wells' syndrome in childhood: case report and review of the literature. J Am Acad Dermatol. 1995;33:857–64.

Eosinophilic Dermatoses: Hypereosinophic Syndrome

374. Kojima K, Maeda J, Mikami S, Yamagishi H, Ide H, Hattori S, Takahashi T, Awazu M. Eosinophilic cystitis presented as a manifestation of hypereosinophilic syndrome: a case report and review of the literature. Nephron Extra. 2013;3:30–5.
375. Wechsler ME, Fulkerson PC, Bochner BS, Gauvreau GM, Gleich GJ, Henkel T, Kolbeck R, Mathur SK, Ortega H, Patel J, Prussin C, Renzi P, Rothenberg ME, Roufosse F, Simon D, Simon H-U, Wardlaw A, Weller PF, Klion AD. Novel targeted therapies for eosinophilic disorders. J Allergy Clin Immunol. 2012;130(3):563–71.
376. Simon H-U, Rothenberg ME, Bochner BS, Weller PF, Wardlaw AJ, Wechsler ME, Rosenwasser LJ, Roufosse F, Gleich GJ, Klion AD. Refining the definition of hypereosinophilic syndrome. J Allergy Clin Immunol. 2010;126(1):45–9.
377. Antoniu SA. Novel therapies for hypereosinophilic syndromes. Neth J Med. 2010;68:304–10.
378. James WD, Berger TG, Elston DM. Andrews' disease of the skin. Clinic dermatology. Philadelphia: Sunders Elsevier; 2011. p. 746–7.
379. Helbig G, Kyrcz-Krzemień S. Diagnostic and therapeutic management in patients with hypereosinophilic syndromes. Pol Arch Med Wewn. 2011;121(1–2):44–52.
380. Amini-Vaughan ZJ, Martinez-Moczygemba M, Huston DP. Therapeutic strategies for harnessing human eosinophils in allergic inflammation, hypereosinophilic disorders, and cancer. Curr Allergy Asthma Rep. 2012;2(5):402–12.
381. Roufosse F, Weller PF. Practical approach to the patient with hypereosinophilia. J Allergy Clin Immunol. 2010;126(1):39–44.
382. Simon H-U, Klion A. Therapeutic approaches to patients with hypereosinophilic syndromes. Semin Hematol. 2012;49(2): 160–70.

Neutrophilic Dermatoses

383. Caucanas M, Heylen A, Rolland F, et al. Associated pyoderma gangrenosum, erythema elevatum diutinum, and Sweet's syndrome: the concept of neutrophilic disease. Int J Dermatol. 2013;52(10):1185–8.
384. Villareal-Villarreal CD, Ocampo-Candiani J, Villarreal-Martínez A. Sweet syndrome: a review and update. Actas Dermosifiliogr. 2016;107(5):369–78.
385. Cohen PR. Sweet's syndrome – a comprehensive review of an acute febrile neutrophilic dermatosis. Orphanet J Rare Dis. 2007;2:34.
386. Marzano AV, Cugno M, Trevisan V, et al. Inflammatory cells, cytokines and matrix metalloproteinases in amicrobial pustulosis of the folds and other neutrophilic dermatoses. Int J Immunopathol Pharmacol. 2011;24(2):451–60.
387. Marzano AV, Cugno M, Trevisan V, et al. Role of inflammatory cells, cytokines and matrix metallopro- teinases in neutrophil-mediated skin diseases. Clin Exp Immunol. 2010;162(1):100–7.
388. Sand FL, Thomsen SF. Off-label use of TNF-alpha inhibitors in a dermatological university department: retrospective evaluation of 118 patients. Dermatol Ther. 2015;28(3):158–65.
389. Kluger N, Gil-Bistes D, Guillot B, et al. Efficacy of anti- interleukin-1 receptor antagonist anakinra (Kineret) in a case of refractory Sweet's syndrome. Dermatology. 2011;222(2):123–7.
390. Xu HH, Xiao T, Gao XH, et al. Ulcerative Sweet syndrome accompanied by interstitial lung disease and myelodysplastic syndrome. Eur J Dermatol. 2009;19(4):411–2.
391. Srisuttiyakorn C, Reeve J, Reddy S, et al. Subcutaneous histiocytoid Sweet's syndrome in a patient with myelodysplastic syndrome and acute myeloblastic leukemia. J Cutan Pathol. 2014;41(5):475–9.
392. Su WPD, Liu H-NH. Diagnostic criteria for Sweet's syndrome. Cutis. 1986;37(3):167–70.
393. Cohen PR, Holder WR, Tucker SB, et al. Sweet syndrome in patients with solid tumors. Cancer. 1993;72(9):2723–31.
394. Rahier JF, Lion L, Dewit O, et al. Regression of Sweet's syndrome associated with Crohn's disease after anti-Tumour Necrosis Factor therapy. Acta Gastroenterol Belg. 2005;68(3):376–9.
395. Marzano AV, Borghi A, Meroni PL, et al. Pyoderma gangrenosum and its syndromic forms: Evidence for a link with autoinflammation. Br J Dermatol. 2016; 175(5): 882–891.
396. Agarwal S, Misra R, Aggarwal A. Interleukin 17 levels are increased in juvenile idiopathic arthritis synovial fluid and induce synovial fibroblasts to produce proinflammatory cytokines and matrix metalloproteinases. J Rheumatol. 2008;35(3):515–9.
397. Marzano AV, Cugno M, Trevisan V, et al. Role of inflammatory cells, cytokines and matrix metalloproteinases in neutrophil-mediated skin diseases. Clin Exp Immunol. 2010;162(1):100–7.
398. Marzano AV, Fanoni D, Antiga E, et al. Expression of cytokines, chemokines and other effector molecules in two prototypic autoinflammatory skin diseases, pyoderma gangrenosum and Sweet's syndrome. Clin Exp Immunol. 2014;178(1):48–56.
399. Dinarello CA. A clinical perspective of IL-1β as the gatekeeper of inflammation. Eur J Immunol. 2011;41(5):1203–17.
400. Marzano AV, Tourlaki A, Alessi E, et al. Widespread idiopathic pyoderma gangrenosum evolved from ulcerative to vegetative type: a 10-year history with a recent response to infliximab. Clin Exp Dermatol. 2008;33(2):156–9.
401. Stichweh DS, Punaro M, Pascual V. Dramatic improvement of pyoderma gangrenosum with infliximab in a patient with PAPA syndrome. Pediatr Dermatol. 2005;22(3):262–5.
402. Bister V, Mäkitalo L, Jeskanen L, et al. Expression of MMP-9, MMP-10 and TNF-α and lack of epithelial MMP-1 and MMP-26 characterize pyoderma gangrenosum. J Cutan Pathol. 2007; 34(12):889–98.
403. Su WPD, Davis MDP, Weenig RH, et al. Pyoderma gangrenosum: clinicopathologic correlation and proposed diagnostic criteria. Int J Dermatol. 2004;43(11):790–800.
404. Pay S, Simşek I, Erdem H, et al. Immunopathogenesis of Behçet's disease with special emphasize on the possible role of antigen presenting cells. Rheumatol Int. 2007;27(5):417–24.
405. Sfikakis PP, Markomichelakis N, Alpsoy E, et al. Anti-TNF therapy in the management of Behçet's disease—review and basis for recommendations. Rheumatology. 2007;46(5): 736–41.
406. Arida A, Sfikakis PP. Anti-cytokine biologic treatment beyond anti-TNF in Behçet's disease. Clin Exp Rheumatol. 2014;32(4 Suppl 84):S149–55.
407. Gul A, Tugal-Tutkun I, Dinarello CA, et al. Interleukin-1β-regulating antibody XOMA 052 (gevokizumab) in the treatment of acute exacerbations of resistant uveitis of Behçet's disease: an open-label pilot study. Ann Rheum Dis. 2012;71(4):563–6.
408. Cantarini L, Lopalco G, Caso F, et al. Effectiveness and tuberculosis-related safety profile of interleukin-1 blocking agents in the management of Behçet's dis- ease. Autoimmun Rev. 2015;14(1):1–9.

Diseases Caused by Genetic or Congenital Defects in the Immune System or Skin Immune System

11

Albert Gutierrez, Mark R. Pittelkow, Liyan Xi, Xiaowen Huang, and Sweta Rai

Contents

A. Gutierrez, MD, PhD • M.R. Pittelkow, MD (✉)
Department of Dermatology, Mayo Clinic, Scottsdale, Arizona, USA
e-mail: pittelkow.mark@mayo.edu

L. Xi (✉) • X. Huang • S. Rai
Department of Dermatology, Sun Yat-sen Memorial Hospital, Sun Yat-sen University, Guangzhou 510120, China
e-mail: xiliyan@mail.sysu.edu.cn

11.1 Skin Manifestations of Primary Immunodeficiency and Hereditary Autoinflammatory Disorders

Albert Gutierrez , MD, PhD and Mark R. Pittelkow, MD

11.1.1 Introduction

PIDDs are a heterogeneous group of diseases that predispose to recurrent, atypical, and often severe infections. These monogenic disorders result from altered immune cell development, homeostasis, or effector function. They can be classified by the arm of the immune system that is disrupted, for example, severe combined immunodeficiency syndrome (SCID) results from at least 20 genetic mutations that alter T- and B-cell development and function [1].

In contrast to the PIDD, HAIDs result from aberrant immune activation leading to a systemic inflammatory state. These monogenic disorders are characterized by episodic fever and severe multiorgan system inflammation including cutaneous eruptions. Many of these disorders result from aberrant activation of inflammasome cytoplasmic complexes or alterations to cytokine signaling pathways [2]. There is significant overlap between autoinflammatory disorders and primary immunodeficiencies due to the fine balance between the inflammatory response and immunoregulation, which prevents the development of autoimmunity. Immunoregulation is often altered in both PIDD and HAIDs and patients share a propensity for autoimmune or inflammatory sequelae.

Cutaneous disease may be the heralding symptom signaling the diagnosis of an HAID or PIDD disorders [3]. Identification of the genetic basis of these disorders has continued to accelerate with the use of genomic sequencing technologies. These disorders are rare, but have characteristic findings allowing physicians to build an appropriate differential diagnosis. Clinicians must be aware of this ever expanding group of conditions and their appropriate evaluation as well as advances in clinical care for these patients.

X.-H. Gao, H.-D. Chen (eds.), *Practical Immunodermatology*, DOI 10.1007/978-94-024-0902-4_11

11.1.2 Common Skin Manifestations of PIDD

11.1.2.1 Eczema and Erythroderma

Aside from cutaneous infection, early onset eczema and erythroderma are the most common cutaneous manifestations of PIDDs [3]. Associated PIDDs include hyperimmunoglobulin E syndrome (HIES), immunodysregulation–polyendocrinopathy–enteropathy–X-linked syndrome (IPEX), Wiskott–Aldrich syndrome (WAS), Omenn syndrome/SCID, immunoglobulin disorders (i.e., selective IgA deficiency and common variable immunodeficiency), and Comèl–Netherton syndrome (Table 11.1). Most of these disorders present early in life with severe eczema and varying predisposition to infection.

Autosomal dominant HIES (also designated as Job's syndrome) (OMIM #147060) is characterized by recurrent cutaneous infections (i.e., candidiasis and staphylococcal "cold abscesses"), sinopulmonary infections, elevated serum IgE levels, and severe atopic dermatitis beginning in infancy. Other clinical manifestations include characteristic course facies, skeletal abnormalities, and an infantile papulopustular eruption in the first months of life that precedes severe eczema [4, 5]. This classical form of HIES is caused by autosomal dominant STAT3 mutation that is predicted to alter protein levels, nuclear localization, and DNA binding [6]. Severe dermatitis is secondary to aberrant immune regulation, as Stat 3 functions downstream of multiple cytokines including IL-6, IL-10, IL-21, IL-22, and IL-23 [7]. T helper 17 cell's differentiation and function are severely impaired giving rise to the predisposition to candidal and bacterial infections. Autosomal recessive forms of HIES also exist with DOCK8 (OMIM #243700) or TYK2 (OMIM #611521) mutations with varied predisposition to viral or mycobacterial infection relative to the classic, autosomal dominant form [8, 9].

WAS (OMIM #301000) is an X-linked recessive disorder characterized by the classic triad of eczema, thrombocytopenia, and recurrent sinopulmonary infection originally described in 1937 by Dr. Alfred Wiskott [10]. Patients pres-

Table 11.1 Cutaneous manifestations and associated primary immunodeficiency disorders (PIDDs)

Cutaneous signs	Associated disorders
Eczema/erythroderma	Omenn syndrome/severe combined immunodeficiency
	Wiskott–Aldrich syndrome
	Immunodysregulation–polyendocrinopathy–enteropathy–X-linked syndrome (IPEX)
	Hyper-IgE syndrome
	Combined variable immunodeficiency
	Comèl–Netherton syndrome
Granulomatous disorders	Chronic granulomatous disease
	Combined variable immunodeficiency
	Severe combined immunodeficiency
	Ataxia telangectasia
Urticaria	Cryopyrin-associated periodic syndromes (CAPS)
	PLCG2-associated antibody deficiency and immune dysregulation (PLAID)
Autoimmune conditions	Omenn syndrome/severe combined immunodeficiency
	Immunodysregulation–polyendocrinopathy–enteropathy–X-linked syndrome (IPEX)
	Autoimmune–polyendocrinopathy–candidiasis–ectodermal dystrophy (APECED)
	Complement deficiency
	Combined variable immunodeficiency
	Wiskott–Aldrich syndrome
Pigment, hair, and nail changes	Comèl–Netherton syndrome
	Chediak Higashi
	Griscelli syndrome type 2
	Hermansky Pudlak type 2
	Dyskeratosis congenita
	Cartilage hair hypoplasia syndrome
	Ectodermal dysplasia with immunodeficiency
Cutaneous infection	Majority of PIDDs

ent in the first week of life with petechiae or ecchymoses prior to the development of an atopic cutaneous eruption. Patients are also at an increased risk of developing autoimmune phenomena and lymphoproliferative disorders later in life. The disorder is caused by mutation in WASP, which regulates actin filament assembly in multiple cell types that are critical for cell trafficking [11]. WAS patients have neutropenia and limited peripheral B-cell and T-cell receptor repertoires [12].

IPEX (OMIM #304790) is an X-linked recessive disorder characterized by severe eczema and numerous autoimmune phenomena including inflammatory enteropathy and polyendocrinopathy (i.e., autoimmune thyroiditis, type 1 diabetes, etc.). FOXP3, which is a critical transcription factor for T regulatory cell development and effector functions, is mutated in this disorder [13]. In the setting of aberrant regulatory T cells, autoimmunity and inflammation are induced and patients present with severe eczema, psoriasiform eruptions, urticarial, and cutaneous autoimmunity [14, 15].

Omenn syndrome (OMIM #603554) presents with early onset generalized eczema or erythroderma. Additionally, patients have lymphadenopathy, hepatosplenomegaly, chronic diarrhea, and failure to thrive that are reminiscent of graft versus host disease [16]. Omenn syndrome is on a clinical spectrum with SCID, Omenn having hypomorphic mutations in SCID associated genes. As a consequence, there is slightly less severe immunodeficiency but more inflammatory or autoimmune sequelae that are observed. Associated genes include recombinase activating enzymes (genes RAG 1, RAG2) and Artemis (gene DCLRE1C), which are involved in B cell and T-cell receptor gene rearrangement [17, 18]. Omenn mutations are "leaky," allowing for the generation of oligoclonal and highly activated T cells that underlie the varied manifestations of this disorder.

Comel–Netherton (OMIM #256500) syndrome is caused by SPINK5 mutation that is characterized by neonatal ichthyosiform erythroderma, severe eczema, and bamboo hairs with trichorrhexis invaginata. Many patients have a mild immunodeficiency leading to sinopulmonary infection along with staphylococcal complicated eczema [19].

11.1.2.2 Cutaneous Granulomatous Disease

Cutaneous granulomatous eruptions are features of common variable immunodeficiency (CVID) and chronic granulomatous disease (CGD). CVID (#607594) is the largest collective group of symptomatic PIDDs with estimated incidence between 1:10,000 and 1:200,000 [20]. CVID is a phenotypically heterogeneous group of disorders characterized by recurrent infections, autoimmunity, lymphoproliferative disease, and granulomatous inflammation (Fig. 11.1). The primary immunologic manifestation is hypogammaglobulinemia but selected patients may also have T-cell-related abnormalities. Associated mutations disrupt B cell signaling, development, and homeostasis pathways with TACI, BAFFR, CD19, CD20, and other genes implicated [21]. The granulomatous reactions of CVID are sarcoidal in nature effecting both cutaneous and internal organs such as spleen, liver, lung, and lymph nodes [22].

Chronic granulomatous disease (CGD) (OMIM #306400) is a group of disorders that result from defective phagocytic cellular killing of pathogens. The disorder is caused by mutations in the NADPH oxidase complex which is composed of five gene subunits: CYBA, NCF4, NCF1, NCF2 (autosomal chronic granulomatous disease), and CYBB (X-linked chronic granulomatous disease). This complex is critical for the respiratory burst, creating reactive oxygen species for the generation of antimicrobial oxidants and bacterial killing [23]. Granulomatous reactions develop as a protective mechanism to contain pathogens. Patients are burdened with severe and recurrent bacterial, mycobacterial, and fungal infections. Cutaneous manifestations include granulomas, dermatitis, folliculitis, lupus-like eruptions, Sweet syn-

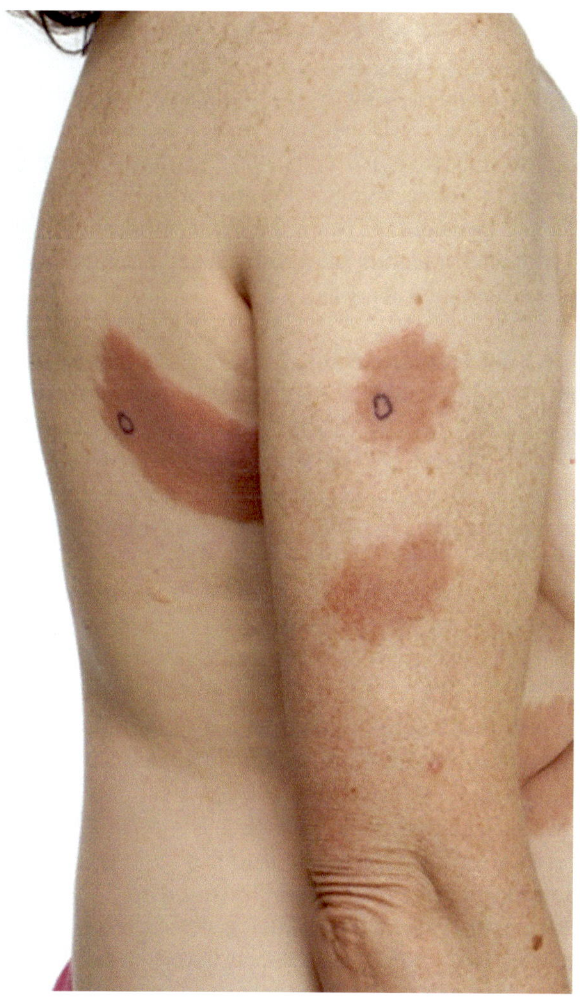

Fig. 11.1 Granulomatous dermatitis of the arm and back of a patient with common variable immunodeficiency

drome, and oral ulcers [24, 25]. Granulomas may occur in lungs, liver, spleen, GI, and GU tracts similar to CVID. Patients with ataxia telangiectasia (AT) and SCID may also present with cutaneous granulomas [26].

11.1.2.3 Cutaneous Autoimmune Eruptions and Vasculitis

Immune dysregulation is a common and unifying characteristic of PIDD. Numerous checkpoints exist during immune cell development, T- and B-cell receptor generation and immune activation that work to prevent autoimmunity. These are lost through various mechanisms in PIDD. T regulatory cells are altered or dysfunctional in Omenn/SCID, IPEX, and autoimmune–polyendocrinopathy–candidiasis–ectodermal dystrophy (APECED) (OMIM #240300) through mechanisms discussed elsewhere in this chapter. Autoreactive T cells are left unabated to promote autoimmunity and systemic inflammation. Patients with complement deficiencies develop systemic lupus erythematosus (SLE) as well as being at increased risk of bacterial infections [27]. In the setting of complement deficiency, clearance of apoptotic debris is impaired leading to presentation of autoantigens (DNA, RNA, etc.) and activation of an autoimmune adaptive response. The immunoglobulin deficiencies, including CVID and selective IgA deficiencies, are at risk for cutaneous and extracutaneous autoimmune phenomena including vitiligo, alopecia, SLE, pernicious anemia, and thyroiditis [21]. Patients with WAS are at risk of autoimmune vasculitis and IgE-mediated reactions such as urticaria and food allergies.

11.1.2.4 Hair and Nails

Nail dystrophy and infection are seen in recurrent candidiasis disorders such as chronic mucocutaneous candidiasis (CMC) (OMIM %114580) and APECED. Comel–Netherton syndrome, discussed above, demonstrates characteristic hair findings with bamboo hairs and trichorrhexis invaginata. X-linked ectodermal dysplasia with immunodeficiency (OMIM #300291), caused by a hypomorphic mutation in NEMO (gene IKBKG), is characterized by hyperhidrosis, recurrent infection, and sparse brittle or absent hair. NEMO is downstream of numerous immunoreceptors regulating NF-κB pathway activation. These patients are susceptible to recurrent pyogenic, mycobacterial, and viral infection [28].

Cartilage hair hypoplasia syndrome (OMIM #250250) is characterized by fine sparse hair that is hypopigmented, immunodeficiency, and short limbed dwarfism [29]. The disorder is due to mutation in RMRP gene which is involved in nucleolar RNA processing. Patients have a varied degree of immunodeficiency with some being categorized as SCID.

Dyskeratosis congenita (DKC) (OMIM #305000) is a clinically heterogeneous group of conditions effecting chromosomal telomeres that leads to nail dystrophy, abnormal reticulate skin pigmentation, and oral leukoplakia among other manifestations. Autosomal dominant, autosomal recessive, X-linked recessive forms of the disorder exist with multiple genes associated with this disorder [30]. The immunodeficiency is most severe in the Hoyeraal–Hreidarsson syndrome variant leading to a SCID-like phenotype [31]. Bone marrow failure and cytopenias are believed to underlie the immunodeficiency seen in this disorder.

11.1.2.5 Syndromic

Many PIDDs present with multiorgan system abnormalities that are characteristic giving clues for accurate diagnosis. The prototypical syndromic PIDD is ataxia telangiectasia (AT) (OMIM #208900), which is characterized initially by cerebellar ataxia, followed by oculocutaneous telangiectasias and recurrent sinopulmonary infection [32]. The disorder is autosomal recessive and caused by mutation in the gene, ATM, a crucial signaling member in the DNA damage response to double-strand breaks and regulation of the cell cycle. This DNA damage signaling pathway is involved in VDJ recombination of T- and B-cell receptors. As well, ATM deficiency leads to telomere shortening and acceleration of the aging process across organs and tissues [33]. Cutaneous telangiectasia have predilection for the ears, eyelids, malar prominence, and V of the neck. Patients are at an increased risk of malignancy and are sensitive to ionizing radiation. Immunodeficiency is characterized by recurrent sinopulmonary infections due to peripheral lymphopenia, humoral deficiencies, and defective T-cell responses that can be demonstrated on delayed hypersensitivity skin testing.

Chediak–Higashi (OMIM #214500) is a disorder of vesicle trafficking that has characteristic pigmentary changes with silvery hair, hypopigmentation, as well as neutropenia and immunodeficiency [34]. The disorder is caused by autosomal recessive mutation in LYST, a gene critical in lysosomal trafficking affecting numerous cell types including melanocytes, leukocytes, and platelets. The decreased pigmentation of hair and eyes was correlated with giant melanosomes and was seen on histopathology. Neutrophil, cytotoxic T cell, and NK cell function are greatly impaired in the setting of aberrant lysosome function. The natural history of the disorder is characterized by predisposition to malignancy as well as early death with an accelerated lymphoproliferative phase that is difficult to treat. This may be remedied by bone marrow stem cell transplantation although neurologic deterioration may still occur [35].

Not infrequently difficult to distinguish from Chediak–Higashi syndrome are Griscelli syndrome (GS) type 2 (OMIM #607624) and Hermansky Pudlak (HP) type 2 (OMIM #608233). GS type 2 is caused by mutation in gene RAB27, and characterized by silvery hair and immunodeficiency with defective cytotoxic T-cell activity [36].

HP type 2 is caused by mutations in gene AP3B1, and characterized by oculocutaneous albinism and immunodeficiency with neutropenia as well as dysfunctional cytotoxic T cells [37].

11.1.2.6 Cutaneous and Systemic Infections

PIDDs have more or less propensity for particular bacterial, fungal, and viral infections. SCID patients are susceptibility to all classes of infectious organisms, even the poorly virulent and live vaccines. The most common genetic forms of SCID are X-linked common gamma chain, ADA, and JAK3 mutations representing 40 %, 20 %, and 6 % of SCID diagnoses, respectively [38, 39]. These mutations affect T- and B-cell development and effector function at various stages as outlined in Fig. 11.2.

11.1.3 Bacterial

The risk of bacterial infection is high in PIDD but most prominent in the setting of defective neutrophils, complement deficiency, and immunoglobulin deficiencies. Defective neutrophil development is seen in severe congenital neutropenia disorders and WAS. Neutrophil function is blocked in CGD and patients are unable to mount a respiratory burst leading to defective bacterial killing. Neutrophils are unable to extravasate into tissues in leukocyte adhesion deficiency (OMIM #116920) caused by mutation in genes ITBG2, FUCT1, or FERMT3. These mutations interfere with integrin- and selectin-mediated leukocyte extravasation [40]. Patients have leukocytosis, delayed wound healing, and recurrent infection. Other commonly associated conditions are listed in Table 11.2.

11.1.3.1 Fungal

Fungal infections are a common manifestation of primary immunodeficiency. Recurrent candidiasis is most prominent in chronic mucocutaneous candidiasis (CMC) but also affects SCID, HIES, APECED, CGD, and complement deficiencies. CMC is a heterogeneous disorder with genetic mutations affecting the antifungal pattern recognition receptor Dectin-1, its downstream signaling member CARD9 or

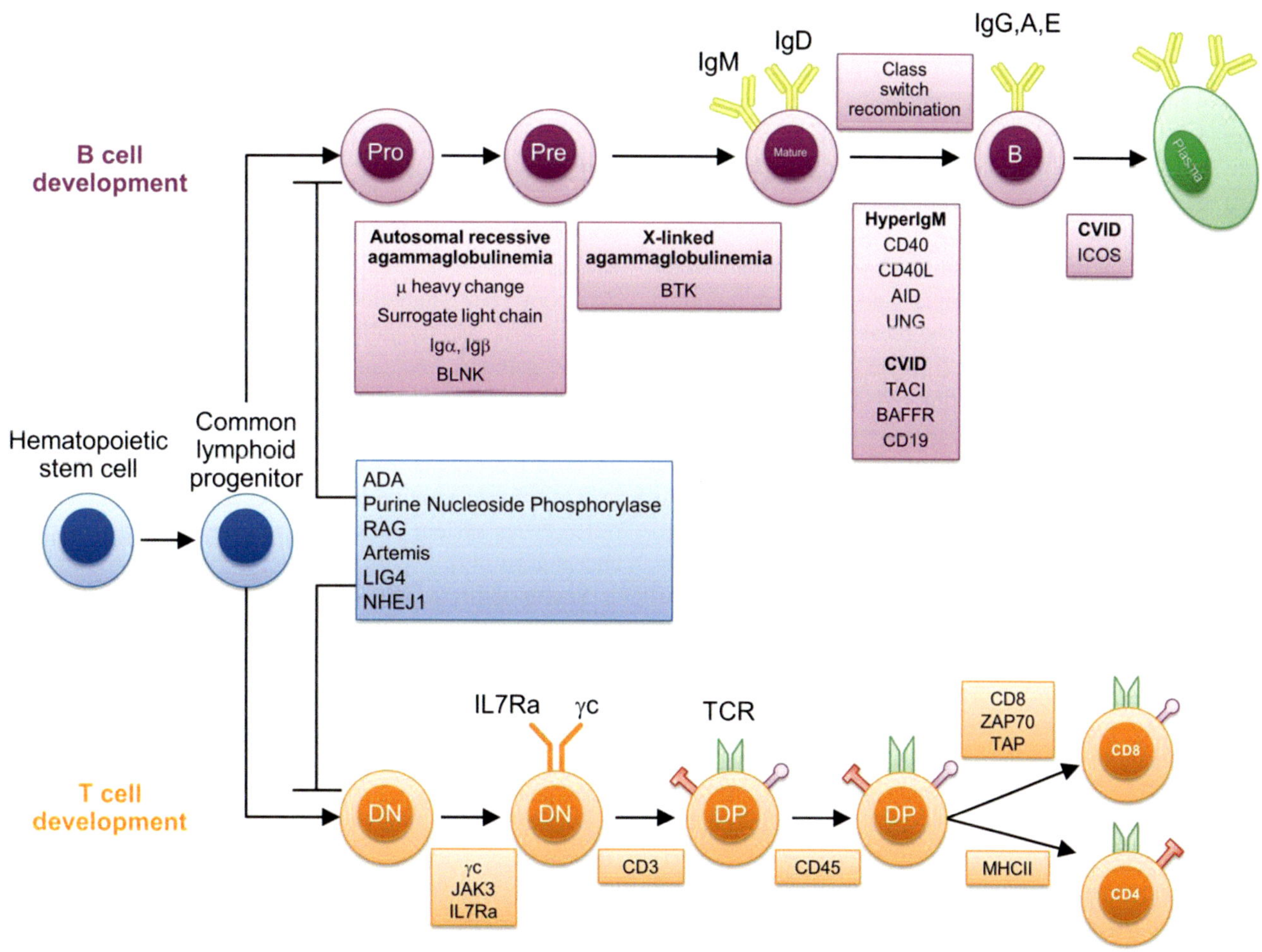

Fig. 11.2 B- and T-cell development and associated primary immunodeficiencies

Table 11.2 Cutaneous infections and associated PIDDs

Recurrent infections	Associated disorders
Bacteria	Severe combined immunodeficiency
	Wiskott aldrich syndrome
	Chronic granulomatous disease
	Leukocyte adhesion deficiency
	HyperIgE syndrome
	Congenital neutropenia
	Combined variable immunodeficiency
	Agammaglobulinemia (X-linked and AR)
	HyperIgM syndrome
	Complement deficiency
Fungal	Severe combined immunodeficiency
	Chronic mucocutaneous candidiasis
	Autoimmune-polyendocrinopathy-candidiasis-ectodermal dystrophy (APECED)
	HyperIgE syndrome
	Chronic granulomatous disease
	Complement deficiency
Virus	Severe combined immunodeficiency
	HyperIgE syndrome (DOCK8)
	Susceptibillity to HSV encephalitis (TLR3)
	Warts, hypogammaglobulinemia, infections, and myelokathexis syndrome
	Epidermodysplasia verruciformis

the IL-17 pathway (i.e., IL-17-RA, IL-17A, IL-17F, STAT1 gain of function) [41]. The patients suffer recurrent bouts of skin, nail, oral, esophageal, and vulvovaginal candidiasis often requiring long-term antifungal therapy. CMC patients also have increased risk of dermatophyte and bacterial infections.

Autoimmune–polyendocrinopathy–candidiasis–ectodermal dystrophy (APECED) is caused by mutation in AIRE, a protein that is critical in prevention of autoimmunity. AIRE mediates peripheral tissue self-antigen expression by thymic antigen presenting cells. This has significant effects on the T-cell repertoire as self-antigen expression is required for positive selection of regulatory T cells and deletion of autoreactive T cells in the thymus [42–44]. As the name of the disorder identifies, patients develop numerous autoimmune sequelae including polyendocrinopathy, alopecia areata, vitiligo, lupus-like panniculitis, and pernicious anemia [45]. Autoimmune endocrine disorders include type 1 diabetes mellitus, hypoparathyroidism, thyroiditis, hypoadrenocorticism, and hypogonadism. Interestingly, the mechanism of recurrent candidal infection is likely also autoimmune in nature as APECED patients have neutralizing autoantibodies to IL-17A, IL-17F, and IL-22 [46]. This is strikingly similar to the defective pathways involved in CMC.

11.1.3.2 Viral

Herpes family viruses (HSV 1 and 2, VZV, EBV, CMV, etc.), human papilloma virus (HPV), and molluscum contagiosum are all common viral infections that present in the setting of adaptive cellular immunodeficiencies. In autosomal recessive hyperimmunoglobulin type E caused by DOCK8 mutation patients suffer from severe herpes simplex virus, molluscum contagiosum, and human papillomavirus infections at a young age [8]. These infections are not seen in the autosomal dominant form of HIES caused by autosomal dominant STAT3 mutation, which is predominated by recurrent bacterial and fungal infections.

The pathogen recognition receptor, Toll-like receptor 3 (TLR3) (OMIM #613002) and UNC93B (OMIM #610551), an endoplasmic reticulum protein involved in TLR activation are critical for immunity to HSV [47, 48]. Mutations in these lead to reduced antiviral IFN-alpha/beta signaling in the central nervous system underlying the predisposition to HSV encephalitis [49].

Susceptibility to HPV infection is seen in epidermodysplasia verruciformis (OMIM #226400) leading to severe disseminated verrucae and risk of oncogenic transformation to squamous cell carcinoma. These are due mutation in TMC6 and TMC8 (aka EVER1 and EVER2, respectively). The exact mechanism leading to susceptibility in these disorders is unknown, although cellular zinc homeostasis appears to play a role [50].

Warts, hypogammaglobulinemia, infections, and myelokathexis syndrome (WHIM) syndrome (OMIM #193670) patients have recurrent bacterial and chronic HPV infection. Impaired chemotaxis causes peripheral neutropenia due to retention of bone marrow neutrophils called myelokathexis

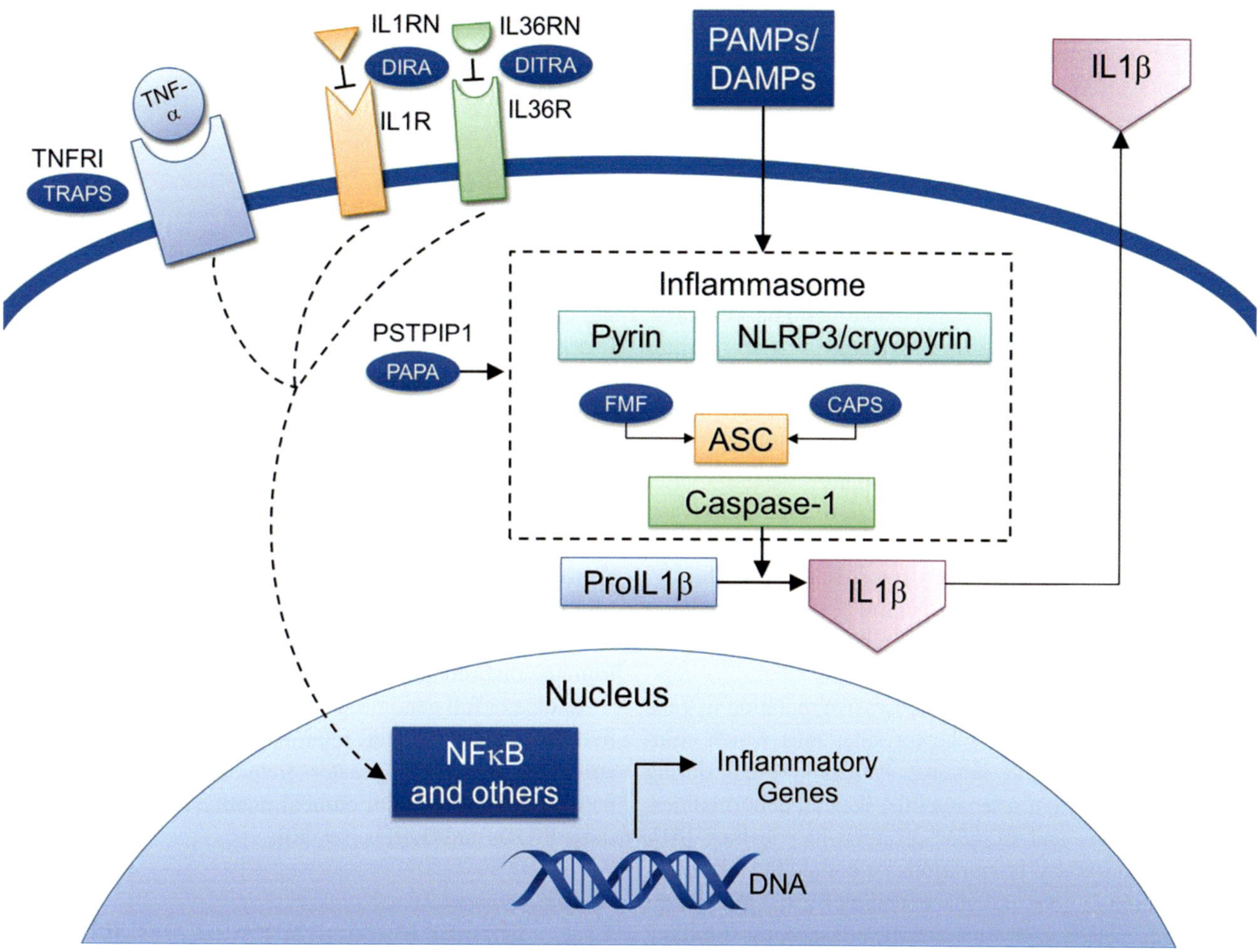

Fig. 11.3 Autoinflammatory signaling and associated disorders

(kathexis = retention). Mutations have been identified in the chemokine receptor, CXCR4 (autosomal dominant), or changes in GRK3 (gene: ADRBK2), which act as a regulator of chemokine signaling [51, 52]. The HPV infection is characterized by severe verruca vulgaris, condyloma accuminata, and cervical infection in females [53].

11.1.4 Hereditary Autoinflammatory Disorders

HAIDs are characterized by aberrant innate immune system activation in the setting of altered inflammatory signaling pathways. These manifest classically with episodic fever, cutaneous eruption, and multiorgan systemic inflammation [54]. This unregulated activation is antigen independent as opposed to autoimmune disorders that are largely mediated by the adaptive immune system. The etiology of aberrant innate activation often centers on pattern recognition receptors (i.e., NOD/NLRP inflammasomes) or inflammatory cytokines (i.e., interleukin-1 [IL-1] and tumor necrosis factor [TNF] alpha families) (Fig. 11.3). As such, monoclonal anti-IL-1 or anti-TNF-alpha biologics have proven efficacious in many HAIDs [55].

Inflammasomes are innate immune complexes that recognize pathogen and danger associated molecular patterns [56]. The cytoplasmic complex NLRP3 inflammasome regulates IL-1β processing and is composed of NLRP3 (aka cryopryin), pyrin, ASC, and caspase 1 [57]. HAIDs associated with this signaling pathway include familial Mediterranean fever (FMF) (OMIM #249100) and cryopyrin-associated periodic fever syndromes (CAPS). CAPS are caused by autosomal dominant mutation in the gene NLRP3, leading to aberrant inflammasome activation. CAPS disorders include familial cold autoinflammatory syndrome (FCAS) (OMIM #120100) type 1, Muckle–Wells (OMIM #191900), and neonatal-onset multisystem inflammatory disease (NOMID) (OMIM #607115). Clinically these disorders present with attacks of fever, urticarial eruption, and arthralgia, although they differ in timing of onset and severity of manifestations, which are outlined in Table 11.3. Patients are at risk for systemic AA amyloidosis, which occurred in 27 % of CAPS patients in one case series [58].

Familial Mediterranean fever (FMF) is caused by mutation in the gene MEFV that encodes pyrin, a regulator of the cryopyrin/NLRP3 inflammasome. Clinically patients present with attacks of fever, abdominal pain, pleurisy, arthralgia, and erysipelas like rash [59]. Again, systemic AA amyloidosis is a potential complication of uncontrolled disease.

Alterations to TNF-alpha or IL-1 family of cytokine signaling lead to systemic inflammation and HAIDs. These disorders include TNF-receptor associated periodic syndrome (TRAPS) (OMIM #142680), deficiency of IL-1 receptor antagonist (DIRA) (OMIM #612852), and deficiency of IL-36 receptor antagonist (DITRA) (OMIM #614204). TRAPS is due to mutation in gene TNFRSF1A, which encodes for TNF-alpha receptor 1. Mutation leads to diminished receptor activation-induced downregulation and decreased levels of cleaved soluble receptor that is antagonistic to circulating TNF-alpha [60]. TRAPS is clinically characterized by episodic fever, painful centrifugal erythematous patches, myalgia, abdominal pain, pleurisy, and conjunctivitis [2].

DIRA is caused by autosomal recessive mutation in gene IL1RN encoding for IL-1 receptor antagonist which competes for IL-1 receptor binding. Patients present during infancy with recurrent osteomyelitis, skeletal abnormalities, failure to thrive, and pustular psoriasis-like lesions [61]. DITRA is caused by homozygous or compound heterozygous mutation in gene IL36RN encoding for IL-36 receptor antagonist, which competes for IL-36 receptor binding. Patients present with severe generalized pustular psoriasis flares that are associated with fever, asthenia, and leukocytosis. The disorder may present in childhood or as an adult and pustular flares were associated with common infectious agents [62].

Hyper-IgD syndrome (HIDS) (aka mevalonate kinase deficiency) (OMIM #260920) patients have mevalonate aciduria due to decreased function of mevalonate kinase. This enzyme is part of the HMG-CoA reductase pathway for cholesterol biosynthesis, and the exact mechanism by which diminished mevalonate kinase induces a proinflammatory state is unknown. Patients have episodic fever, lymphadenopathy, splenomegaly, arthralgia, abdominal pain, and elevated IgD levels [63]. Cutaneous features of HIDS are polymorphic and include acral erythematous macules although papules, plaques, and nodules might also be seen.

HAIDs that have been characterized to date are summarized in Table 11.3. Recent studies have continued to identify new syndromes cataloging the diverse clinical manifestations and genetic basis of these disorders. Newly identified pathways of HAIDs include STING [64], NLRC4 [65, 66], EGFR [67], and ISG15/interferon [68] signaling. Research of HAIDs will continue to accelerate as high-throughput genomic technologies continue to decrease in cost.

11.1.5 Conclusions

Cutaneous eruptions are common manifestations of HAID, PIDD, and associated syndromes. An understanding of the manifestations of these rare disorders is helpful, if not critical, to achieve a timely and accurate diagnosis. Thorough clinical history, detailed review of systems, and complete clinical examination will direct the clinician to the appropriate differential diagnosis and confirmatory laboratory testing required to establish the correct diagnosis. Avoiding diagnostic delays is critical for reducing morbidity and mortality in HAID and PIDD patients. Stem cell transplantation, gene therapies, and targeted biologic therapies have all provided significant advances in the treatment of these challenging and life-threatening immune disorders.

Exome or full genome sequencing has provided definitive molecular diagnosis and appropriate, life-saving treatment strategies with ever greater frequency for undiagnosed patients presenting with clinical manifestations resembling these PIDDs and HAIDs [69, 70].

11.2 Chronic Mucocutaneous Candidiasis (CMC)

Liyan Xi, Xiaowen Huang, and Sweta Rai

Candida spp. (primarily *Candida albicans*) is cosmopolite commensal yeasts colonizing the skin and mucosal surfaces of healthy individuals. However, in some individuals, it causes a persistent infection either by infecting mucosal and/or epidermal surfaces resulting in chronic mucocutaneous candidiasis (CMC) or by disseminating in the blood resulting in systemic candidiasis.

CMC was first described in 1929 by Thorpe and Handley, and followed by more extensive description in the 1950s and 1960s [81–85]. CMC is characterized by a heterogeneous group of clinical syndromes with the unifying feature of susceptibility to chronic or recurrent noninvasive infections. It usually caused by *C. albicans*, localized to the skin, nails, oral, and genital mucous membranes, with early onset (infancy) in most cases (60–80 %), whereas late onset is rare [86–92]. Although the symptoms are not acutely life threatening and rarely associated with disseminated disease, they are disfiguring and debilitating. This disease often affects individuals' life quality. Even more severe secondary com-

Table 11.3 Hereditary autoinflammatory disorders (HAIDs)

	OMIM #	Gene/protein	Inheritance/chromosome	Clinical findings	Cutaneous findings	Tx	Citations
Cryopyrin-associated periodic syndrome (CAPS)							
Familial Cold Autoinflammatory Syndrome (FCAS)	#120100	NLRP3 ; Cryopyrin	AD ; Chrm 1	Episodic fever, arthralgia, myalgia, conjuctivitis, headache	Cold induced urticarial papules and plaques	Anti-IL1 therapy	[57]
Muckle-wells syndrome	#191900	NLRP3 ; Cryopyrin	AD ; Chrm 1	Same as FCAS, sensorineural hearingloss, amyloidosis	Urticarial papules and plaques	Anti-IL1 therapy	[57]
Neonatal-Onset Multisystem Inflammatory Disease (NOMID)	#607115	NLRP3 ; Cryopyrin	AD ; Chrm 1	Infantile onset, skeletal abnormalities, dysmorphic facies, seizures	Urticarial papules and plaques	Anti-IL1 therapy	[57]
Other autoinflammatory syndromes							
Familial Mediterranean Fever (FMF)	#249100	MEFV ; Pyrin	AR ; Chrm 16	Episodic fever, arthralgia, pleuritis, abdominal pain	Erysipeloid erythema and edema	Colchicine, TNF alpha inhibitors, anti-IL1 therapy, thalidomide	[59]
Hyper IgD Syndrome (HIDS)	#260920	MVK ; Mevalonate kinase	AR ; Chrm 12	Episodic fever, arthralgia, myalgia, abdominal pain, lymphadenopathy, HSM, elevated IgD	Erythematous macules and papules; urtcaria	TNF alpha inhibitors, statins, anti-IL1 therapy	[63]
TNF-Receptor Associated Periodic Syndrome (TRAPS)	#142680	TNFRSF1A ; Tumor necrosis factor receptor 1	AD ; Chrm 12	Episodic dever, myalgia, abdominal pain, Pleuritis, conjunctivitis	Painful centrifugal erythematous patches, annular or serpiginous	TNF alpha inhibitors, anti-IL1 therapy	[60]
Deficiency of Il-1 Receptor Agonist (Il-1 RA) known as (DIRA)	#612852	IL1RN ; IL-1R antagonist	AR ; Chrm 2	Fever, neonatal distress, chronic recurrent multifocal osteomyelitis, skeletal abnormalities, HSM	Generalized pustular psoriasis	Anti-IL1 therapy	[61]
Deficiency of IL36R antagonist (DITRA)	#614204	IL36RN ; IL-36R antagonist	AR/AD ; Chrm 2	Episodic fever, asthenia, leukocytosis	Generalized pustular psoriasis	Anti-IL 1 therapy	[62]
Chronic Recurrent Multifocal Osteomyelitis (CRMO)	#609628	LPIN2 ; Lipin 2	AR ; Chrm 18	Fever, chronic recurrent multifocal osteomyelitis, congenital dyserythropoietic anemia	Psoriasis, palmoplantar pustulosis, sweet's syndrome	Prednisone, NSAIDs	[71]
Pyogenic arthritis, Pyoderma gangrenosum, and cystic Acne (PAPA)	#604416	PSTPIP1	AD ; Chrm 15	Juvenile onset destructive arthritis	Pyoderma gangrenosum, nodulocystic acne	Accutane for Acne, Prednisone, TNF alpha inhibitors, Anti-IL1 therapy	[72, 73]
Blau Syndrome	#186580	NOD2 ; CARD15	AD ; Chrm 16	Fever, uveitis, arthritis, joint contractures,	Lichenoid papules, granulomatous dermatitis	Prednisone, TNF alpha inhibitors, Anti-IL1 therapy	[74]

(continued)

Table 11.3 (continued)

	OMIM #	Gene/protein	Inheritance/chromosome	Clinical findings	Cutaneous findings	Tx	Citations
NLRP12 associated autoinflammatory Disorders (NLRP12AD)	#611762	NLRP12	AD ; Chrm 19	Episodic fever, arthralgia, myalgia, sensorineural deafness, headache	Cold induced urticarial papules and plaques	Colchicine, prednisone	[75]
PLCG2-associated antibody deficiency and immune dysregulation (PLAID)	#614468	PLCG2 ; Phospholipase C gamma-2	AD ; Chrm 16	Common variable immunodeficiency, recurrent sinopulmonary infections, atopy, autoimmune disease	Cold induced urticarial papules and plaques, granulomatous dermatitis	Cold avoidance, IVIg	[76]
Chronic Atypical Neutrophilic Dermatosis with Lipodystrophy and Elevated temperature (CANDLE) Syndrome	#256040	PSMB8 ; Proteasome subunit, Beta-type, 8	AR ; Chrm 6	Episodic fever, short stature, failure to thrive, arthralgia, joint contractures, long clubbed fingers, mental retardation, hepatosplenomegaly,	Lipodystrophy (loss of faical subcutaneous fat), panniculitis, erythematous annular plaques	Prednisone, TNF alpha inhibitors, anti-IL1 therapy	[77, 78]
Misc./new							
STING-Associated Vasculopathy, Infantile-Onset syndrome (SAVI)	#615934	TMEM173 ; STING	AD ; Chrm 5	Infantile onset, episodic fever, Systemic vasculopathy, interstitial lung disease, arthritis, lymphadenopathy	Telangiectasia, vesiculopustular eruptions, cutaneous ulcerations	Unknown, clinical trial janus kinase inhibition	[64]
Autoinflammation with Infantile Enterocolitis (AIFEC)	#616050	NLRC4	AD ; Chrm 2	Episodic fever, neonatal-onset enterocolitis, pancytopenia, arthralgia	Erythematous plaques	Dexamethasone, IVIg, cyclosporine,	[65, 66]
Inherited loss-of-function mutation in EGFR	#616069	EGFR ; Epidermal growth factor receptor	AR ; Chrm 7	Diarrhea, Pulmonary disease	Erosions, papules and pustules	Unknown	[67]
Periodic Fever, Aphthous stomatitis, Pharyngitis, and Cervical Adenitis (PFAPA)	Not in OMIM	Unknown	N/A	Periodic fever, aphthous stomatitis, pharyngitis, adenitis (cervical); arthritis	Truncal erythema, aphthous stomatitis	PrednisoneAnti-IL 1 therapy Tonsillectomy	[79]
Pyoderma gangrenosum, Cystic acne, Supprative hidradenitis (PASH)	Not in OMIM	Unknown	N/A	Pyoderma gangrenosum acne supprative hidradenitis	Pyoderma gangrenosum, acne, supprative hidradenitis	Anti-IL 1 therapy	[80]
Interferonopathy caused by ISG15 deficiency	Not in OMIM	ISG15	AR ; Chrm 1	Susceptibility to mycobacterial disease, seizures, basal ganglia calcifications	None reported	Unknown	[68]

plications occur occasionally, such as squamous cell carcinoma, esophageal stricture, and cerebral aneurysms [93–96].

Patients with CMC may present alterations in acquired cellular immunity, remarkably T-cell deficiency. Recently, most studies focus on the defects in interleukin-17 (IL-17). It increases the understanding that IL-17 pathway is critical for regulating antifungal immunity, and defects in IL-17 predispose primarily to infection with *C. albicans* [97–99]. CMC is frequently associated with other acquired infections, immunosuppressive therapies, prolonged antibiotic therapies, diabetes mellitus or various inherited primary T-cell immunodeficiency, and it often presents familial dominant inheritance and autoimmune endocrinopathy [82–84, 87].

11.2.1 Immunopathogenesis and Genetic Susceptibility to CMC

T cells and epithelial cells are essential for the control of mucocutaneous infections [100, 101]. Recently, human genetic studies have revealed the orchestrating role of IL-17 immunity in anti-*Candida* mucocutaneous host defense.

Briefly, *C. albicans* is recognized by several C-type lectin receptors (Dectin-1, Dectin-2, Mincle, etc.) and Toll-like receptors (TLRs) that induce NF-κB and MAPK pathways. It also can be recognized by inflammasomes (NLRP3 and NLRP4) that activate caspases. Then it triggers caspase recruitment domain family member-9 (CARD-9) and induces the production of pro-inflammatory cytokines interleukin-16 (IL-16) and interleukin-23 (IL-23). These cytokines promote the differentiation of T cells toward T helper 17 cells (Th17). A signal transducer and activator of transcription-3 (STAT-3)-dependent process starts [102–106]. However, in the case of signal transducers and activators of transcription (STAT-1) gain-of-function (GOF) mutations, the balance is turned to STAT1 signals which neutralizing Th17 development. Th17 cells secrete IL-17A, IL-17 F and interleukin-22 (IL-22), which then activate epithelial cells to produce neutrophil-recruiting chemokine (e.g., CXCL1 and CXCL8), neutrophil growth factors (G-CSF) and candidacidal antimicrobial peptides (AMPs) (Fig. 11.4) [107–113].

IL-17-mediated recruitment of neutrophils and induction of AMPs at infection sites (mucosal and skin surfaces) represent the primary immune defense mechanism against *Candida* [115–118]. Recent investigations have implicated that the defective maturation of dendritic cells and impairment to Th17 cell-associated signaling pathways are common in immunodeficiency syndromes associated with CMC. The mutation usually happens in CARD-9, STAT-3, STAT-1, IL-17 receptor A gene (IL-17RA), IL-12 receptor B gene (IL-12RB), and IL-17F. The polymorphisms in Dectin-1 and IL-22 encoding genes impair the development of Th17 cells and are associated with susceptibility to candidiasis [119–128].

Familial "Pure" CMC with autosomal dominant (AD) inheritance form can be caused by either STAT-1 GOF mutations that impair IL-17 immunity or IL-17F mutations that lead to IL-17F deficiency. Autosomal recessive (AR) CMC form results from IL-17RA mutations that abolish the function of IL-17RA [129–132]. Studies on autoimmune polyendocrinopathy–candidiasis–ectodermal dystrophy (APECED) patients and individuals with thymoma revealed that the basis for CMC is neutralizing autoantibodies targeting Th-17-associated cytokines (e.g., IL-17A/F, IL-22) [46, 133–137]. It is caused by mutations in autoimmune regulator (AIRE), a transcription factor that mediates thymic and peripheral self-reactive T-lymphocyte deletion [138].

CMC can also be resulted from the defects in the genes encoding dectin-1, a pattern-recognition receptor (PRR) that binds to β-glucan in the *Candida* cell wall and CARD-9 since they act together to activate Th17 response. Inadequate production of IL-23 and overproduction of IL-6, which result in an inefficient IL-17 response, can result in other types of CMC [139–143] Several genetic algorithms along immunological pathway have been shown to cause CMC (Table 11.4) [144].

11.2.2 Clinical Spectrum of CMC

CMC may clinically apparent at any time in life, but it typically presents before 3 years of age (up to 80 %) [85, 87]. Clinical manifestations and severity of CMC can be varied. The disease is more frequently manifested with recurrent oral thrush with erythematous and scaly cutaneous plaques in intertriginous areas, mucosae and nails. Lesions may evolve until the onset of generalized, hyperkeratotic granulomatous crusty plaques. Nails are thick, dystrophic, loose, and brittle, with associated paronychia (Fig. 11.5) [145–147]. Although the initial lesions are identical than the ones seen in the general populations, CMC may characteristically be sequelae to unique disfiguring and debilitating lesions [93–96, 148–151]. Systemic candidiasis is rare while cutaneous dermatophytosis is common.

The secondary illnesses associated in the patients generate the subgroups of CMC as summarized in Table 11.5 [152].

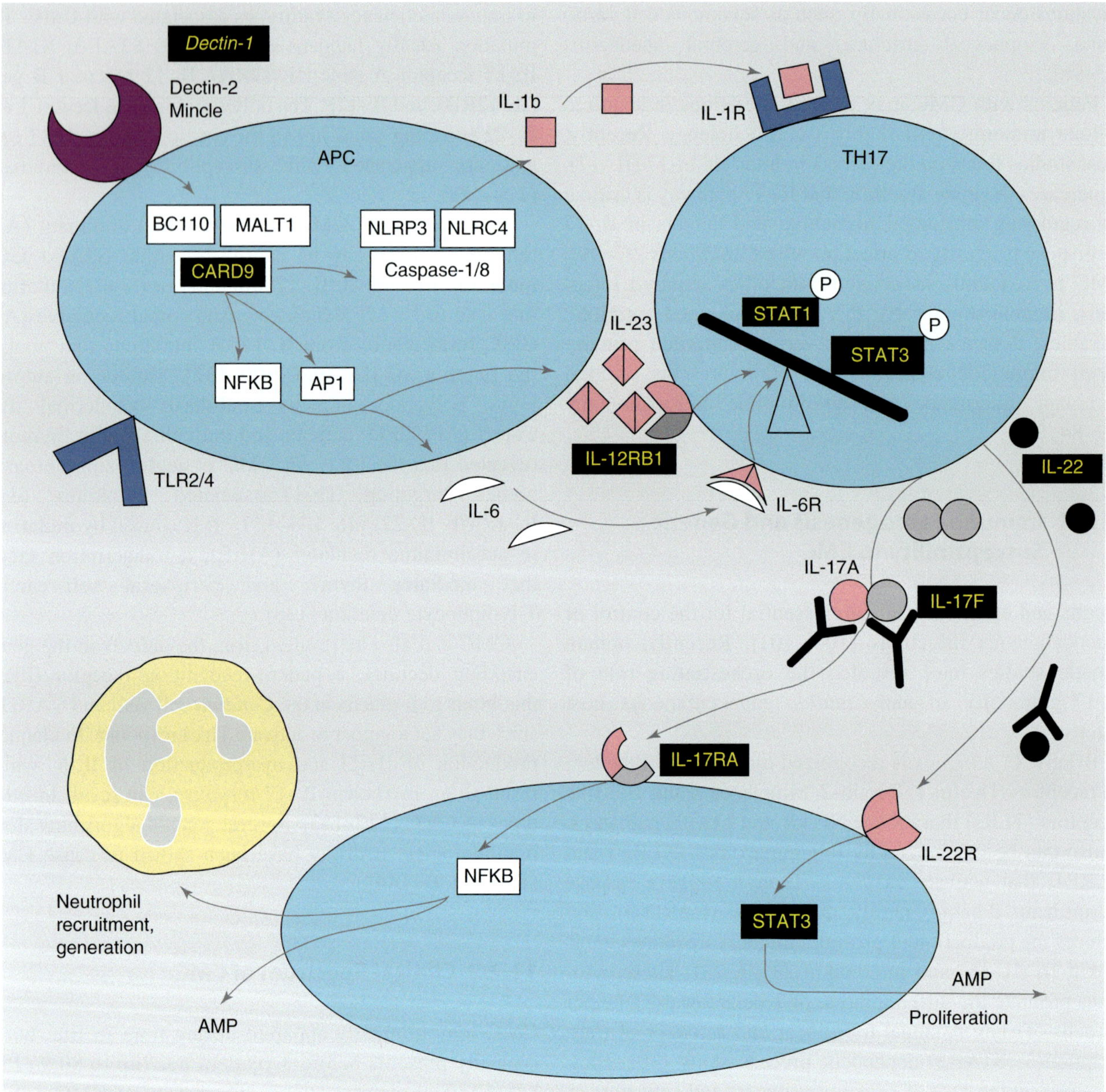

Fig. 11.4 Schematic overview of genetic susceptibility revealing immunopathogenesis of CMC to *Candida albicans* (Reprint with permission from Ref. [114])

11.2.3 Diagnostic Approach of CMC

The diagnosis of this disease is based on the lesions demonstrably caused by *Candida* of chronic evolution. It is necessary to rule out other causes of immunodeficiency, usually refractory to antifungal treatments, and the infection is merely controlled with the use of imidazole derivatives, such as ketoconazole, fluconazole, and itraconazole. The clinical spectrum of the lesions, characterized by noninvasive, chronic, recurrent, and/or persistent in the skin and/or mucous membranes compatible with candidiasis of onset in infancy and research of familial history primarily play core role in establishing the diagnosis of CMC. It is generally associated with autoimmune disorders, the most commonly endocrinopathies. From a diagnostic point of view, the evaluation of patients with suspected CMC is complex and relies on clinical manifestations of the lesions. Kirk Patrick has proposed the following age-based approach for the evaluation of the patients with CMC [85, 87].

Age of onset	Test
Children < 1 year old	CBC with differential, Lymphocyte phenotyping, T-Lyp response to mitogen-stimulated T cells (MT)

Table 11.4 Primary immunodeficiency disorders associated with CMC

Diseases	Molecular defect	Associated gene/transmission
AD-HIES	Dominant-negative effect on multiple intracellular signaling pathways, including impaired generation of Th17 cells, and impaired intracellular signaling by receptors of IL-17 and IL-22	STAT3, AD
APECED	Loss of tolerance, with persistence of auto reactive T cells, including the production of autoantibody to cytokines (e.g., IL-17 and IL-22)	AIRE, AR
SCID	Impaired T cells, with or without accompanying B and NK lymphocytopenia	IL2RG, X-linked; JAK3, AR; IL7Ra, AR; CD3d, AR; CD3e, AR; RAG1, AR; RAG2, AR; ARTEMIS, AR; CD45, AR
AR-HIES	Impaired T-cell activation, possibly impaired maintenance of memory Th17 cells or impaired formation of immunological synapse	DOCK8, AR
IL-12 and IL-23 deficiency	Impaired development of Th17 cells	IL12B, AR; IL12RB1, AR
IL-17 deficiency	Impaired or abolished cellular responses to IL-17, due to either impaired production of or abolished response capacity to IL-17	IL17F, AD; IL17RA, AR
Dectin-1 deficiency	Cell surface expression of the (mutated) receptor is lost, leading to impaired IL-6, IL-17, and tumor necrosis factor alpha (TNF-α) on stimulation in vitro	Dectin-1, AR
CARD-9 deficiency	Impaired function of signal for dectin-1, dectin-2, and other recognition molecules	CARD-9, AR
TYK2 deficiency	Adaptor molecule for several receptor complexes, including IL-23 receptor	TYK2, AR
STAT1 mutations	The mutations in the coiled-coil domain of STAT1	STAT1, AD

AD-HIES autosomal dominant-Hyper-IgE-syndrome, *AIRE* autoimmune regulator element, *APECED* autoimmune polyendocrinopathy–candidiasis–ectodermal dystrophy, *AR* autosomal recessive, *CMC* chronic mucocutaneous candidiasis, *SCID* severe combined immunodeficiency, *TYK2* tyrosine kinase 2

Age of onset	Test
Children > 1 year old	Previously listed tests, plus:
	T-lymphocyte to *Candida*, tetanus and other antigens
	Delayed cutaneous hypersensitivity testing with *Candida*, tetanus, mumps, etc.
	Lymphokine production by antigen or mitogen-stimulated T cells
	Antibodies against endocrine tissues
	Endocrine function tests (calcium, phosphate, TSH, cortisol)
Children with recurrent upper or lower respiratory tract infection	B lymphocyte counts
	Serum IgG, IgA, IgM, and IgE
	IgG subclasses
	Measurement of antibody response
Adults	CBC with differential
	HIV antibody and Western blot
	Lymphocyte phenotyping
	Computed tomography of the chest to rule out thymoma

Detection of microorganisms can be done by direct mycological test, culture, biopsy, or histopathological testing [93]. It helps to rule out malignancies lesions too. The only definitive laboratory test for the diagnosis of CMC is the genetic analysis of the AIRE gene for disease-causing mutations [87, 145]. All patients with chronic candidiasis should be evaluated for primary and secondary immunodeficiency. It includes a complete blood count with differential, immunoglobulin levels containing IgE level and B- and T-cell subsets at a minimum [152, 165]. Assessment of the immune system may identify a selective inability to respond in vitro (T-cell proliferation) or in vivo (cutaneous delayed-type hypersensitivity) to *Candida*, particularly in patients with AIRE deficiency. Humoral immunity may also be affected, including low IgG2 and IgG4.

Other laboratory findings are less definitive, but are still good aids in the diagnosis. The standard laboratory tests for evaluating endocrine disorders, such as hypoparathyroidism and adrenal insufficiency are associated with CMC. Computed tomography of the chest helps to rule out thymoma [94]. Liver function should also be regularly screened to rule out hepatotoxicity, as hepatitis is rarely associated with CMC [153]. Moreover, patients should be evaluated at least annually for the development of endocrinopathies, particularly if there is a family history of CMC or APECED. Serum *Candida* antibodies are not of value in the diagnosis of CMC, nor are skin or serum IgE tests for *Candida*.

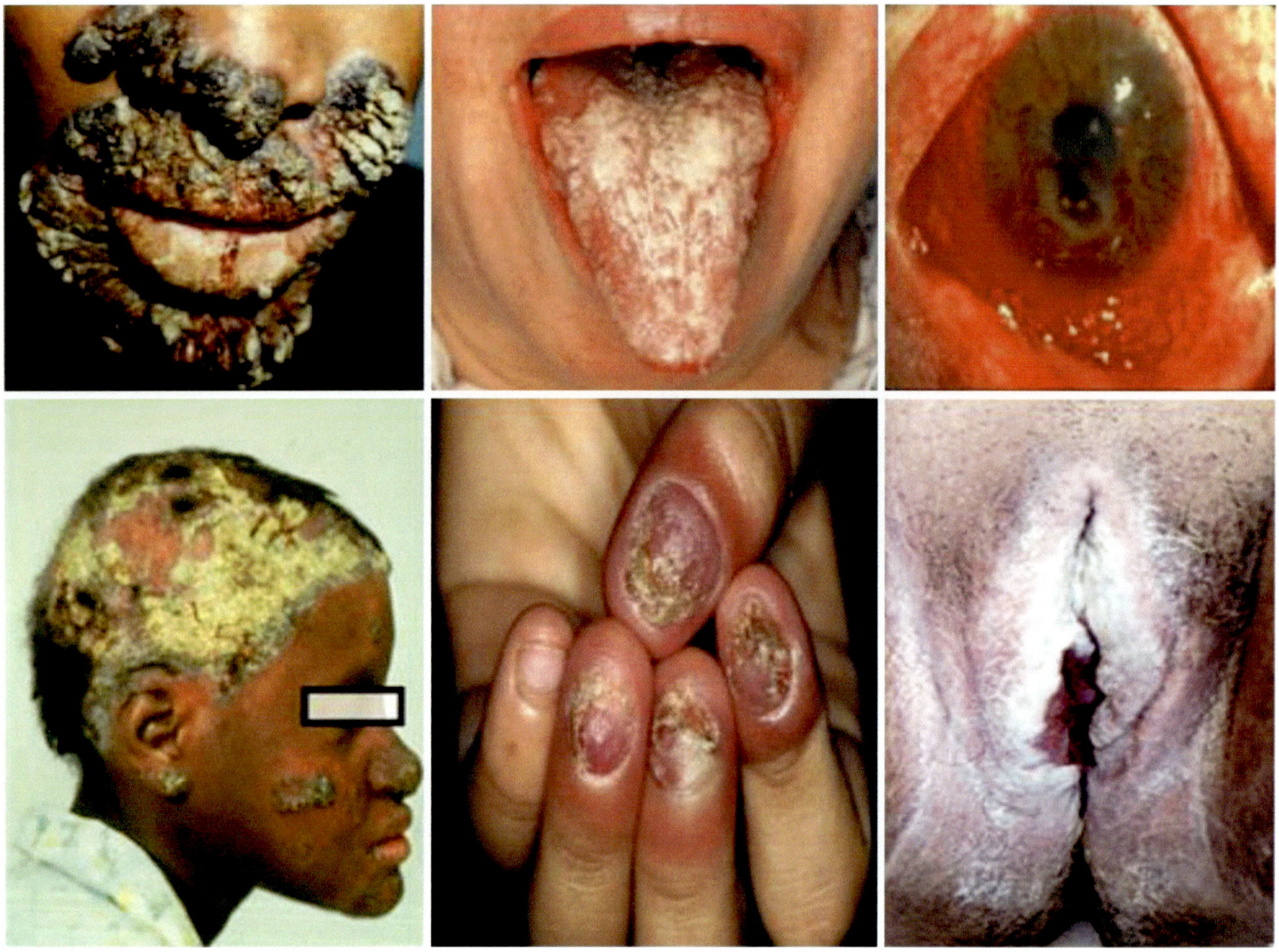

Fig. 11.5 Diverse clinical spectrum of chronic mucocutaneous candidiasis (CMC)

11.2.4 Management of CMC

The management of CMC is complicated for it frequently relapses following the cessation of therapy. The patients with CMC do not respond well to standard topical medications. Current management for CMC principally includes three main categories: systemic antifungal agents, immunologic therapies of associated endocrine and autoimmune abnormalities, and/or combination therapy [154, 155].

The availability of oral antifungal agents, especially azoles antifungal agents has made systemic antifungal therapy as the mainstay of CMC treatment. It may be used alone or in combination with immune-modulator agents. Although chronic suppressive therapy is often required to prevent recurrences, these antifungal agents dramatically cleared candidiasis and changed the patient's quality of life. Ketoconazole was the first agent to be used widely for CMC and proved to be extremely successful when used either continuously or intermittently [154, 156–159]. However, liver toxicity was found to be a limitation [153]. Later, Fluconazole was the preferred treatment as it has good activity against *C. albicans* and lesser side effects. It is also easy to administer and relatively inexpensive [160, 161]. Drug resistance may occur with suppressive therapy and are of concern, but shifting to another azole agents, e.g., itraconazole, voriconazole, or posaconazole can be prolific, besides escalating the dose of previous therapy [162–168]. Amphotericin has been a successfully alternative in severe cases [161]. The drawbacks of systemic antifungal therapy include the risk of adverse effects or toxicity, a failure to correct the underlying immune

Table 11.5 Subgroups and associated secondary illnesses of CMC

Subgroup	Features
Familial "pure" CMC	Autosomal dominant form due to mutations in the STAT-1 gene (which lead to impaired Th17 immunity) or IL-17 F gene. Autosomal recessive form due to mutations in the IL-17 receptor A gene (IL17RA). Oral candidiasis usually begins from 2 years old. Cutaneous and ungual candidiasis is also common but not associated with endocrinopathy
Chronic localized candidiasis	Majority has cutaneous lesions by the age of 5. Thick and adherent crusts most commonly happen on the face and scalp, usually concomitant to oral candidiasis. Histologically, epidermal hyperkeratosis and acanthosis; dermal infiltrates of lymphocytes, plasma cells and giant cells
Autoimmune polyendocrinopathy candidiasis ectodermal dystrophy syndrome (APECED)	Increased prevalence among Finns, Iranian Jews, and Sardinians. Because of the mutations in the AIRE gene, usually with autosomal recessive inheritance. Infections usually begin by the age of 5, and present as granulomas on the face and scalp. Endocrinologic dysfunction may not be apparent until teenage or even adult. An autosomal dominant form of CMC associated with autoimmune thyroid disease may occur due to dominant negative AIRE mutations and has also been linked to chromosome 2p in one family
	Associated autoimmune endocrinopathies: Hypoparathyroidism, hypoadrenocorticism, hypogonadism, thyroid disease, type-1 diabetes mellitus, and hypopituitarism
	Other autoimmune disorders: alopecia areata, vitiligo, lupus-like panniculitis, pernicious anemia, chronic active hepatitis/juvenile cirrhosis, chronic diarrhea and malabsorption (usually associated with hypoparathyroidism, pulmonary fibrosis, keratoconjunctivitis, splenic atrophy, dental enamel hypoplasia)

deficiency, relapse following discontinuation of therapy, and antifungal resistance to some antifungal agents.

Several immunologic therapies have been proposed in an effort to correct the underlying immune deficiency in people with CMC. The most widely and beneficially studied treatment (remission > 10 years) is the use of transfer factor (i.e., a cell-free protein extracted from the T lymphocytes of *Candida* immune donors to defective cell-mediated immunity patients) [169–171]. It has been shown to transfer delayed-type hypersensitivity reactions to patient's earlier anergic to skin testing. Hematopoietic stem cell transplantation, thymus transplantation and leukocyte infusions yielded transient relief in patients with CMC and have been utilized in patients with severe immunologic deficiencies [172, 173].

Potential endocrine abnormalities should be treated with replacement therapy. In cases of hypoparathyroidism, cautious monitoring and supplementing of calcium and magnesium should be specified. Severe antibody deficiency should be treated with immune globulin replacement [174, 175]. The use of corticosteroid (e.g., prednisone) alone or with azathioprine resolves autoimmune panniculitis and autoimmune hepatitis, respectively. In some cases, prednisone, tacrolimus, and mycophenolate mofetil, which are given to prevent renal transplant rejection, reverse multiple autoimmune manifestations and reduce levels of autoantibodies [176].

References

Skin Manifestations of Primary Immunodeficiency and Hereditary Autoinflammatory Disorders

1. Al-Herz W, Bousfiha A, Casanova JL, et al. Primary immunodeficiency diseases: an update on the classification from the international union of immunological societies expert committee for primary immunodeficiency. Front Immunol. 2014;5:162.
2. Drenth JP, van der Meer JW. Hereditary periodic fever. N Engl J Med. 2001;345(24):1748–57.
3. Al-Herz W, Nanda A. Skin manifestations in primary immunodeficient children. Pediatr Dermatol. 2011;28(5):494–501.
4. Freeman AF, Holland SM. Hyper IgE syndrome: review and future directions. Expert Rev Clin Immunol. 2005;1(4):645–51.
5. Eberting CL, Davis J, Puck JM, Holland SM, Turner ML. Dermatitis and the newborn rash of hyper-IgE syndrome. Arch Dermatol. 2004;140(9):1119–25.
6. Holland SM, DeLeo FR, Elloumi HZ, et al. STAT3 mutations in the hyper-IgE syndrome. N Engl J Med. 2007;357(16):1608–19.
7. Freeman AF, Holland SM. Clinical manifestations, etiology, and pathogenesis of the hyper-IgE syndromes. Pediatr Res. 2009;65(5 Pt 2):32R–7.
8. Zhang Q, Davis JC, Lamborn IT, et al. Combined immunodeficiency associated with DOCK8 mutations. N Engl J Med. 2009;361(21):2046–55.
9. Minegishi Y, Saito M, Morio T, et al. Human tyrosine kinase 2 deficiency reveals its requisite roles in multiple cytokine signals involved in innate and acquired immunity. Immunity. 2006;25(5):745–55.

10. Binder V, Albert MH, Kabus M, Bertone M, Meindl A, Belohradsky BH. The genotype of the original Wiskott phenotype. N Engl J Med. 2006;355(17):1790–3.
11. Derry JM, Ochs HD, Francke U. Isolation of a novel gene mutated in Wiskott-Aldrich syndrome. Cell. 1994;79(5):following 922.
12. Petersen SH, Sendel A, van der Burg M, Westerberg LS. Unraveling the repertoire in wiskott-Aldrich syndrome. Front Immunol. 2014;5:539.
13. Bennett CL, Christie J, Ramsdell F, et al. The immune dysregulation, polyendocrinopathy, enteropathy, X-linked syndrome (IPEX) is caused by mutations of FOXP3. Nat Genet. 2001;27(1):20–1.
14. Halabi-Tawil M, Ruemmele FM, Fraitag S, et al. Cutaneous manifestations of immune dysregulation, polyendocrinopathy, enteropathy, X-linked (IPEX) syndrome. Br J Dermatol. 2009;160(3):645–51.
15. Nieves DS, Phipps RP, Pollock SJ, et al. Dermatologic and immunologic findings in the immune dysregulation, polyendocrinopathy, enteropathy X-linked syndrome. Arch Dermatol. 2004;140(4):466–72.
16. Santagata S, Villa A, Sobacchi C, Cortes P, Vezzoni P. The genetic and biochemical basis of Omenn syndrome. Immunol Rev. 2000;178:64–74.
17. Corneo B, Moshous D, Gungor T, et al. Identical mutations in RAG1 or RAG2 genes leading to defective V(D)J recombinase activity can cause either T-B-severe combined immune deficiency or Omenn syndrome. Blood. 2001;97(9):2772–6.
18. Ege M, Ma Y, Manfras B, et al. Omenn syndrome due to ARTEMIS mutations. Blood. 2005;105(11):4179–86.
19. Renner ED, Hartl D, Rylaarsdam S, et al. Comel-Netherton syndrome defined as primary immunodeficiency. J Allergy Clin Immunol. 2009;124(3):536–43.
20. Di Renzo M, Pasqui AL, Auteri A. Common variable immunodeficiency: a review. Clin Exp Med. 2004;3(4):211–7.
21. Salzer U, Warnatz K, Peter HH. Common variable immunodeficiency –an update. Arthritis Res Ther. 2012;14(5):223.
22. Mazzatenta C, Martini P, Luti L, Matteucci L, Domenici R. Granulomatous dermatitis in common variable immunodeficiency with functional T-cell defect. Arch Dermatol. 2006;142(6):783–4.
23. Kuhns DB, Alvord WG, Heller T, et al. Residual NADPH oxidase and survival in chronic granulomatous disease. N Engl J Med. 2010;363(27):2600–10.
24. Dohil M, Prendiville JS, Crawford RI, Speert DP. Cutaneous manifestations of chronic granulomatous disease. a report of four cases and review of the literature. J Am Acad Dermatol. 1997;36(6 Pt 1):899–907.
25. Segal BH, Leto TL, Gallin JI, Malech HL, Holland SM. Genetic, biochemical, and clinical features of chronic granulomatous disease. Medicine (Baltimore). 2000;79(3):170–200.
26. Drolet BA, Drolet B, Zvulunov A, Jacobsen R, Troy J, Esterly NB. Cutaneous granulomas as a presenting sign in ataxia-telangiectasia. Dermatology. 1997;194(3):273–5.
27. Sjoholm AG, Jonsson G, Braconier JH, Sturfelt G, Truedsson L. Complement deficiency and disease: an update. Mol Immunol. 2006;43(1–2):78–85.
28. Hanson EP, Monaco-Shawver L, Solt LA, et al. Hypomorphic nuclear factor-kappaB essential modulator mutation database and reconstitution system identifies phenotypic and immunologic diversity. J Allergy Clin Immunol. 2008;122(6):1169–77. e16.
29. Ridanpaa M, van Eenennaam H, Pelin K, et al. Mutations in the RNA component of RNase MRP cause a pleiotropic human disease, cartilage-hair hypoplasia. Cell. 2001;104(2):195–203.
30. Mason PJ, Bessler M. The genetics of dyskeratosis congenita. Cancer Genet. 2011;204(12):635–45.
31. Cossu F, Vulliamy TJ, Marrone A, Badiali M, Cao A, Dokal I. A novel DKC1 mutation, severe combined immunodeficiency (T+B-NK– SCID) and bone marrow transplantation in an infant with Hoyeraal-Hreidarsson syndrome. Br J Haematol. 2002;119(3):765–8.
32. Cohen LE, Tanner DJ, Schaefer HG, Levis WR. Common and uncommon cutaneous findings in patients with ataxia-telangiectasia. J Am Acad Dermatol. 1984;10(3):431–8.
33. Wong KK, Maser RS, Bachoo RM, et al. Telomere dysfunction and Atm deficiency compromises organ homeostasis and accelerates ageing. Nature. 2003;421(6923):643–8.
34. Kaplan J, De Domenico I, Ward DM. Chediak-Higashi syndrome. Curr Opin Hematol. 2008;15(1):22–9.
35. Tardieu M, Lacroix C, Neven B, et al. Progressive neurologic dysfunctions 20 years after allogeneic bone marrow transplantation for Chediak-Higashi syndrome. Blood. 2005;106(1):40–2.
36. Bizario JC, Feldmann J, Castro FA, et al. Griscelli syndrome: characterization of a new mutation and rescue of T-cytotoxic activity by retroviral transfer of RAB27A gene. J Clin Immunol. 2004;24(4):397–410.
37. Jung J, Bohn G, Allroth A, et al. Identification of a homozygous deletion in the AP3B1 gene causing Hermansky-Pudlak syndrome, type 2. Blood. 2006;108(1):362–9.
38. Buckley RH. The multiple causes of human SCID. J Clin Invest. 2004;114(10):1409–11.
39. Kalman L, Lindegren ML, Kobrynski L, et al. Mutations in genes required for T-cell development: IL7R, CD45, IL2RG, JAK3, RAG1, RAG2, ARTEMIS, and ADA and severe combined immunodeficiency: HuGE review. Genet Med. 2004;6(1):16–26.
40. Hanna S, Etzioni A. Leukocyte adhesion deficiencies. Ann N Y Acad Sci. 2012;1250:50–5.
41. Huppler AR, Bishu S, Gaffen SL. Mucocutaneous candidiasis: the IL-17 pathway and implications for targeted immunotherapy. Arthritis Res Ther. 2012;14(4):217.
42. Abramson J, Giraud M, Benoist C, Mathis D. Aire's partners in the molecular control of immunological tolerance. Cell. 2010;140(1):123–35.
43. Anderson MS, Venanzi ES, Klein L, et al. Projection of an immunological self shadow within the thymus by the aire protein. Science. 2002;298(5597):1395–401.
44. Kekalainen E, Tuovinen H, Joensuu J, et al. A defect of regulatory T cells in patients with autoimmune polyendocrinopathy-candidiasis-ectodermal dystrophy. J Immunol. 2007;178(2):1208–15.
45. Peterson P, Pitkanen J, Sillanpaa N, Krohn K. Autoimmune polyendocrinopathy candidiasis ectodermal dystrophy (APECED): a model disease to study molecular aspects of endocrine autoimmunity. Clin Exp Immunol. 2004;135(3):348–57.
46. Kisand K, Boe Wolff AS, Podkrajsek KT, et al. Chronic mucocutaneous candidiasis in APECED or thymoma patients correlates with autoimmunity to Th17-associated cytokines. J Exp Med. 2010;207(2):299–308.
47. Zhang SY, Jouanguy E, Ugolini S, et al. TLR3 deficiency in patients with herpes simplex encephalitis. Science. 2007; 317(5844):1522–7.
48. Zhang SY, Boisson-Dupuis S, Chapgier A, et al. Inborn errors of interferon (IFN)-mediated immunity in humans: insights into the respective roles of IFN-alpha/beta, IFN-gamma, and IFN-lambda in host defense. Immunol Rev. 2008;226:29–40.
49. Lafaille FG, Pessach IM, Zhang SY, et al. Impaired intrinsic immunity to HSV-1 in human iPSC-derived TLR3-deficient CNS cells. Nature. 2012;491(7426):769–73.
50. Lazarczyk M, Pons C, Mendoza JA, Cassonnet P, Jacob Y, Favre M. Regulation of cellular zinc balance as a potential mechanism of EVER-mediated protection against pathogenesis by cutaneous oncogenic human papillomaviruses. J Exp Med. 2008;205(1):35–42.
51. Balabanian K, Lagane B, Pablos JL, et al. WHIM syndromes with different genetic anomalies are accounted for by impaired CXCR4 desensitization to CXCL12. Blood. 2005;105(6):2449–57.

52. Balabanian K, Levoye A, Klemm L, et al. Leukocyte analysis from WHIM syndrome patients reveals a pivotal role for GRK3 in CXCR4 signaling. J Clin Invest. 2008;118(3):1074–84.
53. Gorlin RJ, Gelb B, Diaz GA, Lofsness KG, Pittelkow MR, Fenyk Jr JR. WHIM syndrome, an autosomal dominant disorder: clinical, hematological, and molecular studies. Am J Med Genet. 2000;91(5):368–76.
54. Ozkurede VU, Franchi L. Immunology in clinic review series; focus on autoinflammatory diseases: role of inflammasomes in autoinflammatory syndromes. Clin Exp Immunol. 2012;167(3): 382–90.
55. Hoffman HM. Therapy of autoinflammatory syndromes. J Allergy Clin Immunol. 2009;124(6):1129–38; quiz 39–40.
56. Latz E, Xiao TS, Stutz A. Activation and regulation of the inflammasomes. Nat Rev Immunol. 2013;13(6):397–411.
57. Beer HD, Contassot E, French LE. The inflammasomes in autoinflammatory diseases with skin involvement. J Invest Dermatol. 2014;134(7):1805–10.
58. Leslie KS, Lachmann HJ, Bruning E, et al. Phenotype, genotype, and sustained response to anakinra in 22 patients with autoinflammatory disease associated with CIAS-1/NALP3 mutations. Arch Dermatol. 2006;142(12):1591–7.
59. Zadeh N, Getzug T, Grody WW. Diagnosis and management of familial Mediterranean fever: integrating medical genetics in a dedicated interdisciplinary clinic. Genet Med. 2011;13(3):263–9.
60. McDermott MF, Aksentijevich I, Galon J, et al. Germline mutations in the extracellular domains of the 55 kDa TNF receptor, TNFR1, define a family of dominantly inherited autoinflammatory syndromes. Cell. 1999;97(1):133–44.
61. Aksentijevich I, Masters SL, Ferguson PJ, et al. An autoinflammatory disease with deficiency of the interleukin-1-receptor antagonist. N Engl J Med. 2009;360(23):2426–37.
62. Marrakchi S, Guigue P, Renshaw BR, et al. Interleukin-36-receptor antagonist deficiency and generalized pustular psoriasis. N Engl J Med. 2011;365(7):620–8.
63. Drenth JP, Haagsma CJ, van der Meer JW. Hyperimmunoglobulinemia D and periodic fever syndrome. The clinical spectrum in a series of 50 patients. International Hyper-IgD Study Group. Medicine (Baltimore). 1994;73(3):133–44.
64. Liu Y, Jesus AA, Marrero B, et al. Activated STING in a vascular and pulmonary syndrome. N Engl J Med. 2014;371(6):507–18.
65. Canna SW, de Jesus AA, Gouni S, et al. An activating NLRC4 inflammasome mutation causes autoinflammation with recurrent macrophage activation syndrome. Nat Genet. 2014;46(10):1140–6.
66. Romberg N, Al Moussawi K, Nelson-Williams C, et al. Mutation of NLRC4 causes a syndrome of enterocolitis and autoinflammation. Nat Genet. 2014;46(10):1135–9.
67. Campbell P, Morton PE, Takeichi T, et al. Epithelial inflammation resulting from an inherited loss-of-function mutation in EGFR. J Invest Dermatol. 2014;134(10):2570–8.
68. Zhang X, Bogunovic D, Payelle-Brogard B, et al. Human intracellular ISG15 prevents interferon-alpha/beta over-amplification and auto-inflammation. Nature. 2014;12:89.
69. Rigante D, Vitale A, Lucherini OM, Cantarini L. The hereditary autoinflammatory disorders uncovered. Autoimmun Rev. 2014;13(9):892–900.
70. Gahl WA, Markello TC, Toro C, et al. The National Institutes of Health Undiagnosed Diseases Program: insights into rare diseases. Genet Med. 2012;14(1):51–9.
71. Ferguson PJ, Chen S, Tayeh MK, et al. Homozygous mutations in LPIN2 are responsible for the syndrome of chronic recurrent multifocal osteomyelitis and congenital dyserythropoietic anaemia (Majeed syndrome). J Med Genet. 2005;42(7):551–7.
72. Wise CA, Gillum JD, Seidman CE, et al. Mutations in CD2BP1 disrupt binding to PTP PEST and are responsible for PAPA syndrome, an autoinflammatory disorder. Hum Mol Genet. 2002;11(8):961–9.
73. Lindor NM, Arsenault TM, Solomon H, Seidman CE, McEvoy MT. A new autosomal dominant disorder of pyogenic sterile arthritis, pyoderma gangrenosum, and acne: PAPA syndrome. Mayo Clin Proc. 1997;72(7):611–5.
74. Alonso D, Elgart GW, Schachner LA. Blau syndrome: a new kindred. J Am Acad Dermatol. 2003;49(2):299–302.
75. Jeru I, Duquesnoy P, Fernandes-Alnemri T, et al. Mutations in NALP12 cause hereditary periodic fever syndromes. Proc Natl Acad Sci U S A. 2008;105(5):1614–9.
76. Ombrello MJ, Remmers EF, Sun G, et al. Cold urticaria, immunodeficiency, and autoimmunity related to PLCG2 deletions. N Engl J Med. 2012;366(4):330–8.
77. Kitamura A, Maekawa Y, Uehara H, et al. A mutation in the immunoproteasome subunit PSMB8 causes autoinflammation and lipodystrophy in humans. J Clin Invest. 2011;121(10):4150–60.
78. Torrelo A, Patel S, Colmenero I, et al. Chronic atypical neutrophilic dermatosis with lipodystrophy and elevated temperature (CANDLE) syndrome. J Am Acad Dermatol. 2010;62(3):489–95.
79. Feder HM, Salazar JC. A clinical review of 105 patients with PFAPA (a periodic fever syndrome). Acta Paediatr. 2010;99(2):178–84.
80. Braun-Falco M, Kovnerystyy O, Lohse P, Ruzicka T. Pyoderma gangrenosum, acne, and suppurative hidradenitis (PASH)–a new autoinflammatory syndrome distinct from PAPA syndrome. J Am Acad Dermatol. 2012;66(3):409–15.

Chronic Mucocutaneous Candidiasis (CMC)

81. Thorpe ES, Handley HE. Chronic tetany and chronic mycelia stomatitis in a child aged four and one half years. Am J Dis Child. 1929;38:228.
82. Craig J, Schiff L, et al. Chronic moniliasis associated with Addison's disease. AMA Am J Dis Child. 1955;89:669.
83. Hung W, Migeon CJ, et al. A possible autoimmune basis for addison's disease in three siblings, one with idiopathic hypoparathyroidism pernicious anemia and superficial moniliasis. N Engl J Med. 1963;269:658.
84. Blizzard RM, Gibbs JH. Candidiasis: studies pertaining to its association with endocrinopathies and pernicious anemia. Pediatrics. 1968;42:231.
85. Hill KC. Chronic mucocutaneous candidiasis: immunology for the pediatrician. Pediatr Infect Dis J. 2001;20:197–206.
86. Kirkpatrick CH. Chronic mucucutaneous candidiasis. Eur J Clin Microbiol Infect Dis. 1989;8:448–56.
87. Kirkpatrick C. Hill. Chronic mucocutaneous candidiasis. In: Bodey GP, editor. Candidiasis: pathogenesis, diagnosis and treatment. New York.: Raven Press, Ltd.; 1993. p. 167–84.
88. Puel A, Cypowyj S, et al. Inborn errors of human IL-17 immunity underlie chronic mucocutaneous candidiasis. Curr Opin Allergy Clin Immunol. 2012;12:616–22.
89. Alcais A, Quintana-Murci L, et al. Life-threatening infectious diseases of childhood: single-gene inborn errors of immunity? Ann N Y Acad Sci. 2010;1214:18–33.
90. Casanova J-L, et al. The genetic theory of infectious diseases: a brief history and selected illustrations. Annu Rev Genomics Hum Genet. 2013;14:215–43.
91. Glocker E, Grimbacher B. Chronic mucocutaneous candidiasis and congenital susceptibility to Candida. Curr Opin Allergy Clin Immunol. 2010;10:542–50.
92. Lilic D. Unravelling fungal immunity through primary immune deficiencies. Curr Opin Microbiol. 2012;15:420–6.
93. Antônio Chambô F, Ingrid Z, et al. Chronic mucocutaneous candidiasis: a case with exuberant cutaneous horns in nipples. An Bras Dermatol. 2014;89(4):641–4.

94. Charles A, Rohrmann JR, et al. Chronic mucocutaneous candidiasis: radiologic abnormalities in the esophagus. Am J Roentgenol. 1978;130:473–6.
95. Koch D, Lilic D, et al. Autosomal dominant chronic mucocutaneous candidiasis and primary hypothyroidism complicated by oesophageal carcinoma. Clin Exp Dermatol. 2009;34:e818–20.
96. Miri SM, TayebiMeybodi A, et al. Fungal granuloma of the brain in a case of chronic mucocutaneous candidiasis. Arch Iran Med. 2012;15(7):452–4.
97. Puel A, Doffinger R, et al. Autoantibodies against IL-17A, IL-17F, and IL-22 in patients with chronic mucocutaneous candidiasis and autoimmune polyendocrine syndrome type I. J Exp Med. 2010;207:291–7.
98. Glocker E-O. BodoGrimbacher; IL-1 7 signalling in fungal infection Mucosal antifungal defence: IL-17 signalling takes centre stage. Immunol Cell Biol. 2011;89:823–6.
99. Huppler AR, Bishu S, et al. Mucocutaneous candidiasis: the IL-17 pathway and implications for targeted immunotherapy. Arthritis Res Ther. 2012;14:217.
100. Wisplinghoff H, Bischoff T, et al. Nosocomial bloodstream infections in US hospitals: analysis of 24 179 cases from a prospective nationwide surveillance study. Clin Infect Dis. 2004;39:309–17.
101. Cua DJ, Tato CM. Innate IL-17-producing cells: the sentinels of the immune system. Nat Rev Immunol. 2010;10:479–89.
102. Cheng SC, Joosten LA, et al. Interplay between Candida albicans and the mammalian innate host defense. Infect Immun. 2012;80:1304–13.
103. Gauglitz GG, Callenberg H, et al. Host defence against Candida albicans and the role of pattern-recognition receptors. Acta Derm Venereol. 2012;92:291–8.
104. Gow NA, van de Veerdonk FL, et al. Candida albicans morphogenesis and host defence: discriminating invasion from colonization. Nat Rev Microbiol. 2012;10:112–22.
105. Zielinski CE, Mele F, et al. Pathogen-induced human TH17 cells produce IFN-gamma or IL-10 and are regulated by IL-1beta. Nature. 2012;484:514–8.
106. Stockinger B, Veldhoen M. Differentiation and function of Th17 T cells. Curr Opin Immunol. 2007;19:281–6.
107. Yang XO, Panopoulos AD, et al. STAT3 regulates cytokine-mediated generation of inflammatory helper T cells. J Biol Chem. 2007;282:9358–63.
108. Ivanov II, McKenzie BS, et al. The orphan nuclear receptor ROR gamma directs the differentiation program of proinflammatory IL-17 þ T helper cells. Cell. 2006;126:1121–33.
109. Eyerich S, Wagener J, et al. IL-22 and TNF-alpha represent a key cytokine combination for epidermal integrity during infection with Candida albicans. Eur J Immunol. 2011;41:1894–901.
110. Iwakura Y, Ishigame H, et al. Functional specialization of interleukin-17 family members. Immunity. 2011;34:149–62.
111. Rutz S, Eidenschenk C, et al. IL-22, not simply a Th17 cytokine. Immunol Rev. 2013;252:116–32.
112. Chang SH, Park H, et al. Act1 adaptor protein is an immediate and essential signaling component of interleukin-17 receptor. J Biol Chem. 2006;281:35603–7.
113. Chang SH, Reynolds JM, et al. Interleukin-17C promotes Th17 cell responses and autoimmune disease via interleukin-17 receptor E. Immunity. 2011;35:611–21.
114. Kai K, Part P. Autoimmune polyendocrinopathy candidiasis ectodermal dystrophy and other primary immunodeficiency diseases help to resolve the nature of protective immunity against chronic mucocutaneous candidiasis. Curr Opin Pediatr. 2013;25:715–21.
115. Hernandez-Santos N, Gaffen SL. Th17 cells in immunity to Candida albicans. Cell Host Microbe. 2012;11:425–35.
116. Liu C, Swaidani S, et al. ACC' loop decoy peptide blocks the interaction between Act1 and IL-17RA to attenuate IL-17- and IL-25-induced inflammation. Sci Signal. 2011;4:ra72.
117. Qian Y, Liu C. The adaptor Act1 is required for interleukin 17-dependent signaling associated with autoimmune and inflammatory disease. Nat Immunol. 2007;8:247–56.
118. Kang Z, Swaidani S, et al. Epithelial cell-specific Act1adaptor mediates interleukin-25-dependent helminth expulsion through expansion of Lin(−)c-Kit(+) innate cell population. Immunity. 2012;36:821–33.
119. Puel A, Cypowyj S, Bustamante J, et al. Chronic mucocutaneous candidiasis in humans with inborn errors of interleukin-17 immunity. Science. 2011;332:65–8.
120. ShrinivasBishu N, Hernández-Santos N, et al. The adaptor CARD9 is required for adaptive but not innate immunity to oral mucosal Candida albicans infections. Infect Immun. 2014;82(3):1173–80.
121. De Beaucoudrey L, Puel A, et al. Mutations in STAT3 and IL12RB1 impair the development of humanIL-17-producing T cells. J Exp Med. 2008;205:1543–50.
122. Renner ED, Rylaarsdam S, et al. Novel signal transducer and activator of transcription 3 (STAT3) mutations, reduced T(H)17 cell numbers, and variably defective STAT3 phosphorylation in hyper-IgE syndrome. J Allergy Clin Immunol. 2008;122: 181–7.
123. De Beaucoudrey L, Samarina A, et al. Revisiting human IL-12R b1 deficiency: a survey of 141 patients from30 countries. Medicine (Baltimore). 2010;89:381–402.
124. van de Veerdonk FL, Plantinga TS, et al. STAT1 mutations in autosomal dominant chronic mucocutaneous candidiasis. N Engl J Med. 2011;365:54–61.
125. Soltész B, Tóth B, Shabashova N, et al. New and recurrent gain-of-function STAT1 mutations in patients with chronic mucocutaneous candidiasis from Eastern and Central Europe. J Med Genet. 2013;50:567–78.
126. Shunichiro T, Masafumi Y, et al. Chronic mucocutaneous candidiasis caused by a gain-of-function mutation in the STAT1 DNA-binding domain. J Immunol. 2012;189:1521–6.
127. Liu L, Okada S, et al. Gain-of-function human STAT1 mutations impair IL-17 immunity and underlie chronic mucocutaneous candidiasis. J Exp Med. 2011;208:1635–48.
128. Smeekens SP, Plantinga TS, et al. TAT1 hyperphosphorylation and defective IL12R/IL23R signaling underlie defective immunity in autosomal dominant chronic mucocutaneous candidiasis. PLoS One. 2011;6:e29248.
129. Uzel G, Sampaio EP, et al. Dominant gain-of-function STAT1 mutationsinFOXP3wild-typeimmunedysregulationpolyendocrinopathy-enteropathy-X-linked-like syndrome. J Allergy Clin Immunol. 2013;131:1611–23, e1613.
130. Casanova J-L, Steven M, Holland SM. Inborn errors of human JAKs and STATs. Immunity. 2012;36(4):515–28.
131. Maysoun Al R, Christine MC, et al. Autosomal dominant cases of chronic mucocutaneous candidiasis segregates with mutations of signal transducer and activator of transcription 1, but Not of toll-like receptor 3. J Pediatr. 2013;163:277–9.
132. Graaf CA, et al. STAT1 mutations in autosomal dominant chronic mucocutaneous candidiasis. N Engl J Med. 2011;365:54–61.
133. Ryan KR, Hong M, Arkwright PD, et al. Impaired dendritic cell maturation and cytokine production in patients with chronic mucocutaneous candidiasis with or without APECED. Clin Exp Immunol. 2008;154:406–14.
134. Ng WF, von Delwig A, Carmichael AJ, et al. Impaired T(H)17 responses in patients with chronic mucocutaneous candidiasis with and without autoimmune polyendocrinopathy-candidiasis-ectodermal dystrophy. J Allergy Clin Immunol. 2010;126:1006–15.
135. Kisand K, Boe Wolff AS, Podkrajsek KT, et al. Chronic mucocutaneous candidiasis in APECED or thymoma patients correlates with autoimmunity to Th17-associated cytokines. J Exp Med. 2010;207(2):299–308.

136. Kisand K, Lilic D. Mucocutaneous candidiasis and autoimmunity against cytokines in APECED and thymoma patients: clinical and pathogenetic implications. Eur J Immunol. 2011;41:1517–27.
137. Adrien Katalin S, Szilvia T, et al. Autoantibodies to IL-17A may be correlated with the severity of mucocutaneous candidiasis in APECED patients. J Clin Immunol. 2014;34:181–93.
138. Liston A, Lesage S, Wilson J, et al. AIRE regulates negative selection of organ-specific T cells. Nat Immunol. 2003;4:350–4.
139. Glocker EO, Hennigs A, Nabavi M, et al. A homozygous CARD9 mutation in a family with susceptibility to fungal infections. N Engl J Med. 2009;361:1727–35.
140. Ferwerda B, Ferwerda G, Plantinga TS, et al. Human dectin-1 deficiency and mucocutaneous fungal infections. N Engl J Med. 2009;361:1760–7.
141. Drewniak A, Gazendam RP, et al. Invasive fungal infection and impaired neutrophil killing in humanCARD9 deficiency. Blood. 2013;121:2385–92.
142. Prando C, Samarina A, et al. Inherited IL-12p40 deficiency: genetic, immunologic, and clinical features of 49 patients from 30 kindred's. Medicine (Baltimore). 2013;92:109–22.
143. Chandesris MO, Melki I, et al. Autosomal dominant STAT3 deficiency and hyper-IgE syndrome: molecular,cellular, and clinical features from a French national survey. Medicine (Baltimore). 2012;91:e1–19.
144. SillevisSmitt JH, Kuijpers TW. Cutaneous manifestations of primaryimmunodeficiency. Curr Opin Pediatr. 2013;25:492–7.
145. Kirkpatrick CH, Windhorst DB. Mucocutaneous candidiasis and thymoma. Am J Med. 1979;66:939–45.
146. Mogensen TH. STAT3 and the Hyper-IgE syndrome Clinical presentation, genetic origin, pathogenesis, novelfidings and remaining uncertainties. JAKSTAT. 2013;2(2):e23435. Landes Bioscience.
147. Mohamad P, Korush R, et al. A child with Polyglandular autoimmune syndrome Type-I and immune thrombocytopenic purpura. Pak J Med Sci. 2011;27(1):223–5.
148. Marcela Kopáčoväl, Stanislav R, et al. Severe gastrointestinal involvement in an adult female patient with chronic mucocutaneous candidiasis. Folia Gastroenterol Hepatol. 2005;3(2):62–6.
149. Kathleen C, Taraneh F, et al. Keratitis, ichthyosis, and deafness (KID) syndrome: a review of infectious and neoplastic complications. J Am Acad Dermatol. 2013;69:127–34.
150. Kalfa VC, Roberts RL, Stiehm ER. The syndrome of chronic mucocutaneous candidiasis with selective antibody deficiency. Ann Allergy Asthma Immunol. 2003;90:259.
151. Hori T, Ohnishi H, et al. Autosomal-dominant chronic mucocutaneous candidiasis with STAT1-mutation can be complicated with chronic active hepatitis and hypothyroidism. J Clin Immunol. 2012;32:1213–20.
152. Bilognia JL, Jorizzo JL, et al. Chap-60. Chronic mucocutaneous candidiasis. In: Dermatology. 3rd ed; 2012.
153. Tkach JR, et al. Severe hepatitis associated with ketoconazole therapy for chronic mucocutaneous candidiasis. Cutis. 1982;29:482–4.
154. Kirkpatrick CH, Rich RR. Treatment of chronic mucocutaneous moniliasis by immunologic reconstitution. Clin Exp Immunol. 1971;9:733–48.
155. Como JA, Dismukes WE. Oral azole drugs as systemic antifungal therapy. N Engl J Med. 1994;330:263–72.
156. Mobacken H, Moberg S. Ketoconazole treatment of 13 patients with chronic mucocutaneous candidiasis. A prospective 3-year trial. Dermatologica. 1986;173:229–36.
157. Montagnani A, Negosanti M, et al. Ketoconazole treatment of chronic mucocutaneous candidiasis. Drugs ExpClin Res. 1986;12:409–12.
158. Leroy D, Dompmartin A, et al. Aneurysm associated with chronic mucocutaneous candidiasis during long-term therapy with ketoconazole. Dermatologica. 1989;178:43–6.
159. Kirkpatrick CH, Petersen EA, et al. Treatment of chronic mucocutaneous candidosis with ketoconazole: preliminary results of a controlled, double-blind clinical trial. Rev Infect Dis. 1980;2:599.
160. Shiraishi S, Murakami S, et al. Oral fluconazole treatment of fungating candidiasis in the keratitis, ichthyosis and deafness (KID) syndrome. Br J Dermatol. 1994;131:904–7.
161. Rautemaa R, Richardson M, et al. Activity of amphotericin B, anidulafungin, caspofungin, micafungin, posaconazole, and voriconazole against Candida albicans with decreased susceptibility to fluconazole from APECED patients on long-term azole treatment of chronic mucocutaneous candidiasis. Diagn Microbiol Infect Dis. 2008;62:182.
162. Davide F, Orietta M, et al. Successful treatment of chronic mucocutaneous candidiasis caused by azole - resistant Candida albicans with posaconazole. Clin Dev Immunol. 2011; Article ID 283239.
163. Fukushima C, Matsuse H, et al. Oral candidiasis associated with inhaled corticosteroid use: comparison of fluticasone and beclomethasone. Ann Allergy Asthma Immunol. 2003;90:646.
164. Hachiya KA, Kobayashi RH, et al. Candida esophagitis following antibiotic usage. Pediatr Infect Dis. 1982;1:168.
165. Husebye ES, Perheentupa J, et al. Clinical manifestations and management of patients with autoimmune polyendocrine syndrome type I. J Intern Med. 2009;265:514.
166. Burke WA. Use of itraconazole in a patient with chronic mucocutaneous candidiasis. J Am Acad Dermatol. 1989;21:1309–10.
167. Tosti A, Piraccini BM, et al. Itraconazole in the treatment of two young brothers with chronic mucocutaneous candidiasis. Pediatr Dermatol. 1997;14:146–8.
168. Kamai Y, Maebashi K, et al. Characterization of mechanisms of fluconazole resistance in a Candida albicans isolate from a Japanese patient with chronic mucocutaneous candidiasis. Microbiol Immunol. 2004;48:937.
169. Ballow M, Hyman LR. Combination immunotherapy in chronic mucocutaneous candidiasis. Synergism between transfer factor and fetal thymus tissue. Clin Immunol Immunopathol. 1977;8:504–12.
170. Aiuti F, Businco L, et al. Reconstitution of T-cell disorders following thymus transplantation. Birth Defects Orig Artic Ser. 1975;11:370–6.
171. Cleveland WW, Fogel BJ, et al. Foetal thymus transplant in a case of DiGeorge's syndrome. Lancet. 1968;2:1211–4.
172. Hoh MC, Lin HP, et al. Successful allogeneic bone marrow transplantation in severe chronic mucocutaneous candidiasis syndrome. Bone Marrow Transplant. 1996;18:797.
173. Buckley RH, Lucas ZJ, et al. Defective cellular immunity associated with chronic mucocutaneous moniliasis and recurrent staphylococcal botryomycosis: immunological reconstitution by allogeneic bone marrow. Clin Exp Immunol. 1968;3:153–69.
174. Sun D, Novotny M, et al. Treatment with IL-17 prolongs the half-life of chemokine CXCL1 mRNA via the adaptor TRAF5 and the splicing-regulatory factor SF2 (ASF). Nat Immunol. 2011;12:853–60.
175. Padeh S, Theodor R, et al. Severe malabsorption in autoimmune polyendocrinopathy-candidosis-ectodermal dystrophy syndrome successfully treated with immunosuppression. Arch Dis Child. 1997;76:532.
176. Ulinski T, Perrin L, et al. Autoimmune polyendocrinopathy-candidiasis-ectodermal dystrophy syndrome with renal failure: impact of posttransplant immunosuppression on disease activity. J Clin Endocrinol Metab. 2006;91:192.

Neoplasms

12

Ke-Hua Li, Thomas Griffin, Neda Nikbakht, Le Qu, Hong-Duo Chen, Chundi He, and Li-Xin Xia

Contents

12.1 Melanoma Immunology and Immune Therapy

Ke-Hua Li, MD, Thomas Griffin, MD, and Neda Nikbakht

12.1.1 Epidemiology

Melanoma is a malignant tumor that arises from melanocytes and has a high potential to metastasize. Melanoma represents less than 2 % of total skin cancer diagnoses, but accounts for an overwhelming proportion of skin cancer deaths. The incidence of melanoma has been increasing in the past 30 years. Between 2006 and 2010, the incidence rate increased by 2.7 % per year. In 2014, the American Cancer Society reported estimated 76,100 new cases of melanoma in the United States and 9710 cases of melanoma mortality [1].

12.1.2 Tumor Immunology and Immunotherapies in Melanoma

There are inherent defense systems to prevent malignant transformation of melanocytes into melanoma tumor cells. These mechanisms are generally regarded as either cell

K.-H. Li, MD (✉) • T. Griffin, MD • N. Nikbakht
Thomas Jefferson University Hospital, Philadelphia, PA, USA
e-mail: kehua_li@yahoo.com

L. Qu (✉) • H.-D. Chen • C. He • L.-X. Xia (✉)
Department of Dermatology, No.1 Hospital of China Medical University, Shenyang 110001, China
e-mail: cmuqule@163.com; xialixin1974@163.com

X.-H. Gao, H.-D. Chen (eds.), *Practical Immunodermatology*, DOI 10.1007/978-94-024-0902-4_12

intrinsic, such as DNA repair mechanisms, or cell extrinsic, mediated by the immune surveillance. The concept of immune response to cancer cells was first introduced by Ehrlich in 1909 and was further postulated into the immune surveillance hypothesis by Burnet [2]. In a series of innovative experiments, Ehrlich demonstrated that immunization of mice with necrotic tumor tissue before transplantation of viable tumor can protect against tumor growth. Half a century later, Burnet proposed malignant cells exhibit traits that can be recognized by innate and adaptive immune cells and result in an immune response.

The ability of malignant cells to elicit an immune response depends on their antigenicity, or the presence of tumor cell surface antigens that can be recognized by adaptive or innate immune responses. Compared to other malignancies, melanoma appears to be a highly immunogenic tumor. Nevertheless, melanoma has evolved mechanisms to escape normal immune surveillance [3]. Recently, significant research has been done to elucidate underlying mechanisms of melanoma's immune escape and to devise new treatment modalities that amplify endogenous tumor immune response to melanoma [4, 5]. The following is a review of our current understanding of melanoma tumor cell immunogenicity as well as existing immunotherapies.

12.1.3 Tumor Immunogenicity in Melanoma

Several clinical observations suggest that melanoma is an immunogenic tumor. Primary melanomas often show areas of depigmentation and exhibit strong lymphocytic infiltration. At times, primary melanomas may spontaneously undergo partial or complete regression. Furthermore, development of halo nevi or vitiligo carries a good prognosis in patients with melanoma while there is a higher incidence of melanoma in immunosuppressed patients [6].

Molecular studies lead to discovery of several melanoma antigens that can elicit cellular or humoral immune responses. The vast majority of these antigens provoke T-cell responses mediated by cytotoxic (CD8) or helper (CD4) T cells. T cells recognize antigens that are processed and presented as peptides coupled with major histocompatibility complex (MHC) on surfaces of cells. Melanoma cells express both classes of MHC on their surface and present antigens coupled to either MHC-I (recognized by cytotoxic T cells) or MHC-II (recognized by helper T cells). Interestingly, the majority of immunogenic epitopes identified on melanoma cells turned out to be "self" epitopes and not mutated or unique to melanoma cells [7].

The first melanoma antigen was discovered using a cytotoxic T-cell clone generated from a patient with melanoma by a group in Brussels and it was named melanoma antigen-1 (MAGE-1) [8]. MAGE-1 was demonstrated to be a nonmutated self antigen, coded by the X chromosome expressed on testicular cells. A family of several similar antigens to MAGE-1 including MAGE-3 and NY-ESO-1 were also discovered as melanoma antigens. Since many of these antigens were found on to be expressed on a variety of tumors as well as normal testicular tissue, they were collectively called cancer testes (CT) or CT antigens [7].

Besides CT antigens, two other classes of antigens are presented as MHC/peptide complexes on surfaces of melanoma cells. First group constitutes antigens found on melanoma cells as well as normal melanocytes. These antigens are referred to as differentiation antigens and include tyrosinase, gp100 (Pmel17), and Melan-A (MART-1). Second group encompasses those unique epitopes that result from melanoma tumor cell mutation and are distinct from self antigens. These melanoma-specific antigens are presented on MHC class I and include cyclin-dependent kinase inhibitor 2A (CDKN2A or p16), cyclin-dependent kinase 4 (CDK4), beta-catenin, and N-ras [7].

The last category of melanoma surface antigens is a group capable of provoking humoral immune responses. Melanoma patients produce antibodies against some cell surface antigens on melanoma cells. Although these antibodies appear to be specific to melanoma cells, the nature of the antigens recognized remains mostly undefined with a few exceptions. Studies in late 1980s defined a number of different types of ganglioside (GM2, GD2, and GD3) on human tumor cell surfaces including melanoma and it was demonstrated that patients with melanoma make antibody responses to gangliosides [9]. Subsequently, the therapeutic potential of gangliosides was utilized in clinical trials using ganglioside vaccines in melanoma treatment [10].

12.1.4 Immune Escape in Melanoma

Immune response to neoplastic cells involves multiple sequential steps including activation, proliferation, and trafficking of immune cells into tumor sites. Melanoma cells have developed multiple strategies to influence and "evade" immune response at all aforementioned stages. As discussed above, melanoma cells express multiple antigens capable of activating melanoma specific T cells. However, melanoma cells develop abilities to modify or downregulate these tumor associated antigens. Furthermore, melanoma cells can prevent presentation of these antigens on MHC surface molecules by downregulating MHC expression on melanoma cell surfaces [11]. Together, these strategies hide melanoma targetable epitopes from T cells leading to impairment of T-cell activation and proliferation.

Melanoma tumor cells are also capable of secreting a number of immunosuppressive cytokines including interleukin (IL)-10 and TGF-β. These cytokines dampen immune response at several stages. Furthermore, they can promote differentiation of CD4+/CD25+ regulatory T cells, a subset of T cells that impede initiation and progression of the immune response [11].

In addition to mechanisms described above, melanoma tumors escape immune response by underexpressing stimulatory ligands and overexpressing inhibitory ligands that regulate immune checkpoints [12]. Regulation of immune response takes place at specific immune checkpoints via counterbalancing stimulatory and inhibitory signals. These signals are relayed through binding of membrane-bound receptors on surfaces of T cells to their corresponding ligands. An example of an inhibitory ligand that is overexpressed on melanoma cells is PD-L1 (B7-H1, CD274). PD-L1 binds to a receptor called programmed cell death-1 (PD-1) on activated T cells and causes apoptosis.

12.1.5 Immunotherapy

Immunotherapy in melanoma is a collection of several therapies that either enhance existing immune response to melanoma tumors or counteract immune evasion of melanoma cells. Some of these therapies are highly specific in targeting melanoma cells while others enhance the immune response in a generalized manner. Therapeutic effects can be achieved by infusing specific cytokines, antibodies, vaccines, or effector cells.

12.1.6 High-Dose Interleukin-2 Treatment

A nonspecific and high-risk approach for inducing a robust boost in T-cell-mediated immunity is administration of high-dose IL-2 in patients with metastatic melanoma. While IL-2 treatment-related toxicity is severe, the US FDA approved this agent for treatment of metastatic melanoma in 1998. Several phase II randomized controlled trials demonstrate that high-dose IL-2 elicited objective response rates about 5–27 % [13]. However, this treatment has not been evaluated in phase III trials.

12.1.7 Cancer Vaccines

A more targeted approach in modifying the immune response to melanoma is to administer vaccines that boost melanoma specific immunity. Melanoma vaccines generally introduce melanoma associated antigens along with immune boosting adjuvants to patients. Melanoma antigens can be prepared in variety of forms, ranging from whole-cell (crude tumor) preparations to DNA, peptide, or viral vectors. Alternatively, antigen presenting dendritic cells that are preexposed to melanoma antigens can be administered as dendritic cell vaccines [14].

Peptide vaccines produced favorable outcomes a phase II trial by Eastern Cooperative Oncology Group (ECOG). The vaccine used in this study was constructed with three peptides derived from melanoma associated antigens tyrosinase, gp100 (Pmel17), and Melan-A (MART-1). Immune responses to melanoma antigens were observed in 35 % of patients in this study. Furthermore, the median overall survival of patients with positive vaccine immune response was longer than that of patients with no immune response [15].

Regarding peptide vaccines, it is important to note the inherent limitation by HLA restriction. As discussed earlier, melanoma antigens are presented in the context of MHC/peptide complexes. Therefore, a particular peptide sequence can only be presented on a specific HLA molecule. In ECOG study, peptides were restricted to HLA-A2; therefore, only patients HLA-A2 positive patients were eligible to participate in this vaccine trial.

12.1.8 Blockade of Immune Checkpoints in Melanoma

Some of the most effective immune therapies in melanoma target immune checkpoints by modifying the interactions of T-cell membrane-bound receptors with inhibitory or stimulatory ligands. Note that such checkpoint immune therapies do not directly target melanoma tumor cells; rather, they interact with T cells to enhance T-cell antitumor response. The two most successful checkpoint immune therapies for melanoma target two receptors on surfaces of T cells: cytotoxic T lymphocyte-associated antigen-4 (CTLA-4) and PD-1 [16].

12.1.8.1 Blockade of CTLA-4 (Ipilimumab and Tremelimumab)

Cytotoxic T lymphocyte-associated antigen-4 (CTLA-4, CD152) is a coinhibitory molecule expressed on T cells. CTLA-4 resembles, with approximately 30 % sequence homology, and antagonizes CD28, a critical costimulatory molecule on T cells. CTLA-4 is expressed on activated T cells and binds to B7-1 (CD80) and B7-2 (CD86) as CD28 does, but with much higher affinity (10- to 40-fold) so that it inhibits CD28-induced T-cell activation. Originally, CTLA-4 blockade in animal studies was demonstrated to enhance T-cell antitumor activities [17], which lead to testing of anti-CTLA-4 antibodies in clinical settings.

Two anti-CTLA-4 fully human monoclonal antibodies, ipilimumab (IgG1 isotype) and tremelimumab (IgG2 isotype), reached clinical trials in treatment of patients with advanced melanoma. A 2010 phase III randomized trial of ipilimumab demonstrated significantly improved overall survival for patients with previously treated unresectable stage III or stage IV melanoma compared to a peptide vaccine

[18]. A subsequent phase III randomized trial for treatment-naïve patients with advanced melanoma showed that ipilimumab plus dacarbazine improved overall survival compared with treatment by dacarbazine alone [19]. These studies led to the FDA approval of ipilimumab for metastatic melanoma patients in 2011. Tremelimumab entered phase III trial for previously untreated patients with promising early phase I and II study results [20]. However, phase III data did not show survival benefit [21].

12.1.8.2 Blockade of PD-1 (Pembrolizumab and Nivolumab)

Programmed cell death-1 (PD-1, CD279) is a type I transmembrane receptor member of the immunoglobulin superfamily, expressed by activated T cells, and binds to two ligands, PD-L1 (B7-H1, CD274) and PD-L2 (B7-DC, CD273), both of which are part of the B7 immunoglobulin superfamily [22]. PD-L1 is expressed on multiple normal tissues and malignant cells, whereas PD-L2 is mainly expressed by antigen presenting cells [23]. The critical role of PD-1 in immune regulatory function has been demonstrated by inhibition of the effector phase of T cells primarily within the tumor microenvironment [24]. Given the selective immune suppressive signals delivered by cancer, it was predicted that the blockade of PD-1/PD-L1 pathway will have greater antitumor activity and fewer side effects compared to CTLA-4 blockade.

Blockade of PD-1 has been tested in animal models such as murine B16 melanoma and demonstrated effective antitumor T-cell responses. These studies confirmed the therapeutic potential of targeting this immune checkpoint and multiple anti-PD-1/PD-L1 antibodies have been evaluated in clinical trials. The first phase 1 clinical trial with an anti-PD-1 antibody showed significant antitumor activity in patients with melanoma, renal cell carcinoma, and lung cancer. This study also provided the first evidence of the correlation of PD-L1 expression and tumor responses [25].

Subsequently, FDA-approved an anti-PD-1 antibody, pembrolizumab, in September of 2014, following reports on the antitumor activity of pembrolizumab in patients who had previously become refractory to ipilimumab [26]. Another anti-PD-1 antibody, nivolumab, gained FDA approval in December 2014 after demonstrating up to 30 % durable response in a phase I study of patients with unresectable stage III or IV melanoma [27].

With the success of the PD-1/PD-L1 blockade, it has become a top priority to identify and characterize the factors in the tumor microenvironment that predict which patients are likely to respond to this therapy. Tumor PD-L1 expression has been pursued as a potential biomarker and studies have demonstrated that PD-L1 baseline expression level showed a strong association with response to anti-PD-1 therapy [28].

12.1.9 Adoptive Cell Therapy

Adoptive cell therapy is by far the most specific melanoma immune therapy and is performed by transferring of antitumor lymphocytes to melanoma patients. The construction of antitumor lymphocytes was pioneered by Steven Rosenberg at National Cancer Institute. Antitumor lymphocytes are generated via a complex process from patient's own lymphocytes. T cells are isolated from peripheral blood or tumor sites in patients. Patient's T lymphocytes are then stimulated by melanoma antigens, activated, and expanded ex vivo. A large number of now primed and activated melanoma specific T cells are then reinfused to donor patient. While this process is labor intensive and time consuming, adoptive cell therapy can generate significant tumor regression (50–70 %) in patients with metastatic melanoma refractory to standard therapies [29, 30].

12.2 Keloids

Le Qu, Hong-Duo Chen, and Chundi He

Wound healing is a complex biological process combining with multiple biological signaling pathways [31]. Deregulation of the wound healing process can lead to excessive scar formation, as seen in keloids [32]. In addition to the aesthetic problems they pose, keloids which forms when excessive scar tissue is deposited within and beyond the boundaries of the wound are often pruritic, painful, and psychologically debilitating. Keloids are common skin lesions that are difficult to treat and are associated with high recurrence rates despite different available treatment options [32].

12.2.1 Pathogenesis

The detailed mechanism of keloid development is poorly understood and the research efforts have been hindered by a lack of reliable animal models, except that the process is known to be induced by skin injury in predisposed individuals. Most of keloids develop within 3 months of the injury that can be secondary to acne, folliculitis, body piercings, burns, lacerations, and surgical wounds, some may occur up to 1 year after skin injury [32]. There are several theories of keloid etiology, most of which are related to fibroblast dysfunction. Keloid fibroblasts overproduce type I procollagen and express higher levels of certain growth factors, such as vascular endothelial growth factor, transforming growth factor βs, and platelet-derived growth factor [32], and these cells in keloid also have lower rates of apoptosis and demonstrate a downregulation of apoptosis-related genes, in comparison with fibroblasts isolated from a normal wound [33].

Recently, studies indicated that a group of non-protein coding gene named micro-RNAs (miRNAs) was involved in keloids development. It suggested that miRNAs expression profile was changed in keloids tissue compared to normal nonkeloid tissue [34]. Another study performed miRNA microarray analysis to compare miRNA expression profiles between keloid-derived and normal fibroblasts. Totally 7 unregulated and 20 downregulated miRNAs were recognized. Among these altered miRNAs, miR-196a showed the highest fold change. Meanwhile, it proved that overexpression or knockdown of miR-196a led to a decreased or increased level of secreted type I/III collagens, correspondingly. Consequently, it suggested that miR-196a could be a new therapeutic target for keloid.

12.2.2 Epidemiology

It is reported that the incidences range from a high of 16% among adults in both black and Hispanic [35] to a low of less than 1% among adults in the United Kingdom [36]. This may explain the sebum hypothesis, generally, Orientals and Blacks have thicker, and more seborrheic skin compared to Caucasians and may account for the higher incidence of keloids in these populations. It is extensively accepted that darker-skinned populations have a higher occurrence of keloids than lighter-skinned populations, with the reported incidence ratio between different groups from 2:1 to 19:1 [37]. The higher rate for earlobe keloids after piercing may be responsible for slight female predominance.

Keloids can happen at any age, but the most are between the age of 11 and 30 years. The average age is 22.3 years for women and 22.8 years for men. It has been suggested that hormones influence keloids formation, as supported by the study showing a higher male hormone level in clinically activated scar tissue. Keloid seem to have an elevated incidence in pregnant women and young boys and girls, which means the compact relationship between keloid and hormone profile, such that increasing neoangiogenesis in pregnancy are probable.

12.2.3 Genetics

There are some cases with documented familial that suggest an autosomal dominant inheritance with incomplete penetrance and variable expression. It has been found that keloid susceptibility loci are on chromosomes 2 and 7 in one large familial study [39], where individuals with mutations at these loci developed keloids.

A multilevel genome-wide association study on 824 individuals with keloid (cases) and 3205 uninfluenced controls in the Japanese population and another study indicated that keloid might have significant associations with four SNP locus in three chromosomal areas: 1q41, 3q22.3–23, and 15q21.3 [40]. However, most cases are sporadic and they do not follow any clear genetic models. Hence, it is impossible that a single candidate gene can answer for most keloids. Some studies suggested that the human leukocytes antigen (HLA) system might be related with the development of keloids and interpret racial differences. It has been suggested that the HLA-DQA1 and DQB1 alleles and haplotypes with keloids in Chinese population had a positive correlation and it also proposed a correlation with the HLA types, HLA-DR5 and HLA DQw3 [41].

12.2.4 Immunology

Immune reactions are likely to take part in keloid development. It was reported that a significantly higher consistence of IgG [41] and IgA and IgM are detected in keloids compared with normal skin [42, 43]. The immunocytes infiltrate in keloids including lymphocytes (CD3+, CD4+, CD45RO+, and HLA-DR+) and dendritic cells (CD1a+, CD36+, HLA-DR+, and ICAM-1+) [44]. What is more, the number of macrophages, epidermal Langerhans cells, and mast cells is increased [45, 46]. The number of mast cells and pruritus decrease in keloids after treatment with silicone gel sheeting and mast cells may promote a high expression of hypoxia-inducible factor 1, alpha (HIF-1α) and vascular endothelial growth factor (VEGF) in keloids [47, 48]. The role of the inflammatory response has not been studied in detail in the formation of keloids and remains to be explored.

12.2.5 Clinical Features

Keloids overgrow the area of the initial wound, invading the normal adjacent tissue and rarely reverse back spontaneously. They often appear after skin trauma and as firm broad nodules, which are itching and painful. Initially, keloids appear pink or red and sometimes with telangiectasias. The scar tissue usually extends in a claw-like appearance beyond the area of the initial skin injury and tends to flatten with time. Strict clinical and histopathological criteria have been used for the differential of keloids and hypertrophic scars (Table 12.1). For some unknown factors, keloids occur more commonly on the chest, shoulders, upper back, back of the neck, and earlobes [49, 50]. This shows the existence of local abnormal cells or tissue factors that led to the formation of keloids. It has been intensively discussed whether keloids occur primarily in the anatomical sites with increased skin tension. This could be an oversimplification [49], for the most commonly affected site, the earlobe, is under minimal tension. However, palms or soles are rarely sites of keloid

Table 12.1 Clinical and histological criteria of keloids and hypertrophic scars [62]

Keloids	Hypertrophic scars
Grow beyond the borders of the original wound	Remain within the boundaries of the original wound
Size varies between a pea and a football; growth may be widespread, vertical, or both	Rarely more than a centimeter in thickness or width
Pruritic and painful	Less pruritic and painful weeks
Appear within several months after initial scar, then gradually proliferate indefinitely	Generally arise within 4 weeks, grow intensely for several months, then regress often within 1 year
Occur often on the chest, shoulders, upper back, back of the neck and earlobes, rarely on the palm or soles	No predominant anatomical site
Do not regress spontaneously	Regress spontaneously
Larger, thicker and more wavy collagen fibers than normal skin, random collagen fiber orientation, increased ratio of type I to type III collagen	Fine collagen fibers oriented parallel to the epidermis
Increased fibroblast density and fibroblast proliferation rate	Increased fibroblast density
Only few α-smooth muscle actin expressing myofibroblasts	Presence of α-smooth muscle actin expressing myofibroblasts is typical

formation, where the skin tension is expected to be significant. All of these suggest that other factors are involved in keloids development.

12.2.6 Treatments

Through the years, therapeutic methods of treating scars have been developed, for example, surgical therapies, intralesional Steroid injections, immunomodulators, radiation therapy, topical silicone gel sheeting, laser therapy, and other physical modalities. Despite the fact that some improvement can be achieved, the therapeutic alternatives illustrates that there is still no single therapy that is 100 % effective and the appearance of the skin cannot completely regress to its pre-wounded condition.

12.2.7 Surgical Excision

Surgical excision of keloids has a close relationship with its high rate of recurrence. It is a well-executed keloid excision that thoroughly removes all abnormal tissue, but this excision may increase the final scar length. Thus, it is possible that keloid recurrence with a longer scar may form a larger keloid [32, 51]. Because excessive wound tension has been proposed as a promoted factor of keloid formation, wound edges should be approximated with just enough tension to close the wound. The surgeon should make incisions along skin tension lines and evert the wound edges during closure [32, 52]. The importance of meticulous technique must be emphasized. As is reported, employing a minimal number of deep absorbable and unabsorbable stitches for skin closure could minimize the inflammatory response during the early period of healing. It should be cautiously undertaken that the recurrence rate of keloids is 45–100 % after surgical excision without adjuvant therapy [32, 53]. In most instances, it should need extra adjunctive therapy such as corticosteroids, pressure, silicone gel sheeting, imiquimod cream, or interferon injections after excising keloids.

12.2.8 Corticosteroid

The injection of triamcinolone is one of the long-term standards of keloid therapy, the most common naturopathy [54]. When administered intralesionally, it decreases inflammation, inhibits fibroblast proliferation, and increases vasoconstriction in a dose-dependent manner [32, 55]. As is commonly reported, side effects involve skin atrophy, hypopigmentation, and telangiectasis. The longer the course of treatment will lead these side effects occur more easily. Triamcinolone can be injected synchronously with lidocaine to relieve injection pain. Before surgical excision, as an adjunct to surgical excision, triamcinolone is best initiated in the preoperative period followed by weekly injections for at least 2 weeks, then monthly injections for up to 3 months [32]. Weekly triamcinolone injections are not necessary if topical imiquimod is used as an adjuvant in the treatment regimen. Topical triamcinolone application is poorly absorbed into dermis.

12.2.9 Imiquimod

Iimiquimod acts as an effective inducer of interferon and cytokine release at the site of skin application. The immunomodulator acts to diminish inordinate collagen production by keloid fibroblasts [32]. Meanwhile, partial application of imiquimod has been shown to upregulate certain apoptosis-related genes in keloid fibroblasts [32, 56]. When formulated as a 5 % cream, imiquimod is a safe and well-tolerated drug. It should be started immediately to use imiquimod after surgery and sustained daily for 8 weeks. Side reactions include skin erosion, exfoliation, flaking, and dropsy at the site of application [32, 57]. Although further studies are needed to illuminate the detailed mechanism of action of imiquimod for keloid management, this therapy appears to have a good clinical benefit when used judiciously.

12.2.10 Interferon-α-2b

Interferon-α-2b (IFN-α2b) specifically has undergone plentiful study for keloid therapy. It has been shown in experimental models to inactivate fibroblasts and to suppress collagen production in a dose-dependent manner [32]. It is typically injected in the lesion in recombinant form either alone or after surgical resection. It was reported that an 18.7 % relapse rate when IFN-α2b injections were given after keloids excision versus a 51 % relapse rate with resection alone and a 58 % relapse rate when treated with resection and postoperative IL triamcinolone [58]. Other researchers have reported similar clinical results.

12.2.11 5-Fluorouracil

5-Fluorouracil (5-FU) is a kind of pyrimidine analog that is widely used for antimetabolite and chemotherapeutic properties. It has been proven that TGF-β signal reduces the rate of type I collagen gene expression in keloid fibroblasts in vitro [32, 59]. Under the 5-FU therapy there are some common side effects such as pain, burning, hyperpigmentation, and ulceration at the injection site. This leads to noncompliance for many patients [32].

12.2.12 Laser

Laser therapy includes the use of a certain wavelength of light energy and pulse duration to ablate targeted tissues. Keloids can be treated with any of several different lasers including fractional carbon dioxide, pulsed dye laser, and neodymium:yttrium–aluminum–garnet (Nd:YAG) lasers [32, 60]. Fractional carbon dioxide lasers have been proven to be highly effective. Laser technology continues to improve, with higher cure rates and fewer postoperative complications [54].

12.2.13 Silicone Gel Sheeting

Silicone gel products have prevailed in the scar therapy [59]. Whereas the accurate mechanism of this function is not clear, meanwhile the effective silicone products must coincide with occlusion, hydration, and add temperature to the cicatrix. Although there are a lot of commercial silicone-containing products, only both the gel sheet and self-drying tube formulations have been connected with enhancing ultimate scar surface. Silicone gel sheeting can be utilized to accomplish reepithelialization as soon as possible and worn for at lowest 12 h every day [38, 54, 59]. These sheets have high prices, however, each one can be cleaned out and reuse to continue to 12 days. The sheets require to be worn all the time in order to achieve better effect; therefore, patient compliance can be a question, especially when the scar lies in an obvious place. Furthermore, they are difficult to maintain in places that are such as joints and the face. There are nonocclusive silicone-based products such as creams that contain silicone oil and have yielded unsatisfying consequences. Similarly, newer formulations containing silicone sprays or foams are invalid owing to the lack of providing occlusion.

12.2.14 Irradiation

Radiation is probably served as a monotherapy or combined with surgery to keep from reappearance of keloids following excision. When used as a monotherapy, radiation is not particularly efficacious and it has a recurrence rate of 50–100 % [54, 60] only if more doses are utilized. Whereas this probably resulted in cutaneous squamous cell carcinoma of the cured positions after 15–30 years [61, 62]. Primary radiation is successful in abating the pruritus, soreness, and tenderness of keloids. Associate preoperative with postoperative radiation has no larger efficiency than postoperative radiation alone. Young children with keloids should either not be irradiated, or if it is the only viable option, the metaphyses should be shielded in order to prevent retardation of bone growth.

12.3 Squamous Cell Carcinoma (SCC)

Thomas Griffin, MD and Kehua Li, MD

12.3.1 Introduction to SCC

Cutaneous squamous cell carcinoma (cSCC) is one of the most common cancers in the United States, second only to basal cell carcinoma [63]. While the incidence of nonmelanoma skin cancer (NMSC) is not reported to the American Cancer Society, it is estimated that cSCC comprises approximately 20 % of the estimated 900,000–3.5 million [64–66] cases of NMSCs diagnosed each year in the United States. cSCC is among the more dangerous of the nonmelanoma skin cancers, with 2500–8791 anticipated deaths each year [63, 64, 69] purportedly due to the propensity for locoregional metastases and perineural spread [67, 68]. It is estimated that anywhere from 1.9 to 5 % of cSCCs will ultimately metastasize [69–71]. Those tumors with "high risk" features, such as tumor size >2 cm, depth >2 mm, and involvement of the nonglabrous lip or anterior ear are at an increased risk for metastases [69, 71]. Nonmelanoma skin cancers are a significant burden to both patients and the health care system at large, with approximately $650 million spent each year on NMSC treatment in the United States alone [72–74].

12.3.2 Causes of SCC

Squamous cell carcinoma arises from the malignant proliferation of keratinocytes. The development of cSCC depends on a variety of gene mutations and subsequent aberrations in cellular functions and signaling processes [93]. Mutations in the tumor suppressor gene, p53, have been identified in as many as 90 % of NMSCs [87, 94]. Disruption of p53 leads to genomic instability, increasing the likelihood of acquiring additional mutations necessary for carcinoma development and growth.

In addition, upregulation of the epidermal growth factor receptor (EGFR) and members of the SRC family of tyrosine kinases (SFKs), such as Fyn, are involved in the development of cSCCs through aberrant keratinocyte proliferation and abnormal differentiation [79–81, 126]. EGFR protein upregulation has been identified in up to 47 % of head and neck SCC [82]. Constitutively active EGFR downregulates the expression of p53 through the effector molecule, c-Jun [83, 84]. This decrease in p53 functioning causes a subsequent decline in Notch1 expression, a protein normally involved in keratinocyte differentiation [85, 86]. This EGFR-mediated decline in Notch1 functioning allows for dysregulated differentiation and subsequent carcinoma development [85, 86, 90]. Fyn activation is also associated with downregulation of p53 and Notch1 [83].

Negative regulators of SFK functioning, such as Srcasm (SRC activating and signaling molecule) are also downregulated in SCC. Srcasm normally functions to block SFK signaling by promoting the lysosomal degradation of SFK proteins [83]. The decreased levels of Srcasm in cSCC promote the consequent upregulation of SFKs, allowing for unchecked tyrosine kinase signaling cascades and cellular proliferation [83, 93].

Additionally, mutations in the Ras oncogene are also implicated in cSCC growth. Ras is a member of the GTP-binding protein family involved in downstream signaling of the EGFR pathway. Activating mutations in the Ras protein can promote SCC development [87] through the induction of cyclin D1, a regulator of cellular proliferation controlling the G1/S cycle transition [93, 126]. Up to 21 % of cSCCs have been found to harbor Ras oncogene mutations [126].

The mutations of essential genes involved in regulation of normal cell cycle progression and cellular functioning are induced by a variety of mechanisms. The most common etiologic factors in the development of cSCC are discussed below.

12.3.3 Ultraviolet Radiation (UVR)

First suggested by Thiersch et al. in 1875, ultraviolet radiation is the most well-described etiologic factor for cutaneous squamous cell carcinoma, particularly the cumulative lifetime dose of UV radiation [75–77]. The vast majority of cSCCs occur in sun-exposed areas, such as the head, neck, upper extremities, and trunk [96, 97]. Based on epidemiologic data, those with low Fitzpatrick skin type number (types I–III) are most susceptible to UVR, presumably due to lower levels of UV-protective melanin in fair skin types [75, 76, 97]. Individuals with darker skin have a significantly reduced incidence of cSCC in sun-exposed areas [96].

UVB radiation, light with wavelengths between 290 and 320 nm, has been shown to be the most carcinogenic due to its ability to directly induce DNA damage [78] as well as inhibit the adaptive immune system [79, 88, 89]. UV radiation causes disruption of the DNA structure, most notably through pyrimidine transitions from cytosine to thymine bases ($C \rightarrow T$). The bulky pyrimidine adducts formed by these pyrimidine substitutions disrupt DNA replication and are believed to be the primary pathogenic mechanism by which ultraviolet light induces cancerous changes in the skin [90–92, 94]. These UVR-induced mutations have been implicated in p53, ras, and EGFR genes as well as other cell cycle regulatory genes [90, 95]. In addition, UVA radiation (320–400 nm) may also contribute to malignant transformation of keratinocytes by the UV-mediated induction of oxidative stress [96].

12.3.4 Immunosuppression

The reduction in immune surveillance due to disruption of the adaptive immune system leads to an increased risk of developing NMSCs, particularly increasing the risk for squamous cell carcinoma [107]. Immune suppression may be endogenous, as in cases of hematologic malignancy, or exogenous as in antirejection therapy in solid organ transplantation. cSCCs in the immunocompromised often develop in sun-exposed areas, similar to immunocompetent patients [96].

Solid organ transplantation has been frequently identified as a major risk factor for the development of cSCC. The risk of developing cSCC is reportedly increased up to 100× in organ transplant recipients (OTRs), with malignant lesions developing on a more rapid time course than in immunocompetent individuals [96, 98]. The chronic use of immunosuppressive medications is likely to blame, with patients receiving longer time courses and higher doses of immunosuppressive therapy suffering a greater burden of cutaneous malignancies [99, 100]. Similarly, patients receiving heart transplants have been noted to have a higher risk of cSCC development compared to kidney transplantation, presumably due to the higher load of immunosuppressive drugs necessary [99, 101].

The specific immunosuppressive regimens used in OTRs also influence the risk of cSCC. For example, the calcineurin inhibitor, cyclosporine increases the risk of cSCC development threefold compared with other agents, such as azathioprine or prednisolone [99, 102]. Additionally, cyclosporine has been shown to have a direct carcinogenic effect independent of its immunosuppressive activity, possibly due to the induction of TGF-B and the disruption of p53-mediated cell senescence [103, 104]. On the other hand, sirolimus, an mTOR inhibitor, has been shown to lower the risk of cSCC through the blockade of intracellular signaling pathways involved in UV-mediated carcinogensis, as well as the inhibition of VEGF secretion [100, 105, 106].

12.3.5 HPV

Human papillomavirus, a double-stranded DNA virus of the papillomaviridae family, has been implicated in the pathogenesis of SCC, more commonly with cancers of the anogenital region, oral mucosa, and cervix [107]. The mucosal "high-risk" HPV subtypes, such as type 16 and 18, have been strongly implicated in cervical SCC through the well-documented mechanism of inactivation of p53 and retinoblastoma tumor suppressors by viral E6 and E7 "early proteins" [87, 107]. Extra-genital Bowen's disease, a form of cutaneous squamous carcinoma *in situ*, has shown a variable presence of intralesional HPV [108, 109]. While HPV DNA has been demonstrated in a high percentage of cSCC lesions, a direct causal mechanism between HPV infection and cSCC development remains unclear [87, 110].

Linkage between HPV and cSCC was initially illustrated in patients with the rare condition epidermodysplasia verruciformis (EV) [111]. The diminished cell-mediated immunity characteristic of EV leads to an increased susceptibility to infection with beta-HPV subtypes and the subsequent development of widespread verrucous lesions, particularly in sun-exposed areas. These numerous flat warts of EV demonstrate an increased risk for development of cSCC [107, 111]. There is some evidence to suggest that beta-HPV subtypes may be associated with cSCC development in immunocompetent individuals, but as above, an exact causal relationship remains elusive [98, 112, 113].

12.3.6 Immunology of SCC

The normal immune response to cancer involves the activation of cell-mediated immunity to provide antitumor cellular destruction [123, 124]. However, the microenvironments of cutaneous squamous cell carcinomas contribute to evasion of immune surveillance through a variety of immunologic mechanisms, thus allowing for uninhibited tumor growth.

As noted previously, UVB radiation causes immunosuppression, mediated by the induction of IL-10 while simultaneously decreasing IL-12 production [125–128]. IL-10 is responsible for shifting the helper T-cell response away from the pro-inflammatory Th1 response, normally responsible for activation of cytotoxic T cells (CD8+) and natural killer (NK) cells through IFN-g and IL-12, toward the suppressive Th2 response [79, 126, 128, 129]. Furthermore, IL-10 inhibits the antigen presenting function of Langerhans cells (LC) within the skin, preventing the stimulation of a Th1 response to tumor antigens [130]. Direct UV radiation similarly disrupts antigen presentation by Langerhans cells, in addition to downregulating the number of LCs in the skin [126, 131]. This reduction in antigen presenting capability in the skin reduces the ability to mount an effective cytotoxic response to tumor antigens.

IL-12 has been implicated in the repair of UV-induced DNA damage, and its downregulation has been associated with rapid tumor growth in mice [132, 133]. These alterations in cytokines, along with the UV-mediated induction of Th2 cells are suspected to be responsible for the immunosuppressive effects of UVB radiation.

Additionally, SCC tumor cells can produce the anti-inflammatory cytokines Il-10 and TGF-B, further downregulating the Th1 cell response [124, 134]. These anti-inflammatory cytokines, specifically TGF-B, can induce the differentiation of T regulatory lymphocytes (Treg, CD4 + CD25+) involved in suppressing normal T-cell activation [124, 127, 135]. These Tregs are normally implicated in the maintenance of self-tolerance by direct, cytokine-independent suppression of T lymphocytes, as well as the downregulation of co-stimulatory molecules on antigen presenting dendritic cells in the skin, such as Langerhans cells [136, 137]. Again, this blockade of dendritic cells prevents the mounting of a T-cell-mediated immune response to tumor antigens allowing for tumor cell immune evasion.

Tregs also express high levels of the transcription factor FOXP3. High levels of FOXP3 expression seem to correlate with more profound immuosuppression [138]. Cutaneous squamous cell carcinomas have been shown to have significant infiltration of FOXP3+ Treg cells, suggesting a mechanism for tumor cell immune evasion through local inhibition of an appropriate cytotoxic T-cell-mediated response [138].

12.3.7 Treatment

Prevention of cSCC centers around the reduction of risk factors, such as use of sunscreens and protective clothing [117, 118]. The avoidance of UV radiation during times of intense sunlight (11 am–3 pm, generally) may also be helpful in preventing cSCC [117, 118]. The use of immunosuppressive medications found to decrease the risk of cSCC, such as sirolimus, may also be helpful in applicable patient populations.

that are specifically associated with a certain disease can be used as ideal biomarkers for diagnosis or to increase the diagnostic accuracy when differentiating several diseases that have overlapped clinical and morphological manifestation. For example, erythrodermic psoriasis is difficult to differentiate from SS by clinical features, but the gene PLS3 which is expressed in SS but not in psoriasis may help. These markers in SS are not always identified in all cases of CTCL, but the high frequent finding rate of these genes and the other associated genes seen frequently in MF/SS hint to a common pathway that becomes dysregulated in the development of MF/SS.

Biomarkers that are not expressed in normal T cells but only on the neoplastic cell are rare, but candidates have been reported in MF/SS. A surface marker that is a member of the killer receptor, KIR3DL2 or CD158, is specific for natural killer (NK) cells, and is not typically expressed on CD4+ T cell. In screening SS patients, Detecting KIR3DL2 in SS T cells can be used to distinguish the malignant clone from multiple clones in peripheral blood. Furthermore, the detection of KIR3DL2 on SS cells has been reported by multiple investigators. However, KIR detected in aged T cells and T cells in autoimmune diseases may increase KIR expression rate. The mechanism of increased KIR receptor expression in aged T cells has been suggested to be epigenetic, hinting to the underlying mechanism in the development of MF/SS.

In addition to surface markers altered, nuclear proteins have been identified abnormal in MF/SS. Dysregulation of genes regulating cytokine expression, with increased STAT3 and loss of STAT4, has been observed in MF/SS. The increased STAT3 may be important in the Th2 phenotype of MF/SS, but the activity of STAT3 is likely to be abnormal based on the observation of the low cytokine expression of SS cells. Genes for nuclear proteins involved in proliferation, such as JunB, JunD, and other cell cycle genes, are increased, but these are not specific for MF/SS and have been detected in other cancers, limiting their use as biomarkers.

Microarray studies have identified additional novel genes in MF/SS. Of note is the manyfold upregulation of genes not normally expressed in T cells, such as TWIST1, DNM3 (dynamin 3), NEDD4L, and PLS3 (T-plastin). The functional role and biologic significance of these genes in MF/SS are unclear, and adaptation of these genetic biomarkers into clinical testing may improve the diagnosis of MF/SS.

12.4.3 Genetic and Epigenetic Alterations in MF/SS

Changes to the genome alters the instructions, which may lead to the disease phenotype of MF/SS and these genomic alterations drive the development of cancer and likely play an important role in the pathogenesis of MF/SS, in altering the phenotype of a normal memory CD4+ T cell to a transformed skin homing T cell. While accumulation of a series of genetic changes via activation of oncogenes has been observed in MF/SS such as Jun, myc, or inactivation of tumor suppressor genes, other mechanisms that affect gene regulation at different levels may be important in the development of MF/SS. It is the totality of expression pattern of additional genes that culminates in MF/SS.

In-depth studies have begun to identify other genetic changes leading to MF/SS. Distinctive and pathognomonic chromosomal translocations such as those seen in B-cell lymphomas and myeloid leukemias have not been identified in MF/SS. Unlike B cells, T cells lack the heavy chain genes which in B cells undergo recombination during maturation and thus the rearrangement increases the susceptibility to aberrant pathognomonic DNA rearrangements and chromosomal translocation. Such genetic maturation does not occur in T cells and recurrent hallmark translocations are infrequent. Nevertheless the inherent developmental program to rearrange T-cell receptor genes by T cells may increase susceptibility to genetic mutations and chromosomes alterations. Indeed numerous studies of CTCL show chromosomal alterations, genomic gains and losses, affecting chromosomes 1, 6, 7, 8, 9, 10, and 17. Recent approaches using comparative genomic hybridization (CGH) have identified more detailed chromosomal changes, with the most common types associated with loss of chromosomal regions (1p, 10p, 10q, and 17p) rather than gain of chromosomal regions (8q and 17q).

As these chromosomal abnormalities are not consistent, their value as diagnostic markers is limited. Rather, studies reveal many chromosomal regions altered, and this hints to an underlying genomic instability in MF/SS. Gene regulation is controlled at multiple levels and the extensive gene expression changes in MF/SS suggest a complex pathogenesis affecting multiple pathways as recurrent specific mutations have not been identified in MF/SS. Evidence suggests that epigenetics play an important role in altered transcriptome in MF/SS. Extensive gene expression changes have been cataloged that are described in MF/SS which are not from alteration of the DNA sequence. In addition, epigenetic changes that include DNA methylation at CpG, alteration of histone, chromosomal breaks also play an important role in the alter gene expression in MF/SS.

With the heterogeneous genetic changes in MF/SS, hypomethylation may be an important mechanism driving the progression of MF to more advanced stages, and increasing genetic instability. The unanswered question is the mechanism responsible for increasing hypomethylation in cancer. Potential pathways include genes involved in regulating DNA methylation, such as DNMT1 which is required for preservation of CpG methylation. Loss of this gene increases the development of cancer in mouse models, especially T-cell lymphoma. However, preliminary analysis has not revealed loss of DNMT1 in MF/SS [163].

12.4.4 Therapy

While numerous therapeutic options are available, no therapy has been shown to be curative. Thus, the goal of therapy is to induce long-term remission without further compromising a patient's immune system or quality of life. In general, MF treatment is divided into two broad categories: skin-directed and systemic therapies. Skin-directed therapy is the key component in management of early disease, while systemic therapy is essential in more advanced cases. Systemic therapy can be either based on the mechanism of action of the systemic agent (e.g., biological modifiers such as interferons, retinoids, and rexinoid; histone deacetylase inhibitors; and traditional chemotherapeutic agents, such as doxorubicin and gemcitabine) or by the number of agents used to treat a patient (e.g., monotherapy vs. multiagent combination therapy).

12.4.5 Skin-Directed Therapies

Various topical agents are not only the mainstay of therapy in cases of CTCL with skin involvement, but also be useful as a palliation treatment in patients with advanced disease. Widely used topical therapies include corticosteroids, nitrogen mustard, carmustine, topical retinoids, and rexinoid (bexarotene), as well as ultraviolet light therapy and body irradiation. These agents/methods may be used alone or in combination. A number of other skin-directed therapies are available, including imiquimod and photodynamic therapy (PDT).

12.4.6 Systemic Therapies

Several novel systemic agents have been recently added to the assortment of therapies available for CTCL.

12.4.7 Histone Deacetylase Inhibitors (HDIs)

Epigenetic modulation is an important mechanism of regulation in gene expression. Histone deacetylase inhibition increases acetylation of lysine residues that form the octomeric histone core of chromatin, thereby decreasing the ability of the histones to bind to DNA. This decreased binding allows chromatin expansion, permitting transcription of the tumor suppressor genes. However, HDIs affect acetylation globally and may have wider effects on various cellular functions.

12.4.7.1 Vorinostat

Vorinostat (suberoylanilide hydroxamic acid, Zolinza) is the first HDI approved by the US FDA in October 2006 for cutaneous manifestations of CTCL in patients with progressive, persistent, or recurrent disease on or following two systemic therapies. The most common drug-related adverse events were diarrhea, fatigue, nausea, and anorexia. Vorinostat is not an immunosuppressive agent, though some degree of bone marrow suppression may occur.

12.4.7.2 Romidepsin

Romidepsin is a cyclic peptide that selectively inhibits histone deacetylase isotypes 1, 2, 4, and 6. Romidepsin, like other HDIs, was shown to induce cell cycle arrest in both G1 and G2/M phases of DNA replication and to trigger apoptosis in several cell lines. Generally, romidepsin is well tolerated; common side effects include fatigue, nausea, vomiting, and transient thrombocytopenia and neutropenia. However, romidepsin monotherapy may not be sufficient for maximal benefit, and hence, the continued search for adjuvant measures capable of providing synergistic effects is needed.

12.4.7.3 Pralatrexate

Pralatrexate is a new antifolate analog that is FDA-approved for relapsed or refractory peripheral T-cell lymphoma. The relative specificity of antifolates for malignant cells is a result of overexpression of their receptor, reduced folate carrier-1 (RFC-1). Pralatrexate was specifically designed to have significantly higher affinity to RFC-1 as compared with other antifolates. In addition, polyglutamylation of pralatrexate secures retention of this drug within the cancer cell. The interference with dihydrofolate reductase affects synthesis of deoxythymidine and the purine DNA nucleotides, which ultimately results in arrest of the cell cycle. Adverse events included mucosal inflammation and thrombocytopenia.

Other agents include Lenalidomide, a thalidomide analog, and the proteasome inhibitor, Bortezomib, and Alemtuzumab that is a humanized IgG1 monoclonal antibody that targets the CD52 antigen.

12.4.8 Extracorporeal Photopheresis

Extracorporeal photopheresis (ECP) is an approved palliative treatment for CTCL. The novel continuous flow separation (CFS) system (THERAKOS™ CELLEX™) has been developed based on the current UVAR®XTS™ device and is designed to reduce treatment times and extracorporeal volumes.

12.4.9 Chemotherapy

Neither single agent nor multiagent therapy is curative in MF. Additionally, single or multiagent chemotherapy results in a higher incidence of transformation to large cell lymphoma, which carries a worse prognosis than the original diagnosis. Because ORR and disease free survival are generally higher after combination therapy, single agent chemotherapy is rarely used. However, use of multiagent chemotherapy results in increased immunosuppression and higher risk of serious infections, leading to death in a majority of patients who develop these complications.

12.4.10 Stem Cell Transplant

The lifetime expectation for transformed MF and Sézary syndrome is less than 2.5 years. Stem cell transplantion (SCT) is a promising approach aimed at providing a cure or increasing life expectancy. Autologous SCT showed very limited efficacy in most patients with CTCL, since 60 % of these patients experienced an early relapse (median time to relapse was 120 days). Nevertheless, SCT carries a risk of significant toxicity and fatal complications, particularly in older patients. Careful patient selection and proper timing of SCT are critical factors in successful therapy [164, 165].

References

Melanoma Immunology and Immune Therapy

1. Siegel R, Ma J, Zou Z, Jemal A. Cancer statistics, 2014. CA Cancer J Clin. 2014;64:9–29.
2. Burnet FM. The concept of immunological surveillance. Prog Exp Tumor Res. 1970;13:1–27.
3. Greenman C, Stephens P, Smith R, Dalgliesh GL, Hunter C, Bignell G, Davies H, Teague J, Butler A, Stevens C, Edkins S, O'Meara S, Vastrik I, Schmidt EE, Avis T, Barthorpe S, Bhamra G, Buck G, Choudhury B, Clements J, Cole J, Dicks E, Forbes S, Gray K, Halliday K, Harrison R, Hills K, Hinton J, Jenkinson A, Jones D, Menzies A, Mironenko T, Perry J, Raine K, Richardson D, Shepherd R, Small A, Tofts C, Varian J, Webb T, West S, Widaa S, Yates A, Cahill DP, Louis DN, Goldstraw P, Nicholson AG, Brasseur F, Looijenga L, Weber BL, Chiew YE, DeFazio A, Greaves MF, Green AR, Campbell P, Birney E, Easton DF, Chenevix-Trench G, Tan MH, Khoo SK, Teh BT, Yuen ST, Leung SY, Wooster R, Futreal PA, Stratton MR. Patterns of somatic mutation in human cancer genomes. Nature. 2007;446:153–8.
4. Miller DM, Flaherty KT, Tsao H. Current status and future directions of molecularly targeted therapies and immunotherapies for melanoma. Semin Cutan Med Surg. 2014;33:60–7.
5. Bruttel VS, Wischhusen J. Cancer stem cell immunology: key to understanding tumorigenesis and tumor immune escape? Front Immunol. 2014;5:360.
6. Nestle FO, Burg G, Dummer R. New perspectives on immunobiology and immunotherapy of melanoma. Immunol Today. 1999; 20:5–7.
7. Mukherji B. Immunology of melanoma. Clin Dermatol. 2013;31: 156–65.
8. Traversari C, van der Bruggen P, Luescher IF, Lurquin C, Chomez P, Van Pel A, De Plaen E, Amar-Costesec A, Boon T. A nonapeptide encoded by human gene MAGE-1 is recognized on HLA-A1 by cytolytic T lymphocytes directed against tumor antigen MZ2-E. J Exp Med. 1992;176:1453–7.
9. Tsuchida T, Saxton RE, Morton DL, Irie RF. Gangliosides of human melanoma. Cancer. 1989;63:1166–74.
10. Livingston PO. Approaches to augmenting the immunogenicity of melanoma gangliosides: from whole melanoma cells to ganglioside – KLH conjugate vaccines. Immunol Rev. 1995;145:147–66.
11. Marincola FM, Jaffee EM, Hicklin DJ, Ferrone S. Escape of human solid tumors from T-cell recognition: molecular mechanisms and functional significance. Adv Immunol. 2000;74: 181–273.
12. Pardoll DM. The blockade of immune checkpoints in cancer immunotherapy. Nat Rev Cancer. 2012;12:252–64.
13. Petrella T, Quirt I, Verma S, Haynes AE, Charette M, Bak K. Single – agent interleukin-2 in the treatment of metastatic melanoma: a systematic review. Cancer Treat Rev. 2007;33:484–96.
14. Lens M. The role of vaccine therapy in the treatment of melanoma. Expert Opin Biol Ther. 2008;8:315–23.
15. Kirkwood JM, Lee S, Moschos SJ, Albertini MR, Michalak JC, Sander C, Whiteside T, Butterfield LH, Weiner L. Immunogenicity and antitumor effects of vaccination with peptide vaccine ± granulocyte – monocyte colony – stimulating factor and/or IFN – alpha2b in advanced metastatic melanoma: Eastern Cooperative Oncology Group Phase II Trial E1696. Clin cancer Res : off J Am Ass Cancer Res. 2009;15:1443–51.
16. Shin DS, Ribas A. The evolution of checkpoint blockade as a cancer therapy: what's here, what's next? Curr Opin Immunol. 2015;33C:23–35.
17. van Elsas A, Hurwitz AA, Allison JP. Combination immunotherapy of B16 melanoma using anti – cytotoxic T lymphocyte – associated antigen 4 (CTLA-4) and granulocyte/macrophage colony – stimulating factor (GM – CSF)-producing vaccines induces rejection of subcutaneous and metastatic tumors accompanied by autoimmune depigmentation. J Exp Med. 1999;190: 355–66.
18. Hodi FS, O'Day SJ, McDermott DF, Weber RW, Sosman JA, Haanen JB, Gonzalez R, Robert C, Schadendorf D, Hassel JC, Akerley W, van den Eertwegh AJ, Lutzky J, Lorigan P, Vaubel JM, Linette GP, Hogg D, Ottensmeier CH, Lebbe C, Peschel C, Quirt I, Clark JI, Wolchok JD, Weber JS, Tian J, Yellin MJ, Nichol GM, Hoos A, Urba WJ. Improved survival with ipilimumab in patients with metastatic melanoma. N Engl J Med. 2010;363:711–23.
19. Robert C, Thomas L, Bondarenko I, O'Day S, Weber J, Garbe C, Lebbe C, Baurain JF, Testori A, Grob JJ, Davidson N, Richards J, Maio M, Hauschild A, Miller Jr WH, Gascon P, Lotem M, Harmankaya K, Ibrahim R, Francis S, Chen TT, Humphrey R, Hoos A, Wolchok JD. Ipilimumab plus dacarbazine for previously untreated metastatic melanoma. N Engl J Med. 2011;364: 2517–26.
20. Camacho LH, Antonia S, Sosman J, Kirkwood JM, Gajewski TF, Redman B, Pavlov D, Bulanhagui C, Bozon VA, Gomez-Navarro J, Ribas A. Phase I/II trial of tremelimumab in patients with metastatic melanoma. J clin oncol : off J Am Soc Clin Oncol. 2009;27:1075–81.
21. Ribas A, Kefford R, Marshall MA, Punt CJ, Haanen JB, Marmol M, Garbe C, Gogas H, Schachter J, Linette G, Lorigan P, Kendra KL, Maio M, Trefzer U, Smylie M, McArthur GA, Dreno B, Nathan PD, Mackiewicz J, Kirkwood JM, Gomez-Navarro J, Huang B, Pavlov D, Hauschild A. Phase III randomized clinical trial comparing tremelimumab with standard – of – care chemotherapy in patients with advanced melanoma. J clin oncol : off J Am Soc Clin Oncol. 2013;31:616–22.
22. Keir ME, Butte MJ, Freeman GJ, Sharpe AH. PD-1 and its ligands in tolerance and immunity. Annu Rev Immunol. 2008;26:677–704.
23. Butte MJ, Keir ME, Phamduy TB, Sharpe AH, Freeman GJ. Programmed death-1 ligand 1 interacts specifically with the B7-1 costimulatory molecule to inhibit T cell responses. Immunity. 2007;27:111–22.
24. Dong H, Strome SE, Salomao DR, Tamura H, Hirano F, Flies DB, Roche PC, Lu J, Zhu G, Tamada K, Lennon VA, Celis E, Chen L. Tumor – associated B7-H1 promotes T-cell apoptosis: a potential mechanism of immune evasion. Nat Med. 2002;8:793–800.
25. Topalian SL, Hodi FS, Brahmer JR, Gettinger SN, Smith DC, McDermott DF, Powderly JD, Carvajal RD, Sosman JA, Atkins

MB, Leming PD, Spigel DR, Antonia SJ, Horn L, Drake CG, Pardoll DM, Chen L, Sharfman WH, Anders RA, Taube JM, McMiller TL, Xu H, Korman AJ, Jure-Kunkel M, Agrawal S, McDonald D, Kollia GD, Gupta A, Wigginton JM, Sznol M. Safety, activity, and immune correlates of anti-PD-1 antibody in cancer. N Engl J Med. 2012;366:2443–54.
26. Robert C, Ribas A, Wolchok JD, Hodi FS, Hamid O, Kefford R, Weber JS, Joshua AM, Hwu WJ, Gangadhar TC, Patnaik A, Dronca R, Zarour H, Joseph RW, Boasberg P, Chmielowski B, Mateus C, Postow MA, Gergich K, Elassaiss-Schaap J, Li XN, Iannone R, Ebbinghaus SW, Kang SP, Daud A. Anti – programmed – death – receptor-1 treatment with pembrolizumab in ipilimumab – refractory advanced melanoma: a randomised dose – comparison cohort of a phase 1 trial. Lancet. 2014;384: 1109–17.
27. Topalian SL, Sznol M, McDermott DF, Kluger HM, Carvajal RD, Sharfman WH, Brahmer JR, Lawrence DP, Atkins MB, Powderly JD, Leming PD, Lipson EJ, Puzanov I, Smith DC, Taube JM, Wigginton JM, Kollia GD, Gupta A, Pardoll DM, Sosman JA, Hodi FS. Survival, durable tumor remission, and long – term safety in patients with advanced melanoma receiving nivolumab. J clin oncol : off J Am Soc Clin Oncol. 2014;32:1020–30.
28. Taube JM, Klein A, Brahmer JR, Xu H, Pan X, Kim JH, Chen L, Pardoll DM, Topalian SL, Anders RA. Association of PD-1, PD-1 ligands, and other features of the tumor immune microenvironment with response to anti-PD-1 therapy. Clin cancer Res : off J Am Ass Cancer Res. 2014;20:5064–74.
29. Dudley ME, Wunderlich JR, Yang JC, Sherry RM, Topalian SL, Restifo NP, Royal RE, Kammula U, White DE, Mavroukakis SA, Rogers LJ, Gracia GJ, Jones SA, Mangiameli DP, Pelletier MM, Gea-Banacloche J, Robinson MR, Berman DM, Filie AC, Abati A, Rosenberg SA. Adoptive cell transfer therapy following non – myeloablative but lymphodepleting chemotherapy for the treatment of patients with refractory metastatic melanoma. J clin oncol: off J Am Soc Clin Oncol. 2005;23:2346–57.
30. Dudley ME, Yang JC, Sherry R, Hughes MS, Royal R, Kammula U, Robbins PF, Huang J, Citrin DE, Leitman SF, Wunderlich J, Restifo NP, Thomasian A, Downey SG, Smith FO, Klapper J, Morton K, Laurencot C, White DE, Rosenberg SA. Adoptive cell therapy for patients with metastatic melanoma: evaluation of intensive myeloablative chemoradiation preparative regimens. J clin oncol : off J Am Soc Clin Oncol. 2008;26:5233–9.

Keloids

31. Gurtner GC, Werner S, Barrandon Y, Longaker MT. Wound repair and regeneration. Nature. 2008;453(7193):314–21.
32. Chike-Obi CJ, Cole PD, Brissett AE. Keloids: pathogenesis, clinical features, and management. Semin Plast surg. 2009;23(3):178–84.
33. Sayah DN, Soo C, Shaw WW, Watson J, Messadi D, Longaker MT, Zhang X, Ting K. Downregulation of apoptosis – related genes in keloid tissues. J Surg Res. 1999;87(2):209–16.
34. Liu Y, Yang D, Xiao Z, Zhang M. miRNA expression profiles in keloid tissue and corresponding normal skin tissue. Aesthetic Plast Surg. 2012;36(1):193–201.
35. Kashiyama K, Mitsutake N, Matsuse M, Ogi T, Saenko VA, Ujifuku K, Utani A, Hirano A, Yamashita S. miR-196a downregulation increases the expression of type I and III collagens in keloid fibroblasts. J Invest Dermatol. 2012;132(6):1597–604.
36. Bloom D. Heredity of keloids; review of the literature and report of a family with multiple keloids in five generations. N Y State J Med. 1956;56(4):511–9.
37. Akoz T, Gideroglu K, Akan M. Combination of different techniques for the treatment of earlobe keloids. Aesthetic Plast Surg. 2002;26(3):184–8.
38. Marneros AG, Krieg T. Keloids – clinical diagnosis, pathogenesis, and treatment options. J Dtsch Dermatol Ges. 2004;2(11): 905–13.
39. Marneros AG, Norris JE, Watanabe S, Reichenberger E, Olsen BR. Genome scans provide evidence for keloid susceptibility loci on chromosomes 2q23 and 7p11. J Invest Dermatol. 2004;122(5): 1126–32.
40. Nakashima M, Chung S, Takahashi A, Kamatani N, Kawaguchi T, Tsunoda T, Hosono N, Kubo M, Nakamura Y, Zembutsu H. A genome – wide association study identifies four susceptibility loci for keloid in the Japanese population. Nat Genet. 2010;42(9): 768–71.
41. Rossi A, Bozzi M. [HLA and keloids: antigenic frequency and therapeutic response]. G Ital Dermatol Venereol. 1989;124(7–8): 341–4.
42. Kischer CW, Shetlar MR, Shetlar CL, Chvapil M. Immunoglobulins in hypertrophic scars and keloids. Plast Reconstr Surg. 1983; 71(6):821–5.
43. Kazeem AA. The immunological aspects of keloid tumor formation. J Surg Oncol. 1988;38(1):16–8.
44. Santucci M, Borgognoni L, Reali UM, Gabbiani G. Keloids and hypertrophic scars of caucasians show distinctive morphologic and immunophenotypic profiles. Virchows Arch : Int J pathol. 2001;438(5):457–63.
45. Niessen FB, Schalkwijk J, Vos H, Timens W. Hypertrophic scar formation is associated with an increased number of epidermal Langerhans cells. J Pathol. 2004;202(1):121–9.
46. Smith CJ, Smith JC, Finn MC. The possible role of mast cells (allergy) in the production of keloid and hypertrophic scarring. J Burn Care Rehabil. 1987;8(2):126–31.
47. Zhang Q, Oh CK, Messadi DV, Duong HS, Kelly AP, Soo C, Wang L, Le AD. Hypoxia – induced HIF-1 alpha accumulation is augmented in a co – culture of keloid fibroblasts and human mast cells: involvement of ERK1/2 and PI-3K/Akt. Exp Cell Res. 2006;312(2):145–55.
48. Eishi K, Bae SJ, Ogawa F, Hamasaki Y, Shimizu K, Katayama I. Silicone gel sheets relieve pain and pruritus with clinical improvement of keloid: possible target of mast cells. J Dermatolog Treat. 2003;14(4):248–52.
49. Seifert O, Mrowietz U. Keloid scarring: bench and bedside. Arch Dermatol Res. 2009;301(4):259–72.
50. Bayat A, Arscott G, Ollier WE, Ferguson MW, Mc Grouther DA. Description of site – specific morphology of keloid phenotypes in an Afrocaribbean population. Br J Plast Surg. 2004;57(2):122–33.
51. Poochareon VN, Berman B. New therapies for the management of keloids. J Craniofac Surg. 2003;14(5):654–7.
52. Chen MA, Davidson TM. Scar management: prevention and treatment strategies. Curr Opin Otolaryngol Head Neck Surg. 2005;13(4):242–7.
53. Mustoe TA, Cooter RD, Gold MH, Hobbs FD, Ramelet AA, Shakespeare PG, Stella M, Teot L, Wood FM, Ziegler UE. International clinical recommendations on scar management. Plast Reconstr Surg. 2002;110(2):560–71.
54. Kelly AP. Medical and surgical therapies for keloids. Dermatol Ther. 2004;17(2):212–8.
55. Alster TS, Tanzi EL. Hypertrophic scars and keloids: etiology and management. Am J Clin Dermatol. 2003;4(4):235–43.
56. Jacob SE, Berman B, Nassiri M, Vincek V. Topical application of imiquimod 5% cream to keloids alters expression genes associated with apoptosis. Br J Dermatol. 2003;149 Suppl 66:62–5.
57. Bilu D, Sauder DN. Imiquimod: modes of action. Br J Dermatol. 2003;149 Suppl 66:5–8.
58. Berman B, Flores F. Recurrence rates of excised keloids treated with postoperative triamcinolone acetonide injections or interferon alfa-2b injections. J Am Acad Dermatol. 1997;37(5 Pt 1):755–7.
59. Wendling J, Marchand A, Mauviel A, Verrecchia F. 5-fluorouracil blocks transforming growth factor – beta – induced alpha 2 type I

collagen gene (COL1A2) expression in human fibroblasts via c – Jun NH2-terminal kinase/activator protein-1 activation. Mol Pharmacol. 2003;64(3):707–13.
60. Liu A, Moy RL, Ozog DM. Current methods employed in the prevention and minimization of surgical scars. Dermatol Surg : off Pub Am Soc for Dermatol Surg. 2011;37(12):1740–6.
61. Borok TL, Bray M, Sinclair I, Plafker J, LaBirth L, Rollins C. Role of ionizing irradiation for 393 keloids. Int J Radiat Oncol Biol Phys. 1988;15(4):865–70.
62. Ehrlich HP, Desmouliere A, Diegelmann RF, Cohen IK, Compton CC, Garner WL, Kapanci Y, Gabbiani G. Morphological and immunochemical differences between keloid and hypertrophic scar. Am J Pathol. 1994;145(1):105–13.

Squamous Cell Carcinoma (SCC)

63. Edge SB, Byrd DR, Compton CC, et al. Cutaneous squamous cell carcinoma and other cutaneous carcinomas. In: AJCC cancer staging manual. Springer, Berlin 2010.
64. Siegel RL, Miller KD, Jemal A. Cancer statistics. CA Cancer J Clin. 2015;65:5–29.
65. Rogers HW, Weinstock MA, Harris AR, Hinckley MR, et al. Incidence estimate of nonmelanoma skin cancer in the United States, 2006. Arch Dermatol. 2010;146:283–7.
66. Diepgen T l, Mahler V. .The epidemiology of skin cancer. Br J Dermatol. 2002;146:1–6.
67. Adams CC, Thomas B, Bingham JL. Cutaneous squamous cell carcinoma with perineural invasion: a case report and review of the literature. Cutis. 2014;93:141–4.
68. Rowe DE, Carroll RJ, Day CL. Prognostic factors for local recurrence, metastasis, and survival rates in squamous cell carcinoma of the skin, ear, and lip. Implications for treatment modality selection. J Am Acad Dermatol. 1992;26:976–90.
69. Jambusaria-Pahlajani A, et al. Evaluation of AJCC tumor staging for cutaneous squamous cell carcinoma and a proposed alternative tumor staging system. JAMA Dermatol. 2013;149:402–10.
70. Brougham NDLS, Dennett ER, Cameron R, Tan ST. The incidence of metastasis from cutaneous squamous cell carcinoma and the impact of its risk factors. J Surg Oncol. 2012;106: 811–5.
71. Brougham NDL, Tan ST. The incidence and risk factors of metastasis for cutaneous squamous cell carcinoma – implications on the T – classification system. J Surg Oncol. 2014;110:876–82.
72. Chen JG, et al. Cost of nonmelanoma skin cancer treatment in the United States. Dermatol Surg. 2001;27:1035–8.
73. Mudigonda T, Pearce DJ, Yentzer BA, Williford P, Feldman SR. The economic impact of non – melanoma skin cancer: a review. J Natl Compr Canc Netw. 2010;8:888–96.
74. Housman TS, et al. Skin cancer is among the most costly of all cancers to treat for the medicare population. J Am Acad Dermatol. 2003;48:425–9.
75. Xiang F, Lucas R, Hales S, Neale R. Incidence of nonmelanoma skin cancer in relation to ambient UV radiation in white populations, 1978–2012: empirical relationships. JAMA Dermatol. 2014;150:1063–71.
76. Brougham NDL, Dennett ER, Tan ST. Non – melanoma skin cancers in New Zealand – a neglected problem. N Z Med J. 2010;123:59–65.
77. Hoy WE. Nonmelanoma skin carcinoma in albuquerque, New Mexico: experience of a major health care provider. Cancer. 1996;77:2489–95.
78. Freeman SE, et al. Wavelength dependence of pyrimidine dimer formation in DNA of human skin irradiated in situ with ultraviolet light. Proc Natl Acad Sci U S A. 1989;86:5605–9.
79. Kripke ML. Immunologic mechanisms in UV radiation carcinogenesis. Adv Cancer Res. 1981;34:69–106.
80. Ayli EE, et al. Activation of Src – family tyrosine kinases in hyperproliferative epidermal disorders. J Cutan Pathol. 2008;35: 273–7.
81. Jost M, Kari C, Rodeck U. The EGF receptor – an essential regulator of multiple epidermal functions. Eur J Dermatol. 2000;10: 505–10.
82. Kalyankrishna S, Grandis JR. Epidermal growth factor receptor biology in head and neck cancer. J Clin Oncol. 2006;24:2666–72.
83. Zhao L, et al. Srcasm inhibits Fyn – induced cutaneous carcinogenesis with modulation of Notch1 and p53. Cancer Res. 2009;69:9439–47.
84. Kolev V, et al. EGFR signalling as a negative regulator of Notch1 gene transcription and function in proliferating keratinocytes and cancer. Nat Cell Biol. 2008;10:902–11.
85. Lefort K, Dotto GP. Notch signaling in the integrated control of keratinocyte growth/differentiation and tumor suppression. Semin Cancer Biol. 2004;14:374–86.
86. Lefort K, et al. Notch1 is a p53 target gene involved in human keratinocyte tumor suppression through negative regulation of ROCK1/2 and MRCKalpha kinases. Genes Dev. 2007;21:562–77.
87. Boukamp P. Non – melanoma skin cancer: what drives tumor development and progression? Carcinogenesis. 2005;26:1657–67.
88. Kripke ML, Fisher MS. Immunologic parameters of ultraviolet-carcinogenesis. J Natl Cancer Inst. 1976;57:211–5.
89. Kripke ML, Morison WL. Modulation of immune function by UV radiation. J Invest Dermatol. 1985;85:62s–5.
90. Ratushny V, Gober MD, Hick R, Ridky TW, Seykora JT. From keratinocyte to cancer: the pathogenesis and modeling of cutaneous squamous cell carcinoma. J Clin Invest. 2012;122:464–72.
91. Brash DE, et al. A role for sunlight in skin cancer: UV induced p53 mutations in squamous cell carcinoma. Proc Natl Acad Sci U S A. 1991;88(22):10124–8.
92. Kubo Y, et al. p53 gene mutations in human skin cancers and precancerous lesions: comparison with immunohistochemical analysis. J Invest Dermatol. 1994;102(4):440–4.
93. Khavari PA. Modelling cancer in human skin tissue. Nat Rev Cancer. 2006;6:270–80.
94. Ziegler A, et al. Sunburn and p53 in the onset of skin cancer. Nature. 1994;372:773–6.
95. Pierceall WE, Goldberg LH, Tainsky MA, Mukhopadhyay T, Ananthaswamy HN. Ras gene mutation and amplification in human nonmelanoma skin cancers. Mol Carcinog. 1991;4: 196–202.
96. Kwa RE, Campana K, Moy RL. Biology of cutaneous squamous cell carcinoma. J Am Acad Dermatol. 1992;26:1–26.
97. Hannuksela-Svahn A, Pukkala E, Karvonen J. Basal cell skin carcinoma and other nonmelanoma skin cancers in Finland from 1956 through 1995. Arch Dermatol. 1999;135:781–6.
98. Harwood CA, et al. Human papillomavirus infection and non – melanoma skin cancer in immunosuppressed and immunocompetent individuals. J Med Virol. 2000;61:289–97.
99. Jensen P, et al. Skin cancer in kidney and heart transplant recipients and different long – term immunosuppressive therapy regimens. J Am Acad Dermatol. 1999;40:177–86.
100. Euvrard S, Ulrich C, Lefrancois N. Immunosuppressants and skin cancer in transplant patients: focus on rapamycin. Dermatol Surg. 2004;30:628–33.
101. Euvrard S, et al. Comparative epidemiologic study of premalignant and malignant epithelial cutaneous lesions developing after kidney and heart transplantation. J Am Acad Dermatol. 1995;33:222–9.
102. Dantal J, et al. Effect of long – term immunosuppression in kidney – graft recipients on cancer incidence: randomised comparison of two cyclosporin regimens. Lancet. 1998;351:623–8.

103. Tanaka T, et al. A novel immunosuppressive drug, FTY720, prevents the cancer progression induced by cyclosporine. Cancer Lett. 2002;181:165–71.
104. Wu X, et al. Opposing roles for calcineurin and ATF3 in squamous skin cancer. Nature. 2010;465:368–72.
105. Yakupoglu YK, Buell JF, Woodle S, Kahan BD. Individualization of immunosuppressive therapy.III sirolimus associated with a reduced incidence of malignancy. Transplant Proc. 2006;38: 358–61.
106. Mathew T, Kreis H, Friend P. Two – year incidence of malignancy in sirolimus – treated renal transplant recipients: results from five multicenter studies. Clin Transplant. 2004;18:446–9.
107. Hofbauer GFL, Bouwes Bavinck JN, Euvrard S. Organ transplantation and skin cancer: basic problems and new perspectives. Exp Dermatol. 2010;19:473–82.
108. Derancourt C, et al. Oncogenic human papillomaviruses in extra – genital Bowen disease revealed by in situ hybridization. Ann Dermatol Venereol. 2001;128:715–8.
109. Zheng S, et al. Human papillomaviruses of the mucosal type are present in some cases of extragenital Bowen's disease. Br J Dermatol. 2005;152:1243–7.
110. Meyer T, Arndt R, Christophers E, Nindl I, Stockfleth E. Importance of human papillomaviruses for the development of skin cancer. Cancer Detect Prev. 2001;25:533–47.
111. De Jong-Tieben LM, et al. High frequency of detection of epidermodysplasia verruciformis – associated human papillomavirus DNA in biopsies from malignant and premalignant skin lesions from renal transplant recipients. J Invest Dermatol. 1995;105: 367–71.
112. Feltkamp MCW, de Koning MNC, Bavinck JNB, ter Schegget J. Betapapillomaviruses: Innocent bystanders or causes of skin cancer. J Clin Virol. 2008;43:353–60.
113. Bavinck JNB, Plasmeijer EI, Feltkamp MCW. β – Papillomavirus Infection and Skin Cancer. J Invest Dermatol. 2008;128:1355–8.
114. Bahner JD, Bordeaux JS. Non – melanoma skin cancers: photodynamic therapy, cryotherapy, 5-fluorouracil, imiquimod, diclofenac, or what?Facts and controversies. Clin Dermatol. 2013;31:792–8.
115. Lansbury L, Bath-Hextall F, Perkins W, Stanton W, Leonardi-Bee J. Interventions for non – metastatic squamous cell carcinoma of the skin: systematic review and pooled analysis of observational studies. BMJ. 2013;347:f6153.
116. Kuflik EG. Cryosurgery for skin cancer: 30-year experience and cure rates. Dermatol Surg. 2004;30:297–300.
117. Green A, et al. Daily sunscreen application and betacarotene supplementation in prevention of basal – cell and squamous – cell carcinomas of the skin: a randomised controlled trial. Lancet. 1999;354:723–9.
118. Thompson SC, Jolley D, Marks R. Reduction of solar keratoses by regular sunscreen use. N Engl J Med. 1993;329:1147–51.
119. Harvey DT, Taylor RS, Itani KM, Loewinger RJ. Mohs micrographic surgery of the eyelid: an overview of anatomy, pathophysiology, and reconstruction options. Dermatol Surg. 2013;39: 673–97.
120. Belkin D, Carucci JA. Mohs surgery for squamous cell carcinoma. Dermatol Clin. 2011;29:161–74.
121. Task Force AH, et al. AAD/ACMS/ASDSA/ASMS 2012 appropriate use criteria for mohs micrographic surgery: a report of the American academy of dermatology, American college of mohs surgery, American society for dermatologic surgery association, and the American society for mohs surgery. J Am Acad Dermatol. 2012;67(531–550).
122. Pugliano-Mauro M, Goldman G. Mohs surgery is effective for high – risk cutaneous squamous cell carcinoma. Dermatol Surg. 2010;36:1544–53.
123. Sakaguchi S, et al. Immunologic self tolerance maintained by T – cell – mediated control of self – reactive T cells: implications for autoimmunity and tumor immunity. Microbes Infect. 2001;3: 911–8.
124. Perrotta RE, Giordano M, Malaguarnera M. Non – melanoma skin cancers in elderly patients. Crit Rev Oncol Hematol. 2011;80: 474–80.
125. Elmets CA, Athar M. Milestones in photocarcinogenesis. Nat Milestones. 2013:E13–7. doi:10.1038/skinbio.2013.179.
126. Grossman D, Leffell DJ. The molecular basis of nonmelanoma skin cancer: new understanding. Arch Dermatol. 1997;133:1263–70.
127. Loser K, et al. IL-10 controls ultraviolet – induced carcinogenesis in mice. J Immunol. 2007;179:365–71.
128. Shreedhar V, Giese T, Sung VW, Ullrich SE. A cytokine cascade including prostaglandin E2, IL-4, and IL-10 is responsible for UV – induced systemic immune suppression. J Immunol. 1998;160:3783–9.
129. Steinbrink K, et al. Interleukin-10-treated human dendritic cells induce a melanoma – antigen – specific anergy in CD8(+) T cells resulting in a failure to lyse tumor cells. Blood. 1999;93: 1634–42.
130. Beissert S, Hosoi J, Grabbe S, Asahina A, Granstein RD. IL-10 inhibits tumor antigen presentation by epidermal antigen – presenting cells. J Immunol. 1995;154:1280–6.
131. Simon JC, Cruz PD, Bergstresser PR, Tigelaar RE. Low dose ultraviolet B-irradiated Langerhans cells preferentially activate CD4+ cells of the T helper 2 subset. J Immunol. 1990;145: 2087–91.
132. Meeran SM, Mantena SK, Meleth S, Elmets CA, Katiyar SK. Interleukin-12-deficient mice are at greater risk of UV radiation – induced skin tumors and malignant transformation of papillomas to carcinomas. Mol Cancer Ther. 2006;5:825–32.
133. Halak BK, Maguire HC, Lattime EC. Tumor – induced interleukin-10 inhibits type 1 immune responses directed at a tumor antigen as well as a non – tumor antigen present at the tumor site. Cancer Res. 1999;59:911–7.
134. Kim J, et al. IL-10 production in cutaneous basal and squamous cell carcinomas A mechanism for evading the local T cell immune response. J Immunol. 1995;155:2240–7.
135. Chen W, et al. Conversion of peripheral CD4+CD25- naive T cells to CD4+CD25+ regulatory T cells by TGF-beta induction of transcription factor Foxp3. J Exp Med. 2003;198:1875–86.
136. Cederbom L, Hall H, Ivars F. CD4+CD25+ regulatory T cells down – regulate co – stimulatory molecules on antigen – presenting cells. Eur J Immunol. 2000;30:1538–43.
137. Shevach EM, McHugh RS, Piccirillo CA, Thornton AM. Control of T-cell activation by CD4+ CD25+ suppressor T cells. Immunol Rev. 2001;182:58–67.
138. Clark RA, et al. Human squamous cell carcinomas evade the immune response by down – regulation of vascular E – selectin and recruitment of regulatory T cells. J Exp Med. 2008;205: 2221–34.
139. Urosevic M, Dummer R. Immunotherapy for nonmelanoma skin cancer: does it have a future? Cancer. 2002;94:477–85.
140. Amini S, Viera MH, Valins W, Berman B. Nonsurgical innovations in the treatment of nonmelanoma skin cancer. J Clin Aesthet dermatol. 2010;3:20.
141. Love WE, Bernhard JD, Bordeaux JS. Topical imiquimod or fluorouracil therapy for basal and squamous cell carcinoma: a systematic review. Arch Dermatol. 2009;145:1431–8.
142. Sauder DN. Immunomodulatory and pharmacologic properties of imiquimod. J Am Acad Dermatol. 2000;43:S6–11.
143. Huang SJ, et al. Imiquimod enhances IFN – gamma production and effector function of T cells infiltrating human squamous cell carcinomas of the skin. J Invest Dermatol. 2009;129:2676–85.
144. Ikić D, et al. Interferon therapy for basal cell carcinoma and squamous cell carcinoma. Int J Clin Pharmacol Ther Toxicol. 1991;29:342–6.

145. Edwards L, et al. Treatment of cutaneous squamous cell carcinomas by intralesional interferon alfa-2b therapy. Arch Dermatol. 1992;128:1486–9.
146. Scaltriti M, Baselga J. The epidermal growth factor receptor pathway: a model for targeted therapy. Clin Cancer Res. 2006;12: 5268–72.
147. Maubec E, et al. Phase II study of cetuximab as first – line single – drug therapy in patients with unresectable squamous cell carcinoma of the skin. J Clin Oncol. 2011;29:3419–26.
148. Bejar C, Maubec E. Therapy of advanced squamous cell carcinoma of the skin. Curr Treat Options Oncol. 2014;15:302–20.
149. Alter M, Satzger I, Mattern A, Kapp A, Gutzmer R. Treatment of advanced cutaneous squamous cell carcinomas with epidermal growth factor receptor inhibitors. Dermatology. 2013;227:289–94.

Mycosis Fungoides

150. Robson A, et al. The pathology of cutaneous T-cell lymphoma. Oncology (Williston Park). 2007;21(2 Suppl 1):9–12.
151. Vowels BR, et al. Aberrant cytokine production by Sezary syndrome patients: cytokine secretion pattern resembles murine Th2 cells. J Invest Dermatol. 1992;99:90–4.
152. Dummer R, et al. Sezary syndrome, T-helper 2 cytokines and accessory factor-1 (AF-1). Leuk Lymphoma. 1998;28:515–22.
153. Berger CL, et al. Cutaneous T-cell lymphoma: malignant proliferation of T-regulatory cells. Blood. 2005;105:1640–7.
154. Wong HK, et al. Increased expression of ctla-4 in malignantT-cells from patients with mycosis fungoides - cutaneousTcell lymphoma. J Invest Dermatol. 2006;126:212–9.
155. Tiemessen MM, et al. Lack of suppressive CD4 + CD25+ FOXP3+ Tcells in advanced stages of primary cutaneousT- cell lymphoma. J Invest Dermatol. 2006;126:2217–23.
156. Vowels BR, et al. Th2 cytokine mRNA expression in skin in cutaneousT-cell lymphoma. J Invest Dermatol. 1994;103: 669–73.
157. Asadullah K, et al. Progression of mycosis fungoides is associated with increasing cutaneous expression of interleukin- 10 mRNA. J Invest Dermatol. 1996;107:833–7.
158. Papadavid E, et al. The relevance of peripheral blood T-helper 1and 2 cytokine pattern in the evaluation of patients with mycosis fungoides and Sezary syndrome. Br J Dermatol. 2003;148: 709–18.
159. Weaver CT, et al. Th17: an effector CD4 Tcell lineage with regulatoryTcell ties. Immunity. 2006;24:677–88.
160. Teunissen MB, et al. Interleukin-17 and interferon – gamma synergize in the enhancement of proinflammatory cytokine production by human keratinocytes. J Invest Dermatol. 1998;111: 645–9.
161. Krejsgaard T, et al. Elucidating the role of interleukin-17F in cutaneous T-cell lymphoma. Blood. 2013;122(6):943–50.
162. Willemze R, et al. Primary cutaneous lymphomas: ESMO Clinical Practice Guidelines for diagnosis, treatment and follow – up. Ann Oncol. 2013;24 Suppl 6:vi149–54.
163. Wong HK, et al. Novel biomarkers, dysregulated epigenetics, and therapy in cutaneous T-cell lymphoma. Discov Med. 2013; 16(87):71–8.
164. Jain S, et al. Novel therapeutic agents for cutaneous T-Cell lymphoma. J Hematol Oncol. 2012;5:24.
165. Akilov OE, et al. Therapeutic advances in cutaneous T-cell lymphoma. Skin Therapy Lett. 2011;16(2):1–5.

Autoimmune Dermatoses

13

Jie Zheng, Meng Pan, S. Gianfaldoni, A.M. D'Erme, T. Lotti, Xingqi Zhang, Peng Zhang, Jin Yuan, Qianjin Lu, Ken Hashimoto, and Fiona Lewis

Contents

J. Zheng (✉) • M. Pan
Department of Dermatology, Rui Jin hospital, School of Medicine, Shanghai Jiao Tong University, 197 Rui Jin Er Road, Shanghai, China
e-mail: jie-zheng2001@126.com

S. Gianfaldoni
Dermatological Department, University of Pisa, Pisa, Italy

A.M. D'Erme
Division of Dermatology, University of Florence, Florence, Italy

T. Lotti (✉)
University of Rome "G. Marconi", Rome, Italy
e-mail: professor@torellolotti.it

X. Zhang (✉)
Department of Dermatology, The First Affiliated Hospital of Sun Yat-sen University, Guangzhou 510080, China
e-mail: xingqi.zhang@aliyun.com

P. Zhang • J. Yuan • Q. Lu (✉)
Department of Dermatology, Hunan Key Laboratory of Medical Epigenomics, Second Xiangya Hospital, Central South University, #139 Renmin Middle Road, Changsha, Hunan 410011, China
e-mail: qianlu5860@gmail.com

K. Hashimoto, MD (✉)
Wayne State University School of Medicine, Detroit, MI, USA

F. Lewis
Wexham Park Hospital, Wexham Street, Slough SL2 4HL, UK

St John's Institute of Dermatology, St Thomas Hospital, Lambeth Palace Road, London SE1 7EH, UK
e-mail: fiona.lewis@fhft.nhs.uk

13.1 Immunobullous Diseases

13.1.1 Pemphigus

Jie Zheng and Meng Pan

Pemphigus is a group of autoimmune blistering diseases of the skin and mucous membranes, with incompletely understood

X.-H. Gao, H.-D. Chen (eds.), *Practical Immunodermatology*, DOI 10.1007/978-94-024-0902-4_13

pathogenic mechanism [1, 2]. Pemphigus usually occurs in the middle and old age, with equal frequency in both sexes. Predisposing genetic background is thought to be essential in the development of pemphigus. To date, the association between HLA class II and pemphigus has been well documented [3–5]. Circulating autoantibodies directed against the cell surface of keratinocytes occured in pemphigus results in acantholysis, the loss of cell–cell adhesion of keratinocytes, and subsequent blister formation. Pemphigus of severe type has been reported in patients with underlying neoplasms.

13.1.1.1 Etiology and Pathogenesis

At present, pemphigus is considered as a group of autoimmune response [6]. The pemphigus autoantibodies found in patients' sera play a pathogenic role in the disease. Patients with pemphigus vulgaris or pemphigus foliaceus have autoantibodies against desmoglein (Dsg)3 and/or Dsg1, which locate in desmosomes on the cell membrane of keratinocytes [7, 8]. The collective action of autoantibodies against self-antigen results in the loss of cell–cell adhesion between keratinocytes, and subsequent blister formation possibly due to collapse and shrinkage of the keratinocytes, IgG-triggered activation of signaling pathways of apoptosis [9, 10].

The onset of paraneoplastic pemphigus is mostly associated with malignant neoplasm [11]. Patients with paraneoplastic pemphigus have a complex of autoantibodies against members of plakin family in addition to desmogleins, including desmplakin-I, envoplakin, periplakin, plectin, and the 230-kDa bullous pemphigoid antigen [12] (Table 13.1).

Drugs may induce or exacerbate pemphigus, especially the drugs containing a sulfhydryl group such as penicillamine, captopril, piroxieam, and rifampicin [13, 14].

13.1.1.2 Clinical Features

According to the clinical features, pemphigus is divided into four major forms: pemphigus vulgaris, pemphigus vegetans, pemphigus foliaceus, and pemphigus erythematosus. Other rare types include pemphigus herpetiformis, IgA pemphigus, paraneoplastic pemphigus (PNP), and drug-induced pemphigus.

Pemphigus Vulgaris

Pemphigus vulgaris is the most frequent type of pemphigus diseases. The lesions may appear in oral mucosa, head, neck, and trunk. The throat, esophagus, conjunctivae, nasal mucosa, vagina, penis, anus, and labia can be involved as well. Over 60% of cases initiate as painful and long-persisting erosions in the oral mucosa. More than half of the patients also develop flaccid blisters and widespread cutaneous erosions. The primary skin lesions of pemphigus vulgaris are flaccid, thin-walled, easily ruptured blisters. They can appear on either normal-appearing skin or erythematous bases. The blisters are fragile and soon rupture to form painful erosions that ooze and bleed easily (Fig. 13.1). During the active phase of pemphigus vulgaris, Nikolsky sign can be

Table 13.1 Types of pemphigus and related self-antigen

Type	Pemphigus vulgaris	Pemphigus vegetans	Pemphigus foliaceus	Pemphigus erythematosus	Paraneoplastic pemphigus
Antigen	Dsg1 Dsg3	Dsg1 Dsg3	Dsg1	Dsg1	Envoplakin Periplakin Desmoplakin I Desmoplakin II

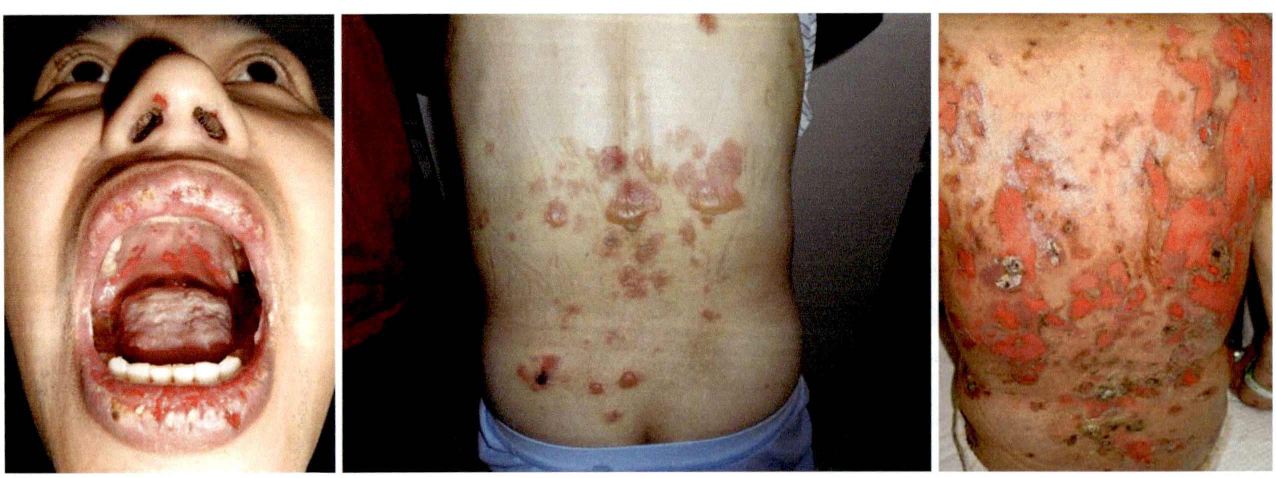

Fig. 13.1 Pemphigus vulgaris

elicited. Without appropriate treatment, pemphigus vulgaris can be fatal because a large area of the skin loses its epidermal barrier function, leading to the failure or secondary bacterial infections.

Pemphigus Vegetans

Pemphigus vegetans is a rare vegetative variant of pemphigus vulgaris. Pemphigus vegetans is characterized by flaccid blisters that become erosions and then form fungoid vegetations or papillomatous proliferations, especially in intertriginous areas (nose lip channel, breast, umbilical fossa, underarms, groin) and on the scalp or face. Pustules rather than vesicles characterize early lesions, but these soon progress to vegetative plaques. The mucous membranes can also be involved (Fig. 13.2).

Pemphigus Foliaceus

Pemphigus foliaceus usually occurs in middle-aged or elderly persons. Lesions of the patients with pemphigus foliaceus usually present as seborrheic distribution, i.e., the face, scalp, and upper trunk. The patients develop scaly, crusted cutaneous erosions, often on an erythematous base. Because the vesicle is so superficial and fragile, often only the resultant crust and scale are seen, below which is a moist, strong smelly surface with a tendency to bleed. The Nikolsky sign is present. The atypically skin lesions are swelling and hyperemia of the local skin, peeling off of the superficial skin with a small amount of exudative erosion, forming a blade shaped crusts, similar to the exfoliative dermatitis. But pemphigus foliaceus do not have clinically apparent mucosal involvement (Fig. 13.3).

Pemphigus Erythematosus

Pemphigus erythematosus is simply a localized benign variant of pemphigus foliaceus. Typical scaly and crusted lesions of pemphigus foliaceus are usually localized on the malar region of the face and in other "seborrheic" areas. Early lesions are scattered superficial blisters in different sizes with positive Nikolsky sign, which are easily broken to form erosion surface with yellow scab or sebaceous scales (Fig. 13.4). Exposure to sun may exacerbate disease activity. Generally, in addition to a slight itching, the patients with pemphigus erythematosus are not severely ill.

13.1.1.3 Other Type of Pemphigus

Herpetiform Pemphigus

This disorder is characterized by erythematous urticarial plaques and vesicles that present in a herpetiform arrangement, with severe itching. Mucous membrane involvement is gentle. Not like other types of pemphigus, the blisters of herpetiform pemphigus are tense. The Nikolsky sign is negative. Some patients with herpetiform pemphigus will evolve into pemphigus foliaceus or vulgaris [15, 16].

IgA Pemphigus

Two distinct types of IgA pemphigus have been described: the subcorneal pustular dermatosis (SPD) type and the intraepidermal neutrophilic (IEN) type. The most common sites of involvement are the axilla and groin, but the trunk and proximal extremities can also be involved. The palms and soles are not always involved, and mucous membrane involvement is rare. Patients with both types of IgA pemphigus present with flaccid vesicles or pustules on either erythematous or normal skin. The pustules tend to coalesce to form an annular or circinate pattern with crusts in the center of the lesion and some blisters in the margin. In IgA pemphigus patients, pruritus is often a significant symptom.

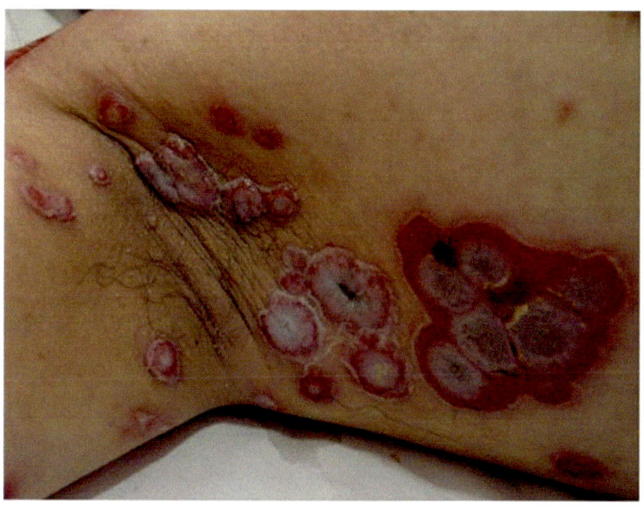

Fig. 13.2 Pemphigus vegetans

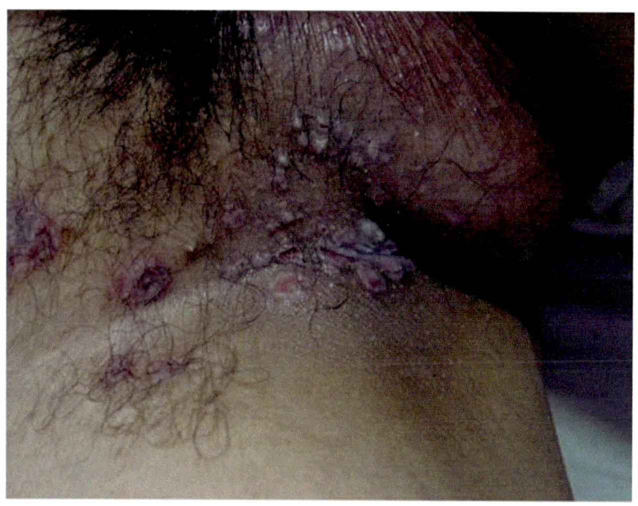

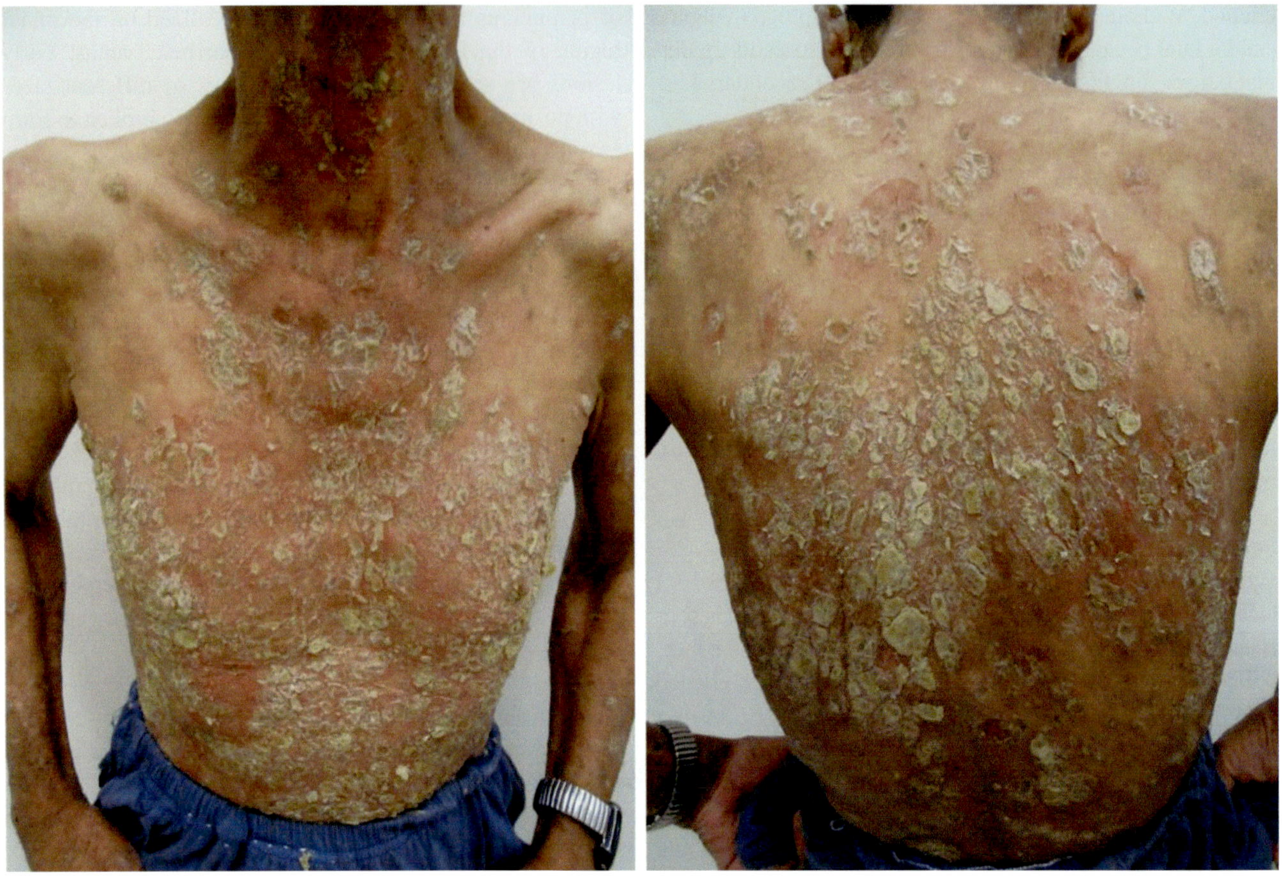

Fig. 13.3 Pemphigus foliaceus

Paraneoplastic Pemphigus (PNP)

Paraneoplastic pemphigus is commonly associated with underlying neoplasms, both malignant and benign, with high rates of mortality, which can occur in all ages. The most commonly associated neoplasms are lymphoproliferative disorders (non-Hodgkin lymphoma, chronic lymphocytic leukemia, Castleman's disease, malignant and benign thymomas, and so on) [17]. Castleman's disease, a very rare lymphoproliferative type, is the most commonly associated neoplasm in PNP patients in China. Other associated tumors include adenocarcinomas of the breast, lung carcinoma, cervical cancer, squamous cell carcinomas, and so on. The most consistent clinical feature of paraneoplastic pemphigus is the presence of severe stomatitis extremely resistant to therapy. This stomatitis consists of erosions, ulcerations, and bleeding that affect all surfaces of the vermilion lip and the oropharynx. Most patients also have a painful ulcerative pseudomembranous conjunctivitis, which may progress to scarring and obliteration of the conjunctival fornices. Esophageal, nasopharyngeal, vaginal, labial, and penile mucosal lesions may also be seen. Cutaneous findings on trunk and extremities are quite polymorphic and may present as erythematous macules, blisters and erosions, scabby and papulosquamous damage, erythema multiforme-like lesions, and lichenoid eruptions on the palms and soles. The pain is often a significant symptom.

Drug-Induced Pemphigus

The onset of drug-induced pemphigus occurs several weeks or months after responsible drug intake. 15–50 % of patients with drug-induced pemphigus recover spontaneously when the drug is withdrawn. Some patients will develop into pemphigus foliaceus or erythematosus.

13.1.1.4 Histopathology and Laboratory Tests

Histopathology: The histopathology of pemphigus typically demonstrates intraepidermal clefts and blisters formation with acantholysis. Blister cavities contain some acantholytic cells. The location of acantholysis in the level of intraepidermal is different in each type of pemphigus [17, 18].

Immunofluorescence: Direct immunofluorescence (DIF) studies of perilesional tissue demonstrate IgG and/or C3 deposited on the surface of keratinocytes [19]. In pemphigus erythematosus, DIF also demonstrates as grainy deposition of IgG and/or C3 along the basement-membrane zone. Indirect immunofluorescence (IIF) studies show circulating antibodies against cell surface of keratinocytes.

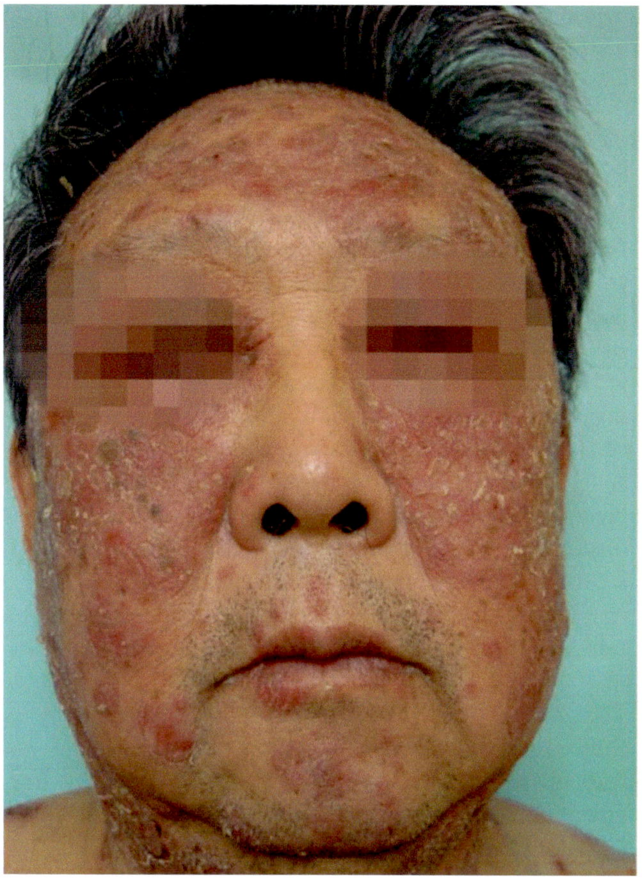

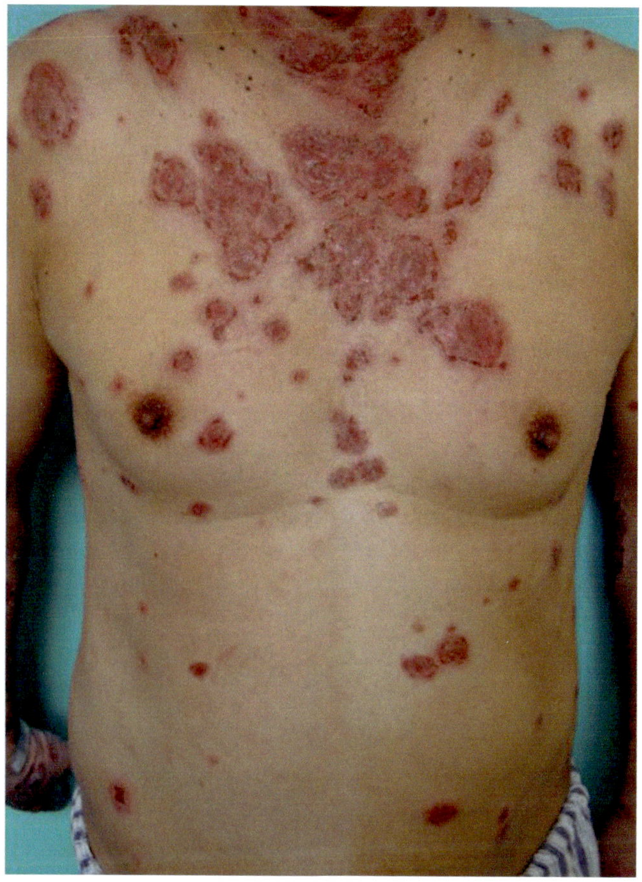

Fig. 13.4 Pemphigus erythematosus

Cytological examination: The smear is taken from a recent lesion by gently scraping with a straight scalpel. The material obtained is smeared onto a microscope slide, air dried, and routinely Gram stained. Single or group of acantholytic cells can be detected. The cells are round, sometimes perfectly circular, intercellular bridge disappeared, showing an abundant basophilic cytoplasm and a single, round hypertrophic nucleus with one or two prominent, viable nucleoli. Characteristically, the cytoplasm basophilic staining is deeper peripherally close to the cell membrane [20].

Enzyme-linked immunosorbent assay (ELISA): Detection of anti-Dsg1 and anti-Dsg3 antibodies can distinguish between pemphigus vulgaris and pemphigus foliaceus. The antibody titers correlate with disease activity. With the improvement of clinical symptoms, antibody titer declines or becomes negative. The specific IgG subtypes are particularly important in the assessment of disease severity and prognosis [21].

13.1.1.5 Diagnosis and Differential Diagnosis

The diagnosis and classification of pemphigus is confirmed by clinical manifestations, histopathology examination, and immunofluorescence test. The differential diagnosis of pemphigus includes bullous pemphigoid, dermatitis herpetiformis, linear IgA bullous disease, epidermolysis bullosa acquisita, erythema multiforme bullosum, subcorneal pustular dermatosis, and familial benign pemphigus. Aphthous ulcer of oral cavity and lichen planus should be considered in the differential diagnosis of the patients with oral lesions.

13.1.1.6 Prevention and Treatment

Patients need high protein and high vitamin diet and should be pay attention to maintain water–electrolyte balance. Side effects inherent to long-term application of glucocorticoids and immunosuppressants should be monitored carefully, including hypertension, diabetes, osteoporosis, aseptic necrosis of femoral head, secondary infection, water and electrolyte disorders, mental nerve symptom and so on.

1. Systemic therapy
   1. Glucocorticoid: At present, systemic corticosteroids are the first choice therapy. Patients should be treated once the diagnosis is established. The initial dose should be enough to control the symptom. It depends on the severity and extent of the disease. If treated and tapered regularity, most patients can be relapse free and stop taking medicine after 4–5 years treatment [22, 23].

2. Immunosuppressive drugs: Azathioprine, cyclophosphamide, methotrexate, cyclosporine, or mycophenolate mofetil combined with corticosteroids can be effective. Patients on these agents can develop side effects such as gastroenteric reaction, bone marrow suppression, hepatic and renal toxicity [24].
3. High-dose intravenous immunoglobulin (IVIg):
   High-dose IVIg is an effective adjunctive therapy in refractory disease or in case of contraindications to immunosuppressants [25].
4. Monoclonal antibody therapy: Alone or in combination with immunosuppressive drugs or intravenous immunoglobulin. Rituximab, an anti-CD20 monoclonal antibody, is usually prescribed for patients with severe pemphigus vulgaris [26].
5. Other treatment: Tripterygium wilfordii, dapsone, thalidomide, nicotinamide, tetracycline, levamizole, chlorambucil or plasma exchange, immunoadsorption therapy, extracorporeal photochemotherapy, all have some effects [27].

2. Topical therapy

Careful nursing is important and can prevent secondary infection. Exposure therapy can be used for treatment of patients with wide range of lesions. Bath or wound dress with 1:8000 liquor potassii permanganatis or 1:1000 benzalkonium bromide is recommended to patients with erosive lesions. Patients with infectious lesions should be treated with effective antibiotics according to the results of bacterial culture. Oral lesions can be treated with mouthwash, tacrolimus ointment, or iodine glycerol [28].

13.1.2 Bullous Pemphigoid

Bullous pemphigoid (BP) is a subepidermal immunobullous disease, mainly affecting the elderly [29]. There are strong evidences indicate that binding of autoantibodies to hemidesmosome antigen plays an important role in the subepidermal blisters formation.

13.1.2.1 Etiology and Pathogenesis

The exact pathogenesis of BP remains unclear. The two major bullous pemphigoid antigens are BP230 and BP180. BP230 is an intracellular composition of hemidesmosome, while BP180 is a transmembrane protein. Patients with BP developed autoantibodies mainly directed to BP180 and BP230. The binding of circulating autoantibodies directed to their target antigens evokes a cascade of events including complement activation, recruitment of inflammatory cells, chemokines and protease releasing, and subsequent subepidermal blister formation [30–33]. The triggering factor of this disease also include drug intake (such as furosemide, penicillamine, fluorouracil, amoxicillin, ciprofloxacin, potassium iodide, phenacetin, captopril, and so on), traumas, burns, ultraviolet light, radiotherapy, and bed ridden [34].

13.1.2.2 Clinical Features

Bullous pemphigoid usually starts with skin itching with/without nonspecific rashes that may be eczema-like, urticaria-like, or excoriation-like lesions. Characteristic lesions of BP include tense blisters or bullae on erythematous or apparently normal skin, and may be accompanied by urticaria-like or infiltrated papule and plaque. The tense blisters can be up to 1–7 cm in diameter, contain clear or bloody fluid (Fig. 13.5). The Nikolsky sign is negative. Erosions can heal rapidly and left hyperpigmentation or hypopigmentation, occasionally milia. Scars are rare. Mucosal lesions occur in 10~30% of the patients, which are mild and transitory.

Clinical variants of BP include pemphigoid nodularis, vesicular pemphigoid, erythrodermic bullous pemphigoid, localized bullous pemphigoid, and so on.

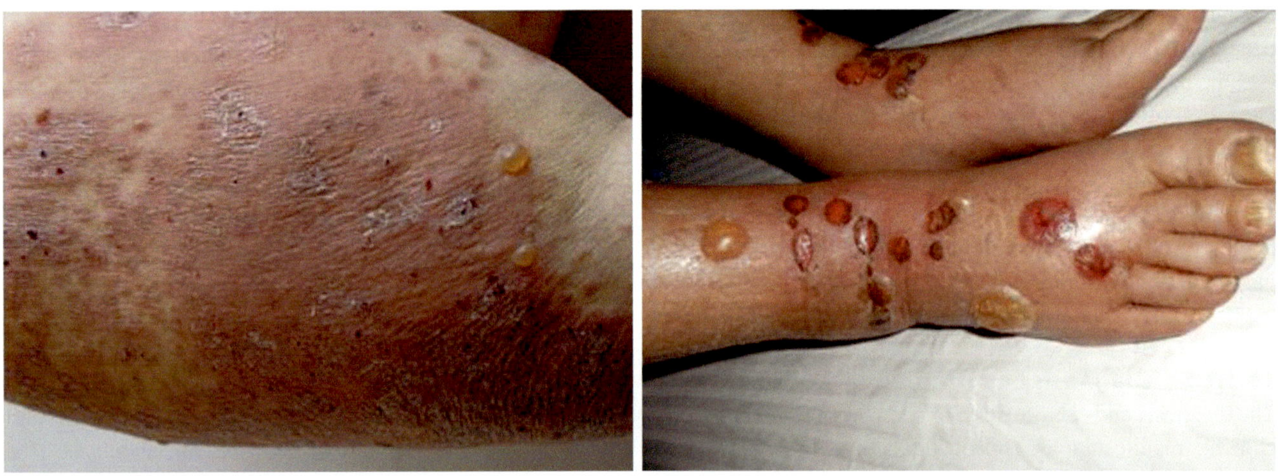

Fig. 13.5 Bullous pemphigoid

13.1.2.3 Histopathology and Laboratory Tests

Histologic features typically demonstrate as subepidermal blisters accompanied a dermal inflammatory infiltrate composed of eosinophils and mononuclear cells.

A perilesional biopsy specimen for direct immunofluorescence can typically demonstrate as linear deposition of IgG and/or C3 along the basement-membrane zone in most patients. When the perilesional specimen is treated with 1 mol/L sodium chloride (salt-split skin), immune deposits can be found in the epidermal side or in both the epidermal side and dermal side of the split.

The process of ELISA techniques to detect antibodies against specific antigens of BP180 and BP230 is found to be convenient and very sensitive in the diagnosis of BP. It has been shown that the serum levels of IgG and IgE autoantibodies to BP180 correlate with the disease severity [30–32, 35–37].

13.1.2.4 Prevention and Treatment

BP follows a chronic course. Severe itches and blisters result to a poor quality of life in BP patients. Severe BP can be fatal [38, 39]. Thus, it is necessary to control the disease in time. Disease severity, complications, and patients' persistence in topical therapy all over the body should all be taken into consideration when making treatment plans.

Evidence shows that both systemic and topical corticosteroids have efficacy in BP and either one can be used alone or as adjunct therapies of other treatments. There are suggestions that systemic antibiotics may be much safer to those patients with diabetes or hypertension or to children need more samples to be confirmed [40–42]. Immunosuppressive drugs, high-dose IVIg, and plasma exchange are also be used in severe patients.

13.2 Vitiligo

S. Gianfaldoni, A.M. D'Erme, and T. Lotti

13.2.1 Introduction

Vitiligo is an acquired pigmentary cutaneous disease, characterized by the progressive loss of melanocytes, resulting in hypopigmented skin areas which progressively become amelanotic.

Clinically, vitiligo is characterized by asymptomatic milk-white macules and patches, with well-defined borders. The color contrast between the healthy pigmented skin and the vitiliginous patches, results in a leopard-like skin appearance [43].

13.2.2 Vitiligo Clinical Presentation and Autoimmunity

Lesions may be singular or multiple, varying in form and size. At the beginning, they are usually small, round, or oval in form, affecting limited skin areas. As the disease progress, lesions tend to enlarge and to involve new tegumental areas. Vitiliginous patches may also coalesce into bigger sized lesions.

An uncommon form of vitiligo is the red form (also known as inflammatory vitiligo), characterized by an erythematous halo surrounding the white patches.

Another rare variant of vitiligo is the trichrome variant [44], which is characterized by a hypopigmented area between the central amelanotic zone and the peripheral normal skin. In darker skin phototypes, a quadrichrome vitiligo has been also described. It is characterized by the presence of repigmentation foci at the follicular ostia. Rare is the pentachrome vitiligo, in which lesions show the occurrence of five shades of color from white to black [45].

Finally, there is a blue vitiligo, characterized by a bluish color appearance of the skin, as a result of the presence of dermal melanophages [46].

Skin lesions may affect any part of the body, however, they are more often localized on the body folds, periorificial, and sun-exposed sites. Characteristic lesions of vitiligo is the Koebner's phenomenon (or "isomorphic response"), referring to the development of new skin lesions on trauma sites.

Mucosal regions may be affected similarly to the cutaneous regions. Moreover, a variable percentage of patients have a damage of the melanocytes within the hair follicles, which result in a depigmentation of hair (leukotrichia).

In addition to such more common clinical features, vitiligo patients may show extracutaneous abnormalities of the melanocytes, like eyes, ears, brain, heart, and lungs [47].

13.2.3 Classification

Vitiligo can be classified into localized (focal, unilateral/segmental, and mucosal), generalized (vulgaris, acrofacial, and mixed), and universal (including also special forms such as trichrome vitiligo, quadrichrome vitiligo, and inflammatory vitiligo) according to the extension of the involved areas [48–56].

Furthermore, on the basis of the clinical features and natural history, vitiligo has been classified as segmental or non-segmental [52–56].

Segmental vitiligo (SV) is characterized by one or more vitiliginous patches in a linear or flag-like pattern of mosaicism with a unilateral dermatomal distribution. It is characterized by rapid onset and involvement of the hair follicle pigmentary system. A dysfunction of sympathetic nerves has been hypothesized in its pathogenesis. In the basis of the lesions' localization, SV may be classified as unisegmental, bisegmental, or multisegmental. Among these, the unisegmental type is the most commonly described. It consists of a singular or multiple white macules localized on one side of the body, usually respecting the body midline.

Segmental vitiligo is usually described in children, where it tends to remain localized. Unlike the nonsegmental forms, the association to autoimmune diseases is uncommon. A particular common manifestation of SV is poliosis, which clinically characterized by a patch of white hair and poor treatment responses [49–52].

Nonsegmental vitiligo (NSV) is the most common form of vitiligo and it is characterized by the involvement of several parts of the body, usually with a symmetrical pattern. Clinically, NSV is represented by a heterogeneous group of pigmentary disorders with different localization. Among these, the most commonly described is the generalized vitiligo, also known as common type or vitiligo vulgaris, characterized by multiple lesions in a symmetrical pattern. Even if common vitiligo may affect any part of the cutaneous areas, it is most commonly seen on the face, the digits and the trauma-exposed areas.

Another form of nonsegmental vitiligo is the acrofacial form, characterized by white macules and patches localized on the face, the head and on the distal end of extremities, where it usually involves the fingers. Over the time, acrofacial vitiligo may evolve and become widespread.

Particular is the mixed vitiligo, characterized by the combination of segmental and nonsegmental lesions.

Universal vitiligo is another variant of NSV, consisting in the complete or nearly complete skin depigmentation (80–90 % body's surface). Scalp hair involvement is common, and some patients may also show mucosal lesions. Universal vitiligo is the most common type in adulthood, and usually represents the evolution of the common form.

More rarely, a mucosal vitiligo has been described, where lesions are localized on the oral and genital mucosa. Lesions may be isolated or associated with more common types of lesions.

Finally, there are rare variants such as the punctata, the minor, or the follicular variant. The former is characterized by small, punctuate-like, depigmented macules. Minor vitiligo is a particularly rare condition, described in dark-skinned individuals, characterized by a partial defect in pigmentation.

Also rare is the follicular vitiligo, a form of generalized vitiligo involving the follicular reservoir with poor cutaneous lesions.

Recently, the *Vitiligo Global Issues Consensus Conference 2011–2012 (VGICC)* has introduced a third group of lesions that are the undetermined lesions [48]. Undetermined vitiligo comprises the focal and the mucosal forms. The former is characterized by small isolated lesions without segmental localization, and not evolving into NSV after a period of at least 2 years. Moreover, the latter is characterized by lesions affecting only one mucosa.

13.2.4 Autoimmunity Comorbidities

Various studies suggest that vitiligo's patients have an increased risk of developing autoimmune and endocrine diseases [53]. Among these, the association with autoimmune thyroid disorders is well known. Other endocrinologic disorders less commonly associated to vitiligo include hypoparathyroidism, Addison's disease, polyglandular syndrome type I and type II, and diabetes mellitus. Vitiligo has been also described in association with hematologic disorders (e.g. autoimmune hemolytic anemia, pernicious anemia) and several skin diseases (e.g. pemphigus vulgaris, alopecia areata, morphea). Of particular interest is the correlation between vitiligo and melanoma. The development of the depigmentary disorders in melanoma's patients seems to lead to more favorable prognosis maybe as a sign of an active immune response direct versus melanocytes.

Recent data support the linkage of vitiligo with systemic inflammatory disorders, such as obesity and the metabolic syndrome [54].

13.2.5 Pathophysiology and Autoimmunity

The etiopathogenesis of vitiligo is best described as multifactorial, polygenic and with incomplete penetrance [49, 55]. Despite new researches and progresses, the pathogenesis of vitiligo is still enigmatic. It remains unclear what represent an environmental trigger or other triggers that might induce localized dysfunction, damage, and subsequent death of melanocytes in predisposed patients [56].

Several theories regarding etiology have been proposed in vitiligo but they are not so strongly supported. Nowadays the most evidence support an autoimmune phenomenon associated with underlying genetic predisposition; even genetic studies are not so contributory at the moment [56, 57]. In fact, most of the cases of vitiligo are sporadic and up to 20 % of patients report an affected relative [58, 59]. The incidence of concordance of vitiligo in monozygotic twins is only 23 % [58]. This low concordance indicates that vitiligo is inherited in a non-Mendelian, multifactorial, and polygenic pattern, with incomplete penetrance and underlie how the environmental factors can be important for the development of vitiligo [55, 56, 58].

Regarding the vitiligo genetic/individual susceptibility, recent studies have investigated the role of human leukocyte antigen (HLA) haplotypes [60, 61].

Some studies have pointed out the frequent elevation of major histocompatibility complex classes I and II (HLAs-A2, -DR4, -DR7, and -DQB1*0303) among vitiligo patients and suggesting an implication of cellular and humoral immunity [49, 62–65].

The strongest associations of vitiligo with particular HLA haplotypes appear to be in patients and families with various vitiligo-associated autoimmune/autoinflammatory syndromes, further supporting an autoimmune diathesis [57, 66].

Other susceptibilities have been studied with regards to a small nucleotide polymorphisms in cytotoxic T lymphocyte antigen 4, a negative feedback regulator of T cell activation and proliferation, associated with patients with both vitiligo and concomitant autoimmune disease [57, 67].

Nonreceptor type 22 encoding the gene for lymphoid protein tyrosine phosphatase and mannose-binding lectin are among other factors studied recently in vitiligo [57, 68].

Nevertheless, the etiopathogenesis of vitiligo is largely unknown, it is likely to be multifactorial in nature, or rather being an amalgamation of different combinations of pathophysiological theories, including autoimmunity, neurogenic dysregulation, autocytotoxicity, biochemical dysregulation, oxidative stress, melanocytorrhagy, and frail melanocyte viability [49, 56, 57].

It is still not known what roles these pathophysiological mechanisms have in the different forms of vitiligo. In this chapter we are going to analyze deeply the immunological process in vitiligo, even a role of other kind of process can have an outstanding role in the vitiligo lesions' development.

13.2.6 (Auto)Immune Mechanisms in Vitiligo

There is substantial evidence for the immune-mediated destruction of melanocytes. As reported before, this evidence starts from the clinical coexistence of melanocyte destruction with the presence of autoimmune diseases, particularly autoimmune endocrinological disease (thyroid) [49, 69–81].

Furthermore, patients suffering from melanoma who develop hypopigmentation during their follow-up have a better prognosis, indicating that a common immune response to melanocytes is responsible for both hypopigmentation and tumor control [56, 57, 72].

A humoral immunity involvement in vitiligo patients has been highlighted by the presence of the circulating antibodies versus melanocyte antigens which denoted and categorized as antibodies to cell surface pigment cell antigens (as VIT40, VIT75, and VIT90), intracellular pigment cell antigens, and nonpigment cell antigens (common tissue antigens). For example, the antibodies to cell surface pigment cell antigens are present in 83 % of vitiligo patients in comparison to 7 % of controls [49, 57, 73–75].

Furthermore antibodies against tyrosinase and tyrosinase-related proteins 1 and 2 (TRP-1 and TRP-2) and SOX9 and SOX10 (transcription factors involved in the differentiation of cells derived from the neural crest) have been reported in vitiligo patients with different incidence [82-86].

These antibodies may activate antibody-dependent cytotoxic pathways that can lead to the melanocytes apoptosis [47, 49, 66–76].

Altered cellular immunity is also present and can have a role in vitiligo, in addition or in combination with a humoral response [57].

In perilesional skin, a high number of epidermotropic T cells exerting antimelanocytic cytotoxic activity against Melan-A/MART1, tyrosinase, and gp100 have been shown to be frequently juxtaposed to the remaining melanocytes. They present an increased CD8/CD4 ratio, express adhesion and activation molecule [87, 88].

Moreover studies have shown that Melan-A specific CD8+ T cells are highly present in peripheral blood of vitiligo patients in a proportional number to the severity and extension of the disease [47, 89–91].

The involvement of genetic, immunologic, autoimmunologic, cytotoxic, neuronal, autocytotoxic, biochemical, oxidative, melanocyte, and inflammatory factors has been supported by several intriguing but not always proven researches. The autoimmune hypothesis remains as one of the more interesting hypotheses [49–52, 56, 57].

Nonsegmental vitiligo represents a spectrum of many different disorders with different etiologies and pathogeneses causing a common phenotype: the loss of melanocytes and/or their products [56].

13.2.7 Practical Immunology in Vitiligo

Because of several autoimmune comorbidities, it is recommended to rule out the presence of associated diseases through the autoimmune antibodies and clinical laboratory data, as reported in Table 13.2 [50–52, 89].

At the moment there are no available laboratory biomarkers to evaluate the vitiligo severity and the possible association with autoimmune comorbidities [53].

13.2.8 "Immune" Therapy

In the last years, several therapeutic options [90], both medical and surgical, have been proposed for vitiligo. Surgical therapies are recommended in patients who have a stable vitiligo and not responding to medical treatments. Among these, corticosteroids, calcineurin inhibitors, and phototherapies are still the mainstay of medical treatment of vitiligo.

The therapeutic efficacy of corticosteroids as anti-inflammatory and immunosuppressant agents has been known for many years. Topical steroids are recommended for the treatment of limited areas of vitiligo. They are quite safe but their use should be limited for 2–4 months to avoid

Table 13.2 first and second line autoantibodies to be checked in a patient with vitiligo

Circulating autoantibodies to be checked	
Routine	
	Anti-thyroid peroxidase Ab (ATPO)
	Anti-thyroglobulin Ab (ATG)
	Anti-thyroid
	Anti-parietal gastric cell antibody
	Total IgE
Second line	
	Anti-nuclear Ab (ANA)
	Additional autoantibodies (only if patient's history, family history and/or laboratory parameters highlight a strong risk of additional autoimmune disease or if endocrinologist/immunologist advice if multiple autoimmune syndrome detected
Laboratory data	
Thyroid stimulating hormone (TSH)	
Eosinophil count	
Vitamin B12	
Folic acid	

Routine laboratory data to be checked [52, 89, 90]

percutaneous adsorption and local side effects (e.g. skin atrophy, striae, telangiectasia, hypertrichosis, acneiform eruption). Systemic steroids are useful in vitiligo patients with rapid course to stop the progression of the disease and to induce repigmentation.

A valid alternative to corticosteroids in the treatment of vitiligo are the calcineurin inhibitors (tacrolimus and pimecrolimus), which are immunosuppressant agents. They are usually applied twice a day, alone or in combination with corticosteroids or phototherapy. Recent studies suggest how calcineurin inhibitors have the same efficacy to topical corticosteroids without the risk of cutaneous atrophy in the long-term use [91].

Finally there is phototherapy; the last four decades have seen significant technological advances in the field of phototherapy which evolved from PUVA to the introduction of narrowband UVB (NB-UVB) [47].

PUVA therapy consists of oral medication of a photosensitizing psoralen followed by exposure to photoactivating UVA light (320–400 nm). Treatment is done two to three times a week, increasing the dose of UVA according to patient's response. The treatment is not always safe and the side effects are due to both radiations (erythema, pruritus, xerosis, phototoxic reactions, chronic actinic damage, and carcinogenesis) and psoralens (e.g. gastric and ocular damage). The most common short-time side effects are erythema, pruritus, xerosis, and phototoxic reactions. Long-term side effects include chronic actinic damage and carcinogenesis.

Better results in terms of efficacy and safety profile have been achieved with the more recent narrow-band UVB (311 nm). The treatment of the exposure to NB-UVB starts at the dose 0.1 mJ/cm^2, followed by 20 % increasing dose of UVR on a weekly basis according to response. Treatment is generally well tolerated, but the side effects due to radiation are well described (e.g. pruritus, erythema, photodamaging).

More recent is the target phototherapy, which consists of the treatment limited just to the affected vitiliginous areas, avoiding exposure to unaffected skin. Target phototherapy acts as the same modalities of classical phototherapy but in a more precise way because of treating only the skin lesions, the operator can use more appropriate dose of energy in a safer way. New encouraging results are coming from a new UVA1–355 nm laser therapy, which has been proved to be efficacious facing the inflammatory immune response in psoriasis and eczema [92].

13.3 Alopecia Areata

Xingqi Zhang

13.3.1 Overview of Alopecia

Alopecia is a group of diseases with prominent feature of hair loss. They can be divided into congenital and acquired disorders. The later can also be divided into scarring/cicatricial (primary and secondary) and nonscarring alopecia. Nonscarring alopecias are the most commonly found hair loss disorders in hair clinics, including alopecia areata and androgenic alopecia, etc.

Primary scarring alopecias are a group of rare diseases of the inflammation specifically targeting hair follicles [93]. These disorders destroy the hair follicles, result in permanent hair loss, and often lead to discomfort and serious psychological distress in patients. The commonly used classification is proposed by the North American Hair Research Society, which divides the entities into lymphocytic group (e.g., chronic cutaneous lupus erythematosus and lichen planopilaris), neutrophilic group (e.g., folliculitis decalvans), mixed group, and nonspecific group according to the histopathologic features [94]. Secondary scarring alopecias are a group of diseases or physical and chemical factors affecting scalp and hair follicles.

Here we focus on alopecia areata (AA), a commonly seen nonscarring alopecia.

13.3.2 Definition and Epidemiology

AA is a recurrent, inflammatory nonscarring hair loss condition that affects people of all ages without sex predilection. The condition affects 0.1–0.2 % of humans, with a calculated lifetime risk of approximately 2 %, making it one of the most prevalent autoimmune diseases [95, 96]. Owing to its devastating effects on a patient's quality of life and self-esteem, AA is not simply a "cosmetic problem" [97]. Although

AA usually occurs in apparently healthy individuals without skin disorders, there is a higher risk of developing allergic diseases such as allergic rhinitis, asthma, eczema, and atopic dermatitis among AA patients than normal people [98, 99].

13.3.3 Pathogenesis

The pathogenesis of AA is still largely unknown, but studies revealed that genetic linkage and environmental factors are involved [100–102]. Currently, evidence points to a T cell–driven immune reaction inducing fast regression of hair follicles [103, 104]. Autoimmunity, loss of immune privilege in hair follicle, stress and neuroendocrine etc., all take part in the pathogenesis of AA [105, 106].

Clinical clues include presence of autoantibodies against HF, higher prevalence of autoimmune diseases such as thyroiditis and vitiligo in AA patients [107], and correlation with certain types of HLA subtypes [108, 109]. One study involving 513 cases of AA showed that severe AA subtypes (alopecia totalis/alopecia universalis or AT/AU) could possibly be associated with familial autoimmunity and thyroid disease [110]. Recently, allergy to common allergens is also investigated in AA, with the finding that sIgE to dust mite is elevated in AA patients with early onset and severe types [111].

13.3.4 Clinical Features

AA is characterized by sudden onset of hair loss in the form of round or oval patches with a clear margin, without much of discomfort. Hair loss is usually complete with a smooth skin surface. Extension of hair loss lesion usually occurs at peripheral of the lesion, or new hair loss patches elsewhere. In half of the cases, there is a tendency to be self-limited, i.e., hair regrowth starts spontaneously without any intervention. However, in a minority of patients, the course progresses, resulting in loss of all the scalp hairs (AT), or together with all of the body hairs (AU).

Clinical subtypes include patchy (single and multiple), reticular (extensive patchy), ophiasis, diffuse AA/AA incognita [112], AT, and AU (Fig. 13.6). Clinical stages include progressive, stable, and recovery stage. Positive in pull test is characteristic for progressive stage.

Loss of eyebrow and eyelashes can be affected alone or together with scalp hairs, but usually occurs in patients with severe hair loss. Nail pits also present in patients with severe types of AA.

Comorbidity profile includes disorders of autoimmunity such as vitiligo, autoimmune thyroid diseases, and connective tissue diseases such as Sjogren's syndrome and lupus erythematosus. Also, higher frequency of atopic diseases including atopic dermatitis and allergic rhinitis was found in AA patients [113].

13.3.5 Pathological Features

The major histological features of AA are the regression of hair follicles and the peribulbar and intrabulbar mononuclear cell infiltrate, which can be considered to be a diagnostic feature [114, 115] (Fig. 13.7a, b). The presence of eosinophils was found to be a helpful diagnostic feature of alopecia [116] (Fig. 13.7c).

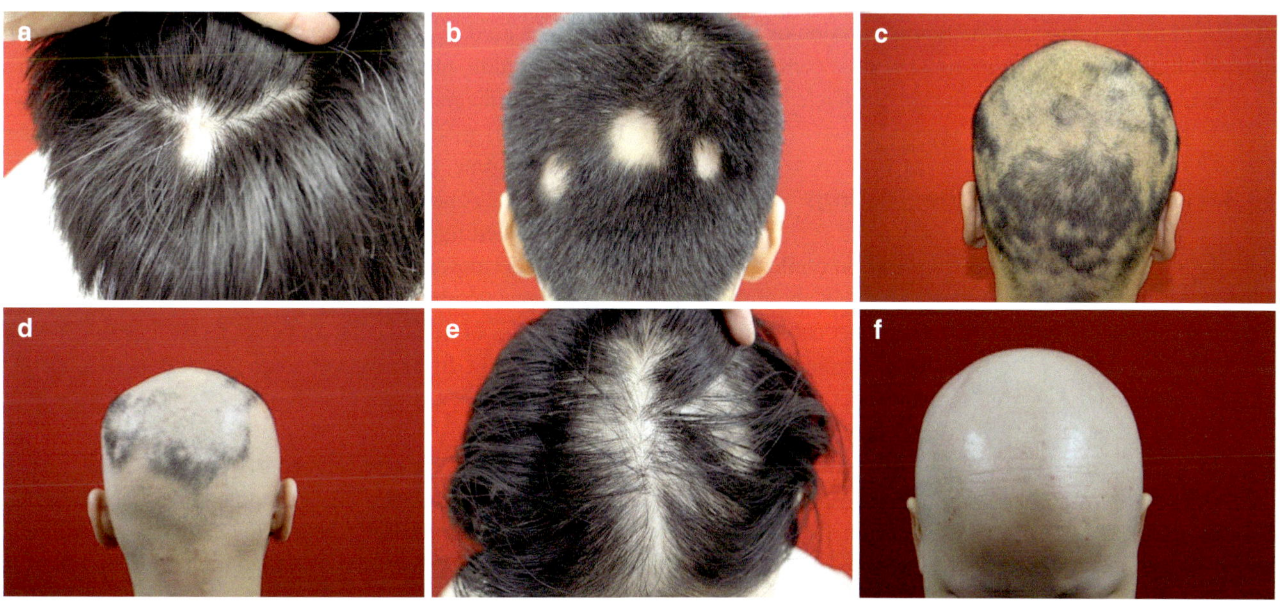

Fig. 13.6 Clinical subtypes of alopecia areata. Clinical subtypes include single patchy (**a**), multiply patchy (**b**), reticular (extensive patchy, **c**), Ophiasis (**d**), diffuse AA/AA incognita (**e**), AU (alopecia universalis, **f**)

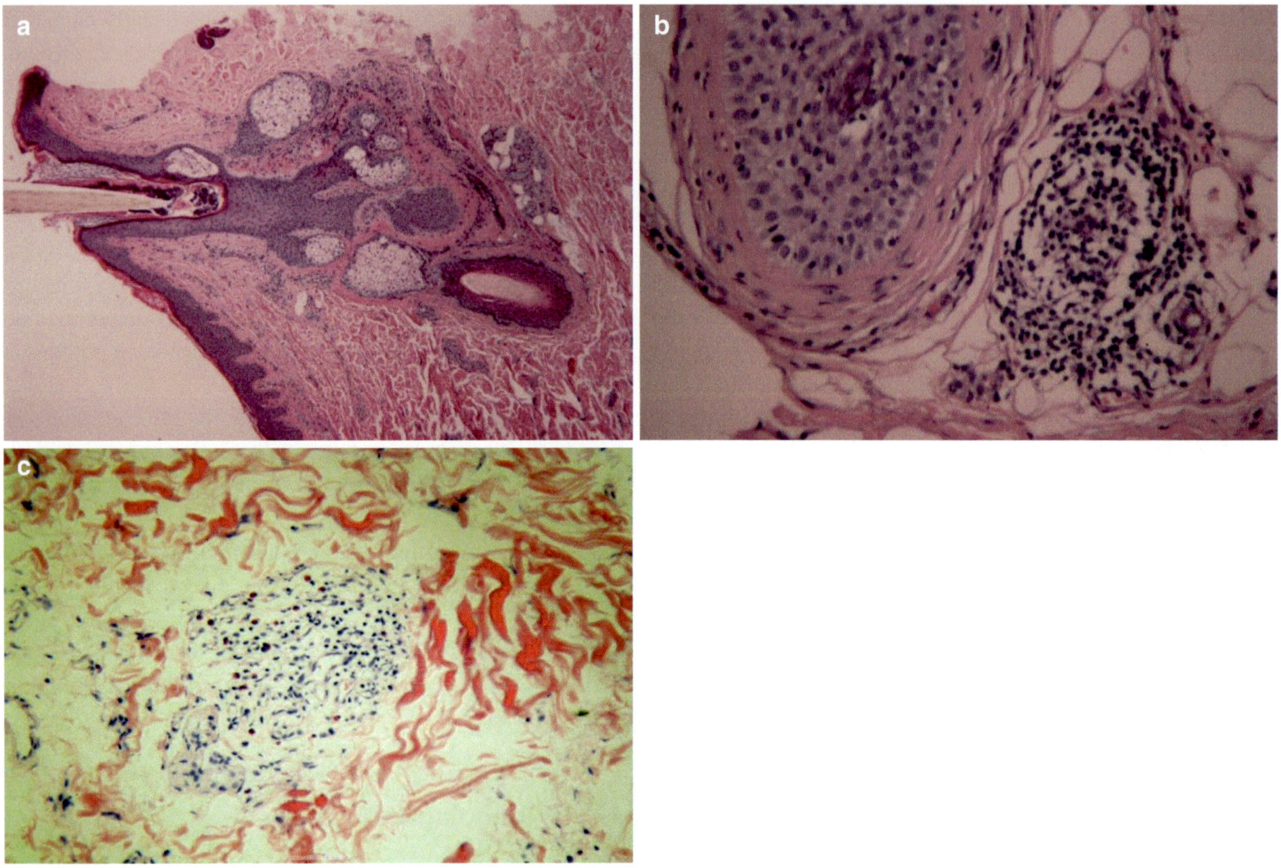

Fig. 13.7 Histopatological changes of alopecia areata. Histopatological changes of alopecia areata are regression of hair follicles (**a**, ×40), perifollicular mononuclear cell infiltrate (**b**, ×400), and presence of eosinophils in rapid progression lesion (**c**, ×400).

We found that early AA is histologically characterized as vascular dilation, edema, perifollicular and perivascular infiltration of mononuclear cells and mast cells in upper dermis, damage of upper HF, accompanied by morphological changes of ORS in the infundible of HF, and regression of lower follicle. Infiltration of T cells in upper dermis consists of both $CD4^+$ and $CD8^+$ T cells inside the upper follicle [117, 118].

13.3.6 Laboratory and Other Testings

Usually, diagnosis of AA can be based on clinical features and dermoscopy. However, if there is a doubt about the diagnosis, the following laboratory tests are needed: fungal culture, biopsy and histopathology, serology test for autoantibodies and syphilis, thyroid function tests, serum IgE, allergen tests, level of ferritin.

13.3.6.1 Dermoscopy

Specific dermoscopic patterns can be found from hair-loss region in patients with AA, i.e., yellow dots, short vellus hair, black dots, broken hairs, irregular hairs, exclamation mark hairs, and uneven thickness of hair shafts [119]. It facilitates diagnosis, evaluation of disease activity and effectiveness of therapies of AA. Yellow dots are highly sensitive and can be used as a preliminary screening marker. Existence of exclamation mark hairs, black dots and broken hairs confirm the diagnosis of AA and indicate disease activity. This provides guidance to the clinician in choosing proper treatment regime. Broken hairs, numeral black dots or short broken hairs in one follicular unit, splitting or curling of broken ends, bleeding dots are commonly seem in trichotillomania. Also, dermoscopy proves to be a useful tool in diagnosis of androgenetic alopecia, syphilis alopecia, and in differential diagnosis of nonscarring alopecia, as well as in discerning the cause in diffuse type of acute alopecia.

13.3.7 Diagnosis and Differential Diagnosis

In most cases, diagnosis can be made by clinical observation. Diseases need to differential excluded include trichotillomania, tinea capitis, pseudo Palada in scarring alopecia, androgenic alopecia, patchy hair loss in systemic lupus erythematosus and syphilis alopecia, etc. Dermoscopy and sometimes histopathologic examination are required to make a correct diagnosis.

13.3.8 Management

13.3.8.1 Baseline of Treatment Option

There is still no cure for AA currently due to unrevealed pathogenesis. The aim of management is set to enhance hair regrowth and reduce relapse, but not to eradicate it. An effective treatment modality is composed of anti-inflammatory and inducement of hair follicle to enter anagen to start the process of hair regrowth. Early intervention is encouraged to prevent turning into severe form and relapse, although it is controversial in the Western world, where many hold 'wait and see' policy due to spontaneous remission in part of the AA patients.

One of references to design an effective treatment model is that the disease is not detrimental to the general health and important organs, although it is a strong psychological stress. Besides, no cure for AA is present at the moment. Therefore, it is not recommended to use medications with severe side effects. Systematic corticosteroids is usually effective for parts of cases, but it is not recommended to maintain hair regrowth for its severe side effects, weakening response of repeated use and relapse of AA after cessation of administration.

British Dermatology Association published a guideline for AA management in 2013 [120]. It recommended topical and intralesional injection of steroids for patchy hair loss; contact immunotherapy and hair piece/wig for extensive hair loss (AT/AU).

13.3.8.2 Counseling and General Management

Counseling is vital in clinical setting to explain the nature of the disease, and what treatment outcome patients should be expected. Avoidance of stress and effective stress management, quality sleep and balanced diet, physical exercise are all encouraged to facilitate a satisfactory treatment outcome. For patients with severe types and seasonal relapse, allergen detection and desensitization may have some help.

13.3.8.3 Treatment Modalities

Current AA treatment modalities mainly include topical and systemic corticosteroids, T-cell inhibitors, topical hair follicle stimulants, and topical immunotherapy [121, 122].

1. Mild type.

   Single patch of hair loss with short disease duration can be intervened with only oral corticosteroids and potent topical steroids and minoxidil.
2. Extensive, progressive, and severe types.

   For these cases and for AT/AU with disease duration shorter than 2 years, short-term systematic steroids can be used, best with tapered amount starting from prednisone of 0.5 mg/kg/day for a total of around 3 months. We used three to four intramuscular injection of long acting steroids with an interval of 3 weeks.
3. Chronicity and relapse.

   For those patients with recurrent relapse, only treat those with unfulfilled need for outlook. It is best to avoid using systemic steroids in recurrent and frequent relapsing cases. Contact immunotherapy or wig can be considered here.
4. Childhood AA.

   Childhood AA are fast progressive and easy to enter AT/AU status. We use potent topical steroids in occlusion, and it is effective in 90 % of cases. Side effects include folliculitis, atrophy of skin, and hypertrichosis.
5. Contact immunotherapy.

   Topical contact immunotherapy is reserved for patients with extensive hair loss, especially for AT/AU. It was first introduced as a treatment for AA in 1978 treated with dinitrochlorobenzene and has already been used for more than 30 years. Squaric acid dibutylester and diphenylcyclopropenone (DPCP) have since been used extensively as contact sensitizers for AA [123]. DPCP is a nonmutagenic chemical substance with a high sensitization potency, which does not react with other contact allergens; therefore it has been the common agent used in the treatment of severe types of AA. DPCP treatment has been found to have an efficacy rate ranging from 5 to 85 %, with a relapse rate ranging from 10.6 to 68.9 % [124]. In our group of 63 patients treated with DPCP, the efficacy was 61 % and relapse rate was 28 %.
6. New drugs and others.

   Prostaglandin $F_2\alpha$ analog is effective in treating AA patients with eyebrow loss, but other bio and immune suppressors seems to be not effective. Laser, PUVA, Botox, and platelet-rich plasma had been reported effective in AA treatment.
7. No treatment.

   No treatment is a good choice for those with severe types and long disease duration, due to the psychological and financial burden to the patients and repeated cycles of hair regrowth and loss.
8. Wig and hair piece.

   For patients with severe types and long disease duration, prosthesis is a good choice.

13.3.9 Prognosis

Patients usually have a poor prognosis if with a long disease course, young age at onset, large hair loss area, AD, and nail change.

13.4 Lupus Erythematosus

Peng Zhang, Jin Yuan, and Qianjin Lu

13.4.1 Introduction

Lupus erythematosus (LE) is generally regarded as a spectrum-like chronic, autoimmune disorder, ranging from a purely cutaneous form to a life-threatening systemic type, with a common feature that the immune system becomes hyperactive and harmful to normal, healthy tissues. Originally, the word *lupus* means *wolf* in Latin, as the destructive injuries caused by LE are similar to the bites caused by the wolf. There are four main types of lupus erythematosus: systemic, discoid, drug-induced, and neonatal, of which systemic lupus erythematosus (SLE) is the most common and serious type.

In this chapter, we will focus on the pathogenesis, clinical presentations, as well as treatments of various types of LE.

13.4.2 Epidemiology

According to recent studies, the incidence of cutaneous LE (CLE) in Sweden and USA is around 4/100,000 inhabitants [125, 126]. The incidence of SLE in the USA is 5.1 per 100,000 per year [127]. Although the prevalence of SLE is varied in different counties, the highest is reported in Italy, Spain, and Martinique population [128]. Gender is a strong risk factor for lupus. The incidence of SLE is up to 10 times more common in women than in men, and generally has a predilection for women in their childbearing years. Discoid LE (DLE) patients also show female predominance with female-to-male ratio of about 3:1 [125]. Besides gender, ethnicity is also a risk factor for SLE. In USA, SLE is more common in African Americans, Hispanics, and Asians than in Caucasians [128].

13.4.3 Etiology/Pathogenesis

The underlying etiology of lupus erythematosus is still incompletely known, and some factors are believed to play important roles in its pathogenesis, such as genetic background, virus infection, drugs, UVB exposure, and hormone. Therefore, it is generally believed that the pathogenesis of lupus is a genetic predisposition triggered by environmental factors.

Twin studies initially indicated the importance of genetic factors, and genome screening has highlighted a number of potential loci of interest [129]. Several candidate genes are found to be associated with SLE, such as *PTPN22*, *FcγRIIA/Fcγ*, *RIIIA*,*FasL*,*CTLA-4*, *PDCD-1*, *HLA-DR2/DR3*, *C4*, *IRF5*, *MBL*, *Fas*, and *Dnase1* [130]. However, the mode of inheritance of SLE is not completely clear yet.

Environmental factors are also important risk factors that can exacerbate the development of LE. Ultraviolet (UV) irradiation can upregulate GADD45a expression and induce DNA methylation, and finally trigger lupus flares [131]. Smoking is another important cause associated with CLE. The prevalence of DLE is statistically higher in smokers than in nonsmokers [132, 133]. Hormonal factors, like estrogens, are thought to be capable of exacerbating or increasing the risk of developing LE, which helps explain the phenomenon of the female predominance in LE. Besides, drugs such as *terbinafine*, *TNF-α inhibitors*, *antiepileptic*, and proton-pump inhibitors (PPIs) are reported to be relevant with the development of subacute CLE [134].

However, genetics alone cannot elucidate the pathogenesis of LE, as the prevalence of LE is not 100 % in twins who have the identical genetic background. In recent years, epigenetics evoked a great interest since it can provide a potential link between genetic and environmental factors. DNA hypomethylation may play an important role in the pathogenesis of SLE as decreased global DNA methylation levels were seen in the T cells of patients with active lupus [135, 136]. Histone modifications are also involved in the pathogenesis of SLE, with global histone H3 and H4 acetylation as well as global histone H3 lysine9 (H3K9) methylation reduced in SLE CD4+ T cells [137]. Moreover, abnormal miRNA(microRNA) expressions also contribute to DNA hypomethylation, T-cell activation, breakdown of T- and B-cell tolerance, and autoantibody production in SLE [138]. These findings demonstrate critical importance of epigenetics in the pathogenesis and development of LE.

13.4.4 Clinical Symptoms

Localized cutaneous LE and severe systemic LE are the two ends of the spectrum of LE, both of which may exist simultaneously or separately. According to the American dermatologists Gilliam and Sontheimer, the cutaneous manifestations of LE can be grouped into LE-specific and LE-nonspecific skin manifestations based on their different histopathological findings [139]. LE-specific skin manifestations can be further subdivided into acute CLE (ACLE), subacute CLE (SCLE), and chronic CLE (CCLE). Furthermore, CCLE can be subcategorized into localized DLE, generalized DLE, hypertrophic LE, lupus panniculitis, lupus erythematosus tumidus, and chilblain lupus. DLE is the most common form of CCLE and rarely associated with SLE, when it is only confined to the head and neck. The LE-nonspecific skin manifestations includes a wide range of symptoms with different histopathological changes, which are not exclusive to LE but are often seen in patients with active SLE and other autoimmune diseases. Importantly, LE-nonspecific symptoms may indicate systemic organ damage and progression to SLE [126, 140].

13.4.4.1 ACLE

ACLE is closely related with systemic disease and mostly occurs on the fair-skinned female in her 30s. The lesions can be localized (concentrated above the neck) or generalized. The most localized lesion is malar rash or butterfly erythema, which often comes after sun exposure and lasts for hours to days. Postinflammatory hyperpigmentation is common but scarring does not happen. The generalized lesions of acute CLE are rare and associated with a previous sun exposure and preferably located to sun-exposed areas [127, 139] (Fig. 13.8).

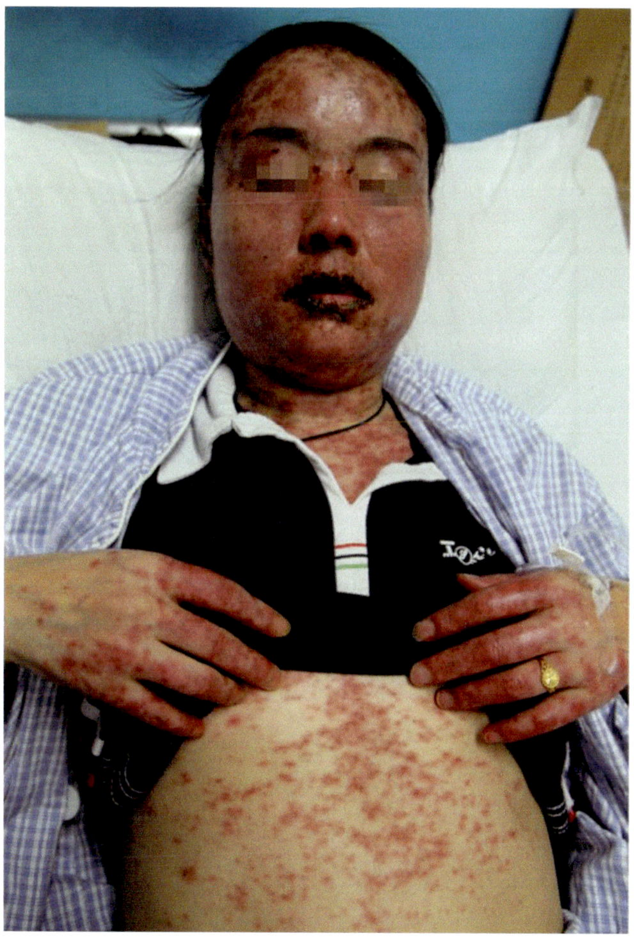

Fig. 13.8 Patient of acute CLE. Generalized ACLE patient presents with widespread erythema and maculopapular eruptions on the face, neck, trunk, and hands. Usually, the lesions are nonscarring

13.4.4.2 SCLE

SCLE mainly occurs in young and middle-aged women [141]. SCLE is the most photosensitive major subset of CLE, with 70–90 % of patients meeting the American College of Rheumatology (ACR) definition of abnormal photosensitivity [142]. The lesions start as erythematous papules or small plaques covered with fine scales and then expand and merge into retiform arrays of papulosquamous lesions or clear centrally to produce annular, polycyclic arrays. Most patients have predominantly one type, while some may exhibit both papulosquamous and annular lesions [143]. Sun-exposed areas are the most susceptive areas of lesions, including the upper thorax ("V" distribution), upper back, and the extensor surfaces of arms and forearms. Central face and scalp, however, are usually spared and lesion below the waist is seldom seen [141] (Fig. 13.9). The cutaneous lesions can cause pigmentary changes and telangiectasias, but typically without dermal atrophy or scarring. Patients with SCLE usually present mild systemic diseases, in which musculoskeletal symptoms are common, and severe systemic symptoms, such as systemic vasculitis, nephritis, and central nervous system (CNS) lupus occur in less than 10 % [144].

13.4.4.3 CCLE

Here, we will mainly discuss the three different forms of CCLE: discoid LE (DLE), LE profundus (LEP), and chilblain LE (CHLE).

13.4.4.4 DLE

DLE can be classified into two forms: localized form (above the neck), usually accounting for 70 % of DLE, and the generalized form (lesions both above and below the neck, with the extensor forearms and hands typically involved) for the rest 30 % [141, 143]. Classic DLE lesions start as a well-defined, scaly, erythematous macule or papule that gradually develops into a coin-shaped (discoid) plaque, with adherent scales difficult and painful to be removed [145]. Then, the lesions expand and form areas of peripheral inflammation and hyperpigmentation, leaving a central region of scarring with hypopigmentation and telangiectasia [146] (Fig. 13.10). Photosensitivity can be seen in most DLE patients (about 70 %), with sun-exposed areas, such as face, scalp, and ears commonly involved [140]. Adherent scale usually extends into hair follicles, leading to changes in hair pigment and even permanent alopecia. Mucosal involvement is also common, with inner cheeks and lips most frequently affected [146].

According to a recent study, almost 25 % of newly diagnosed DLE patients already obtain a primary diagnosis of SLE. And the probability of DLE patients receiving an additional diagnosis of SLE is 9.8 % after the first year and 16.7 % after 3 years [125].

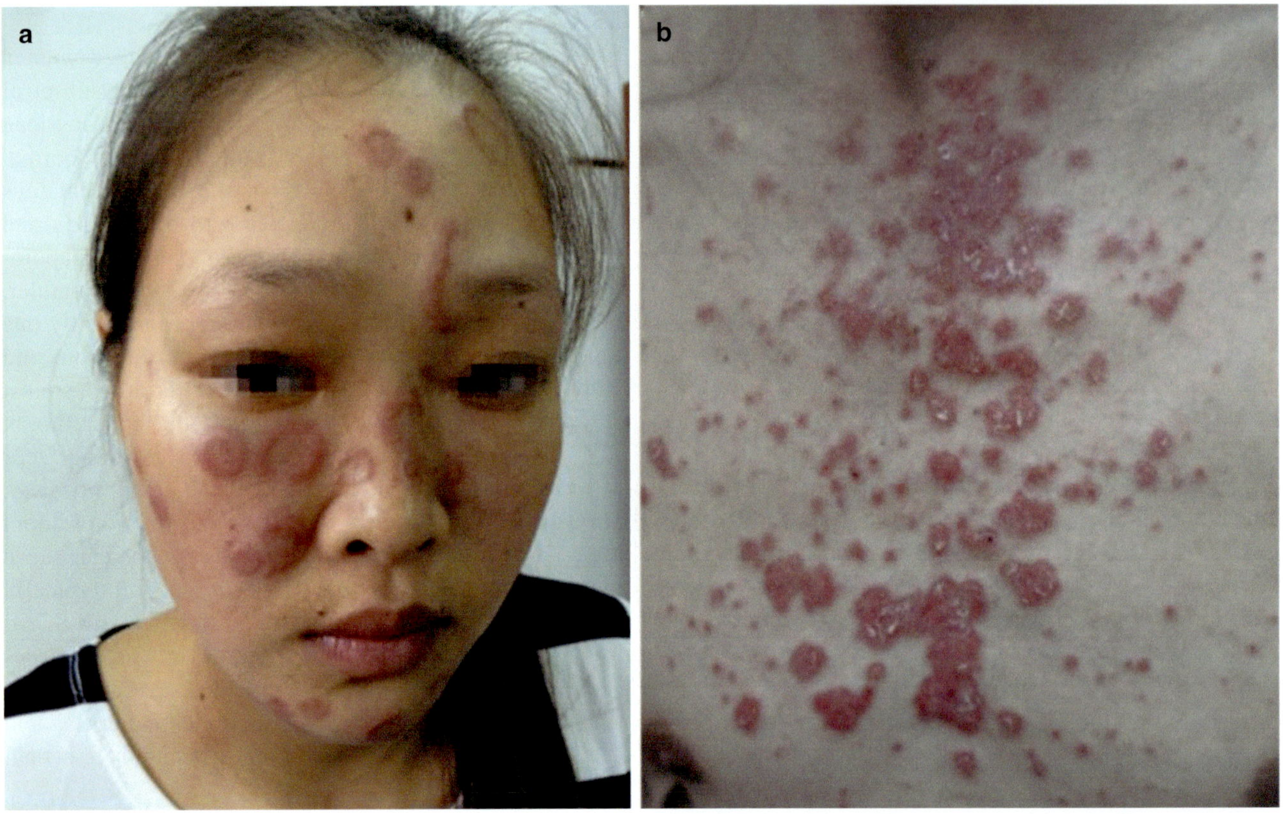

Fig. 13.9 Patients of SCLE. Annular lesions on the faces of SCLE (**a**). The primary lesion of SCLE is an erythematous papule or a small plaque with a slight scaling. Primary lesions expand and may merge and eventually form plaques with scaling (**b**)

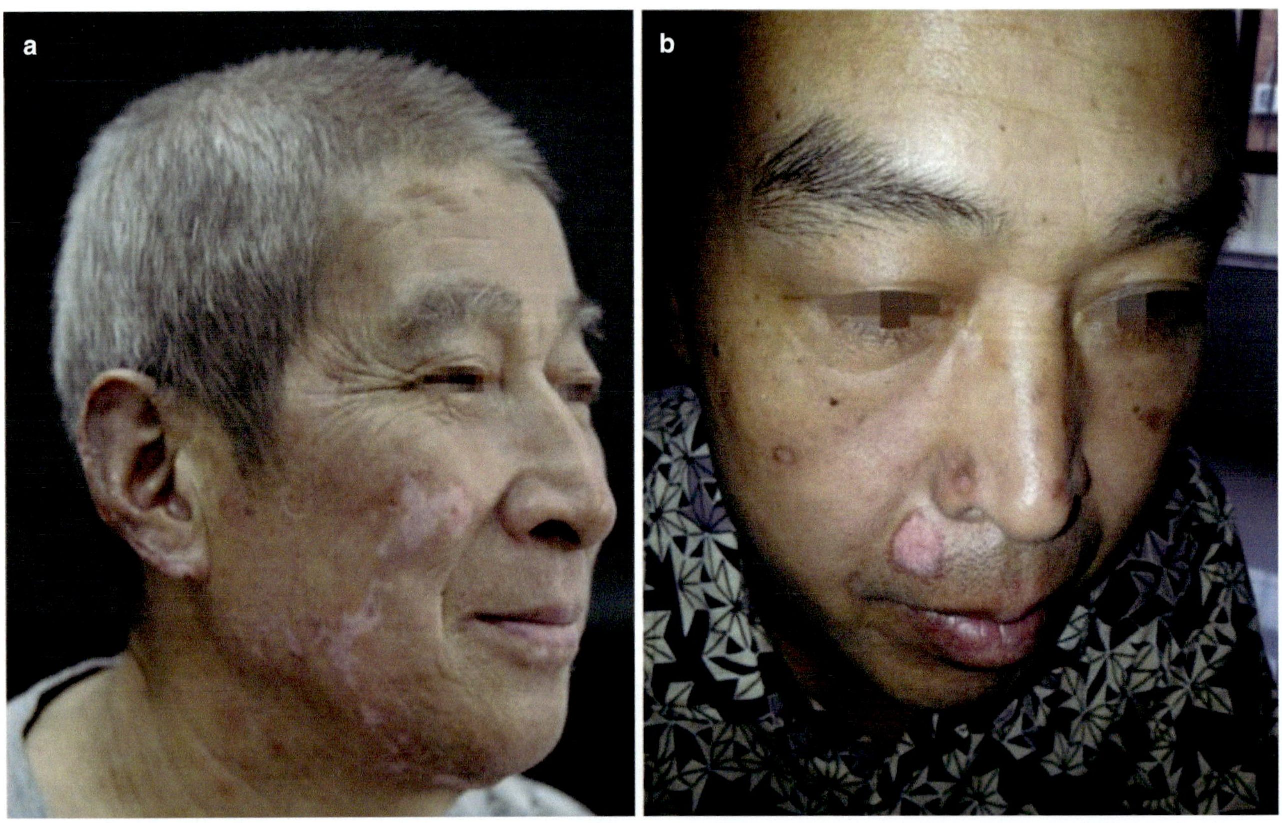

Fig. 13.10 Patients of DLE. The most affected areas are sun-exposed, such as the cheeks, nose, ears, upper back, neck, and the backs of hands. Red scaly patches develop which leave pigmentation, atrophy, and white scars

13.4.4.5 LEP

LEP, also known as lupus panniculitis, typically appears as multiple firm and painful (later asymptomatic) subcutaneous nodules and plaques within the deep dermis and underlying adipose tissue. Areas with increased fat deposition, such as the gluteal region, thighs, upper arms, face, and breasts are the predominantly affected areas. Occasionally, periorbital edema is the initial symptom before the typical skin changes occur [147]. The course of LEP tends to be chronic, with both remission and aggravation, and finally forms atrophic scars [143].

13.4.4.6 CHLE

CHLE is a rare form of CCLE, which is characterized by painful, violaceous plaques, and nodules in cold-exposed areas. Central erosions or ulcerations sometimes can be seen on the affected acral surfaces, especially the fingers, toes, heels, nose, and ears [145]. CHLE lesions are generally triggered or exacerbated by exposure to cold and damp environment, especially when there is an evident drop in temperature. It is usually difficult to distinguish CHLE from frostbite. As reported, about 20 % of SLE patients could present features of chronic chilblain lupus [148].

13.4.4.7 SLE

SLE is a severe and life-threatening form of LE with various organ damages, such as skin, lung, joint, kidney, nerve system, and so on.

Skin Involvement Skin lesions are also very common in SLE, which can present as the classic malar or discoid rashes, as well as more generalized photosensitive rashes. Oral or nasal ulcers (usually painless) are often seen during disease flares (Fig. 13.11).

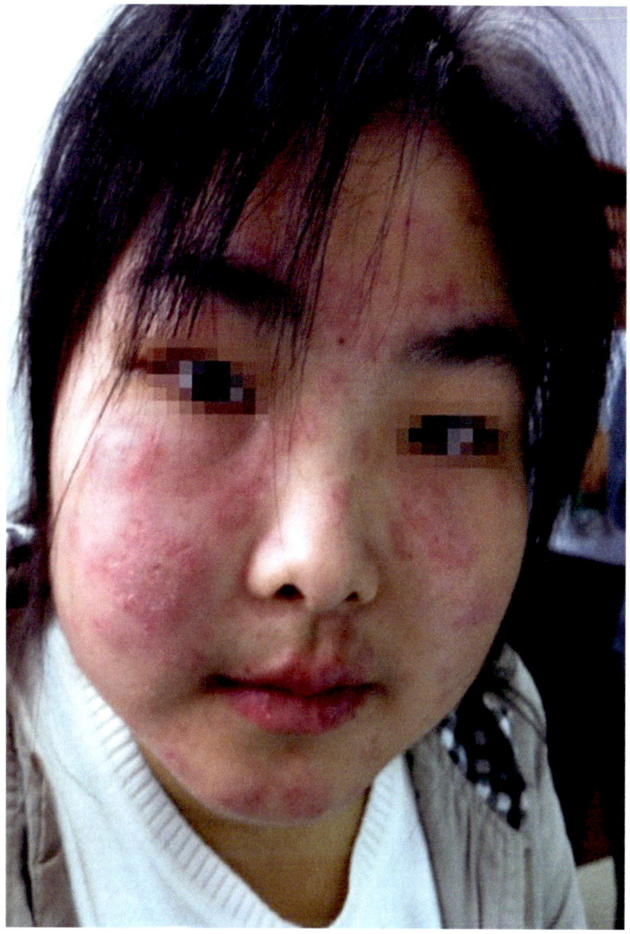

Fig. 13.11 Patient of SLE. The classic malar rash is also known as a butterfly rash, with distribution over the cheeks and nasal bridge. Note that atypical lesions often occur

Pleuritis Pleuritis is the most common pulmonary feature of SLE, which causes chest pain, cough, and breathlessness [149]. Pleural effusions are often exudates, with low levels of complement, and test positive for antinuclear antibodies (ANA). Other complications include pneumonia, pulmonary embolism, pulmonary hypertension, and pulmonary hemorrhage.

Musculoskeletal Symptoms Arthritis and arthralgia can be present in most patients. Joint pain, particularly the small joints of the hands and wrists followed by larger joints, is the most common symptom. Joint deformity that is caused by "Jaccoud's arthropathy" may occur later in the disease course. Morning stiffness and muscle pain can also be seen in some patients [141].

Renal Damage Renal damage occurs in about 50 % of SLE patients, and still remains the most dangerous, life-threatening complication of SLE. The clinical manifestation includes persistent hematuria (not criteria), proteinuria (>0.5 g/24 h), or cellular casts. As it is often asymptomatic, especially at the beginning, regular urinalysis and blood pressure monitoring are suggested. Renal biopsy is also recommended as it is very important for the classification of nephritis and its prognosis and further treatments [150, 151].

Neuropsychiatric Lupus (NPSLE) NPSLE is a significant factor of morbidity and mortality in SLE, which affects about 20 % patients. The manifestations are diverse, ranging from central nervous system disease causing headache and seizures, or psychiatric disorders including psychosis and depression, to cognitive impairment and peripheral neuropathy. Among them, seizures or psychosis are considered as the most characteristic CNS features and were included as criteria of SLE [150, 151].

Gastrointestinal Involvement Nonspecific abdominal pain and dyspepsia are the common presentations when gastrointestinal system is involved. Mesenteric vasculitis and lupus enteritis, although rare, are thought to cause the abdominal pain, and may lead to intestinal necrosis and perforation that can be life-threatening [150, 152].

Hematological Features Hematologic lupus includes normocytic normochromic anemia, leukopenia, lymphopenia, and thrombocytopenia.

Constitutional Symptoms Except for those specific organ involvements, fatigue, weight loss, and fever also present in most SLE patients. Though not life-threatening, these symptoms can significantly impact their quality of life.

13.4.5 Laboratory Findings

Over 90 % of patients with SLE have positive anti-nuclear antibodies (ANA). Significant titers are accepted to be of 1:80 or greater. ANA, although sensitive, is not specific for SLE. Positive ANA is also seen in many other disorders including systemic sclerosis and polymyositis, as well as some chronic infections. All patients should be screened for extractable nuclear antigens (ENAs). Different ENAs are associated with different clinical manifestation. For instance, anti-Sm is associated with renal involvement, and anti-Ro is associated with secondary Sjogren's syndrome.

As with SLE, cutaneous LE also has similar immunological changes. Positive ANA is found in 95 % of ACLE patients, anti-double-stranded DNA (anti-dsDNA) and anti-Sm antibodies are also detected in a majority of ACLE patients [153]. In SCLE, 60–80 % patients are ANA positive, and 70–90 % patients have anti-Ro/SSA antibodies while anti-La/SSB antibodies are found in 30–50 % patients. High-titer ANA is positive in about 5 % DLE patients. There are generally no anti-dsDNA antibodies and rarely antibodies to Ro/SSA in patients with DLE [147]. However, the presence of ANA and anti-dsDNA antibodies in DLE usually correlates with a more active and progressive disease with poorer prognosis [154].

In addition to serologic antibodies, cutaneous histopathology is of great importance in the diagnosis of LE. Histopathological features of ACLE lesions include liquefaction degeneration of the basal layer, edema of the upper dermis, perivascular, and periadnexal lymphocytic infiltrate. But these findings are often less pronounced than other forms of CLE [145]. Direct immunofluorescence (DIF) is able to detect the deposition of immunoglobulin (Ig) G, IgM, and IgA and complement component fractions at the dermoepidermal junction. This test is also called the "lupus band test" (Fig. 13.12). 60–100 % of DIF display a lesional lupus band, but this can commonly be seen in sun-damaged skin from healthy individuals. SCLE characteristically shows hydropic degeneration of the basal keratinocytes and dermal edema, whereas adherent hyperkeratosis, follicular plugging, and superficial inflammatory infiltrate are less striking [143]. Positive DIF (direct immunofluorescence) occurs in 30–60 % cases. The histology of active DLE lesions typically exhibits hyperkeratosis, follicular plugging, vacuolar degeneration of the epidermal basal layer and follicular epithelium, epidermal atrophy, and inflammatory dermal infiltrate. Dermal atrophy with postinflammatory pigmentation and scarring are generally shown in chronic inactive DLE [146]. In SLE, fibrinoid necrosis at dermoepidermal junction with liquefactive degeneration and atrophy of epidermis can be seen. And there is more mucin deposition in reticular dermis than discoid lupus. Edema, small hemorrhages, and a mild infiltrate of inflammatory cells, principally lymphocytes, are in upper dermis. Eosinophils could be found in drug-induced cases and urticarial lesions. Fibrinoid material is deposited in the dermis around capillary blood vessels, on collagen and in the interstitium. In nonbullous cases, neutrophils are sometimes present in the upper dermis, both perivascular and interstitial with leukocytoclasis (Fig. 13.13). Besides, IgG, IgM, and C5b-C9 by DIF are positive in clinically involved skin as an irregular band at dermoepidermal junction. However, IgG and IgM could be positive in 50 % of cases in normal skin.

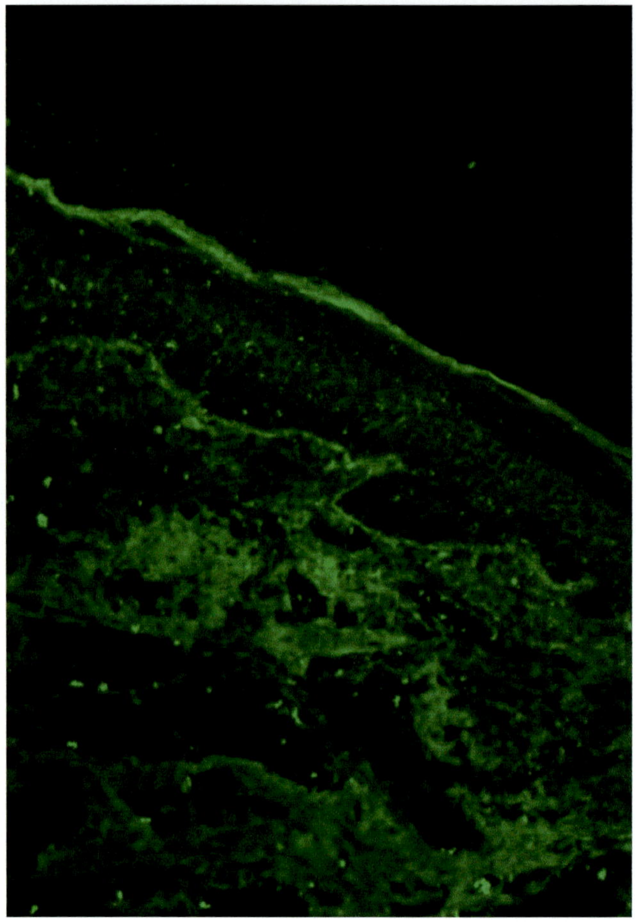

Fig. 13.12 Lupus band test

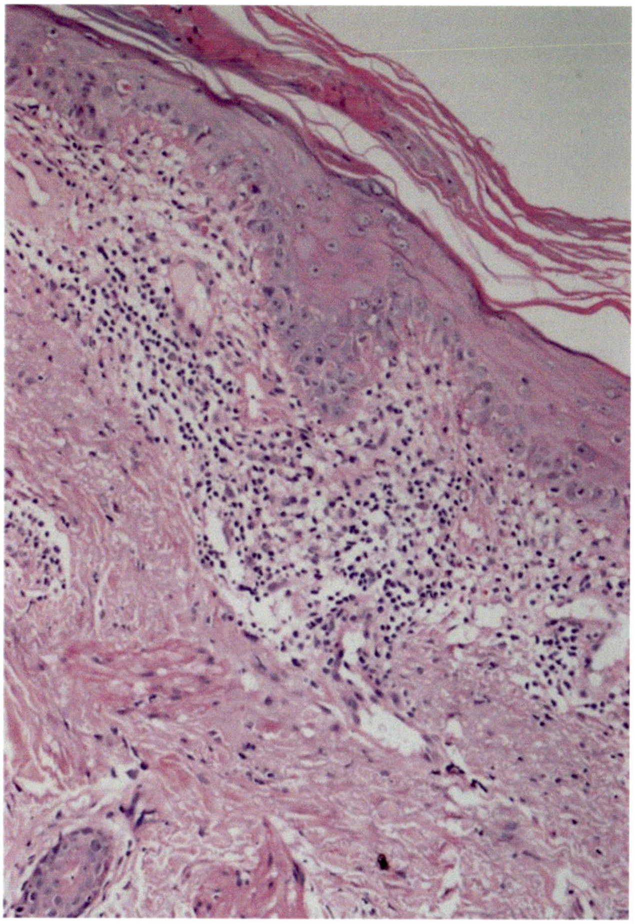

Fig. 13.13 Histopathology of skin lesions in SLE patients

13.4.6 Diagnosis

Diagnosis of LE depends on medical history, clinical examination, serological tests, and histopathological findings. When taking the patients' histories, physicians should pay attention to family history, UV exposure, drugs, smoking, as well as history of exposure to estrogen-containing contraceptives. A detailed description of the initial occurrence and evolution of the skin lesions is also useful for the diagnosis. Careful skin examination is crucial for determining the CLE clinical subtypes by referring to their typical features described before. Meantime, complete physical examination for extracutaneous manifestations is also required to differentiate from SLE.

Skin biopsy is another option to make the diagnosis of LE. Direct immune fluorescence (DIF) of skin lesions can be used to supplement the diagnosis when the histology is not definitive. Although DIF examination is usually found positive in CLE lesions, a negative test does not exclude the diagnosis. Similarly, a positive DIF test does not secure the diagnosis, as false positive tests can occur in other skin diseases. Generally, clinical and histologic findings can provide sufficient information for diagnosing CLE. Therefore, DIF is not necessary [145]. Assessment of the autoantibody is useful in determining the presence of SLE. In addition, a full blood count, renal function test, and erythrocyte sedimentation rate (ESR) should also be performed to rule out systemic involvements associated with SLE.

As for diagnosis of SLE, 4 of 11 criteria are required based on the ACR recommendations [155]. The ACR criteria include butterfly rash, discoid rash, photosensitivity and oral ulcers, arthritis, serositis, renal, neurological, hematological or immunological disorder, as well as detection of antinuclear antibody. However, as 4 of the 11 criteria are skin or mucosa manifestations, the diagnosis of SLE can be made with cutaneous symptoms alone, which leads to overdiagnosis of SLE. To improve clinical associations, the Systemic Lupus International Collaborating Clinics (SLICC) revised and validated the ACR SLE classification criteria recently, and identified 17 clinical and immunologic criteria. The SLICC criteria for diagnosing SLE required: (1) achieve ≥ 4 criteria, with at least one clinical criterion and one immunologic criterion; or (2) biopsy confirmed lupus nephritis in the presence of SLE autoantibodies as the sole clinical criterion [156]. The SLICC criteria showed less falsely classified SLE patients and greater sensitivity for the diagnosis of SLE compared to the ACR criteria [156].

13.4.7 Treatments

Any type of LE is a relapsing and remitting disease, and they can only be managed but not cured so far.

13.4.7.1 Treatments for CLE

Treatment Treatment options are very similar in different CLE subtypes. Managements of CLE include prevention, topical, and systemic treatment according to the activity and progression of the disease.

Prevention Patients should avoid exposure to sunlight and artificial UV radiation, as well as excessive heat, cold, or trauma. Broad-spectrum sunscreen with high sun-protection factor (SPF) should be applied daily at least 20–30 min before sun exposure. Photoprotective clothing is also encouraged as an additional protection. Smoking and drugs, such as *terbinafine*, *TNF-α inhibitors*, *antiepileptic*, and *PPIs*, are recommended to be avoided. As sunlight is required in the synthesis of *vitamin D*, patients who are actively avoiding sun and routinely using sunscreen are recommended to supplement at least 400 IU of vitamin D3 per day [157].

Topical Treatment Topical *corticosteroids* are the mainstay of treating all subtypes of CLE. Potency and vehicle of the topical steroid should be taken into consideration when making choices of the treatment. The potency should be chosen depending on the location of the skin lesions. A low potency steroid can be used at thin areas of skin (e.g., face). For the trunk and extremities, a mid-potency steroid is a good option. And a high potency steroid is often required for thick areas of skin [158]. The choice of vehicle is usually related to occlusion and physician or patient preference, with creams commonly applied initially. Because of the side effects, such as skin atrophy, telangiectasias, and steroid-induced rosacea, treatment with steroid should be time-limited and intermittent to make steroid-free intervals for the skin. Topical calcineurin inhibitors like *tacrolimus* and *pimecrolimus* have also showed great efficacy in treating CLE. And because topical *calcineurin* inhibitors have no steroid-associated systemic side effects, they are playing a more important role in treating some CLE subtypes. Intralesional *triamcinolone acetonide* injections can be chosen when lesions do not respond to topical therapy, and should use the minimum possible dose. Some other topical medications include *R-salbutamol*, *imiquimod*, and topical *retinoids*, which also show significant effect in treating DLE lesions. Physical treatments, such as laser therapy, cryotherapy, and dermabrasion, can be applied only after a comprehensive discussion on the risks and benefits of these measures [158].

Systemic treatment: Systemic therapy is indicated when the skin lesions are widespread, scarring, or topical therapies alone are ineffective for the disease. CLE patients presenting extracutaneous symptoms also need systemic therapies. Oral *antimalarials* still remain the first-line agents in the systemic treatment for all CLE subtypes. The currently used *antimalarials* are *hydroxychloroquine*, *chloroquine*, and *quinacrine*, with *hydroxychloroquine* being the first line as its lower retinal toxicity compared to *chloroquine* [159]. It is important to notice that *antimalarials* take 6–8 weeks to take effect. High doses or prolonged treatment with *hydroxychloroquine* or *chloroquine* can cause retinal toxicity, so it requires patients and physicians to keep an eye on any potential side effects. *Quinacrine* can be added to either *hydroxychloroquine* or *chloroquine* to improve efficacy, without an increased risk of retinopathy. Systemic corticosteroids can only be applied in patients with severe and highly acute skin lesions due to their well-known side effects, including osteoporosis and Cushing syndrome. The suggested dose of corticosteroids is 0.5–1 mg/kg/day and tapered over 2–4 weeks or 3-day intravenous pulse therapy of methylprednisolone [157]. Meanwhile, other regimens may be administered in progressive or generalized type, or localized disease refractory to other therapies. For example, in lupus panniculitis, corticosteroids can be applied along with antimalarial therapy to prevent lipoatrophy [157].

Immunosuppressants such as *cyclosporine*, *methotraxate*, *mycophenolate mofetil*, and *azathioprine* have been shown to be effective in treating refractory CLE as steroid-sparing agents. Immunomodulators, like *dapsone* and *thalidomide*, are also useful therapeutic alternatives in the management of some CLE subtypes, but should be used in low doses due to the potential severe side effects. Other systemic treatments, including intravenous *immunoglobulins* (IVIG) and *rituximab*, can be used for patients who are refractory to various combinations of *antimalarials* and immunosuppressives or immunomodulators [158].

13.4.7.2 Treatments for SLE

Treatments for SLE aim at managing acute stage of potential life-threatening diseases, preventing flares during relatively stable periods, and controlling the less life-threatening but severely impacting life quality symptoms [150].

SLE flares, which mean periods of increased disease activity, are generally classified as mild/moderate or severe based on the severity of symptoms and are helpful in guiding treatments [151]. In mild/moderate flares (e.g., rashes, oral ulcers, arthritis, fatigue, and fever), *hydroxychloroquine*, nonsteroidal anti-inflammatory drugs (NSAIDs), and low doses oral *steroids* are commonly used. Immunosuppressants, such as *methotrexate* or *azathioprine*, maybe applied to SLE patients who need more than 10 mg prednisone to control diseases. *Belimumab*, a monoclonal antibody targeted against a soluble B lymphocyte survival factor, has been found beneficial for patients of mild/moderate flares [151]. Severe flares can present as organ or life-threatening state, such as disseminated ulcerating rashes, severe nephritis, central nervous system involvement, or serious hematological disease. Treatments for these severe symptoms include continued *hydroxychloroquine* 400 mg with consideration of pulse steroid and high dose prednisone 1–2 mg/kg/day [151]. Immunosuppressive treatments, such as cyclophosphamide, azathioprine, and *mycophenolate mofetil* can be used as maintenance therapy. Biologic therapies are now being developed in the treatment of severe SLE. Rituximab is a monoclonal antibody targeting against CD20 on B cells and their precursors, which is previously used in the treatment of lymphoma, and it is now showing substantial effect for patients with severe disease who were not responsive to conventional treatments [160]. In addition, IVIG and stem cell transplantation may also be tried for the refractory cases [161].

13.4.8 Conclusions

LE is an important autoimmune disease comprising a wide range of clinical manifestations, from localized CLE to severe SLE. The etiology of LE is regarded as a genetic predisposition triggered by environmental factors. The diagnosis of LE can be challenging due to various presentations, and medical history, clinical examination, and histological findings are of great value. Protection against UV radiation and topical therapies with *corticosteroids* and *calcineurin* inhibitors is the most important means in the management of CLE. Besides, treatments for SLE, especially severe lupus nephritis and lupus encephalopathy, can be much more challenging. Thus, improving the quality of life and minimizing the side effects of systemic drugs are the major objectives in the treatment of SLE.

13.5 Dermatomyositis

Ken Hashimoto, MD

13.5.1 Dermatomyositis

Incidence: Dermatomyositis (DM) is a rare disease. The generally accepted incidence rate is 1 in 1 million. The ratio between male and female is 1:2. This figure will change to 1:5 if juvenile patients are counted. It could be said that DM is a disease of young girls (Fig. 13.14). Regarding the age of onset there are two peaks; juvenile type at 6 ~ 8 years old and adult type between 40 and 60 years of age [162, 163].

In some patients myositis is absent; this variant could have a full blown skin manifestations of DM but no sign or laboratory evidence of myositis. This type is called DM sine myositis, amyopathic DM, or clinically amyopathic DM (CADM). In other instances dermatitis is absent and only polimyositis is the presenting symptom. Additional subtypes include cancer-associated DM and overlap types DM, such as sclerodermatomyositis. Calcinosis of skin is more frequent in juvenile type than in adult patients.

Etiology: Clinical observations, episodic events, and anecdotal incidence sometimes give clues for diseases etiology. In DM, the following factors may play etiological role: (1) Vigorous use of muscles. (2) Drugs causing DM-like side effects include penicillamine, NSAIDS, carbamazapine, tamoxifen, and progesterone. (3) Infections with toxoplasma and streptococcus. Myosin and type C protein of streptococcus have a common antigen; streptococcus infection could trigger the production of antimyosine antibody by molecular mimicry. Other incriminated agents are parvovirus for adult DM and group B coxsackie virus in juvenile DM. (4) HLA prolifes are not strong enough to suggest genetic background in DM. HLA-DR3 and B8 are associated with juvenile DM [164]. DM-specific antibody, e.g., Jo-1 linked to HLA-DR52 and Mi-2 is associated with HLA-DRT and DRW 53. Jo-1 and Mi-2 are the major autoantibodies of DM.

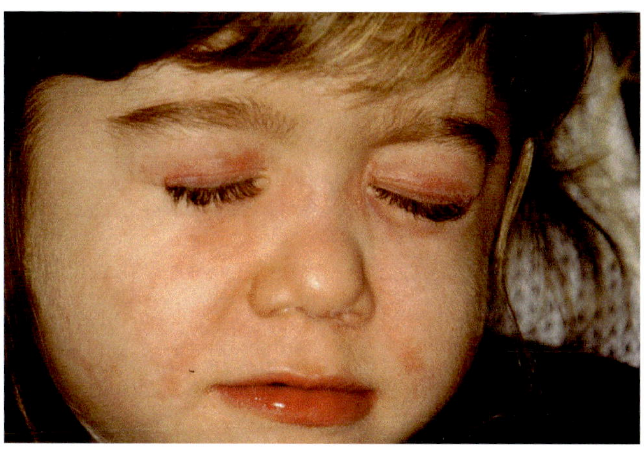

Fig. 13.14 Juvenile DM, eyelids, especially upper ones, are swollen and dyscolored to violaceous or heliotrope pink. The center of the face and cheeks are similarly affected but less intensely. The distribution of the involved areas (butterfly lesion) suggested photosensitivity

13.5.2 Autoantibodies (Table 13.3)

It is believed that DM patients have lost control over the immune tolerance. As a result many unrelated autoantibodies are produced in DM, whereas in SLE only several DNA- and RNA-related autoantibodies are allowed to produce by the host. It has been shown that DM patient's blood lymphocytes are myotoxic as demonstrable by mixing cultured muscle cells with lesional lymphocytes, conversely patient's lymphocytes exhibit transformation when mixed with cultured muscle cells.

Aminoacyl t-RNA synthetases (ARS) or simply synthetases are enzymes concerned with protein synthesis. The best-known antibody in this group, called ARS autoantibodies, is Jo-1. Others are listed in Table 13.3. Some of those are specifically related to clinically amyopathic DM and diffuse interstitial pulmonary fibrosis. NXP-2 is associated with malignancies. If a patient has one of the ARS autoantibodies and chronic interstitial pneumonitis, myositis, arthritis or Raynaud's phenomenon, this patient has anti-ARS (antisynthetase) syndrome.

Clinical symptoms: In one large series of case study, 20 % of DM patients followed for 10 years never developed myositis [164]. This variant is called amyopathic DM (CADM). There are several diagnostic signs. (1) Edema and dusky purplish discoloration (heliotrope rash) of eyelids, especially the upper eyelid (Fig. 13.14). (2) Nose and cheeks are red and mildly scaly. This looks like butterfly lesion of photosensitive SLE. Patient appears sad, sullen, and unhappy (Fig. 13.14). (3) Dorsal skin of finger joints (knuckles) is thickened and pigmented. Similar change occurs on the knees and elbows. This is called Gottron's sign. If papules and small nodules arise within the thickened patches; these are referred to as Gottron's papules (Figs. 13.15 and 13.16). The skin of distal dorsal fingers and posterior nailfolds are red and either thickened or thinned. There are telangiectasia (Fig. 13.17). (4) The upper back (Fig. 13.18), V of neck,

Table 13.3 Autoantibodies in dermatomyositis

Autoantibodies in dermatomyositis			
Autoantibodies	Frequency	Antigens	Clinical correlation
With high specificity			
P155	20–80 %	Transcriptional intermediary factor 1 gamma (T1FIr)	Classic DM, CADM[a], malignancy association
MDA5[C]/CADM-140	10–15 %	IF1H1[b]/MDA5[c]	CADM, rapidly progressive lung disease, palmar papule vasculitis to ulcers
Jo-1	20 %	Histit-RNA synthetase	Antisynthetase syndrome
Mi-2	15 %	Helicase nuclear proteins	
PL-12	3 %	Alanyl t-RNA synthetase	Antisynthetase syndrome
PL-7	5 %	Threonyl t-RNA synthetase	Antisynthetase syndrome
SRP	5 %	Signal recognition particle	Fulminant DM/PM
With low specificity			
ANA(nucleolar; discrete speckled pattern or centromeric)	40 %		CADM (65 %)
ssDNA	40 %	Single stranded DNA	SIE, SSC, morphea
PM-Scl(PM1)	10 %	Ribosomal RNA processing enzyme	Overlap with Scl
U1RNP	10 %	Splicesome RNP	Overlap with other autoimmune connective tissue diseases

[a]Clinically amyopathic DM
[b]IFN-induced with helicase C domain proteins
[c]Melanoma differentiation-associated gene 5

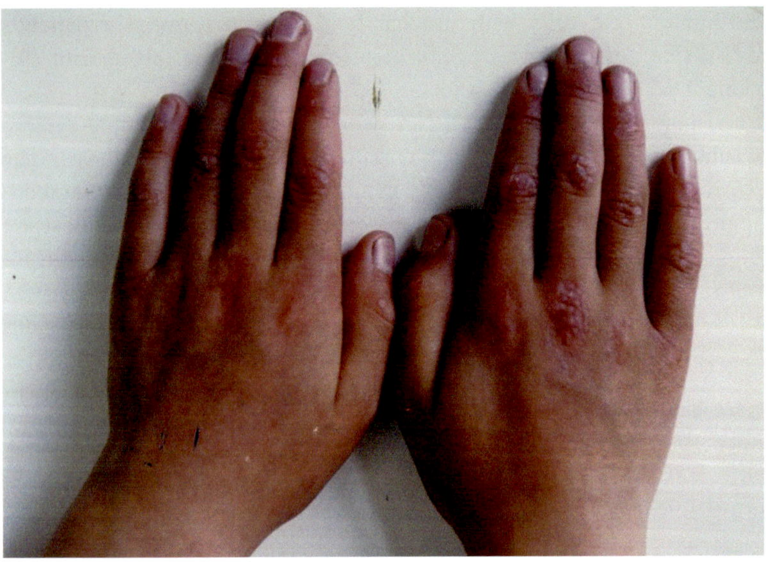

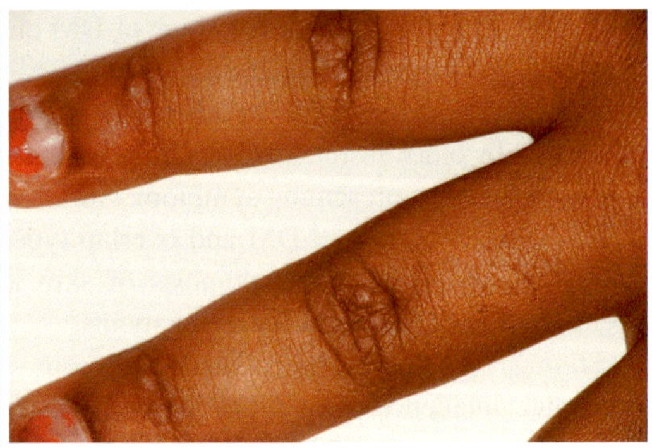

Figs. 13.15 and 13.16 Gottron's papule. Knuckle pad-like erythematous patches, periungual edema, and erythema are shown. These discolored patches are either elevated to form flat plaque or multiple papules. These are called Gottron's papules. Gottron's sign and Gottron's papules are often present in the same lesion

nape, and the skin areas usually covered with a shawl become erythematous and mildly scaly is called shawl sign. (5) Poikiloderma. Shawl sign areas or sun-exposed parts become pigmented as well as depigmented (Fig. 13.19). Pigmentation is not homogeneous but variegated or retiform (net-like) and of variable densities. (6) Flagella erythoma are linear red lines or bands on the back or extremities (Fig. 13.20). The configurations of these lesions are like excoriations or whipped skin marks. (7) Mechanic's hand. Hand looks like automechanic's hand. Areas of the hand subject to constant pressure from hand-hold instruments become callus (Fig. 13.17). This change is a part of ARS syndrome. DM lesions tend to develop on the sun-exposed areas, e.g., heliotrope sigh and poikiloderma. The friction sites (Gottron's

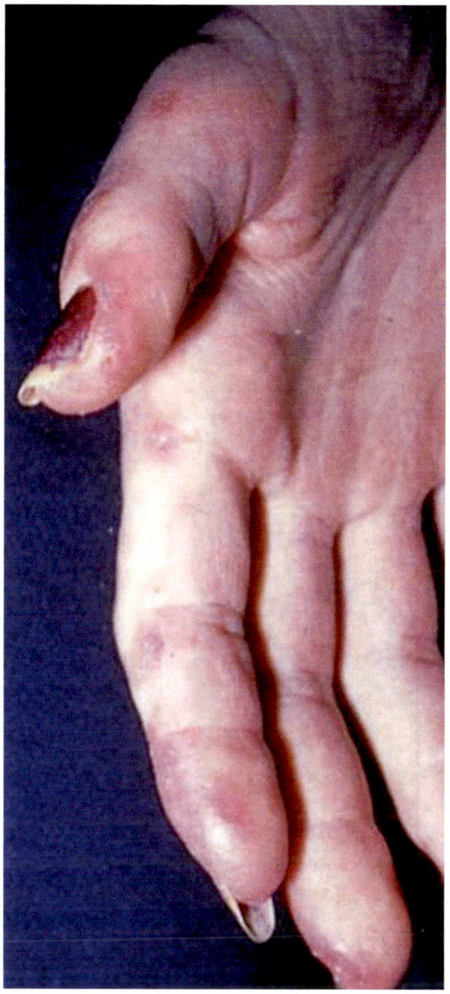

Fig. 13.17 DM, mechanic's hand. Hypertrophic patches are seen on the spots of pressure and friction of dexterous right hand as if automechanic has used hand-held instruments for a long time. Other hallmarks of DM, such as the hyperemia, edema, and erythema of distal fingers and posterior nailfolds are also present. DM is a friction- and pressure-sensitive skin disease

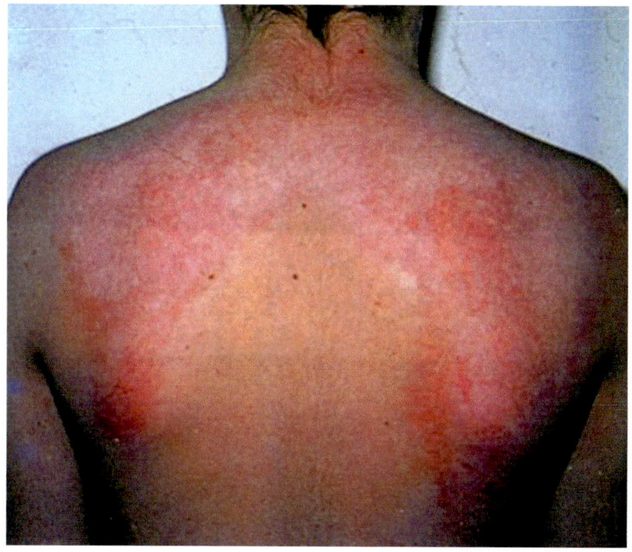

Fig. 13.18 DM, shawl sign, shoulder, upper back, nape, and V of the neck are covered with erythema. These areas coincide with sun-exposed sites, and the areas to be covered with shawl, hence this erythema has been called shawl sign

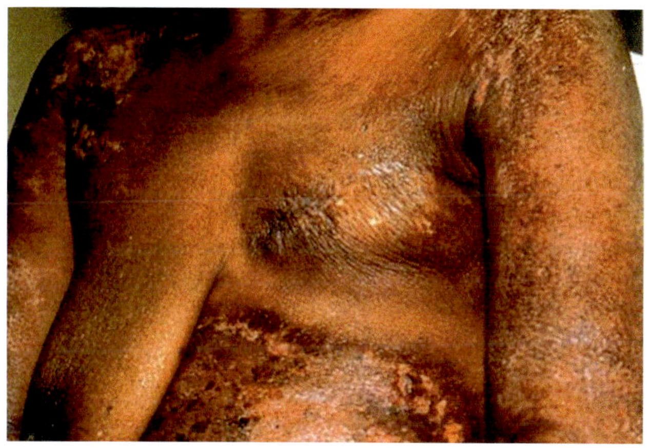

Fig. 13.19 DM, cancer and poikiloderma. After breast cancer and mastectomy DM began. After erythematous rashes subsided, net-like pattern of hyperpigmentation, multiple small patches of depigmentation and telangiectasia occurred. DM is a photosensitive disease

papules and mechanic's hand) produce pressure-related lesions.

Systemic Diseases: If a patient has one of the aminoacyl-tRNA synthetase antibody, he may have antisynthetase syndrome (ASS) now or in future. The target antigen of the synthetase antibodies is engaged in the synthesis of cellular proteins. Clinical symptoms of this syndrome include myositis, arthritis, fever, Reynaud's phenomenon, and interstitial pneumonitis. Skin manifestations of this syndrome are Gottron's papules and mechanic's hand. ASS syndrome does not respond well to corticosteroids.

Proximal extensor muscles, such as triceps and quadriceps muscles, are affected at an early stage of the disease. Patients cannot stand up from squatted position with both arms outstretched; this is named Gower's sign. Usually skin eruptions precede the muscle symptoms. If the myositis is the first sign, it is not easy to determine if it is a part of the DM or other banal myositis. DM may involve small muscles and bring about serious paralyses. Myositis of cricopharyngeal muscle causes dysphagia, weakness of pharyngeal muscles may evoke dysphonia, and hoarseness. Diffuse interstitial fibrosis of the lung is the most serious complication of DM, it could induce an acute respiratory distress that does not respond well to corticosteroids as in ASS syndrome.

Malignancies in DM: Only adult DM is associated with malignant neoplasms (10–50 %). Amyopathic DM seems to be more frequently associated with malignant tumors than other types. Ovarian and colon cancers are the most common varieties. Nasopharyngeal carcinomas are predominant

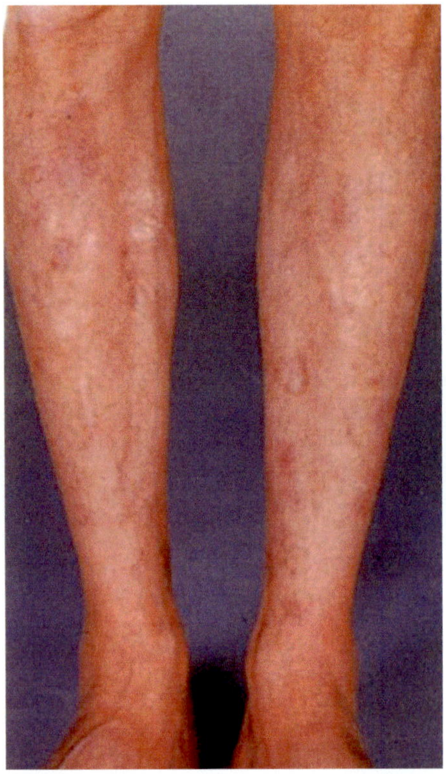

Fig. 13.20 DM, flagellate erythema. A few linear erythema with fine scales appear like excoriation marks or sin marks after whipping

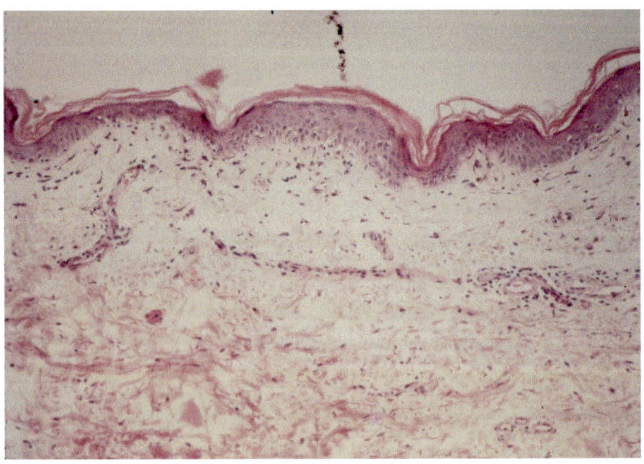

Fig. 13.21 DM. The dermal edema is severe in the upper dermis. A few small venules are marked surrounded with inflammatory cells which also invading the epidermis focally to cause vacuolization of the basal cells. The dermal edema shows a bluish grey tinge, suggesting the presence of mucins

DM-related cancers in Southeast Asia [165]. NK/T-cell lymphoma also develop in the nose (nasal type) in this regional group. It is suspected that this regional population is generally predisposed to develop nasal neoplasms.

Laboratory studies: Muscle enzyme level in the peripheral blood indicates the extent of muscle damages. Creatine phosphokinase (CK) for instance will be elevated in 95 % of DM patients [164]. The enzyme levels go parallel with the disease activities. Commonly checked muscle enzymes are aldolase, lactic dehydrogenase, aspartic and alanine transaminases and CK. When creatine is ordered, isotype 3 should be specified because it is more sensitive to the muscle injuries. If urine creatine is elevated, there is a possibility of myoglobinuria which might lead to renal failure.

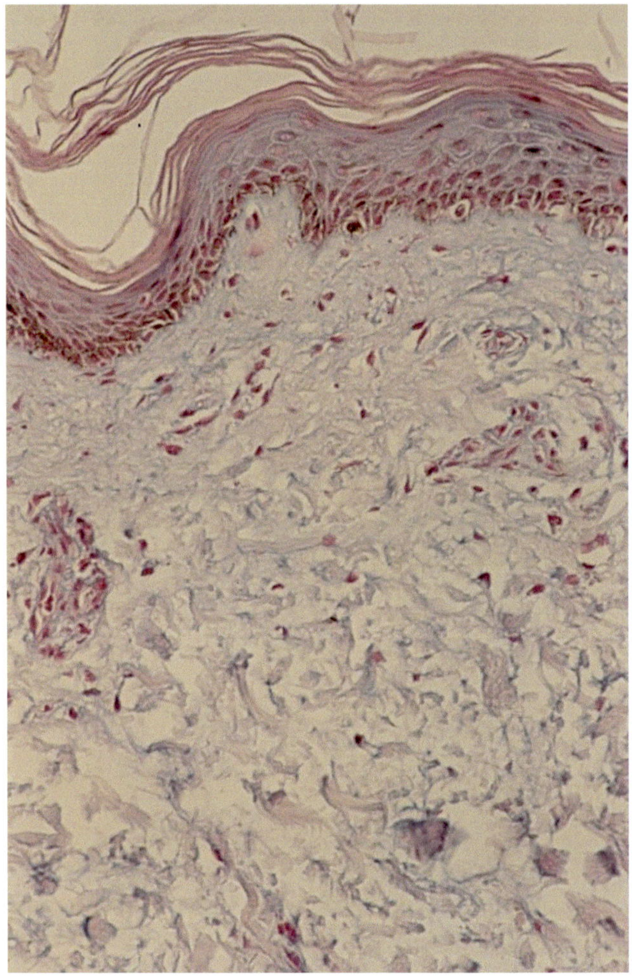

Fig. 13.22 DM, mucin deposition. Alcian blue stain (pH 2.5), the epidermis does not have rete ridges and has thin areas at left edge. The marked edema in the upper dermis is stained light blue indicating the presence of non-sulfated acid muco-polysaccharides, mainly hyaluronic acid; a pretreatment of the section with hyaluronidase with abolish most of the Alcian blue stain

Histopathology: Abnormal features are similar to changes; in early inflammatory stage with heliotrope rash perivascular and interstitial diffuse infiltration of lymphocytes are the main findings in the edematous dermis (Fig. 13.21). The edema is induced by water retaining capability (hygroscopic power) of hyaluronic acid produced as mucin by mucoblasts (modified fibroblast). We do not know why fibroblasts are specialized in mucin production but we can show that the accumulating edema fluid contains hyaluronic acid by means of Alcian blue stain (pH 2.5) (Fig. 13.22). The blue color representing the positive reaction could be abolished by incubation of the tissue reactions on the slide with hyaluronidase.

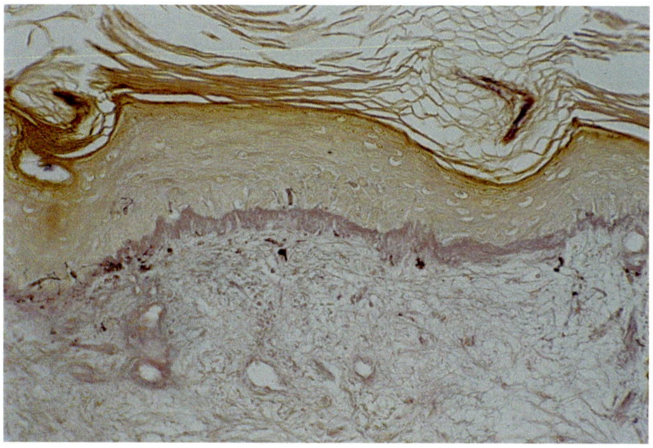

Fig. 13.23 DM, Alcian blue-PAS stain. The tissue section was pretreated with diastase (amylases) to remove glycogen. The reactive substances along the dermo-epidermal (DE) junction or so-called basement membrane zone are mainly neutral mucopolysaccharrides, fibrin, type IV and type VII collagens and others. These materials have traditionally been called "fibrinoid"

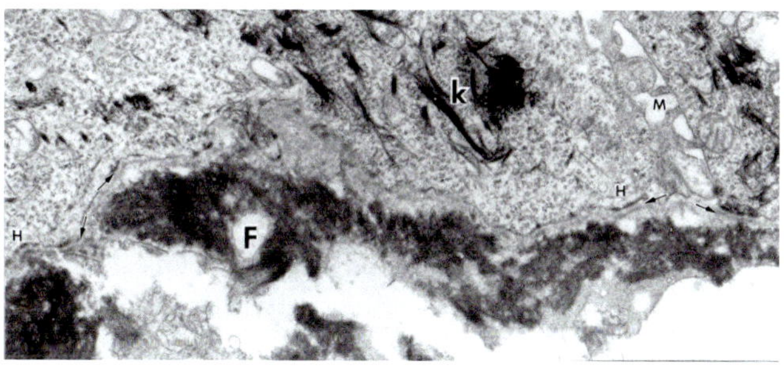

Fig. 13.24 DM, D-E junction. Electron dense, amorphous, substance (*F*) is located just beneath the lamina densa (*arrow*) or continuous to it. This substance is an admixture of multiplicated lamina densa, immunoglobulins, complements C3, anchoring fibrils, fibrin, fibrillin and many other fibrous proteins. The basal cell above this deposit shows no cellular damage; it has intact cell membrane (*M*), keratin fibrils (*K*), and hemidesmosomes (*H*)

Dermo-epidermal junction (D-E junction) of old lesion is thickened by a deposition of PAS positive, diastase (amylase) nondigestible (or resistant) neutral mucopolysaccharides (Fig. 13.23).

Direct immunofluorescence (DIF): This is the test to check if immunoglobulin and/or complement (C3) are deposited in the lesional skin. Fluorescein-conjugated antihuman IgM is used assuming that immunoglobulin antibody is IgM class as most other DM cases.

In DM, IgM deposition occurs along the D-E junction. If peroxidase-conjugate is used, the surrounding structures, such as the epidermis, is visible and the tissue orientation of the positive band is easier. It seems that IgM, other Ig and C3, which may be positive are not pathogenic but caught by the fine network of filament in the papillary dermis because there is no sign of structural damage in the vicinity of the immunoglobulin deposit (Fig. 13.24). The filaments in this

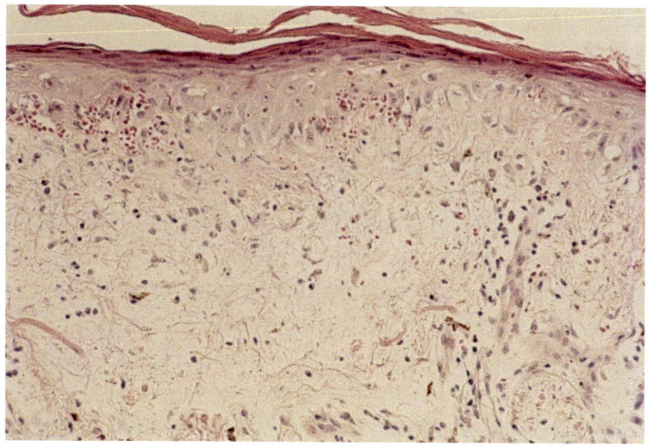

Fig. 13.25 DM. The epidermis became thin and lost rete ridges. The basal cells are focally vacuolated and lymphocytes are seen around the vacuolated foci. In the papillary dermis capillaries are dilated in the edematous upper dermis. Red blood cells are leaking out of the ruptured capillaries

region comprise type IV and VII collagens, laminin fibrillin, and reticulum fibers. They work together as molecular sieve and Ig, particularly large IgM molecules are caught passively and nonimmunologically. Pemphigus autoantibodies destroy desmogleins and therefore are pathogenic [166].

Poikilodermatous lesions (Fig. 13.19) show similar features to those seen in poikiloderma atrophicans vasculare of Jacobi. This type of poikiloderma is also seen in SLE, mycosis fungoides, and dyskeratosis congenita, like in DM, these conditions develop vacuolization or sustain severe damages to the basal cells (Fig. 13.25). Melanin granules are released from damaged basal cells and melanocytes. The epidermis is atrophic within the poikiloderma lesion. The epidermis in the Gottron's papules maintains normal thickness of knuckles.

Electron Microscopy: You may be curious about the components of Alcian blue stained, PAS (+) band along the D-E junction. Also what ultrastructural components are the targets of those immunoglobulins and complement C3? The answer to those questions is under the immunoelectron microscopy (Fig. 13.24). This method is the same with the direct immunofluorescence (DIF), except that antihuman immunoglobulins are conjugated with peroxidase. Peroxidase is a protein and therefore electron dense by itself. In a low magnification the thickened basal lumina, anchoring fibrils and others are positively labeled. In high magnification mostly a morphous, electron-dense materials whose density is enhanced by peroxidase were revealed to be deposited below or continuously to the basal lamina (Fig. 13.24). The amorphous materials are an admixture of multiplicated lamina dense (basal lamina), filamentous structures of D-E junction (anchoring fibrils, fibrillin), and peroxidase-Ig conjugates. The structural alterations are rather hyperplastic than degenerative and mild; basal cells are intact and normal basal lamina and hemidesmosomes are visible between the dense amorphous deposits (Fig. 13.24). These observations suggest that these Igs are not toxic to the structures of this junction and nonpathogenic in the skin. These DE junction deposit materials correspond to fibrinoid material of DE junction as seen and defined in the light microscopy pathology (Fig. 13.23).

When the muscle biopsy is required, triceps is preferred to deltoid and others because the chances to encounter the pathological changes are greater with the triceps. Muscle changes are mainly so-called lymphocytic myositis consisting of infiltration of myotoxic lymphocytes between muscle fibers. Muscle fibers lose striations and are fragmented (Fig. 13.26).

Differential diagnosis: (1) Psoriasis resembles DM with thick knee and elbow lesions. Sebo-psoriasis presents similar lesions to Fig. 13.14. However, heliotrope-colored eyelids telangiectasia and erythema of distal dorsal fingers and posterior nailfold (Fig. 16) are absent. (2) SLE shares the butterfly lesion and photosensitivity, nailfold erythema and telangiectasia with DM. Histology of SLE is almost identical including atrophy of the lesional epidermis, fibrinoid deposit along the D-E junction and dermal mucin accumulation. Gottron's papules look like verruca vulgaris. Elevated muscle enzymes and Jo-1, Mi-2 antibodies are in favor of DM.

Treatments: DM is a rare disease and double blind tests of new drugs are difficult. However, empirically and small number of controlled studies identified several drugs which are currently being used. The mainstay of DM treatment is prednisone (1 mg/kg/day). Keep patient on this dose until remission and then taper to find out the minimum required dose. Steroid sparing drugs such as methotrexate may be added (up to 20 mg/wk). Several drugs have been used to reduce prednisone or as an independent medications. A few examples are azathioprine (2–3 mg/kg/day), IVIg (2 g/kg/month), cyclosporin (3–5 mg/kg/day), and chlorambucil (4 mg/day). Anti-TNFa was used with variable results. There is no doubt that biologics continue to be invented and if an effective one should be found, it may give an insight to the pathogenesis of DM.

13.6 Scleroderma

Ken Hashimoto, MD

13.6.1 Scleroderma

13.6.1.1 Systemic Scleroderma

In the first edition of Lever's *Histopathology of the Skin* (1949), scleroderma was simply divided into two types, i.e., circumscribed (morphea) and systemic (generalized) [167]. For about 25 years since then, the term "progressive systemic scleroses (PSS)" enjoyed popularity. Morphea has never changed the name and in the meantime has established its brand name. As it happens in many diseases of unknown etiology, scleroderma has adjusted to comply with the most popular concept of the time limited systemic sclerosis (lSSc) and diffuse systemic sclerosis (dSSc) [168] are the current ones. The latter variant is generalized and more severe form than the former. The details of this classification criteria are listed in Table 13.3, one of the advantages of this classification is that many signs, symptoms, and autoantibodies could be divided and assigned either to limited or diffuse group. For example, tendon friction rubs, interstitial pulmonary fibrosis, renal crisis, and SCL-70 autoantibodies are more frequently seen in dSSc, whereas calcimosis, mat telangiectasia (Figs. 13.34 and 13.35) and anticentromere autoantibodies (Fig. 13.27) are more frequently encountered in lSSc

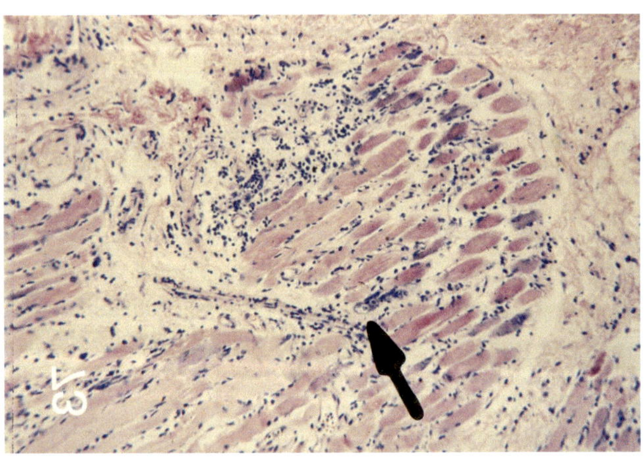

Fig. 13.26 DM, myositis. Muscle fibers are damaged and fragmented, probably due to toxic proteins secreted by the infiltrating cells including CD8 cytotoxic T cells. Basophilic thin fibers (*arrow*) represent regenerating young fibers

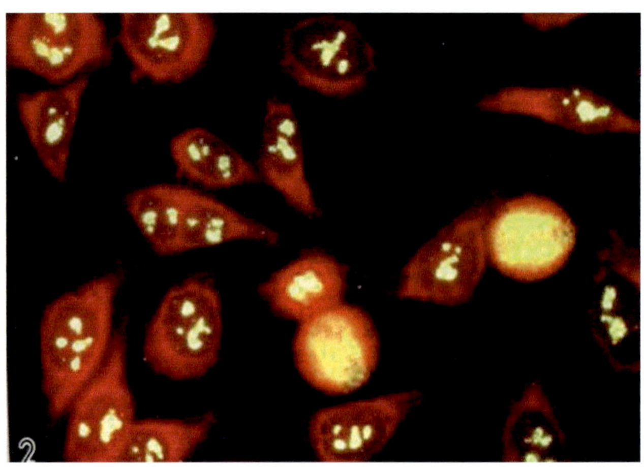

Fig. 13.27 FANA. Centromeric pattern, also called discrete speckled pattern. Each nucleus has 46 speckles, the numbers of chromosomes. The antigen showing fluorescence is CENP-1 protein of centromere. The presence of this antibody reliable predict that the patient has lSSc

Table 13.4 Criteria for limited (lSSc) and diffuse (dSSc) systemic sclerosis

Diffuse cutaneous SSc (dSSc)	
1	Internal between the episodes of Reynaud's phenomenon and the first appearance of the skin signs must be shorter than one year
2	Involved areas expand from distal extremities forward trunk beyond elbows and knees
3	Tendon friction rubs
4	Renal crisis (decreased with advent of ACE inhibitors)
5	Pulmonary fibrosis, interstitial pneumonitis, cardiomyopathy, small intestine involvements, esophageal dysmotility
6	Telangiectasia and hemorrhage of posterior nail fold
7	CREST syndrome
8	Higher positive rate of certain autoantibodies; e.g. Scl-70 (20–60)
9	Survival rates(5 years) 70 %; (10 years) 50 %
Limited cutaneous SSc (lSSc)	
1	Interval between the Reynaud's phenomena occurrence and the start of sclerosis is longer than 1 year
2	Skin sclerosis is limited to the periphery such as hands, feet and face. It does not spread proximally beyond elbows and knees
3	Calcinosis of the skin
4	Mat telangiectasia on face, palms and lips. These also appear like vascular spiders, capillary loop and/or hemorrhage in posterior nail folds
5	CREST syndrome
6	Late onset pulmonary hypertension
7	Anti-centromere antibody or discrete speckled pattern IIF (50–90 %)
8	ANA is positive in 90 % of both lSSc and dSSc
9	Survival rates (5 years) 90 %, (10 years) 70 %

(Table 13.4). Both lSSc and dSSc begin with Reynaud's phenomenon and swelling of fingers and toes. The ensuing sclerosis does not advance proximally beyond elbows and knees in lSSc. In dSSc, the sclerosis expands beyond elbows and knees.

Incidence and prevalence rate in the United States, these are 20 and 250/million, respectively [169]. As in other autoimmune connective tissue diseases female/male ratios are 3–4/1 [169]. The age of onset is between 30 and 50; racially, blacks have earlier onset and more diffuse types (dSSc). Japanese dSSc patients [170] develop less renal crisis and pulmonary hypertension than USA and European dSSc counterpart.

SSc and autoantibodies [171] 90 % of SSc patients have antinuclear autoantibodies (ANA). The expression of these autoantibodies precedes Reynaud's phenomenon, the earliest symptom of SSc. Several autoantibodies are helpful to establish the diagnosis and predict the course of the patient. Centromeric (discrete speckled pattern) (Fig. 13.27) and nuclear pattern (Fig. 13.28) in IIF strongly suggest SSc or morphea. SCL-70 patient may develop dSSc and interstitial pulmonary fibrosis (Table 13.4). It is unknown why Scl-70 (topoisomerase 1), which unwind double-stranded DNA, causes severe fibroplasia in the skin and lung. Further analysis of autoantibodies may yield more information if these antoantibodies are pathogenic. Some autoantibodies are truly pathogenic; e.g., anti-desmoglein 3 antibodies that exhibit nuclear IIF pattern (Fig. 13.28), are specific for dSSc

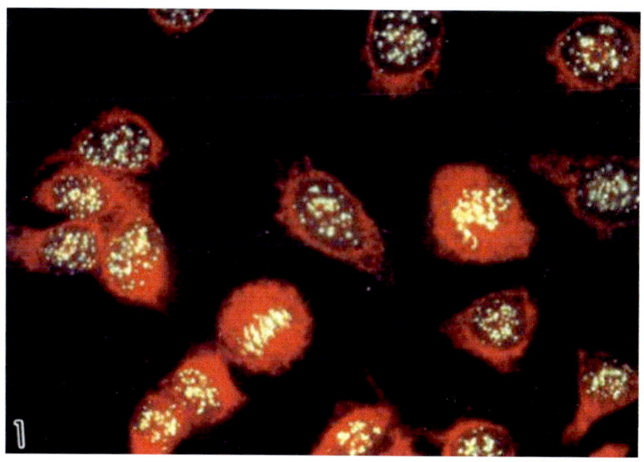

Fig. 13.28 FANA. Nucleolar pattern. The antigens are Th/To and U3RNP of nucleolus. If this is singly (exclusively) positive, it is likely that the patient has SSc. The positive rate is 5 % of SSc. Fluorescent particles are larger in size but smaller in number* than those of centromeric pattern (Fig. 13.27)

if they are positive singly without other positive autoantibodies [172]. In Japan U3RNP(ribonucleoprotein) and Th/To antibodies are found in 5 % of SSc.

A. *Anti-topoisomerase-1 (topo-1):* Topo-1 is a representative marker of dSSc. Topo-1 autoantibodies are found in severe cases of widespread cutaneous sclerosis and pulmonary fibrosis. Patient's clinical course is variable;

Table 13.5 Disease-type specific autoantibodies of SSc [174]

Autoantibodies	Frequency	Clinical correlation
Scl-70(topoisomerase 1)	30–40 %	Wide-spread sclerosis (dSSc) Poor peripheral circulation-Finger-tip ulceration Pulmonary fibrosis
Centromere	30–40 %	Sclerosis is limited to distal extremities (lSSc) Pulmonary fibrosis, renal crisis, severe internal diseases are rare Telangiectasia and calcinosis are common Pulmonary hypertension may start after along course
RNA polymerase III	5 % (lSSc) 45 % (dSSc)	Rapid progress of wide-spread sclerosis A high degree of cutaneous sclerosis -contracture of fingers Interstitial pneumonitis is uncommon Disturbance of peripheral circulation is mild Oral corticosteroid is effective
PM-Scl	5–15 %	PM-SSc overlap syndrome
n-RNP	15 %	Overlap with SLE and arthritis Mixed connective tissue diseases

some patients progress rapidly and other slowly. In white and black SSc patients, 15–30 % are topo-1 positive, but in Japanese patients the positive rate is up to 65 %. IIF pattern of topo-1 is mainly homogenous.

B. *Centromere antibody:* This is the marker of lSSc which is generally less severe than dSSc; the sclerosis is limited to the face and distal extremities below the knees and elbows (Table 13.5). Sometimes mitochondrial antibodies (PDC-E1) are produced; this combination is found in some primary biliary cirrhosis. Anticentromere autoantibody can be demonstrated on cultured Hep-2 cell. This cell line was established from a human laryngeal cancer. If patient serum contains antibody to centromere, it combines to 46 centromeres of mitotic Hep-2 cell (Fig. 13.27). The TTF pattern of centromere antoantibody is "discrete speckled" (Fig. 13.27).

   Indirect immunofluorescence

   The precise antigenic molecules in the centromere are CENPA, B, C; any one of these three gives the same fluorescence pattern.

C. Antinucleolar autoantibody: If this antibody is singly positive without others, the possibility of SSc is high. In Japan approximately 5 % of SSc patients carry this antibody. The singly positive nucleolar antibodies include anti-U3RNP and Th/To antibodies [172]. IIF pattern is similar to centromere's speckled image, but number of nucleolus is much smaller than 46 centromeres. However, the individual sizes of speckles are larger in nucleolar (Fig. 13.28) than those of centromeric (Fig. 13.27) pattern.

D. *Anti-RNA polymerase autoantibody:* RNA polymerase functions in RNA duplication. Antibody against this protein, i.e., RNAPI, II, III, are more often found in elderly male patients of late onset. Renal diseases are common but pulmonary fibrosis and peripheral vascular problems are not frequent. Overall the prognosis is good. IIF pattern is nucleolar probably because RNA is concentrated in nucleoli (Fig. 13.28).

E. *Anti-UIRNP (Th/To) autoantibody*: This has been best known for mixed connective tissue disease (MCTD) but also found in SSc and SLE. The patients who have this antibody demonstrate a limited spread of sclerotic (Table 13.5). UIRNP molecule is made from UI-A, UI-C,UI70KD. Despite the mild and limited involvement of the skin, this subset presents with severe pulmonary fibrosis and inflammatory arthritis. U1RNP antibody positive patients manifest symptoms similar to those of anticentromere positive patients with much less gastrointestinal symptoms. Antigens are 40-kDa protein that is bound to 7-2 RNA (To RNA) *and* 8-2 RNA (Th RNA).

   Indirect immunofluorescence. Microscope should be equipped with the lamp capable to emit 495 nm wave length ray. 495 nm is the absorption spectrum of fluorescein.

F. *Anti-infibrillarin (U3RNA) autoantibody*: The antigen of this antibody is present in the fibrillar center of nucleolus, i.e., 34-kDa submit of U3RNP. In white population this antibody is associated with dSSc and the patients exhibit pitted ulcers of fingertips, calcinosis, myopathies, small intestinal disease, and primary pulmonary hypertension.

G. Anti-PM-Scl autoantibody: This was initially thought specific for polymyositis-SSc overlap syndrome, only later to discover cases of SSc without myositis. The antigen is a compound protein of granular region of nucleolus. Most patients who have PM-Scl antibody experience a mild lSSc but some patients suffer from muscle weakness with elevated muscle enzymes.

H. Antinuclear antibodies (ANA): If fluorescein is used in anti-human IgG* conjugate, the method is called FANA. All autoantibodies whose antigens reside in the nucleus and nucleolus are ANA. By means of molecular mimicry (antigen crossing) extranuclear material may serve as antigen of ANA. It does not matter where the antigen is located; it is important where the fluorescence occurred within the boundary of nuclear membrane. In the routine use of ANA, however, we usually look for more specific antibodies. If FANA is positive, i.e., the nucleus or nuclear component with homogeneous are peripheral pattern we report that ANA is positive. In this case the nuclear antigen is commonly ssDNA, namely the denatured DNA. ssDNA antibody is found in all autoimmune connective tissue diseases (SLE, DLE, SSc, morphea, DM/PM, MCTD, SjS, and RA).

Etiology: There seems to be three major areas of investigations; autoantibodies as pathogenic agents, a damaged vascular endothelial cell, and increased collagen synthesis. As I have discussed above that SSc patient has lost control over the production of autoantibodies of miscellaneous and nucleolar components. Nucleolar antibodies if occur singly, specifies SSc, there is no evidence that the nucleoli of SSc patient are destroyed by those antibodies. This is different from antidesmoglein 3 antibody that is toxic to the desmosomes by attacking extracellular molecule of desmoglein 3 [173].

Perhaps, we are producing millions of abnormal, damaged cellular organelles but we dispose them properly, so that autoantibodies of high titers are not found in our sera, SSc patient's surveillance system or immune tolerance is dysfunctional at least. Vascular endothelial cells are injured repeatedly by some unknown anoxia. The anoxia thus created in the tributary of the damaged vessels contribute to anoxic or hypoxic fibrosis. Perivascular lymphocytes are somehow stimulated to produce IL-4 and TGF-b that stimulate fibroblast to produce collagen [174].

Additionally, dermal fibronectin, proteoglycan, and fibrillin increase in the dermis, connective tissue growth factor contribute to the deposition and maintenance of collagen through the stimulation of fibroblasts. There are many exciting theories and some data to support his favorite story or pet hypothesis. Unfortunately, we have not seen really convincing one yet.

Clinically presentations: The difference between lSSc and dSSc is not only the dimensions of affected skin areas but also the signs and symptoms are different types and severities of internal organ involvements are also different between lSSc and dSSc (Table 13.5). Single nucleolar IIF strongly suggests SSc. The presence of centromere antibody suggests lSSc, whereas Scl-70 often predicts dSSc. Clinical symptoms of a disease comprise a few major changes and additional abnormalities. In scleroderma, both lSSc and dSSc have several major lesions in common.

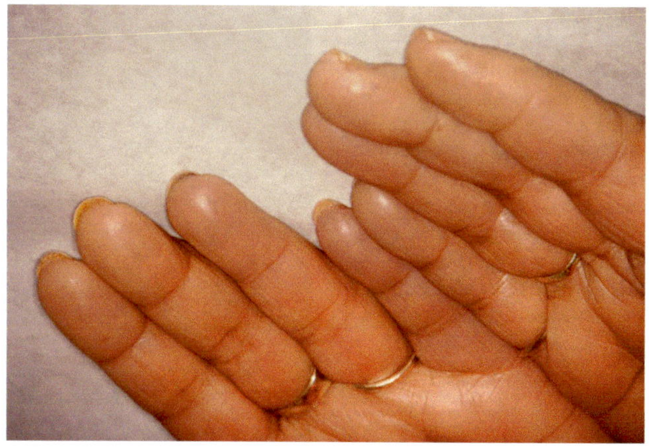

Fig. 13.29 Reynaud's phenomenon. An early stage symptom of SSc. Hands and fingers blanch when the patient is exposed to cold weather, cold water, or when he smokes. The edema is one of the early sign of SSc

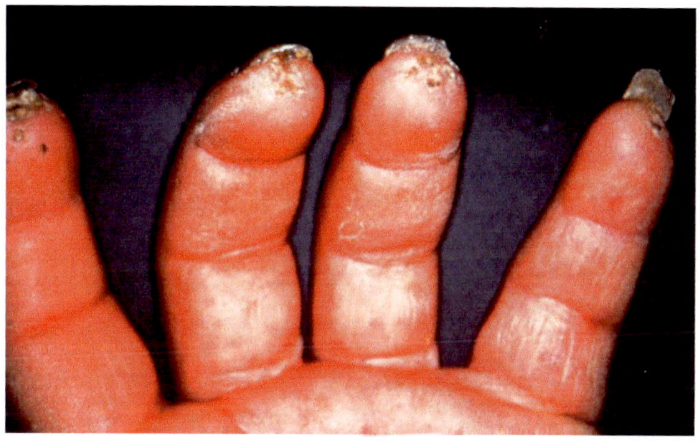

Fig. 13.30 Finger-tip ulcerations and telangiectasia. The edema is persisting

A. Raynaud's phenomenon and vascular dysfunction: Between the attacks of vasoconstriction the edematous skin of fingers and toes is dark-purple due to cyanosis. Vasoconstrictive reaction immediately begins when hands and fingers are immersed in an ice-cold water. Swollen fingers blanch and often the distal parts of the blanched fingers feet pain. Repeated attacks to the vascular endothelial cells induce fibrotic repair and intimal proliferation, luminal occlusion, and hypoxia. Hypoxia causes fibrosis of connective tissues. Poor circulation is maximized at the tips of fingers and toes (Figs. 13.29, 13.30, 13.31, 13.32, and 13.33) and spontaneous ulceration follows (Figs. 13.30 and 13.32). The dorsal skin of interphalangeal joints also undergo ulceration (Fig. 13.30). The joint capsules, tendon, and small fingers muscles are hardened. The position of fingers is set and fixed in contracture (Fig. 13.32). The same vascular dysfunctions occur in the toes (Fig. 13.33). The

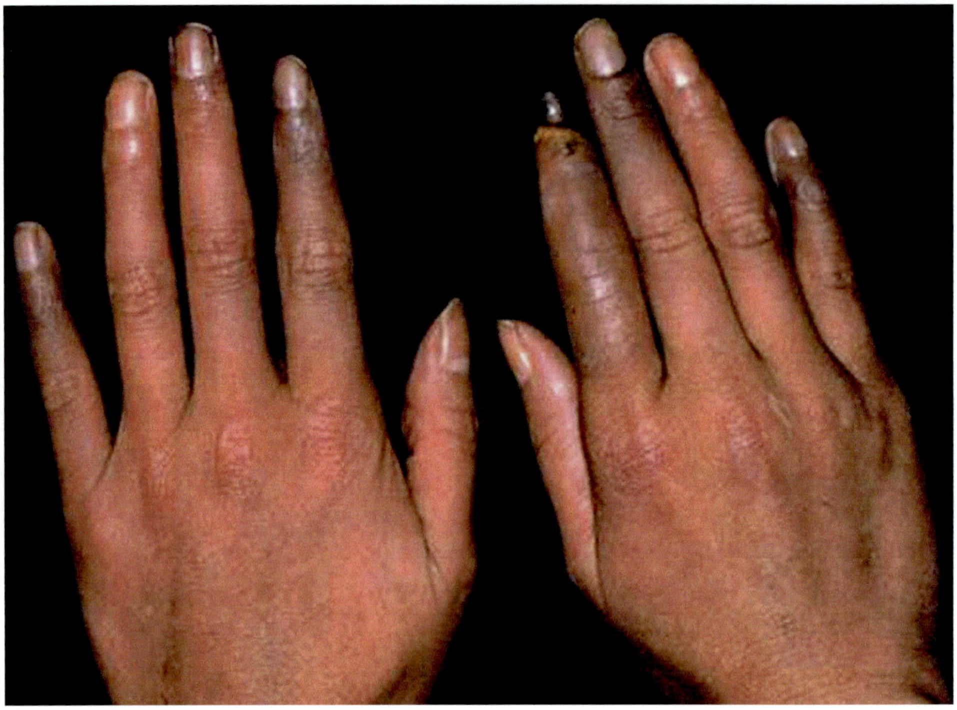

Fig. 13.31 Acrosclerosis or sclerodactyly. The skin of hands and fingers is pulled down to deep dermis and looks tight. Compare Fig. 13.31 with early edematous phase (Fig. 13.29); hands and fingers are because in the sclerotic stage subcutaneous fat and muscles are reduced and collagen fibers are compacted (Fig. 13.46). Over the knuckles the epidermis is hypertrophic and may be ulcerated

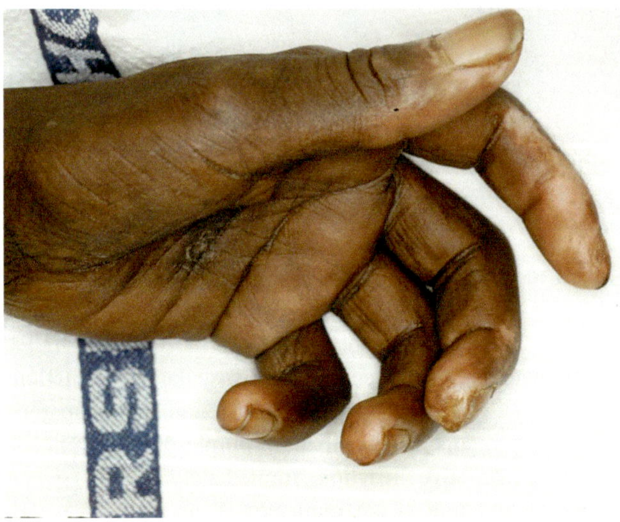

Fig. 13.32 Sclerodactyly. Sclerosis has advanced to fascia, muscle, and small tendons and restrict to the movements of interphalangeal joints of fingers causing ankylosis of joints in contracture position (claw hands)

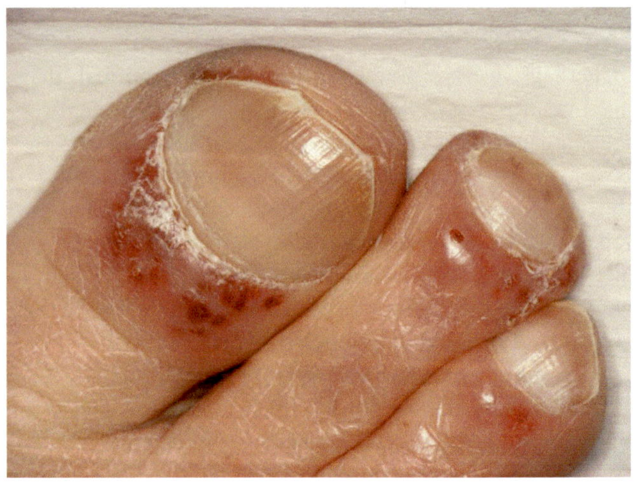

Fig. 13.33 Capillary dilation and hemorrhage in proximal nail folds. *Dark red* discoloration indicates the rupture of capillary and small hemorrhages. *The maximum number of nucleoli per Hep-2 cell is 4–5 (Fig. 13.28)

connective tissue sclerosis advances and capillaries upper dermis are squeezed between increasing collagen fibers. Between the constrictions superficial capillaries are dilated and produce capillary loops and hemorrhages in the proximal nail folds (Fig. 13.33). On the face the mat telangiectasia is seen (Figs. 13.34 and 13.35). It may also be present on the lips and palms.

B. Sclerosis: As the disease progresses edematous and soft skin of fingers and toes become hardened and could not be pinched with fingers. As collagen and other connective tissue components increase, the epidermis is pushed up from below and wrinkles are stretched. Wrinkles-free or reduced facial skin reflect light straight back without deflection or scattering. The patients appear young for their ages (Fig. 13.34).

C. Shiny skin: Edematous skin of Reynaud's stage SSc (Fig. 13.29 and 13.31) is replaced by tightly bound down hard skin (Fig. 13.30). Fingers appear thin (Fig. 13.30) and the face looks like wearing mask (Fig. 13.34) because

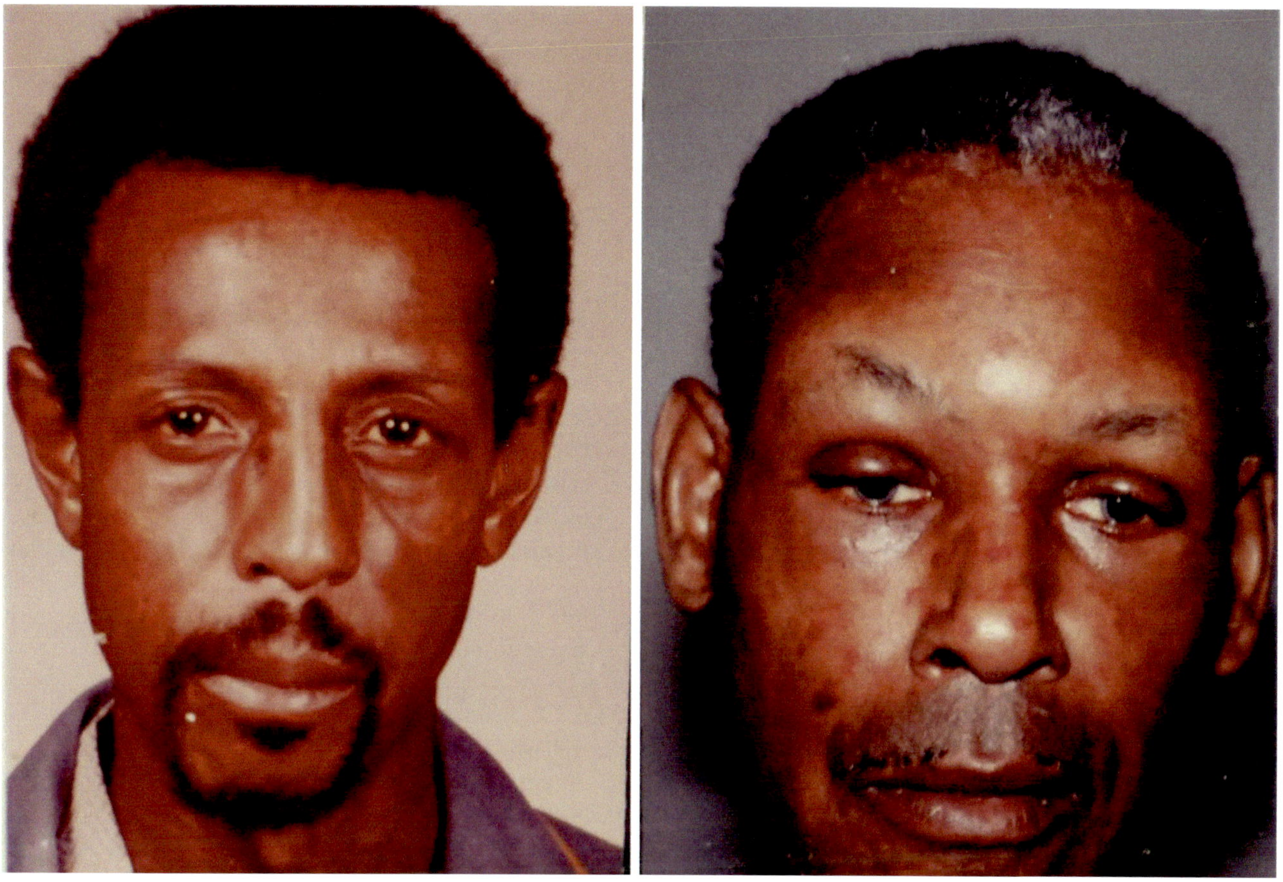

Fig. 13.34 Shiny face. The increased collagen edema and a mild inflammation stretched facial wrinkles to make the facial skin wrinkle free to make patient's face look younger. The patient on the right has numerous telangiectasia: These are called mat telangiectasia [5] but some of these appear more like vascular spiders with pulsating central feeding arteriole

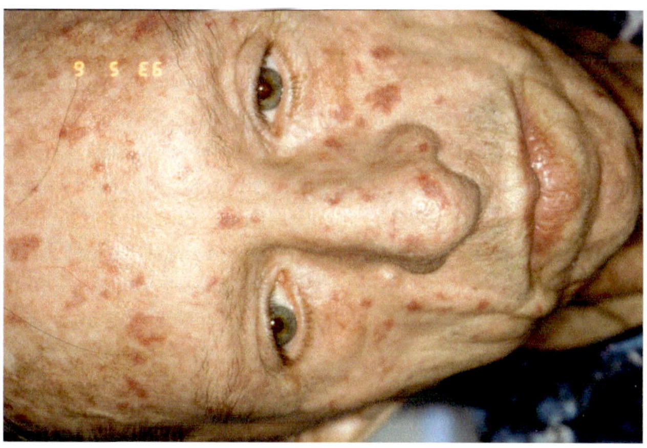

Fig. 13.35 Telangiectasia and vascular spider. This patient also had finger-tip ulceration

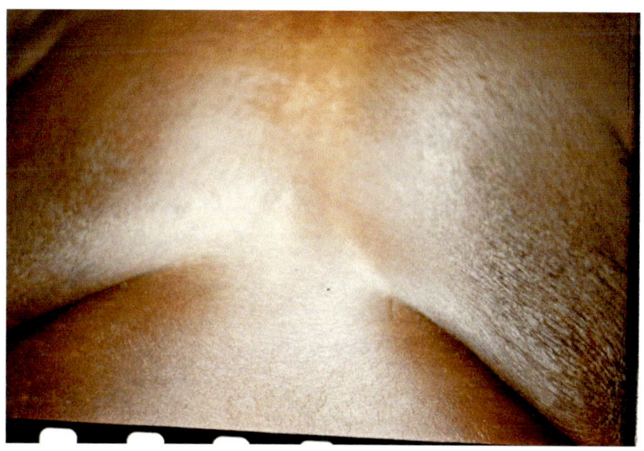

Fig. 13.36 Shiny skin. The skin of chest and breasts is stretched and shiny because skin surface is smooth and reflects light more efficiently without scattering

the skin is tout, wrinkle-free, and shiny. The patient looks younger than his or her real ages. Shiny skin is also seen on the trunk and breast (Figs. 13.35 and 13.36).

D. Dyspigmentation: Melanocytes are injured or stimulated by the stretching forces from underneath. Hypopigmentation or macular leukoderma is produced if melanocytes are damaged (Figs. 13.36, 13.37, and 13.38). Hyperpigmentation will be the result of melanocyte stimulation (Fig. 13.39). Incontinence of melanin granules released from damaged

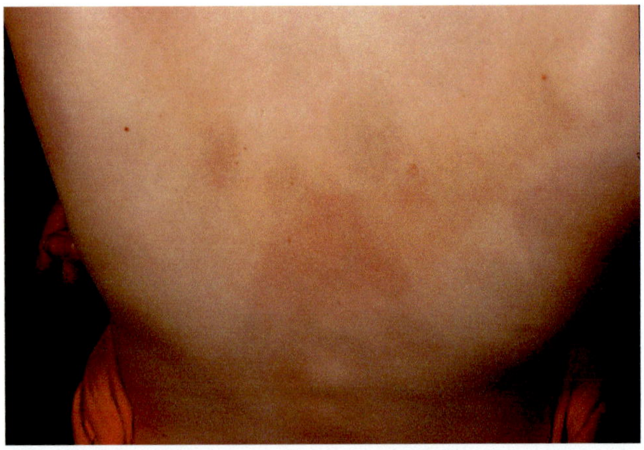

Fig. 13.37 Multiple morphea. This young patient has already had 10 plaque type morphea. This could progress to generalized morphea, probably by the similar mechanism to the dissemination of multiple DLE to SLE with ANA expression. Morphea to SSc conversion is accompanied by the production of autoantibodies, e.g., Scl-70

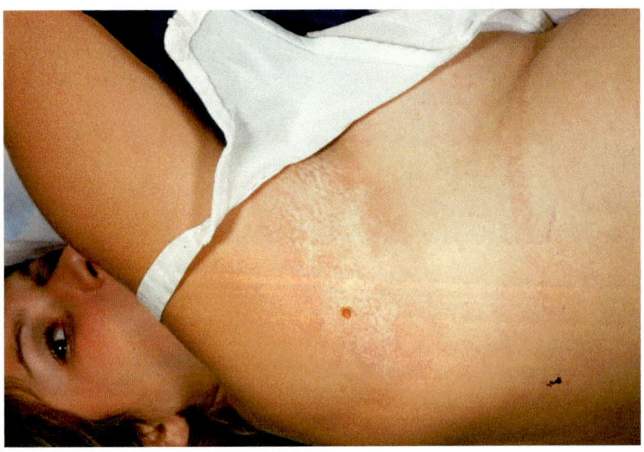

Fig. 13.38 Morphea plaque type. Ivory white center is slightly depressed. The irregular periphery is surrounded with purplish red layer or lilac ring. Without biopsy this lesion cannot be differentiated from lichen sclerosus et atrophicus

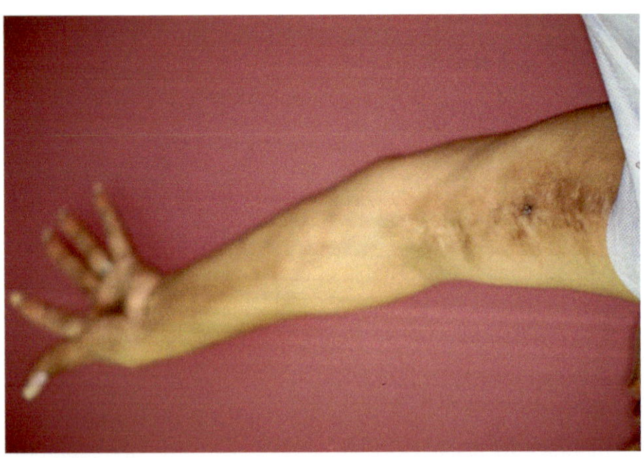

Fig. 13.39 Linear morphea. Extremities, especially extensor side is the favored site for linear morphea. Sclerotic skin appear pulled down from below. This is an old lesion and as usual pigmented

melanocytes and epidermal basal cells draw a picture of "salt and pepper". Salt and pepper pattern of skin discoloration also occurs in the early recovery stages of vitiligo when intraepidermal hair canal (acrotrickium) initiate repigmentation*. If poikiloderma-like change should occur, it is identical to that of dermatomyositis (seen Fig. 7 of chapter 13).

E. CRST and CREST syndrome: This is a subset of lSSc and the patient exhibits subcutaneous calcinosis, *R*eynaud's phenomenon, *s*clerosis, multiple telangiectasia (Figs. 13.34 and 13.35). If the patient has in addition esophageal dysfunction, it is called CREST syndrome.

F. Unusual variants: We discussed above the most common features of SSc. There are a few rather unusual variants: sclerosis sine scleroderma is reminiscent of dermatomyositis sine myositis. In some rare cases the sclerosis begins on the trunk and spread later over the extremities. Perioral sclerosis narrows opening of the mouth or pulls lips away to expose denture. This is one of the most severe cosmetic problems for SSc patients.

13.6.1.2 Morephea

Morephea is a well-defined sclerotic skin plague (s) of up to 15–20 cm in diameters. Multiple plague type, generalized plague type, linear type, and profound type exist. Regardless of the clinical types, the histopathological changes are similar to each other. Systemic symptoms are related to lung and kidney diseases and vascular dysfunction such as Reynaud's phenomenon are absent. The age of onset is younger (36 years) than SSc (42 years) [175]. The age distribution of the patients ranges from infants to the elderly. The plaque type is most common (Fig. 13.38). Generalized type is not just an increased number of plaques but numerous lesions develop with positive SSc autoantibodies. Normal skin remains between individual plaques, a distinguishing feature from SSc. Linear type affects extremities (Fig. 13.40). Linear type persists but plaque type may regress spontaneously after several years. A survey study from Olmsted County, Minnesota, between 1960 and 1993 revealed annual incidence rate of 27 per million. Women/men ratio was 2.6:1 [174]; as in other autoimmune connective tissue diseases morphea is a female predominant disease. Autoantibodies in morphea are either absent or of low titers equivalent to that of normal population. Exceptions are antibodies against single-stranded DNA (ssDNA), topoisomerase IIa, phospholipid, fibrillarin, and histone. It is obvious that these antibodies do not possess pathogenic effects on their antigens as desmoglein I autoantibody has on desmoglein I of desmosomes in pemphigus foliaceous [173]. High titers of ANA are found in linear type of juvenile morphea and in patients with generalized morphea [174]. It has been postulated that PDGFR on fibroblast is stimulated by autoantibodies and produce collagen [174]. Special variants of morphea are "sclerodermie en coup de sabre" meaning scleroderma of

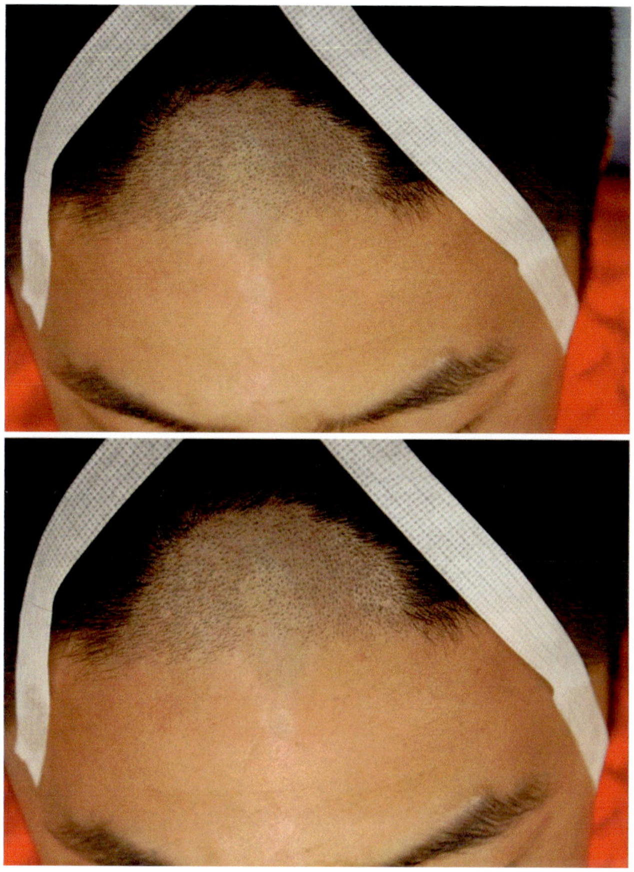

Fig. 13.40 Linear morphea of forehand and scalp, so-called sclerodermie en coup de sabre. The lesion expanded linearly into the scalp to causing linear alopecia

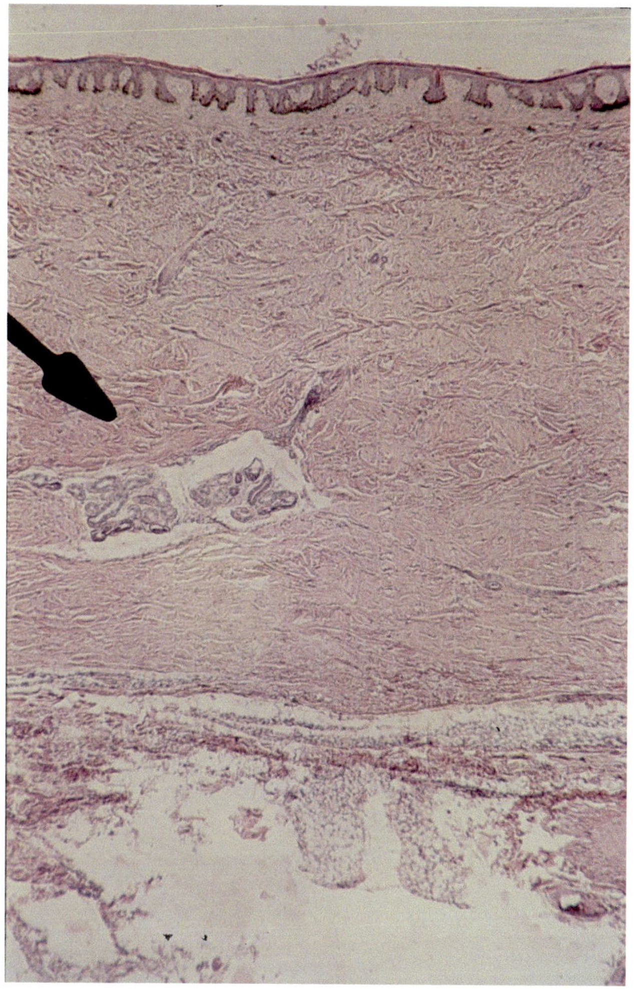

Fig. 13.41 Histology of SSc. Morphea and its variants show essentially the same abnormalities. Figure 13.41 is a relatively early lesion with scattered lymphocytic infiltration in the dermis and along the border between dermis and subcutaneous fat. Ecrrine gland (*arrow*) is pushed up by newly synthesized collagen. Periglandular space is not as tight as that of late stage compare with Fig. 13.43. The epidermis has preserved rete ridges

saber strike (Fig. 13.41) and hemiatrophie facei progressive in which the sclerosis affects the right or left half of the face. It may destroy bones.

Morphea does not have disease-specific autoantibodies like Sm of SLE, Jo-1 of DM, and Scl-70 of dSSc. In 50 % of morphea ssDNA antibody is positive, particularly so in linear morphea. If ssDNA antibody titers are measured with ELISA, ELISA scores (titers) fluctuate parallel with disease activities; the scores are predictive for flares and relapses. In SSc ELISA scores are useful to adjust oral corticosteroid dosage. Antihistonantibody is also positive in 50 % of morphea. Expression of this antibody seems to depend on the dimension of affected areas. FANA pattern of histone antibody is homogeneous because histone equals DNA in quantity and omnipresent within the nucleus. Mild cases of linear morphea have anti-P80 coilin antibody in place of ssDNA antibody. FANA pattern is like that of anticentromere antibody, i.e., discrete speckled pattern. Late-onset morphea of elderly patients often have antimitochondria antibody. This is rather rare (5 %) antibody in the whole morphea population.

A. *Clinical presentations*: Plaque type morphea begins as a small macule of light brown. The periphery of the expanding macule is often purplish red and referred to as a lilac ring or lichen sclerosus at atrophicus when the center of the macule is whitish, if not porcelain or ivory white (Fig. 13.39). The color of the lesion varies greatly depending upon the original color of patient's skin. As the lesion expands peripherally, the macule gains thickness and becomes a plaque of various density and colors. The center of the plaque appears depressed (Fig. 13.38) and feels hard in consistency. Some patients develop several plaques lesions, i.e., multiple plaque type, whereas other patients are covered with numerous plaques of various sizes; this type is called generalized morphea.

Patients who have symmetrical morphea on the extremities may eventually progress to SSc. Morphea rarely combines with SSc. In generalized morphea SSc-like symptoms and SSc-like autoantibodies appear; thus

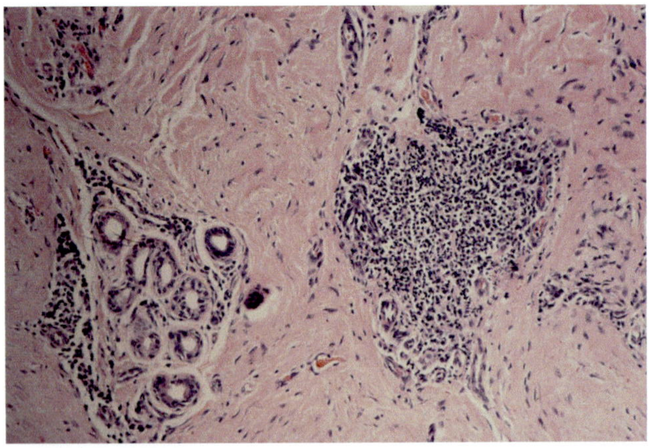

Fig. 13.42 Early lymphocytic stage. One of the eccrine glands is heavily infiltrated with lymphocytes. Other gland is spared from this infiltration but squeezed by increased new collagen

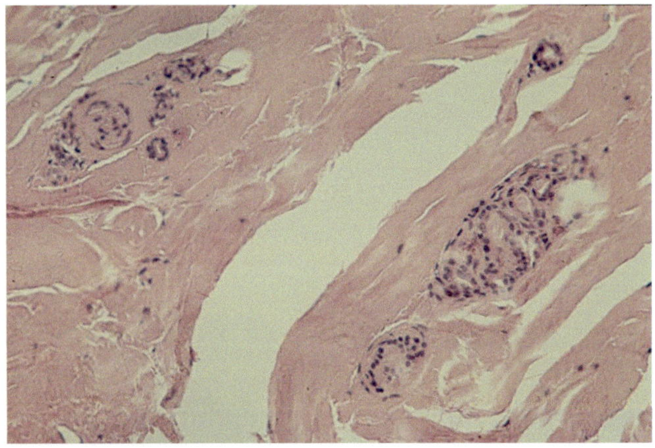

Fig. 13.43 Increased and hyalinized collagen are invading ecrrine glands to replace them with fibrosis. Rigid, inflexible collagen splits, and cracks in many places

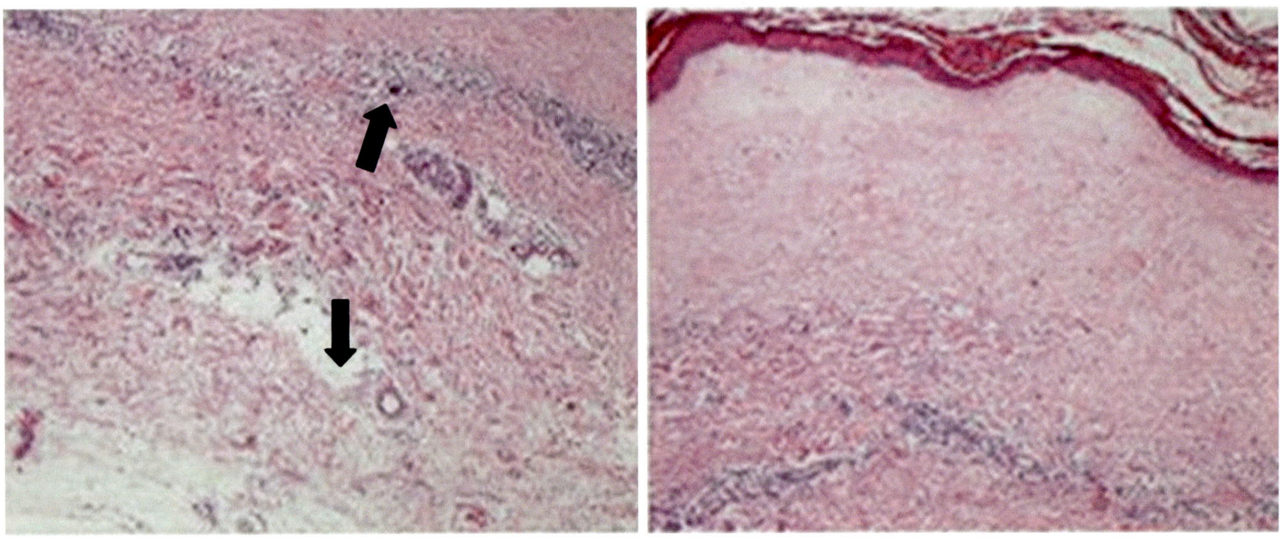

Fig. 13.44 Late stage lesion. Hyalinized collagen occupied entire dermis diffusely. Eccrine gland is pushed up (*left picture*). Arterioles show fibrotic thick wall (*arrow*) and transformation into hyalinized strand (*arrowhead*) (*right picture*)

arthralgia with positive RA factor, anti-histone autoantibody, and ssDNA may become positive.

B. *Linear morphea*: Predilection sites are extremities (Fig. 13.40), forehead to scalp (Fig. 13.41) and mandibular angle. The linear band is depressed, hard, and sometimes shiny. The surface appearance is a "plaque lesion made linear". Forehead scalp lesion takes the configuration of a stroke of a sabre or in original French "sclerodermie en couple de sabre". Scalp portion of this stroke causes a linear alopecia (Fig. 13.40).
C. *Morphea profunde* or subcutaneous morphea: This is an ill-defined and hard feeling plaque that is fixed firmly to the subcutaneous structures such as muscle, tendon, or fascia. The covering skin is smooth and shiny.

Histopathology: lSSc, dSSc, morphea, and their variants show essentially the same histological abnormalities but of different severity. Significant differences exist between the same clinical types according to the ages of individual lesions. Early lesions of all clinical types are characterized by a moderate infiltration of lymphocytes, most heavily surrounding the appendages (Fig. 13.42), particularly in and surrounding the eccrine gland (Fig. 13.42). Collagen deposition seems to occur where the inflammation has subsided, as surrounding eccrine gland (Figs. 13.42 and 13.43). Collagen synthesis takes place also in the subcutis and replaces subcutaneous fat tissue after the panniculitis (Figs. 13.41, 13.42, and 13.43).

New collagen deposition filled loosely woven periglandular spaces and pushes eccrine gland upward (Fig. 13.41). Squeezed glands also anoxic, disappear, or pushed up to the mid-dermis (Fig. 13.41). The wall of blood vessels are thickened and sclerotic but endothelial cells are often hypertrophic (Fig. 13.44 and 13.45). In late stage, the lesion has

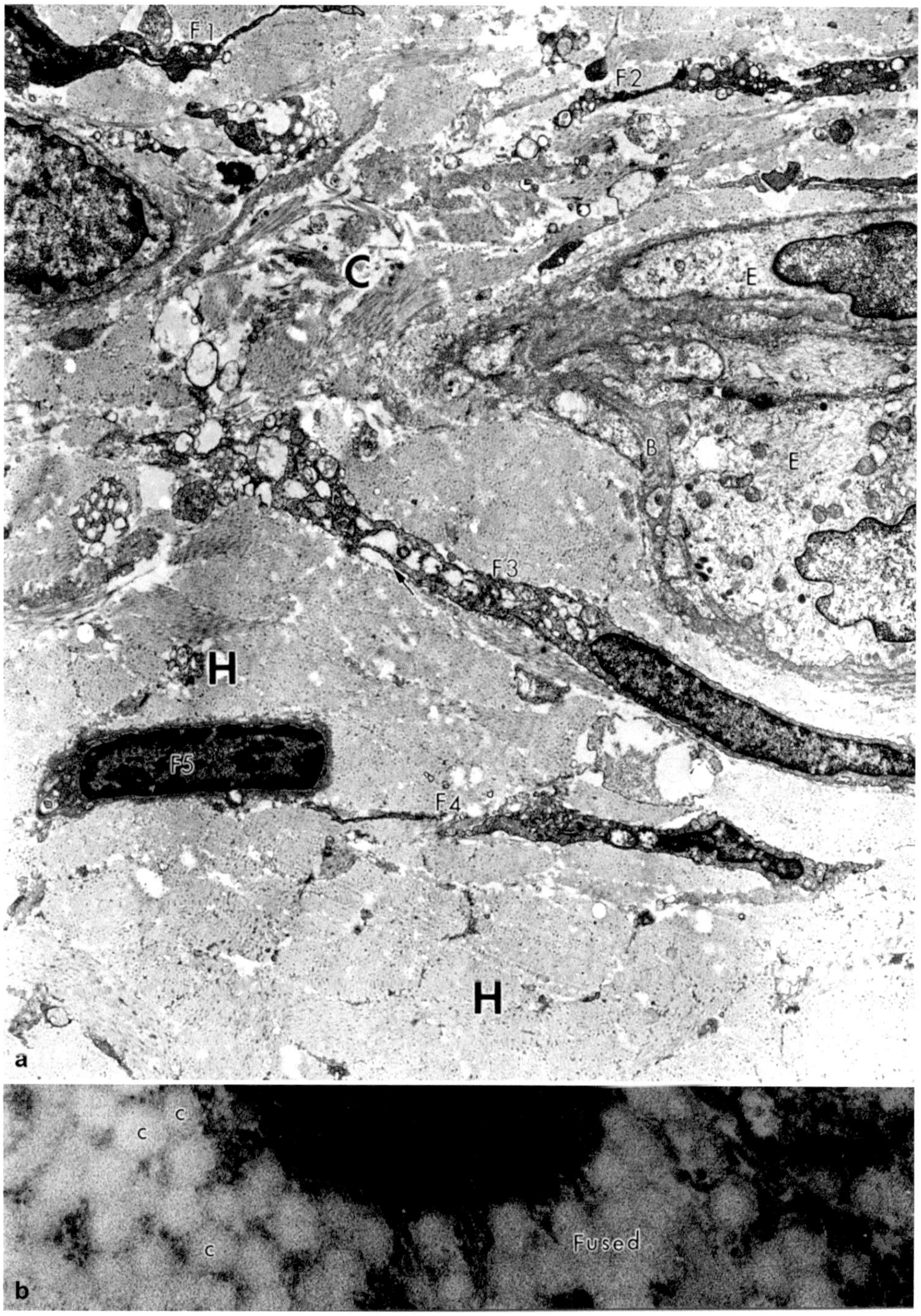

Fig. 13.45 Electron microscopy of scleroderma. Hyalinized collagen fibers (*H*) are poorly stained with osmium-uranyl/acetate-lead salt, the standard method of electro-staining. These hyalin collagen fibrils (*C*) are often fused to make a sheet of electron-light fibrous mass (*H*). Fibroblast (*F1–F5*) are not totally lost; they are squeezed between hyalinized collagen islands (*H*) and vacuolated. They extend thin trailing tail (*F1*). Fibroblast#5 has lost everything but nucleus. Small number of normal collagens are occasionally found (large lotten *C*). One fibroblast (*F3*) shows rough endoplasmic reticulum indicating that it is active in collagen production. (*B*) Fused collagen fibrils (Fused) and non-fused recognizable individual collagen unifibril (*C*) are recognized. Vascular endothelial cells are swollen (*E*) and surrounded with multiplicated basal lamina (*B*) and thin collagen fibrils

almost nothing but tightly bound hyalinized collagen (Figs. 13.43, 13.44, 13.45, and 13.46).

Histology of deep linear type and morphea profoundly show lymphedema due to pressure occlusion of lymphatic vessels. Fibrotic changes may be seen in the striated muscles and fascia.

Electron microscopy: Established lesion contains tightly packed or fused collagen fibrils (Figs. 13.45 and 13.46), degenerated fibroblasts (Fig. 13.45) and thick-walled blood vessels (Figs. 13.44 and 13.45). The dermal elements are squeezed between large islands of collagen fibrils. These collagen unit fibrils have lost periodical banding pattern of

67 nm (Fig. 13.47). Type I collagen unit fibrils vary their diameters from 30 to 150 nm in tendon and 50 to 55 nm in reticulum fiber. In sclerodermas of all types the diameters of these fibrils are smaller than normal. The most striking feature is the compaction of fibrils leaving little elbow rooms between unit fibrils (Fig. 13.46) under the light microscope, these matted fibers appear poorly stained with HE. These packed collagen masses are shiny and glassy, i.e., hyalinized (Figs. 13.44 and 13.45).

Treatments: During early stage when Reynaud's phenomenon and edema of hands and fingers are present, patients respond well to calcium channel blockers because the vascular motility is still maintained. Nifedipine is commonly prescribed. Inhibitors of angiotensin II receptor, e.g., Losartan, are used alone or in combination with others. Angiotensin II receptor blockers may be given alone or in combination. Phosphodiesterase type 5 inhibitor, e.g., sildenafil and tadalafil, which affect nitric oxide mediated vasodilatation, gave a mixed result. D-penicillamine has not met the initial expectation. Methotrexate, interferon, and photopheresis have had good days and bad days. Currently, UVA1 (340–400 nm) seems to be effective on morphea. Unlike SSc, morphea may eventually self-resolve. In the treatment of morphea self-resolution must be considered. Also, any treatment that leaves permanent skin color changes or scars must be avoided.

13.7 Lichen Sclerosus

Fiona Lewis

13.7.1 Introduction

Lichen sclerosus (LS) is one of the most common dermatoses to affect the anogenital skin and has a predilection at this site in both males and females. It is a chronic inflammatory disorder with unique features.

13.7.2 Etiology

Several theories have been proposed but the exact etiology of lichen sclerosus remains unclear.

13.7.2.1 Immunology

The skin immune system is involved throughout the epidermis and dermis [176] and the cytokines seen in LS may vary with early or late progression of lesions. It has been suggested that increased levels of interleukin-4 with respect to fibrogenesis may be implicated in the sclerosis that is seen in the disease [177]. Proinflammatory cytokines

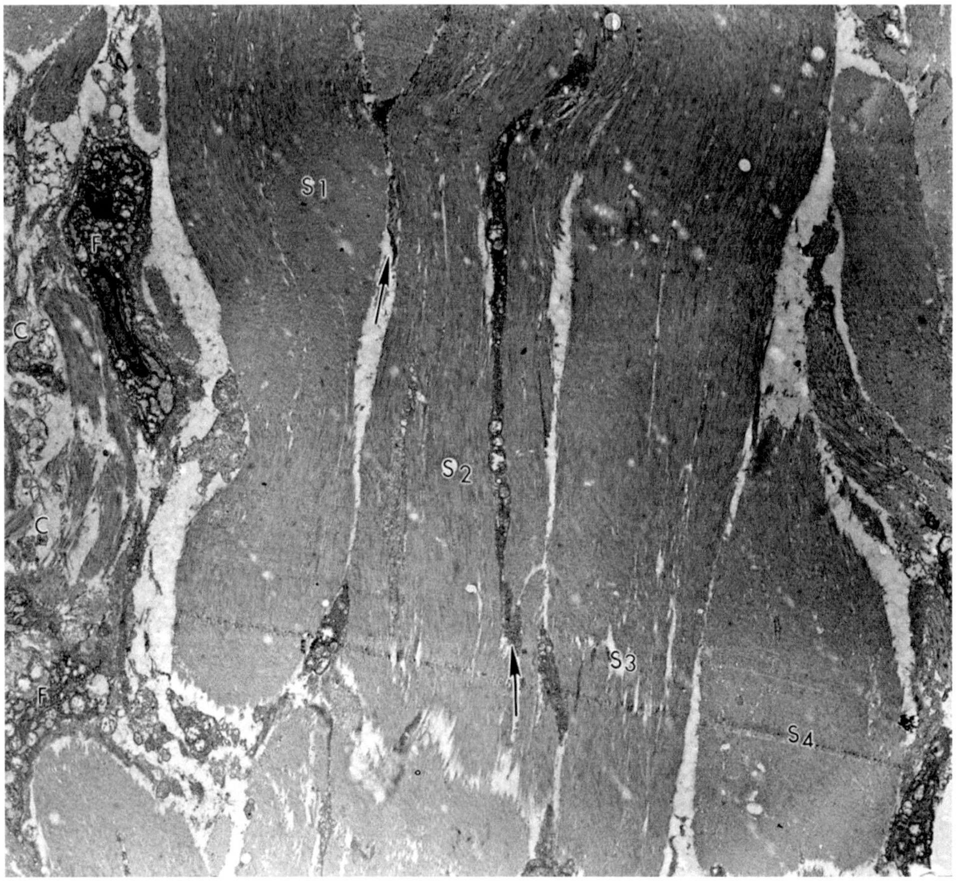

Fig. 13.46 Late stage SSc. Collagen fibrils are tightly packed to make collagen strands (*S1–S4*). Vasculated fibroblasts (*F*) interpose into the space between the strands. Some fibroblasts have slender, trailing cell bodies (*arrow*). Normal collagen (*C*) makes smaller strands in which nonfused individual fibrils are visible

specific for Th1 interferon-gamma induced immune response have been shown to be significantly increased in patients with lichen sclerosus [178]. The antibody to extracellular matrix protein 1 is raised in both females [179] and in males [180]. It is very interesting to investigate the circulating autoantibodies to the basement membrane zone [181] but their role is unclear as other studies have not confirmed these findings [182].

There does appear to be a strong association of LS in females with circulating autoantibodies or coexisting autoimmune disease. Antibodies in tissue have been reported in 40–75 % women [183–185] and up to 34 % may have at least one coexisting autoimmune disease. However, this link does not seem to occur in males [186].

13.7.2.2 Genetics

Women with lichen sclerosus have been investigated and show raised levels of DQ7 antigens of the HLA system compared with controls [187]. These are also raised in men, together with DR11 and DR12 [188].

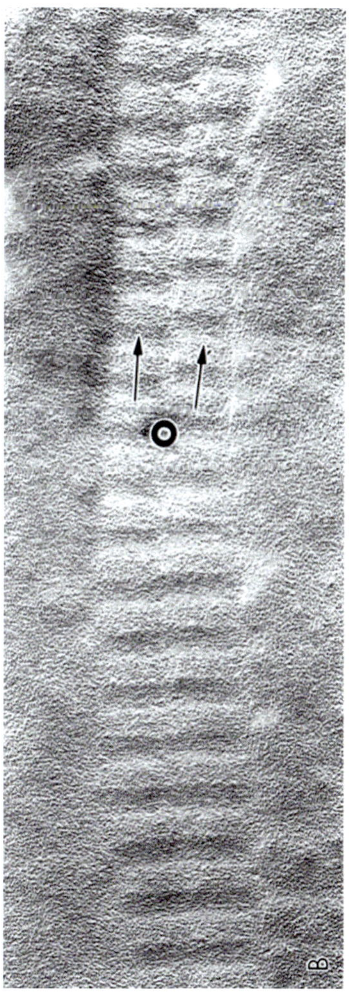

Fig. 13.47 Fusion (*o*) and separation (*arrows*) of 2 unit fibrils of collagen are seen in freeze fractured SSc skin

13.7.2.3 Infection

There has been interest in the role of *Borrelia burgdorferi* in lichen sclerosus but different studies have reported conflicting results and the high prevalence cited in some reports may just reflect the endemic incidence. There is no role of human papilloma virus (HPV) infection.

13.7.2.4 Hormones

Studies have shown a decrease in androgen receptors in lichen sclerosus [189] and this may explain the inefficacy of topical testosterone as treatment.

13.7.2.5 Trauma

Chronic exposure to urine is postulated as a factor in the development of lichen sclerosus in males [190, 191]. It is extremely rare for a male who has been circumcised at birth to develop LS.

13.7.3 Incidence

The prevalence is unknown and quoted figures vary depending on the population studied. They range from 0.0014 % in a large male population [192] to 1.7 % in women attending a general gynecological practice [193]. It is known that there is a bimodal peak of incidence in both sexes. In females, the symptoms of LS will start in the prepubertal age group, usually last for 3–5 years and the other modal peak is in postmenopause. However, the recurrence of symptoms occurs in 42 % of patients [194]. In males, the two peaks are in boys and the fourth decade [186].

13.7.4 Histology

The histopathological features of LS are a thinned epidermis overlying a dense homogenous band of collagen and an

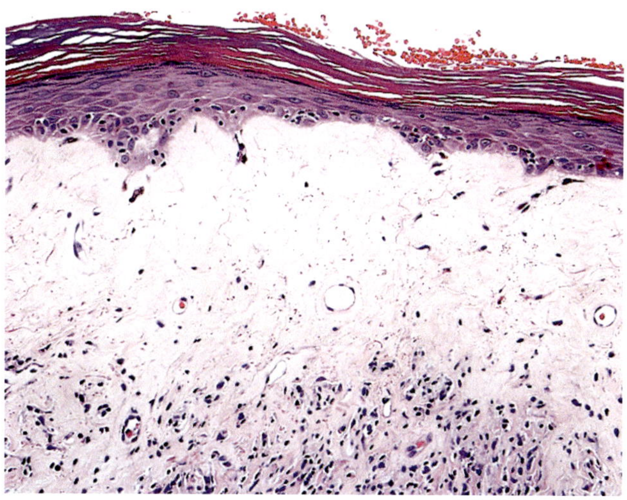

Fig. 13.48 Histology of lichen sclerosus (Courtesy of Dr Eduardo Calonje)

inflammatory infiltrate in dermis, admixed with predominant lymphocytes (Fig. 13.48). In early disease there may be difficulty in distinguishing LS from lichen planus as inflammatory cells infiltrate is denser in the dermis. Dermal edema and areas of hemorrhage are sometimes seen, corresponding to the ecchymosis seen clinically. It is important to note a thickened epithelium as these patients often have more recalcitrant disease and a higher risk of malignant changes.

13.7.5 Clinical Features

Lichen sclerosus is characterized by white sclerotic plaque. At extragenital sites, these may be thickened and follicular delling visible. Ecchymosis (purpura) is a frequent sign in active period of disease (Fig. 13.49).

13.7.5.1 Females

Pruritus is the predominant symptom in vulval LS and this may be severe enough to affect sleep. The resultant scratching can lead to excoriation and result in soreness and discomfort. Dyspareunia results from fissuring and introital narrowing. For children, constipation is a common symptom and is supposed to be a reason of perianal fissuring and discomfort. Dysuria is also common in children.

The inner labia majora and minora are the most frequently affected sites (Fig. 13.50) and the clitoral hood is also a common site. Perianal involvement as a "figure of eight" pattern is observed in about 30 % of females. Extragenital lesions have been reported in 13 % of patients [195].

Without treatment, there is a progressive alteration in the normal vulval structure. The labia minora is resorbed and the clitoral hood is sealed, eventually it can lead to burial of the clitoris. A pseudocyst can develop from the build-up of smegma and secretions under the clitoral hood. Anterior and posterior fusion of the labia can cause introital narrowing, resulting in dyspareunia and problems with micturition in severe cases. These patients need expert surgical management.

In children, the symptoms tend to improve at puberty but any structure change of skin may persist [196].

13.7.5.2 Males

In males, the prepuce and glans are the most commonly affected by lichen sclerous [186]. Urethral and meatal disease leads to stenosis and obstruction. Perianal and extragenital disease is rare in males. Phimosis is the most frequent presenting feature and is found in 40 % boys with lichen sclerosus [197]. Sexual dysfunction is common.

13.7.6 Treatment

The first line treatment for lichen sclerosus is an ultrapotent topical steroid [198], and clobetasol propionate 0.05 % is generally used on a three month induction regimen and then as required [199]. The same treatment is suitable for children [200]. Improvement of symptoms occurs in the majority of women and children with this therapy [201]. Clobetasol propionate 0.05 % will be helpful in the management of male genital lichen sclerosus but up to 40 % will also require circumcision [186, 202].

There are few comparative studies of different topical corticosteroids or regimens used but a recent study has shown that mometasone furoate may be effective in vulval LS [203]. There has been interest in the topical calcineurin inhibitors but they

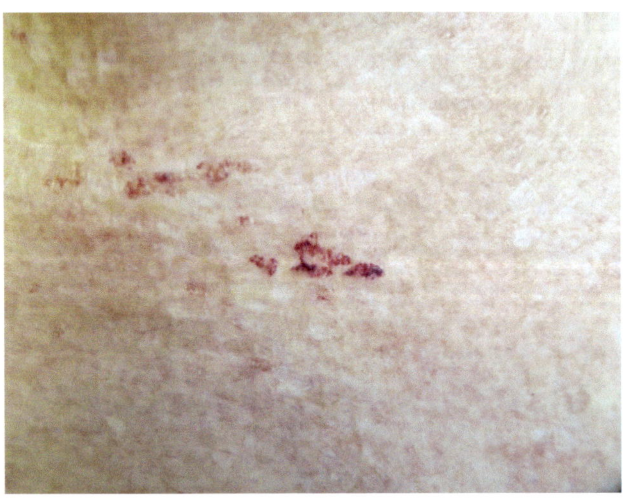

Fig. 13.49 Purpura in extra genital lichen sclerosus

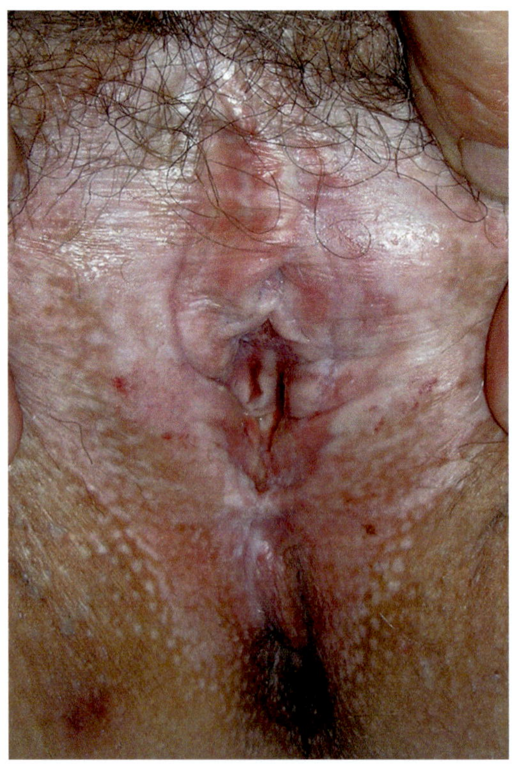

Fig. 13.50 Vulval lichen sclerosus

are not as effective as topical steroids in improving symptoms [204] or altering inflammatory histological features [205].

In females, surgery is only used for patients with severe scarring, or those who have suffered from vulval intraepithelial neoplasia or SCC. Conversely, in males, circumcision can be extremely useful, and other surgical procedures are sometimes necessary for achieving good results [206]. Few patients will require ultrapotent steroid as alternative treatment.

Other treatment options have been reported, including phototherapy, retinoids and photodynamic therapy [199, 207, 208].

13.7.7 Malignancy

The risk of developing squamous cell carcinoma (SCC) is quoted at 4–5 % of women with lichen sclerosus [209]. The risk appears to be greater in those suffered from hyperkeratotic disease. Studies of patients with vulval SCC have demonstrated lichen sclerosus is presented in the surrounding tissue in up to 32 % patients [210–212]. Differentiated vulval intraepithelial neoplasia (VIN) is a precursor of vulval SCC and may be observed at the edge of the tumor. This is not generally associated with HPV. Similarly in males, LS has been found in 55 % of patients with penile SCC [213].

13.7.8 Summary

Lichen sclerosus is a common disease and if managed well and early, it should lead to good control of symptoms and cessation of any further scarring. It is important for good patient education and detecting abnormal signs and any neoplastic change early. This is especially important in those with atypical or difficult to control disease.

References

Pemphigus

1. Amagai M. Pemphigus: autoimmunity to epidermal cell adhesion molecules. Adv Dermatol. 1996;11:319–52.
2. Kasperkiewicz M, Zillikens D, Schmidt E. Pemphigoid diseases: pathogenesis, diagnosis, and treatment. Autoimmunity. 2012; 45(1):55–70.
3. Ahmed AR, et al. Major histocompatibility complex haplotype studies in Ashkenazi Jewish patients with pemphigus vulgaris. Proc Natl Acad Sci. 1990;87:7658–62.
4. Niizeki H, et al. HLA-DQA1, -DQB1 and -DRB1 genotyping in Japanese pemphigus vulgaris patients by the PCR-RFLP method. Tissue Antigens. 1994;44:248–51.
5. Veldman C, et al. Dichotomy of autoreactive Th1 and Th2 cell responses to desmoglein 3 in patients with pemphigus vulgaris (PV) and healthy carriers of PV-associated HLA class II alleles. J Immunol. 2003;170:635–42.
6. Hertl M, Veldman C. Pemphigus–paradigm of autoantibody-mediated autoimmunity. Skin Pharmacol Appl Skin Physiol. 2001;14:408–18.
7. Stanley JR. Autoantibodies against adhesion molecules and structures in blistering skin diseases. J Exp Med. 1995;181:1–4.
8. Daneshpazhooh M, et al. Desmoglein 1 and 3 enzyme-linked immunosorbent assay in Iranian patients with pemphigus vul garis: correlation with phenotype, severity, and disease activity. J Eur Acad Dermatol Venereol. 2007;21(10):1319–24.
9. Shapiro L, et al. Structural basis of cell-cell adhesion by cadherins. Nature. 1995;374:327–37.
10. Pan M, Liu X, Zheng J. The pathogenic role of autoantibodies in pemphigus vulgaris. Clin Exp Dermatol. 2011;36(7):703–7.
11. Anhalt GJ, et al. Paraneoplastic pemphigus an autoimmune mucocutaneous disease associated with neoplasia. N Engl J Med. 1990;323:1729–35.
12. Anhalt GJ. Paraneoplastic pemphigus. J Invest Dermatol Symp Proc. 2004;9:29–33.
13. Brenner S, Bialy-Golan A, Ruocco V. Drug-induced pemphigus. Clin Dermatol. 1998;16:393–7.
14. Brenner S, Goldberg I. Drug-induced pemphigus. Clin Dermatol. 2011;29(4):455–7.
15. Jablonska S, et al. Herpetiform pemphigus, a variable pattern of pemphigus. Int J Dermatol. 1975;14:353–9.
16. Kasperkiewicz M, Kowalewski C, Jabłońska S. Pemphigus herpetiformis: from first description until now. J Am Acad Dermatol. 2014;70(4):780–7.
17. Virendra N, et al. Paraneoplastic pemphigus/paraneoplastic autoimmune multiorgan syndrome. Int J Dermatol. 2009;48: 162–9.
18. Tsuruta D, Ishii N, Hashimoto T. Diagnosis and treatment of pemphigus. Immunotherapy. 2012;4:735–45.
19. Ferguson CD, Taybos GM. Diagnosis and treatment of pemphigus. Quintessence Int. 1985;16:473–6.
20. Enrique Acosta Gio A. Immunofluorescence in the diagnosis and treatment of pemphigus vulgaris. Pract Odontol. 1986;7:6–8.
21. Ruocco E, Brunetti G, Del Vecchio M, Ruocco V. The practical use of cytology for diagnosis in dermatology. J Eur Acad Dermatol Venereol. 2011;25:125–9.
22. Cheng SW, Kobayashi M, Kinoshita-Kuroda K, Tanikawa A, Amagai M, Nishikawa T. Monitoring disease activity in pemphigus with enzyme-linked immunosorbent assay using recombinant desmogleins 1 and 3. Br J Dermatol. 2002;147:261–5.
23. Hertl M, Jedlickova H, Karpati S, et al. Pemphigus. S2 Guideline for diagnosis and treatment – guided by the European Dermatology Forum (EDF) in cooperation with the European Academy of Dermatology and Venereology (EADV). J Eur Acad Dermatol Venereol. 2015;29(3):405–14.
24. Joly P, Bernard P, Bedane C, Prost C, Ingen-Housz-Oro S. [Pemphigus. Guidelines for the diagnosis and treatment. Centres de reference des maladies bulleuses auto-immunes. Societe Francaise de Dermatologie]. Ann Dermatol Venereol. 2011;138:252–8.
25. Yeh SW, Ahmed B, Sami N, Razzaque AA. Blistering disorders: diagnosis and treatment. Dermatol Ther. 2003;16:214–23.
26. Czernik A, Toosi S, Bystryn JC, Grando SA. Intravenous immunoglobulin in the treatment of autoimmune bullous dermatoses: an update. Autoimmunity. 2012;45:111–8.
27. Kasperkiewicz M, Schmidt E, Zillikens D. Current therapy of the pemphigus group. Clin Dermatol. 2012;30:84–94.
28. Sinha AA, Hoffman MB, Janicke EC. Pemphigus vulgaris: approach to treatment. Eur J Dermatol. 2015;25(2):103–13.

Bullous Pemphigoid

29. Korman N. Bullous pemphigoid. J Am Acad Dermatol. 1987;16(5 Pt 1):907–24.
30. Schmidt E, Obe K, Brocker EB, Zillikens D. Serum levels of autoantibodies to BP180 correlate with disease activity in patients with bullous pemphigoid. Arch Dermatol. 2000;136:174–8.

31. Charneux J, Lorin J, Vitry F, et al. Usefulness of BP230 and BP180-NC16a enzyme-linked immunosorbent assaysin the initial diagnosis of bullous pemphigoid: a retrospective study of 138 patients. Arch Dermatol. 2011;147:286–91.
32. Tsuji-Abe Y, Akiyama M, Yamanaka Y, et al. Correlation of clinical severity and ELISA indices for the NC16a domain of BP180 measured using BP180 ELISA kit in bullous pemphigoid. J Dermatol Sci. 2005;37:145–9.
33. Liu Z, Diaz LA. Bullous pemphigoid: end of the century overview. J Dermatol. 2001;28(11):647–50.
34. Lo Schiavo A, Ruocco E, Brancaccio G, Caccavale S, Ruocco V, Wolf R. Bullous pemphigoid: etiology, pathogenesis, and inducing factors. Facts and controversies. Clin Dermatol. 2013;31:391–9.
35. Pomponi D, Di Zenzo G, Zennaro D, Calabresi V, Eming R, Zuzzi S, Bernardi ML, Scala E. Detection of IgG and IgE reactivity to BP180 using the ISAC microarray system. Br J Dermatol. 2013;168(6):1205–14.
36. Fania L, Caldarola G. IgE recognition of bullous pemphigoid (BP)180 and BP230 in BP patients and elderly individuals with pruritic dermatoses. Clin Immunol. 2012;143(3):236–45.
37. Yayli S, Pelivani N. Detection of linear IgE deposits in bullous pemphigoid and mucous membrane pemphigoid: a useful clue for diagnosis. Br J Dermatol. 2011;165(5):1133–7.
38. Roujeau JC, Lok C, Bastuji-Garin S, et al. High risk of death in elderly patients with extensive bullous pemphigoid. Arch Dermatol. 1998;134(4):465–9.
39. Thomas TP. The complications of systemic corticosteroid therapy in the elderly. A retrospective study. Gerontology. 1984;30(1):60–5.
40. Joly P, Roujeau JC, Benichou J, et al. A comparison of oral and topical corticosteroids in patients with bullous pemphigoid. N Engl J Med. 2002;346(5):321–7.
41. Culton DA, Diaz LZ. Treatment of subepidermal immunobullous diseases. Clin Dermatol. 2012;30:95–102.
42. Schiavo AL, Puca RV, Ruocco V, Ruocco E. Adjuvant drugs in autoimmune bullous diseases, efficacy versus safety: Facts and controversies. Clin Dermatol. 2010;28:337–43.

Vitiligo

43. Lotti T, Hanna D, Buggiani G, Urple M. The color of the skin: psyco-anthropologic implications. J Cosmet Dermatol. 2005;4(3): 219–20.
44. Lee DY, Kim CR, Lee JH. Trichrome vitiligo in segmental type. Photodermatol Photoimmunol Photomed. 2011;27(2):111–2.
45. Sehgal VN, Srivastava G. Vitiligo: compendium of clinico-epidemiological features. Indian J Dermatol Venereol Leprol. 2007;73(3):149–56.
46. Chandrashekar L. Dermatoscopy of blue vitiligo. Clin Exp Dermatol. 2009;34(5):e125–6.
47. Huggins RH, Janusz CA, Schwartz RA. Vitiligo a sign of systemic disease. Indian J Dermatol Venereol Leprol. 2006;72:68–71.
48. Ezzedine K, Lim HW, Suzuki T, et al. Revised classification/nomenclature of vitiligo and related issues: the Vitiligo Global Issues Consensus Conference. Pigment Cell Melanoma Res. 2012;25(3):E1–13.
49. Lee BW, Schwartz RA, Hercogová J, Valle Y, Lotti TM. Vitiligo road map. Dermatol Ther. 2012;25 Suppl 1:S44–56.
50. Lotti TM, Hercogová J, Schwartz RA, et al. Treatments of vitiligo: what's new at the horizon. Dermatol Ther. 2012;25 Suppl 1:S32–40.
51. Valle Y, Lotti TM, Hercogova J, Schwartz RA, Korobko IV. Multidisciplinary approach to R&D in vitiligo, a neglected skin disease. Dermatol Ther. 2012;25 Suppl 1:S1–9.
52. Lotti T, Hautmann G, Hercogovà J. Vitiligo: disease or symptom? From the confusion of the past to current doubts. In: Lotti T, Hercogovà J, editors. Vitiligo. Problems and solutions. New York/Basel: Marcel Dekker, Inc.; 2004. p. 1–14.
53. Hercogová J, Schwartz RA, Lotti TM. Classification of vitiligo: a challenging endeavor. Dermatol Ther. 2012;25 Suppl 1:S10–6.
54. Pietrzak A, Bartosińska J, Hercogová J, et al. Metabolic syndrome in vitiligo. Dermatol Ther. 2012;25 Suppl 1:S41–43.
55. Sun X, Xu A, Wei X, et al. Genetic epidemiology of vitiligo: a study of 815 probands and their families fromsouth China. Int J Dermatol. 2006;45(10):1176–81.
56. Lotti T, D'Erme AM. Vitiligo as a systemic disease. Clin Dermatol. 2014;32(3):430–4.
57. Alikhan A, Felsten LM, Daly M, Petronic-Rosic V. Vitiligo: a comprehensive overview Part I. Introduction, epidemiology, quality of life, diagnosis, differential diagnosis, associations, histopathology, etiology, and work-up. J Am Acad Dermatol. 2011;65(3):473–91.
58. Alkhateeb A, Fain PR, Thody A, et al. Epidemiology of vitiligo and associated autoimmune diseases in Caucasian probands and their families. Pigment Cell Res. 2003;16:208–14.
59. Nath SK, Majumder PP, Nordlund JJ. Genetic epidemiologyof vitiligo: multilocus recessivity cross-validated. Am J Hum Genet. 1994;55:981–90.
60. Prignano F, Pescitelli L, Ricceri F, et al. The importance of genetical link in immuno-mediated dermatoses: psoriasis and vitiligo. Int J Dermatol. 2008;47(10):1060–2.
61. Abu Tahir M, Pramod K, Ansari SH, et al. Current remedies for vitiligo. Autoimmun Rev. 2010;9(7):516–20.
62. Jin Y, Ferrara T, Gowan K, et al. Next-generation DNA re-sequencing identifies common variants of TYR and HLA-A that modulate the risk of generalized vitiligo via antigen presentation. J Invest Dermatol. 2012;132(6):1730–3.
63. Zhang XJ, Chen JJ, Liu JB. The genetic concept of vitiligo. J Dermatol Sci. 2005;39(3):137–46. 73.
64. Liu JB, Li M, Chen H, et al. Association of vitiligo with HLAA2: a meta-analysis. J Eur Acad Dermatol Venereol. 2007;21(2): 205–13.
65. Majumder PA. Genetics and prevalence of vitiligo vulgaris. In: Hann SK, Nordlund J, editors. Vitiligo: a monograph on the basic and clinical science. Oxford: Blackwell Science Ltd; 2000.
66. Spritz RA. The genetics of generalized vitiligo. Curr Dir Autoimmun. 2008;10:244–57.
67. Birlea SA, Laberge GS, Procopciuc LM, et al. CTLA4 and generalized vitiligo: two genetic association studies and a meta-analysis of published data. Pigment Cell Melanoma Res. 2009;22:230–4.
68. Canton I, Akhtar S, Gavalas NG, et al. A single-nucleotide polymorphism in the gene encoding lymphoid protein tyrosine phosphatase (PTPN22) confers susceptibility to generalised vitiligo. Genes Immun. 2005;6:584–7.
69. Spritz RA. Shared genetic relationships underlying generalized vitiligo and autoimmune thyroid disease. Thyroid. 2010;20(7):745–54.
70. Colucci R, Lotti F, Dragoni F, et al. High prevalence of circulating autoantibodies against thyroid hormones in vitiligo and correlation with clinical and historical parameters of patients. Br J Dermatol. 2014;24.
71. Arunachalam M, Colucci R, Berti S, et al. Autoimmune signals in non-segmental vitiligo patients are associated with distinct clinical parameters and toxic exposures. J Eur Acad Dermatol Venereol. 2013;27(8):961–6.
72. Nordlund JJ, Kirkwood JM, Forget BM, et al. Vitiligo in patients with metastatic melanoma: a good prognostic sign. J Am Acad Dermatol. 1983;9:689–96.
73. Bystryn JC. Serum antibodies in vitiligo patients. Clin Dermatol. 1989;7:136–45.
74. Cui J, Harning R, Henn M, Bystryn JC. Identification of pigment cell antigens defined by vitiligo antibodies. J Invest Dermatol. 1992;98:162–5.

75. Cui J, Arita Y, Bystryn JC. Characterization of vitiligo antigens. Pigment Cell Res. 1995;8:53–9.
76. Song YH, Connor E, Li Y, Zorovich B, et al. The role of tyrosinase in autoimmune vitiligo. Lancet. 1994;344:1049–52.
77. Baharav E, Merimski O, Shoenfeld Y, et al. Tyrosinase as an autoantigen in patients with vitiligo. Clin Exp Immunol. 1996;105: 84–8.
78. Xie Z, Chen D, Jiao D, Bystryn JC. Vitiligo antibodies are not directed to tyrosinase. Arch Dermatol. 1999;135:417–22.
79. Okamoto T, Irie RF, Fujii S, Huang SK, et al. Anti-tyrosinase-related protein-2 immune response in vitiligo patients and melanoma patients receiving activespecific immunotherapy. J Invest Dermatol. 1998;111:1034–9.
80. Kemp EH, Gawkrodger DJ, Watson PF, et al. Immunoprecipitation of melanogenic enzyme autoantigens with vitiligo sera: evidence for cross-reactive autoantibodies to tyrosinase and tyrosinase-related protein-2 (TRP-2). Clin Exp Immunol. 1997;109:495–500.
81. Kemp EH, Waterman EA, Gawkrodger DJ, Watson PF, Weetman AP. Autoantibodies to tyrosinase-related protein-1 detected in the sera of vitiligo patients using a quantitative radiobinding assay. Br J Dermatol. 1998;139:798–805.
82. Hedstrand H, Ekwall O, Olsson MJ, et al. The transcription factors SOX9 and SOX10 are vitiligo autoantigens in autoimmune polyendocrine syndrome type I. J Biol Chem. 2001;276:35390–5.
83. Ruiz-Argüelles A, Brito GJ, Reyes-Izquierdo P, et al. Apoptosis of melanocytes in vitiligo results from antibody penetration. J Autoimmun. 2007;29(4):281–6.
84. Le Poole IC, van den Wijngaard RM, Westerhof W, et al. Presence of T cells and macrophages in inflammatory vitiligo skin parallels melanocyte disappearance. Am J Pathol. 1996;148:1219–28.
85. Badri AM, Todd PM, Garioch JJ, et al. An immunohistological study of cutaneous lymphocytes in vitiligo. J Pathol. 1993;170: 149–55.
86. Ogg GS, Rod Dunbar P, Romero P, et al. High frequency of skin-homing melanocyte-specific cytotoxic T lymphocytes in autoimmune vitiligo. J Exp Med. 1998;188:1203–8.
87. Palermo B, Campanelli R, Garbelli S, et al. Specific cytotoxic T lymphocyte responses against Melan-A/MART1, tyrosinase and gp100 in vitiligo by the use of major histocompatibility complex/peptide tetramers: the role of cellular immunity in the etiopathogenesis of vitiligo. J Invest Dermatol. 2001;117:326–32.
88. Lang KS, Caroli CC, Muhm A, et al. HLA-A2 restricted, melanocyte-specific CD8(+) T lymphocytes detected in vitiligo patients are related to disease activity and are predominantly directed against MelanA/MART1. J Invest Dermatol. 2001;116(6):891–7.
89. Taieb A, Alomar A, Böhm M, et al. Guidelines for the management of vitiligo: the European Dermatology Forum consensus. Br J Dermatol. 2013;168(1):5–19.
90. Colucci R, Lotti T, Moretti S. Vitiligo: an update on current pharmacotherapy and future directions. Expert Opin Pharmacother. 2012;13:1885–99.
91. Coskun B, Saral Y, Turgut D. Topical 0.05% clobetasol propionate versus 1% pimecrolimus ointment in vitiligo. Eur J Dermatol. 2005;15:88–91.
92. Gianfaldoni S, Zarrab Z, Lotti T. Phototherapy and Vitiligo Re-pigmentation: From PUVA to Micro-focused Phototherapy. Pigmentary Disorders. 2014;1:102. doi:10.4172/jpd.1000102.

Alopecia Areata

93. Qi S, Zhao Y, Zhang X, Li S, Cao H, Zhang X. Clinical features in primary cicatricial alopecia in Chinese patients. Indian J Derm Venereol Leprol. 2014;80(4):306–12.
94. Olsen EA, Bergfeld WF, Cotsarelis G, et al. Summary of North American Hair Research Society (NAHRS)-sponsored Workshop on Cicatricial Alopecia, Duke University Medical Center, February 10 and 11, 2001. J Am Acad Dermatol. 2003;48(1): 103–10.
95. Safavi K. Prevalence of alopecia areata in the First National Health and Nutrition Examination Survey. Arch Dermatol. 1992;128:702.
96. Gilhar A, Etzioni A, Paus R. Alopecia areata. N Engl J Med. 2012;366:1515–25.
97. Picardi A, Pasquini P, Cattaruzza MS, et al. Psychosomatic factors in first-onset alopecia areata. Psychosomatics. 2003;44:374–81.
98. Huang KP, Mullangi S, Guo Y, et al. Autoimmune, atopic, and mental health comorbid conditions associated with alopecia areata in the United States. JAMA Dermatol. 2013;149:789–94.
99. Chu SY, Chen YJ, Tseng WC, et al. Comorbidity profiles among patients with alopecia areata: The importance of onset age, a nationwide population-based study. J Am Acad Dermatol. 2011;65(5):949–56.
100. Petukhova L, Duvic M, Hordinsky M, et al. Genome-wide association study in alopecia areata implicates both innate and adaptive immunity. Nature. 2010;466:113–7.
101. Petukhova L, Cabral RM, Mackay-Wiggan J, et al. The genetics of alopecia areata: What's new and how will it help our patients? Dermatol Ther. 2011;24:326–36.
102. Petukhova L, Christiano AM. The genetic architecture of alopecia areata. J Investig Dermatol Symp Proc. 2013;16(1):S16–22.
103. McElwee KJ, Gilhar A, Tobin DJ, Ramot Y, Sundberg JP, Nakamura M, Bertolini M, Inui S, Tokura Y, King Jr LE, Duque-Estrada B, Tosti A, Keren A, Itami S, Shoenfeld Y, Zlotogorski A, Paus R. What causes alopecia areata? Exp Dermatol. 2013;22(9): 609–26.
104. Bertolini M, Gilhar A, Paus R. Alopecia areata as a model for T cell-dependent autoimmune diseases[J]. Exp Dermatol. 2012; 21(6):477–9.
105. Paus R, Ito N, Takigawa M, et al. The hair follicle and immune privilege. J Investig Dermatol Symp Proc. 2003;8:188–94.
106. Paus R, Arck P. Neuroendocrine perspectives in alopecia areata: does stress play a role? J Invest Dermatol. 2009;129:1324–6.
107. Hordinsky M, Ericson M. Autoimmunity: alopecia areata. J Investig Dermatol Symp Proc. 2004;9:73–8.
108. Xiao FL, Yang S, Lin GS, et al. HLA haplotypic association with different phenotype of alopecia areata in Chinese Hans. J Dermatol Sci. 2007;45:206–9.
109. Entz P, Blaumeiser B, Betz RC, et al. Investigation of the HLA-DRB1 locus in alopecia areata. Eur J Dermatol. 2006;16:363–7.
110. Goh C, Finkel M, Christos PJ, et al. Profile of 513 patients with alopecia areata: associations of disease subtypes with atopy, autoimmune disease and positive family history. J Eur Acad Dermatol Venereol. 2006;20:1055–60.
111. Shuifeng Li, Xiaoting Zhang, Shiling Qi, Yanting Ye, Hui Cao, Yuqing Yang, Kevin J. McElwee, Xingqi Zhang. Allergy to dust mites may contribute to early onset and severity of alopecia areata. Clin Exp Dermatol. 2015; 40(2): 171-6.
112. Rebora A. Alopecia areata incognita. J Am Acad Dermatol. 2011;65(6):1228.
113. Chu SY, Chen YJ, Tseng WC, Lin MW, Chen TJ, Hwang CY, Chen CC, Lee DD, Chang YT, Wang WJ, Liu HN. Comorbidity profiles among patients with alopecia areata: the importance of onset age, a nationwide population-based study. J Am Acad Dermatol. 2011;65:949–56.
114. Whiting DA. Histopathologic features of alopecia areata: a new look. Arch Dermatol. 2003;139:1555–9.
115. Dy LC, Whiting DA. Histopathology of alopecia areata, acute and chronic: Why is it important to the clinician? Dermatol Ther. 2011;24(3):369–74.

116. Elston DM, McCollough ML, Bergfeld WF, et al. Eosinophils in fibrous tracts and near hair bulbs: A helpful diagnostic feature of alopecia areata. J Am Acad Dermatol. 1997;37:101–6.
117. Bin Zhang, Ying Zhao, Zeming Cai, Sillani Caulloo, Kevin J McElwee, Mei Yu, Xiaohong Chen, Jian Yang, Wenna Chen, Xuhua Tang, Xingqi Zhang. Early stage alopecia areata is associated with inflammation in the upper dermis and damage to the hair follicle infundibulum. Aust J Derm. 2013;54(3):184–91.
118. Zhao Y, Zhang B, Caulloo S, Chen X, Yang L, Zhang X. Diffuse Alopecia Areata is associated with intense local inflammatory infiltration and CD8+ T cells in hair loss region and an increased IgE level. Indian J Derm Venereol Leprol. 2012;78(6):709–14.
119. Miteva M, Tosti A. Hair and scalp dermatoscopy. J Am Acad Dermatol. 2012;67(5):1040–8.
120. Messenger AG, McKillop J, Farrant P, McDonagh AJ, Sladden M. British Association of Dermatologists' guidelines for the management of alopecia areata. Br J Dermatol. 2012;166(5):916–26.
121. Miteva M, Tosti A. Treatment options for alopecia: an update, looking to the future. Expert Opin Pharmacother. 2012;13(9):1271–81.
122. Garg S, Messenger AG. Alopecia areata: evidence-based treatments. Semin Cutan Med Surg. 2009;28(1):15–8.
123. Happle R, Hausen BM, Wiesner-Menzel L. Diphencyprone in the treatment of alopecia areata. Acta Derm Venereol. 1983;63(1):49–52.
124. Sotiriadis D, Patsatsi A, Lazaridou E, et al. Topical immunotherapy with diphenylcyclopropenone in the treatment of chronic extensive alopecia areata. Clin Exp Dermatol. 2007;32(1):48–51.

Lupus Erythematosus

125. Gronhagen CM, et al. Cutaneous lupus erythematosus and the association with systemic lupus erythematosus: a population-based cohort of 1088 patients in Sweden. Br J Dermatol. 2011;164(6):1335–41.
126. Durosaro O, et al. Incidence of cutaneous lupus erythematosus, 1965–2005: a population-based study. Arch Dermatol. 2009;145(3):249–53.
127. Naleway AL, et al. Epidemiology of systemic lupus erythematosus in rural Wisconsin. Lupus. 2005;14(10):862–6.
128. Danchenko N, Satia JA, Anthony MS. Epidemiology of systemic lupus erythematosus: a comparison of worldwide disease burden. Lupus. 2006;15(5):308–18.
129. Nath SK, Kilpatrick J, Harley JB. Genetics of human systemic lupus erythematosus: the emerging picture. Curr Opin Immunol. 2004;16(6):794–800.
130. Arbuckle MR, et al. Development of autoantibodies before the clinical onset of systemic lupus erythematosus. N Engl J Med. 2003;349(16):1526–33.
131. Li Y, et al. Overexpression of the growth arrest and DNA damage-induced 45alpha gene contributes to autoimmunity by promoting DNA demethylation in lupus T cells. Arthritis Rheum. 2010;62(5):1438–47.
132. Miot HA, Bartoli Miot LD, Haddad GR. Association between discoid lupus erythematosus and cigarette smoking. Dermatology. 2005;211(2):118–22.
133. Gallego H, et al. Report of an association between discoid lupus erythematosus and smoking. Cutis. 1999;63(4):231–4.
134. Gronhagen CM, et al. Subacute cutaneous lupus erythematosus and its association with drugs: a population-based matched case–control study of 234 patients in Sweden. Br J Dermatol. 2012;167(2):296–305.
135. Corvetta A, et al. 5-Methylcytosine content of DNA in blood, synovial mononuclear cells and synovial tissue from patients affected by autoimmune rheumatic diseases. J Chromatogr. 1991;566(2):481–91.
136. Richardson B, et al. Evidence for impaired T cell DNA methylation in systemic lupus erythematosus and rheumatoid arthritis. Arthritis Rheum. 1990;33(11):1665–73.
137. Hu N, et al. Abnormal histone modification patterns in lupus CD4+ T cells. J Rheumatol. 2008;35(5):804–10.
138. Amarilyo G, La Cava A. miRNA in systemic lupus erythematosus. Clin Immunol. 2012;144(1):26–31.
139. Gilliam JN, Sontheimer RD. Distinctive cutaneous subsets in the spectrum of lupus erythematosus. J Am Acad Dermatol. 1981;4(4):471–5.
140. Cardinali C, et al. The spectrum of cutaneous manifestations in lupus erythematosus--the Italian experience. Lupus. 2000;9(6):417–23.
141. Walling HW, Sontheimer RD. Cutaneous lupus erythematosus: issues in diagnosis and treatment. Am J Clin Dermatol. 2009;10(6):365–81.
142. Callen JP, Klein J. Subacute cutaneous lupus erythematosus. Clinical, serologic, immunogenetic, and therapeutic considerations in seventy-two patients. Arthritis Rheum. 1988;31(8):1007–13.
143. Fabbri P, et al. Cutaneous lupus erythematosus: diagnosis and management. Am J Clin Dermatol. 2003;4(7):449–65.
144. Sontheimer RD. Subacute cutaneous lupus erythematosus. Clin Dermatol. 1985;3(3):58–68.
145. Okon LG, Werth VP. Cutaneous lupus erythematosus: diagnosis and treatment. Best Pract Res Clin Rheumatol. 2013;27(3):391–404.
146. Mackay IR, Rose NR. Encyclopedia of medical immunology, vol. 3. Springer Science; Berlin, 2013.
147. Kuhn A, Sticherling M, Bonsmann G. Clinical manifestations of cutaneous lupus erythematosus. J Dtsch Dermatol Ges. 2007;5(12):1124–37.
148. Yell JA, Mbuagbaw J, Burge SM. Cutaneous manifestations of systemic lupus erythematosus. Br J Dermatol. 1996;135(3):355–62.
149. Paran D, Fireman E, Elkayam O. Pulmonary disease in systemic lupus erythematosus and the antiphospholpid syndrome. Autoimmun Rev. 2004;3(1):70–5.
150. Manson JJ, Rahman A. Systemic lupus erythematosus. Orphanet J Rare Dis. 2006;1:6.
151. Askanase A, Shum K, Mitnick H. Systemic lupus erythematosus: an overview. Soc Work Health Care. 2012;51(7):576–86.
152. Janssens P, et al. Lupus enteritis: from clinical findings to therapeutic management. Orphanet J Rare Dis. 2013;8:67.
153. Tebbe B, et al. Markers in cutaneous lupus erythematosus indicating systemic involvement. A multicenter study on 296 patients. Acta Derm Venereol. 1997;77(4):305–8.
154. Callen JP, Fowler JF, Kulick KB. Serologic and clinical features of patients with discoid lupus erythematosus: relationship of antibodies to single-stranded deoxyribonucleic acid and of other antinuclear antibody subsets to clinical manifestations. J Am Acad Dermatol. 1985;13(5 Pt 1):748–55.
155. Hochberg MC. Updating the American College of Rheumatology revised criteria for the classification of systemic lupus erythematosus. Arthritis Rheum. 1997;40(9):1725.
156. Petri M, et al. Derivation and validation of the Systemic Lupus International Collaborating Clinics classification criteria for systemic lupus erythematosus. Arthritis Rheum. 2012;64(8):2677–86.
157. Kuhn A, Ruland V, Bonsmann G. Cutaneous lupus erythematosus: update of therapeutic options part I. J Am Acad Dermatol. 2011;65(6):e179–93.
158. Chang AY, Werth VP. Treatment of cutaneous lupus. Curr Rheumatol Rep. 2011;13(4):300–7.
159. Tripp JM, Maibach HI. Hydroxychloroquine-induced retinopathy: a dermatologic perspective. Am J Clin Dermatol. 2006;7(3):171–5.

160. Leandro MJ, et al. An open study of B lymphocyte depletion in systemic lupus erythematosus. Arthritis Rheum. 2002;46(10):2673–7.
161. Merrill JT. Treatment of systemic lupus erythematosus: a 2012 update. Bull NYU Hosp Jt Dis. 2012;70(3):172–6.

Dermatomyositis

162. Bende Wald MJ, Welter DA, Li X, Davis MD. Incidence of dermatomyositis and clinically amyopathic dermatomyositis. A population based study in Olmsted County Minnesota. Arch Dermatol. 2010;146:26–30.
163. Mc Cann LJ, Juggin SAD, Maillard SM, et al. The Juvenile dermatomyositis. National Registry and Repository (UK and Irland) -Clinical characteristics of children within the first 5 years. Rheumatology (Oxford). 2006;45:1255–60.
164. JOrrizzo JK, Vleugels RA. Dermatomyositis. In: Bolognia JL, Jorrizo JL, Schafter JW, editors. Dermatology. 3rd ed. Elsevierp; Netherlands, 2012. 631–91.
165. Nuang YL, Chm YJ, Lim MW, et al. Malignancies associated with dermatomyositis and polymyositis in Taiwan. A nation-wide, population based study. Br J Dermatol. 2009;161:854–60.
166. Amagai M, Hashimato T, Shimizu H, et al. Asorption of pathogenic autoantibodies bythe extracellular domain of pemphigus vulgaris antigen(Dsg 3) produced in vaculovirus. J Clin Invest. 1994;94:55–7.

Scleroderma

167. Lever WF. Histopathology of the skin. 1st ed. Philadelphia: J.B. Lippincott Co.; 1949. p. 260–4.
168. Le Roy EC, Black C, Fleischmajer R. Scleroderma (systemic sclerosis), classification and pathogenosis. J Rheumatol. 1988;15:202–5.
169. Silver RM, Medsger TA Jr, Bolster MB. Systemic sclerosis and scleroderma variants. In: Kooperman NJ, Moorland LW, editors. Arthritis and allied conditions. 15th ed. Baltimore: Lippincott, Williams-Wilkins; 2005. p. 1635–80.
170. Sato S. Classification of SSc and early diagnosis. Jpn J Dermatol. 2008;118:2745–9. (Japanese).
171. Connolly MK. Systemic sclerosis(scleroderma) and related disorders. In: Bolognia J Jr, Jorrizzo JL, Schaffer JV, editors. Dermatology. 3rd ed. Elsevier; Netherlands, 2013. p. 643–55.
172. Amagai M, Hashimoto T, Shimiza H, et al. Absorption of pathogenic autoantibodies by the extracellular domail of pemphigus vulgaris antigen(Dsg3)produced by vacuovirus. J Clin Invest. 1994;94:55–7.
173. Asano Z. Detection and interpretation of autoantibodies in collagen vascular diseases Japan. J Dermatol. 2014;124:1533–8 (In Japanese).
174. Peterson LS, Nelson AM, Su WP, et al. The epdemiology of morphea (localized scleroderma) in Olmsted county 1960–1993. J Rheumatol. 1997;24:73–80.
175. Rocken M, Ghoreschi K. Morphea and lichen sclerosus. In: Bolognia JL, Jorrizzo JL, Schaffer JV, editors. Dermatology. 3rd ed. Elsevier; Netherlands, 2013. p. 657–70.

Lichen Sclerosus

176. Farrell AM, Marren P, Dean D, et al. Lichen sclerosus: evidence that immunological changes occur at all levels of the skin. Br J Dermatol. 1999;140:1087–92.
177. Carli P, Moretti S, Spallanzani A, et al. Fibrogenic cytokines in vulvar lichen sclerosus. J Reprod Med. 1997;42:161–5.
178. Terlou A, Santegoets LAM, van der Meijden WI, et al. An autoimmune phenotype in vulval lichen sclerosus and lichen planus: a Th1 response and levels of microRNA-155. J Invest Dermatol. 2012;132:658–66.
179. Oyama N, Chan I, Neill SM, et al. Autoantibodies to extracellular matrix protein 1 in lichen sclerosus. Lancet. 2003;362:118–23.
180. Edmonds EV, Oyama N, Chan I, et al. Extracellular matrix protein 1 autoantibodies in male genital lichen sclerosus. Br J Dermatol. 2011;165:218–9.
181. Howard A, dean D, Cooper S, et al. Circulating basement membrane zoen antibodies are found in lichen sclerosus of the vulva. Australas J Dermatol. 2004;45:12–5.
182. Gambichler T, Hoxtermann S, Skrygan M, et al. Occurrence of circulating anti-bullous pemphigoid antibodies in patients with lichen sclerosus. J Eur Acad Dermatol Venereol. 2011;25:369–70.
183. Goolamali SK, Barnes EW, Irvine WJ, et al. Organ specific antibodies inpaients with lichen sclerosus. Br Med J. 1974;4: 78–9.
184. Harrington CI, Dunsmore IR. An investigation into the incidence of auto-immune disorders in patients with lichen sclerosus et atrophicus. Br J Dermatol. 1981;104:563–6.
185. Meyrick-Thomas RH, Ridley CM, McGibbon DH, et al. Lichen sclerosus et atrophicus and autoimmunity: a study of 350 women. Br J Dermatol. 1988;118:41–6.
186. Edmonds EV, Hunt S, Hawkins D, et al. Clinical parameters in male genital lichen sclerosus: a case series of 329 patients. J Eur Acad Dermatol Venereol. 2012;26:730–7.
187. Marren P, Yell J, Charmock FM, et al. The association between lichen sclerosus and antigens of the HLA system. Br J Dermatol. 1995;132:197–203.
188. Azurdia RM, Luzzi GA, Byren I, et al. Lichen sclerosus in adult men: a study of HLA assocaitions and susceptibility to autoimmune disease. Br J Dermatol. 1999;140.79–83.
189. Clifton MM, Garner IB, Kohler S, et al. Immunohistochemical evaluation of androgen receptors in genital and extragenital lichen sclerosus: evidence of loss of androgen receptors in lesional epidermis. J Am Acad Dermatol. 1999;41:43–6.
190. Gupta S, Malhotra AK, Ajith C. Lichen sclerosus: role of occlusion of the genital skin in the pathogenesis. Indian J Dermatol Venereol Leprol. 2010;76:56–8.
191. Edmonds EV, Bunker CB. Nuclear magnetic resonance spectroscopy of urine in male genital lichen sclerosus. Br J Dermatol. 2010;163:1355–6.
192. Nelson DM, Peterson AC. Lichen sclerosus: epidemiological distribution in an equal access health care system. J Urol. 2011;185:522–5.
193. Goldstein AT, Marinoff SC, Christopher K, et al. Prevalence of vulvar lichen sclerosus in a general gynaecologypractice. J Reprod Med. 2005;50:477–80.
194. Meyrick-Thomas RH, Ridley CM, McGibbon DH, et al. Anogenital lichen sclerosus in women. J Roy Soc Med. 1996;89:694–8.
195. Simpkin S, Oakley A. Clinical review of 202 patients with vulval lichen sclerosus: a possible association with psoriasis. Australas J Dermatol. 2007;48:28–31.
196. Smith SD, Fischer G. Childhood onset vulvar lichen sclerosus does not resolve at puberty: a prospective case series. Pediatr Dermatol. 2009;26:725–9.
197. Kiss A, Kiraly L, Kutasy B, et al. High incidence of balantitisxeroticaobliterans in boys with phimosis: prospective 10-year study. Pediatr Dermatol. 2005;22:305–8.
198. Chi CC, Kitschig G, Baldo M, Brackenbury F, Lewis F, Wojnarowska F. Topical interventions of genital lichen sclerosus (Review). Cochrane Database Syst Rev. 2011;7(12), CD008240.

199. Neill SM, Lewis FM, Tatnall FM, Cox N. British Association of Dermatologists' guidelines for the management of lichen sclerosus 2010. Br J Dermatol. 2010;163:672–82.
200. Fischer G, Rogers M. Treatment of childhood vulvar lichen sclerosus with potent topical corticosteroid. Pediatr Dermatol. 1997;14:325–8.
201. Cooper SM, Gao XH, Powell JJ, et al. Does treatment of vulvar lichen sclerosus influence its prognosis? Arch Dermatol. 2004; 140:702–6.
202. Dhalman-Ghozlan K, Hedblad MA, von Krogh G. Penile lichen sclerosusetatrophicus treated with clobetasoldipropionate cream: a retrospective clinical and histopathological study. J Am Acad Dermatol. 1999;40:451–7.
203. Virgili A, Borghi A, Toni G, et al. First randomized trial on clobetasol propionate and mometasonefuroate in the treatment of vulvar lichen sclerosus: results of efficacy and tolerability. Br J Dermatol. 2014;171:388–96.
204. Funaro D, Lovett A, Leroux N, Powell J. A double-blind, randomized prospective study evaluating topical clobetasol propionate 0.05% versus topical tacrolimus 0.1% in patients with vulvar lichen sclerosus. J Am Acad Dermatol. 2014;71:84–91.
205. Goldstein AT, Creasey A, Pfau R, et al. A double-blind, randomized controlled trial of clobetasol versus pimecrolimus in patients with vulvar lichen sclerosus. J Am Acad Dermatol. 2011;64: e99–104.
206. Kulkarni S, Barbagli G, Kirpekar D, et al. Lichen sclerosus of the male genitalia and urethra: surgical options and results in a multicenter international experience with 215 patients. Eur Urol. 2009;55:945–56.
207. Fistarol SK, Itin PH. Diagnosis and treatment of lichen sclerosus. Am J Clin Dermatol. 2013;14:27–47.
208. Lewis FM. Lichen sclerosus. In: Lebwohl MG, editor. The treatment of skin disease. 4th ed. Elsevier; Netherlands, 2014. p. 399–401.
209. Wallace HJ. Lichen sclerosusetatrophicus. Trans St John's Hosp Dermatol Soc. 1971;57:9–30.
210. Zaki I, Dalziel KL, Solomons FA, et al. The under-reporting of skin disease in association with squamous cell carcinoma of the vulva. Clin Exp Dermatol. 1997;21:334–7.
211. Derrick EK, Ridley CM, Kobza-Black A, et al. A clinical study of 23 cases of female anogenital carcinoma. Br J Dermatol. 2000; 143:1217–23.
212. Chiesa-Vottero A, Dvoretsky PM, Hart WR. Histopathologic study of thin vulvar squamous cell carcinomas and associated cutaneous lesions: a correlative study of 48 tumors in 44 patients with analysis of adjacent vulvar intraepithelial neoplasia types and lichen sclerosus. Am J Surg Pathol. 2006;30: 310–8.
213. Powell J, Robson A, Cranston D, et al. High incidence of lichen sclerosus in patients with squamous cell carcinoma of the penis. Br J Dermatol. 2001;145:85–9.

Part IV

Immuno-Techniques, Immuno-Diagnosis and Immunotherapy in Dermatology

1.1 Overview

Immunohistochemical study of skin diseases is becoming a routine to aid in the diagnosis of several infectious diseases, autoimmune skin diseases, tumors of different cellular origins. Skin is rich in cellular resources. Separation, acquisition, characterization and manipulation of individual cells in the skin is a basic requirement for the study of skin immunology. In the first chapter, the authors details the techniques in handling different cells in the skin. Based on the understanding of mechanistic cellular or molecular pathways, the last chapter describes the use of immunobiologics in skin diseases, as exemplified in psoriasis and lupus.

Tissue or Cell-Based Techniques

14

Tammie Ferringer, Dirk Elston, Jang-June Park, Leihong Xiang, Yuling Shi, Matthew Weiland, Ruiqun Qi, and Zhenghong Di

Contents

T. Ferringer, MD
Geisinger Medical Center, Danville, PA, USA

D. Elston, MD (✉)
Ackerman Academy of Dermatopathology, New York, NY, USA
e-mail: DElston@ameripath.com

J.-J. Park
Perelman School of Medicine at the University of Pennsylvania,, Philadelphia, PA, USA
e-mail: janpark@mail.med.upenn.edu

L. Xiang
Department of Dermatology, Huashan Hospital, Fudan University, Shanghai 200040, China
e-mail: flora_xiang@vip.163.com

Y. Shi
Department of Dermatology, Shanghai Tenth People's Hospital, Tongji University School of Medicine, Shanghai, China
e-mail: shiyuling1973@tongji.edu.cn

M. Weiland
DeVos Cardiovascular Research Program, Van Andel Research Institute, Grand Rapids, MI, USA

Department of Dermatology, Henry Ford Health System, Detroit, MI, USA
e-mail: matthew.weiland@vai.org

R. Qi
Department of Dermatology, No.1 Hospital of China Medical University, Shenyang, China
e-mail: xiaoqiliumin@163.com

Z. Di
Department of Dermatology, Shengjing Hospital of China Medical University, Shenyang, China
e-mail: dizh2005@163.com

X.-H. Gao, H.-D. Chen (eds.), *Practical Immunodermatology*, DOI 10.1007/978-94-024-0902-4_14

14.1 Immunohistochemistry

Tammie Ferringer, MD and Dirk Elston, MD

14.1.1 Introduction

Immunohistochemistry (IHC) is a commonly used method to identify the lineage or histogenesis of tissue cells in paraffin-fixed processed tissue. Various methods are employed to bind a chromogen to a target epitope within the tissue (Table 14.1). The chromogens attach via antibody-binding or protein–ligand binding utilizing avidin–biotin or streptavidin–biotin affinities. Commonly used chromogen methods employ alkaline phosphatase (AP) or horseradish peroxidase (HRP), resulting in a red or brown chromogen.

IHC is widely used in the practice of pathology to differentiate between types of tumors, distinguish benign from malignant tumors, and to classify hematopoietic malignancies. Quantitative IHC allows for the identification of therapeutic targets or predictors of biological response and can be important in directing therapy for malignancies.

14.1.2 Procedure

Tissue sections are cut at 5–7 μm in thickness and placed on a charged slide. Antigen retrieval is required because epitopes in tissue are masked by protein linkage that occurs during formalin fixation. Antigen retrieval methods typically rely on heat-induced epitope retrieval (HIER), but proteolytic enzymatic retrieval (PIER) is still occasionally used. HIER is commonly performed on charged slides, whereas PIER may require glued sections. In this method, 10% Elmer's glue is added to the water bath, and the sections are dried thoroughly prior to processing to ensure adherence.

Horseradish peroxidase or calf alkaline phosphatase catalyze conversion of colorless chemicals into the final chromogen. A brown chromogen forms when 3,3′-diaminobenzidine tetrahydrochloride (DAB) interacts with horseradish peroxidase. Red chromogens include amino ethylcarbazole (AEC) and Fast Red TR. Secondary antibodies are used to amplify the signal and result in greater sensitivity, and also introduce more opportunities for technical error.

The avidin–biotin complex (ABC) method takes advantage of the strong and irreversible binding between egg white avidin and biotin. Endogenous biotin present in tissue must be blocked when this method is used. Tissues particularly high in endogenous biotin include lymph nodes, kidney, liver, the gastrointestinal tract, and lung, but blocking is good practice for all tissue types.

Polymer-based detection methods use antibodies bound to a dextran backbone. Modern 3 step polymer detection methods are highly sensitive but have the disadvantage of steric hindrance because of the large molecular size of polymer conjugates. Micropolymer systems have been used to overcome this problem.

Heat-induced antigen retrieval (HIER) uses microwaves or high temperature to induce cleavage of the protein–protein cross-links produced during the process of formalin fixation. Heating up to at least 100 ° C for a brief period is generally superior to using lower temperatures for a longer time. Heating by autoclave and microwave is commonly used, and careful attention must be paid to the pH of the retrieval solution, as this can have a profound effect on the final staining results. As a general rule, high pH increases staining intensity of cell membrane or cytoplasmic antigens, while low pH retrieval solutions preserve tissue morphology and are superior for nuclear targets, but individual antibody systems vary widely. Ki-67, smooth muscle actin (SMA), desmin, CD3, CK7, and CK20 demonstrate greater staining at extremes of pH, but staining intensity decreases with intermediate pH. HMB-45, S100, and CEA demonstrate more intense staining with increasing pH [1, 2]. Citrate buffering is often used to control pH [3]. Recommended pH ranges are listed in Table 14.2, but each lab must validate the procedure and determine the optimal antigen retrieval pH for each antibody protocol.

Table 14.1 Immunohistochemical techniques

Method	Description
Peroxidase antiperoxidase	Horseradish peroxidase is used with anti-HRP antibodies to produce stable immune complexes
Alkaline phosphatase antialkaline phosphatase	Alkaline phosphatase (AP) forms complexes with anti-AP antibodies
Avidin–biotin	Biotinylated antibodies form avidin–biotin complexes
Streptavidin–biotin	Biotinylated antibodies form complexes with streptavidin
Polymer method	Enzymes and antibodies attached to dextran backbone

14.1.3 Specific Applications

14.1.3.1 Pagetoid Intraepidermal Proliferations

Pagetoid intraepidermal lesions include melanoma, Paget's disease, Bowen's disease, and hidroacanthoma simplex. Staining for cytokeratin (CK) 7 has been used to differentiate

Paget's disease from pagetoid Bowen disease, but reports of CK7 expression in Bowen's disease suggest that this practice should be reevaluated [4, 5]. Expression of CEA, diastase-resistant sialomucin, and BerEP4 favors Paget's disease, while p63 expression favors Bowen's disease [6]. While there is considerable overlap in staining of Paget's

Table 14.2 Recommended initial pH for IHC validation

Antibody	Supplier	Recommended initial pH
Melan-A	Dako Clone A103	High pH
S100	Dako	High pH
Melanosome/ HMB-45	Dako	High pH
MITF	Dako, Clone D5	Citrate buffer pH 6.1
SOX-10	Leica	Citrate buffer pH 6
Cytokeratin	Dako, Clone AE1/AE3	Citrate buffer pH 6.1
CD4	Leica, Clone 1 F6	EDTA buffer pH 8
CD3	Leica Clone LN10	EDTA buffer pH 9
CD31	Pierce Clone 1A10	EDTA buffer pH 9
CK7	Leica Clone OV-TL 12/30	Citrate buffer pH 6
Ki-67	Dako M7240	Low pH
KBA.62	Ventana	Citrate buffer, pH = 6.5

disease of breast and extramammary Paget's disease (EMPD), CDX2 reactivity has only been reported in EMPD associated with underlying gut carcinoma [7].

14.1.4 Sclerosing Epithelial Neoplasms (Paisley Tie Pattern Neoplasms)

IHC may be helpful to distinguish between superficial biopsies of desmoplastic trichoepitheliomas (DTE), morpheaform basal cell carcinoma (BCC), and microcystic adnexal carcinoma, but data are still evolving, and the best method to confirm the diagnosis remains a deeper biopsy. CK20-positive Merkel cells may be identified within DTE but not BCC and microcystic adnexal carcinoma, but they can be few in number, and serial sections may be required to demonstrate them [8]. Nuclear androgen receptor expression favors BCC over DTE [9]. Staining for p75 nerve growth factor favors DTE over BCC, but microcystic adnexal carcinoma can also stain strongly with this marker. Strong PHLDA1 staining also favors DTE [10]. BCL-2 and CD34 staining are of little value in small specimens.

14.1.5 Cutaneous Spindle Cell Neoplasms

The list of differential diagnosis for an atypical spindle cell neoplasm abutting the epidermis includes atypical fibroxanthoma (AFX), spindle cell melanoma, spindled squamous cell carcinoma, and leiomyosarcoma (LMS). A panel of IHC markers can be helpful to confirm the diagnosis. AFX commonly stains for CD10, S100A6, and procollagen I, but no marker appears to be specific for this lesion, and AFX remains a diagnosis of exclusion [11–14]. Positive staining for any of the listed markers may be nonspecific and should be interpreted in the context of negative staining for each of the entities in the differential diagnosis. Spindle cell melanomas do not stain reliably with Melan A or HMB-45, but S100 and SOX10 are fairly reliable markers [15, 16]. Neither will distinguish spindle cell melanoma from malignant peripheral nerve sheath tumor, and care should be taken not to confuse S100-positve Langerhans cells colonizing other tumors with true positivity of the atypical spindle cell population. Spindled squamous cell carcinoma stains for polyclonal pancytokeratin, a mix of monoclonal keratins 1 and 3 (AE1/3), high molecular weight keratin (cytokeratin 903), and p63 [17–19]. No single immunostain is completely reliable in this setting, and at least two are recommended in spindle SCC if strongly suspected. LMS stains for desmin, caldesmon, actin, and smooth muscle actin. Desmin and h-caldesmon offer greater specificity compared to actin and smooth muscle actin [20].

14.1.6 Small Blue Cell Tumors

The differential diagnosis of small blue cell tumors includes Merkel cell carcinoma (MCC), Ewing sarcoma/primitive neuroectodermal tumor (EWS/PNET), metastatic small cell carcinoma of the lung, neuroblastoma, lymphoma, small cell endocrine carcinoma, and melanoma. MCCs express neuroendocrine markers, including chromogranin, neuron specific enolase, and synaptophysin as well as a characteristic paranuclear dot pattern with CK20. Merkel cell polyoma virus can be detected via IHC with the antibody CM2B4 or via PCR assay [21].

Metastatic small cell carcinoma of the lung is typically negative for CK20 and positive for CK7 and thyroid transcription factor 1 (TTF-1). Lymphomas stain for leukocyte common antigen (CD45). Like MCC, EWS/PNET can express neuron-specific enolase, chromogranin, and synaptophysin. CD99 expression is characteristic of EWS/PNET, but can also be noted in lymphoblastic lymphoma, carcinoid tumors, and melanoma [22]. FLI1 antibody is utilized as a nuclear marker for EWS/PNET. It is also expressed in vascular tumors, MCC, melanoma, and some lymphomas [23]. CK20 expression has not been reported in EWS/PNET. Panels of IHC markers can typically distinguish between the tumors, but if necessary, cytogenetic analysis for the characteristic EWS/PNET translocation t(11;22) can be used.

14.1.7 Fibrohistiocytic Tumors

IHC can be helpful to distinguish cellular dermatofibroma (DF) from dermatofibrosarcoma protuberans (DFSP). DFSP generally expresses CD34, while DF expresses factor XIIIa. CD34 also stains solitary fibrous tumor, spindle cell lipoma, superficial acral fibromyxoma, sclerotic fibroma, endothelial tumors, neurofibroma, trichilemmoma, scleromyxedema, and nephrogenic systemic fibrosis. Nestin is expressed in DFSP, and stromelysin 3 is expressed in DF [24, 25]. These stains can be helpful in equivocal cases. Fluorescence in situ hybridization for COL1A1–PDGFB translocation can also be used to identify DFSP.

14.1.8 Hematopoietic Neoplasms

CD20 is generally used as a B cell marker, but is rarely expressed in T cell lymphomas and is not expressed is the early and late stages of B cell development [26]. Expression may be lost in lymphomas treated with the anti-CD20 antibody rituximab. CD79a is expressed throughout the B cell life cycle, including in plasma cells. BCL-2 is expressed in normal marginal zone cells, marginal zone lymphoma (MZL), about 15 % of primary cutaneous follicle center cell lymphomas (PCFCCL), and in many systemic lymphomas. BCL-6 is a reliable marker for follicle center lineage. CD10 is also expressed, but is lost in PCFCCL with a diffuse growth pattern. CD21 and CD35 can be used to demonstrate the normal follicular dendritic cell network which is prominent in benign follicle centers. Benign follicle centers also express a high proliferative fraction (>90 %) with Ki-67. PAX5 is a nuclear marker expressed in early B cell development and is not expressed in plasma cells. In contrast, CD138 (syndecan-1) is expressed in plasma cells. In MZL, light chain restriction can often be demonstrated by IHC or chromogenic in situ hybridization. Diffuse large B cell lymphoma, leg-type, commonly expresses MUM-1 as well as CD20 and BCL-2, while BCL-6 staining is variable.

Normal T cells express CD3, CD2, CD5, and CD7. Loss of pan-T cell markers can occur in mycosis fungoides [27]. CD30-positive cells present in sheets and large clusters are a feature of anaplastic large cell lymphoma (ALCL), lymphomatoid papulosis, and large cell transformation of mycosis fungoides. In the setting of ALCL, ALK1 expression suggests systemic disease. Subcutaneous panniculitis-like T cell lymphoma is typically positive for βF-1, TIA-1, granzyme B, and perforin.

Myeloperoxidase (MPO), CD68 (KP1), CD4, and lysozyme commonly stain myeloid cells [28]. Blastic plasmacytoid dendritic cell neoplasm is a form of leukemia that frequently presents skin involvement with a dense monomorphous infiltrate of blastic cells that are commonly positive for CD4, CD56, and CD123, but negative for CD3, CD20, and CD79a.

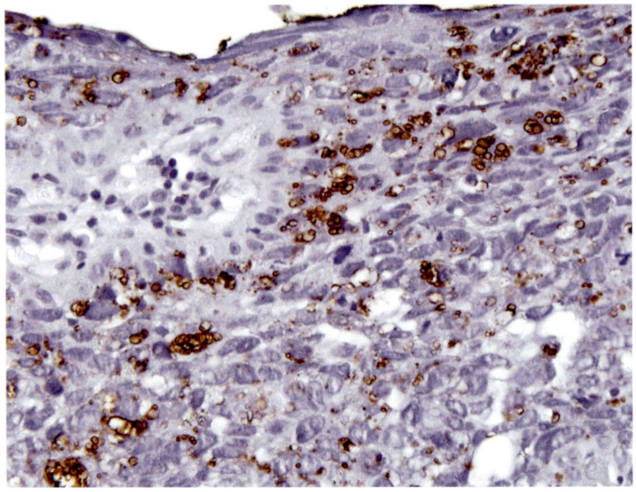

Fig. 14.1 Sebaceous carcinoma (Adipophilin 200X)

14.1.9 Sebaceous Tumors

Membranous vesicular expression of EMA and adipophilin (Fig. 14.1) in sebaceous tumors distinguishes these tumors from basal cell and squamous cell carcinomas that are typically negative, or if reactive, only show rare granular staining [29]. Similarly, androgen receptor (AR) marks sebaceous tumors but not squamous cell carcinomas, and only stains focally in BCC, if present [30].

Diagnosis of a sebaceous gland tumor should raise the concern of underlying microsatellite instability associated with genitourinary and gastrointestinal malignancies in Muir–Torre syndrome. IHC stainings for mismatch repair genes, such as MSH2 and MLH1, can be used to screen for this syndrome. Loss of nuclear staining suggests the need for additional investigation, possibly including genetic testing [31].

14.1.10 Primary Cutaneous Adnexal Neoplasms Versus Metastatic Adenocarcinoma

Reactivity with p63, CK5/6, D2-40, and CK15 is seen in primary cutaneous adnexal tumors with glandular differentiation, but is absent in most metastatic adenocarcinomas to the skin [32].

14.1.11 Cutaneous Metastases of Unknown Origin

Differential staining of CK7 and CK20 with additional IHC markers can help determine the origin of most metastases to skin. Colorectal carcinomas are typically CK7-negative/CK20-positive and also show nuclear expression with CDX-2. Lung carcinomas are CK7-positive/CK20-negative and react with

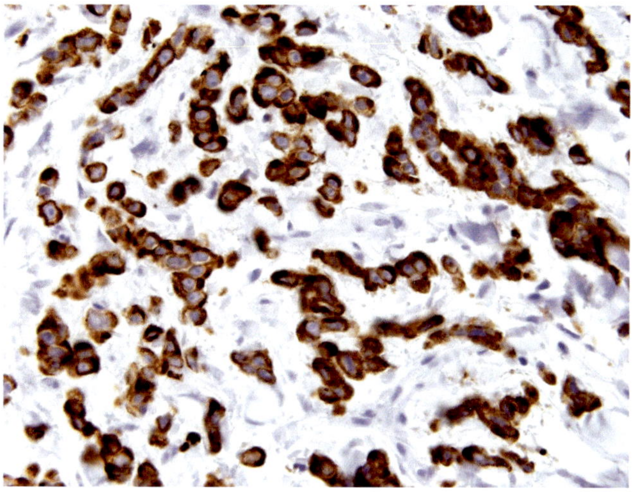

Fig. 14.2 Metastatic breast carcinoma (CK7400X)

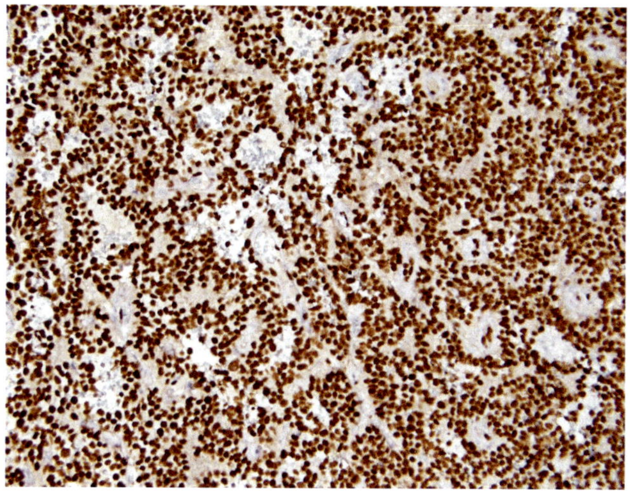

Fig. 14.3 Angiosarcoma (ERG 200X)

thyroid transcription factor-1 (TTF-1). Metastatic breast cancer is also CK7-positive/CK20-negative (Fig. 14.2), but does not show expression of TTF-1. Renal cell carcinoma marker (RCC-Ma), PAX8, and CD10 can be used to identify renal cell carcinoma metastatic to the skin. However, CD10 is not specific, and stains various other clear cell tumors of the skin [33].

14.1.12 Vascular Tumors

Endothelial markers include CD34, CD31, and most recently, the nuclear markers, FLI1 and ERG. CD34 is a sensitive vascular marker but stains numerous other fibrohistiocytic tumors. ERG is reportedly the most specific and sensitive marker for angiosarcoma (Fig. 14.3) [34]. Although heterogeneity of expression has been noted, Prox1, D2-40, and LYVE-1 have been investigated in the differentiation of blood vessel from lymphatic endothelial cells [35].

Histopathological distinction of vascular proliferative lesions from static vascular malformations can be difficult, but is important in determining appropriate management. Vascular proliferative lesions such as infantile hemangiomas show reactivity with GLUT1 and WT1, unlike stable vascular malformations [36].

MYC amplification, a notable finding in postradiation angiosarcomas, differentiates it from atypical vascular lesions in the same group of patients. Good concordance has been noted with MYC IHC in separating these problematic lesions [37].

14.1.13 Melanocytic Lesions

The brown chromogen, DAB, can be difficult to identify in a heavily pigmented lesion. Alternatives include use of the red chromogen AEC or Fast Red TR, melanin bleach, or replacement of the hematoxylin counterstain with azure B to convert melanin to a green-blue color [38]. Several markers are available to identify tumors of melanocytic lineage. S100 is highly sensitive but not particularly specific for these lesions. S100-positive Langerhans cells in the epidermis can be particularly problematic when interpreting an intraepithelial component. Similarly, S100-positive follicular dendritic cells complicate interpretation of sentinel lymph nodes for evaluation of metastatic melanoma. MART-1 and Melan-A antibodies recognize the same gene product common to most melanocytic cells. Unlike S100, these antibodies are not reliable in desmoplastic melanoma and fail to identify a small proportion of metastatic melanomas. Rarely, nonspecific MART-1 or Melan-A staining can be noted in clusters of cells at the junction in lichenoid interface dermatitis. These pseudonests are not melanocytes but may mimic a melanocytic proliferation [39].

More recently, nuclear melanocytic markers have become popular. SOX10 is one example that shows similar sensitivity to S100 but greater specificity limited to melanocytes and Schwann cells. Nuclear expression avoids the distracting staining of melanocytic dendrites that encircle keratinocytes seen in sections stained with cytoplasmic markers, thus complicating interpretation of intraepidermal melanocytic proliferations. SOX10 has the advantage over another nuclear melanocytic marker, MITF, of also reacting with any underlying desmoplastic melanoma (Fig. 14.4) [40]. The issue of background S100-positive dendritic cells in lymph nodes can also be avoided with SOX10.

HMB-45 is an organelle-specific melanosome marker, thus often used as a surrogate for maturation with staining limited to the junctional and superficial dermal component of nevi. Blue nevi are an exception, since they contain premelanosomes at all levels and lack a maturation gradient histologically. Melanomas, in contrast, may lack HMB-45

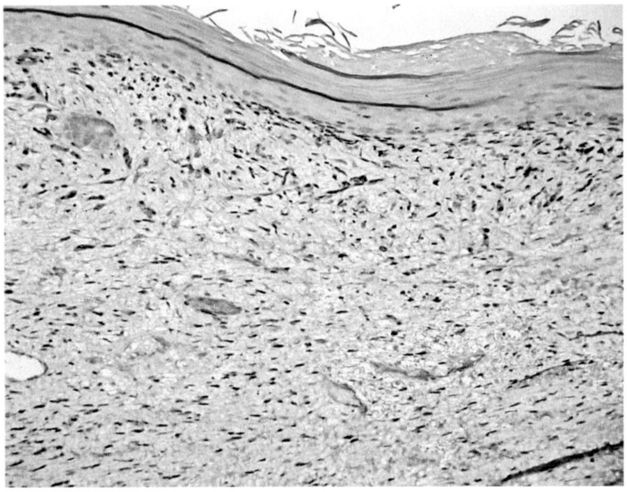

Fig. 14.4 Desmoplastic melanoma (SOX10 100X)

expression, or, if positive, shows a uniform distribution with no gradient or a random distribution. Ki-67 is a marker of cell proliferation that can also be useful in distinguishing benign from malignant melanocytic lesions. A proliferation index over 10 % favors a melanoma, while an index below 2 % favors a nevus [41]. Similar to HMB-45, Ki-67 typically highlights proliferating melanocytes only at the junction or superficially, if present, in nevi but shows more random proliferation in melanomas. Care is required, since Ki-67 is not melanocyte-specific and will highlight any proliferating cell. Dual staining with a cytoplasmic melanocytic marker with a contrasting chromogen can improve identification.

Clear distinction between benign and malignant spitzoid melanocytic proliferations can be difficult. HMB-45 and Ki-67may be useful, as described above. In addition, the cell cycle inhibitor, p16, is commonly lost in spitzoid melanomas [42]. S100A6, a S100 subtype, strongly and diffusely marks Spitz nevi, but is weak, patchy, or negative in spitzoid melanomas [43].

Immunoreactivity of desmoplastic melanoma differs from other subtypes of melanoma. Desmoplastic melanoma lacks HMB-45 and MART-1 expression in most cases. Strong staining with either of these antibodies argues for desmoplastic nevus over melanoma. SOX10 and S100 are the most sensitive markers for this type of melanoma [44].

IHC may also help determine prognosis in melanomas. D2-40 or CD31 can enhance identification of lymphatic or vascular invasion [45]. Similarly, pHH3 facilitates identification of mitotic figures that can be easily missed or confused with apoptotic, hyperchromatic, or pyknotic nuclei [46]. pHH3 is not lineage-specific; so, it is often paired with a cytoplasmic melanocytic marker. While IHC improves reproducibility of mitotic counts, the current American Joint Commission of Cancer guidelines are based on a mitotic rate determined on hematoxylin and eosin-stained sections.

Advent of targeted therapy for melanoma rely on an understanding of the underlying molecular pathways. IHC is helpful to select melanoma patients who may benefit from such treatments. For example, antibody to BRAF V600E (VE1) has been proved to be a sensitive and specific marker to identify melanomas with the BRAF V600E mutation that are candidates for BRAF inhibitors [47].

14.2 Acquisition and Culture of Primary Keratinocytes from Human Skin

Zheng-Hong Di

14.2.1 Introduction

The in vitro culture of keratinocytes is an important tool in the study of skin biology, disease, and pharmacology. The following method aims to provide plenty of keratinocytes for research. The combination use of Dispase II and trypsin digestion can separate the epidermis from dermis completely and result in high rate of living keratinocytes and shortened time for confluence growth without contamination [48]. The keratinocytes grow steadily and rapidly in the serum-free, bovine pituitary extract-free, and feeder cell-free culture media, maintaining the normal morphological characteristics for about five to six passages [49, 50].

14.2.1.1 Materials

Medium can be purchased from companies and must be of cell-culture reagent grade. All procedures must be carried out in clean bench using aseptic technique.

14.2.1.2 Key Reagents

Defined keratinocyte culture medium (Gibco. USA, containing insulin, epidermal growth factor, fibroblast growth factor, 0.09 mM calcium), antihuman cytokeratin monoclonal antibody.

14.2.1.3 Equipment and Supplements

CO_2 incubator
Inverted phase contrast microscope
Clean bench
Cryogenic refrigerator
Refrigerated centrifuge
Hemocytometer
Petri dish
Glass beaker 10 ml
Tissue culture flask
Tissue culture plate
Pipette
Six-well plate

Tubes
Forceps
Scissors
Scalpel
Nylon mesh with 100 μm pores

14.2.1.4 Reagents Setup

0.25 % Dispase II in PBS
0.25 % typsin and 0.02 % EDTA in PBS
100 U/ml penicillin and 100 μg/ml streptomycin in PBS
10 % fetal calf serum (FCS)
0.4 % Trypan Blue solution

14.2.1.5 Rinsing Buffer

1 × PBS (without calcium and magnesium)

14.2.2 Methods

14.2.2.1 Culture of Primary Keratinocytes

1. Samples: Human keratinocytes are isolated from the basal layer of skin epidermis as described by Barlow and Aliquot [51]. Normal foreskin specimens can be obtained from plastic surgery, and those from donors of young age are preferred.
2. Digestion and isolation:

   The keratinocytes are isolated by using two-step combined dissociation with Dispase II and trypsin. The skin should be treated as soon as possible after excision. Samples are rinsed with PBS containing 1 % penicillin and streptomycin. Fatty tissue is scraped off with a scalpel, and the connective tissue is removed using sterile scissors and forceps in a petri dish. Samples are cut into 0.5 cm × 0.5 cm pieces in a new sterile petri dish. The pieces of samples are incubated overnight at 4 °C in 0.25 % Dispase II solution. Then, the epidermis is separated from the dermis with fine forceps to avoid the contamination of fibroblasts. The pieces of epidermis are cut into small pieces by scissors and put in the 0.25 % trypsin–EDTA solution at 37 °C for 15–30 min in a glass beaker. After that, the small pieces of epidermis are blown gently by using a pipette for about 5 min to obtain single cells in the solution. Then, 10% FCS is added to stop the digestion. The remaining epidermal pieces and cell suspension are pipetted and filtered through a100 μm pore nylon mesh into a 15 ml tube, centrifuged for 5 min at 1000 rpm at 4 °C. The supernatant is discarded, and the pellet is resuspended in 5 ml PBS, and this step is repeated for two more times.
3. Cell counts

   An equal volume of cell suspension and 0.4 % Trypan Blue solution are mixed and kept at room temperature for 5 min, and the live cell numbers are counted using a hemocytometer.
4. Seed of the primary keratinocytes

   The suspended cells are diluted in serum-free defined keratinocyte-SFM (containing 0.09 mM calcium), supplemented with defined keratinocyte-SFM growth supplementand with 1 % penicillin/streptomycin and seeded at a density of 1×10^5/ml in a culture flask in an incubator, at 37 °C and 5 % CO_2. Cells are allowed to adhere for 24–48 h and then change the medium for the first time. Small aggregates of cells could be observed within about 5 days. Cultured cells usually reach confluence within 1–2 weeks. The medium is changed every two or three days, in accordance with the growing speed.

14.2.2.2 Passage

Keratinocytes are passaged after the primary cultures reach confluence. The flask with confluent cells is washed twice with PBS; then, 0.25 % trypsin is added with 0.02 % EDTA solution, and incubated at 37 °C for 5 min. The cells are dispersed into solution by tapping the flask vigorously. Digestion is stopped by the addition of 10 % FCS. The suspended cells are harvested by centrifuging for 5 min at 1000 rpm at 4 °C. The pellet is resuspended and washed in PBS for three times. Cells are seeded at 1×10^5/ml and cultured for 5–7 days when cells reach 60–80 % confluence. The third or fourth passage of keratinocytes is usually used in subsequent experiments [52].

14.2.2.3 Quality Control

The cultured cells in serum-free media are identified by morphology and immunohistochemistry, and the quality is evaluated by growth curve analysis.

1. The morphology of the keratinocytes is inspected by inverted phase contrast microscope every day. Keratinocytes show typical pavement-like structure as cultures approach confluence (Fig. 14.5).

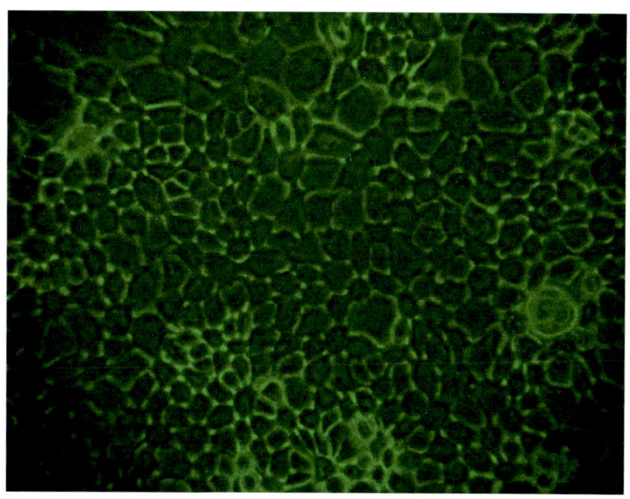

Fig. 14.5 Typical keratinocytes show pavement-like structure.

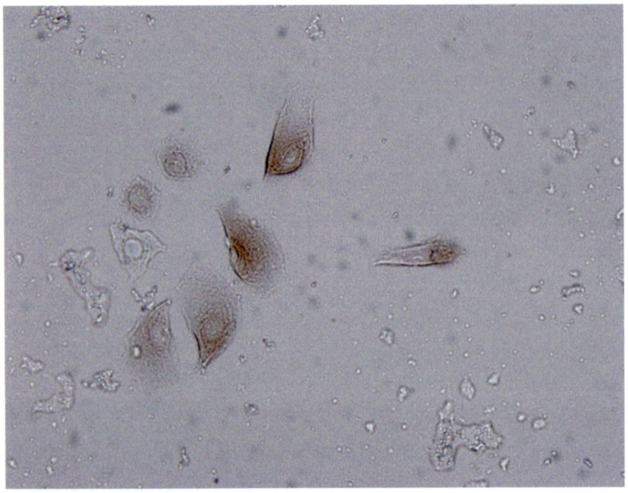

Fig. 14.6 Keratin expression of primary keratinocytes (DAB stain, ×400)

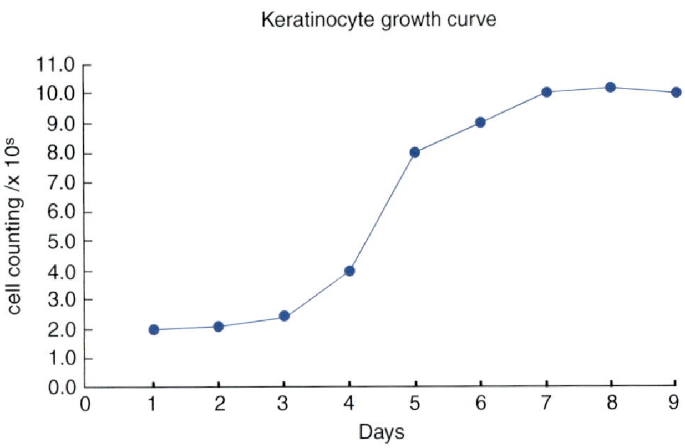

Fig. 14.7 The growth curve of keratinocytes

2. Detection of keratin in keratinocytes by immunocytochemistry. The keratinocytes are seeded on the sterile cover glass in a petri dish and cultured. 10 % FCS is added into the medium, and differentiation and keratin expression are induced. Then, immunohistochemistry is performed on the cover glass according to the manufacturer's instructions. Keratinocytes are confirmed by the positive staining with antihuman cytokeratin monoclonal antibody, as shown in Fig. 14.6.
3. Growth curve analysis

The passed keratinocytes after primary culture are seeded at 1×10^5/ml in a six-well plate, 2 ml/well. The cells are counted every day after trypsin–EDTA digestion by inverted phase contrast microscope, and the growth curves are plotted, as shown in Fig. 14.7.

14.3 Isolation of Epidermal Cells: Keratinocytes, Langerhans Cells, and Gamma/Delta T Cells

Rui-Qun Qi and Xing-Hua Gao

14.3.1 Introduction

The major resident cell populations of the epidermis are mainly keratinocytes (KCs), Langerhans cells (LCs), melanocytes, gamma/delta T (gdTs) cells (note: gdTs are absent from human epidermis). KCs represent the largest population, serving to establish the primary barrier against external (environmental) insults. LCs and gdT cells are smaller in number, and in the mouse, 1–3 % of epidermal cells are LCs and 2–6 % are gdT cells [53]. However, they play important roles in skin immunity [54]. Epidermal LCs are immature skin-homing dendritic cells (DCs) that have long been considered prototypic "sentinel" DCs [55]. LCs have the ability to traffic centrally, with acquired antigens, to skin-draining lymph nodes where they present processed antigens to T cells, thereby initiating adaptive immune responses. Recent data suggest LCs may have immunoregulatory function as well [56–58].

Skin gdT cells are a population of dendritic-like T cells in the epidermis (Fig. 14.8 b). The function of gdT cells remains largely unknown. Accumulating data has shown that skin gdT cells play important roles in immune response in some skin diseases [59–61].

Isolation of specific cell populations is the first step in experimental studies of the skin. In mice (C57BL/6), Langerin (CD207), the main molecular component of intracellular Birbeck granules, is a useful marker for LCs in both the epidermis and skin-draining lymph nodes [62, 63]; however, Langerin molecules are expressed intracellularly, and their use for cell identification requires permeabilization of the cells. Thus, Langerin is not suitable for live cell studies [64]. Two other markers allow discrimination of keratinocyte, Langerhans cells, and gdT cells, without damaging the target cells: the hematopoietic marker CD45.2 and MHC class II molecules. Using these markers, we can distinguish three cell populations as shown in Fig. 14.8a. LCs are MHC $II^{+}CD45.2^{+}$ double positive, gdT cells are MHC $II^{-}CD45.2^{+}$ single positive, and KCs are MHC $II^{-}CD45.2^{-}$ double negative. When epidermis is employed to isolate these cells, MHC class II may be replaced by CD11c.

In human skin, Langerin and CD1a are used to identify LC in the epidermis. Dermal DC are typical myeloid DCs that can be identified by DC-SIGN/CD209, CD11c, and BDCA-1/CD1c. Few plasmacytoid DC are identified by IL-3R/CD123 and BDCA-2/CD303 [65, 66].

The technique of isolating mouse epidermal cells is described as follows:

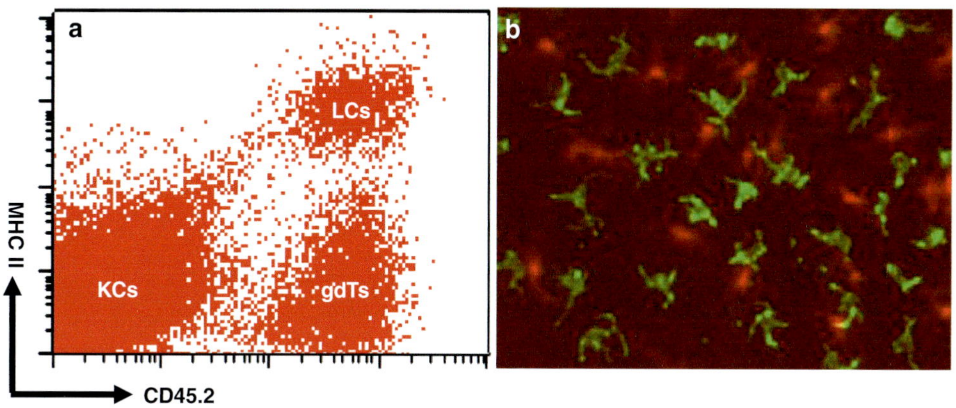

Fig. 14.8 (**a**) FACS data show three populations of mouse epidermal cells that are stained with anti-MHC II and anti-CD45.2. (**b**) Epidermal sheet is stained with anti-MHC II-PE and anti-CD3-FITC. *Red*: LCs, *Green*: gdTs

Materials

Reagents

- Anti-MHC II-APC
- Anti-CD45.2-PE
- Stain buffer
- Anti-PE MicroBeads
- FcR blocking reagent
- DPBS
- FBS
- EDTA
- Alcohol 75%
- DNase I
- RPMI 1640 with L-glutamine
- 2-mercaptoethanol (1×1000)
- Sodium bicarbonate (7.5%)
- MEM sodium pyruvate (100 mM)
- nonessential amino acids (1×100)
- HEPES Buffer
- Penicillin and Streptomycin
- Trypsin EDTA 0.25%

Equipment

- Hemocytometer
- Forceps (Roboz RS-5130)
- Scissors, curved (Fine science tools Cat.#14085-08)
- Scalpel 1 in. (Fisher Cat#08 920A)
- T-Finisher Trimmer (Oster)
- Petri dish 60×15 mm
- Tissue culture dish 60×15 mm
- Tissue culture dish 94×16 mm
- Incubator
- Reciprocal shaking bath
- Invertoskop 40°C
- AutoMACS separator
- AutoMACS column
- BDFACS Aria II
- Pipette
- Cell strainer 40 µm
- FACS tubes 5 ml
- Tubes 15 ml, 50 ml
- Sorvall Legend RT+ Centrifuge
- Microscope for cell counting
- Weighing scales

Reagents setup

Dispase solution 0.25–0.5% Dispase in 1×PBS without calcium and magnesium

Tripsin–DNase solution 1.5 ml 0.25% trypsin–EDTA and 1 ml DNase I in 5 ml 1×DPBS

Complete media RPMI 1640 with L-glutamine, 10% heat-inactivated FBS, 5×10^{5} M 2-mercaptoethanol (1×1000), 0.15% sodium bicarbonate (7.5%), 1 mM MEM sodium pyruvate (100 mM), 1× nonessential amino acids (1×100), 100 U/ml penicillin (10,000 U/ml), 100 µg/ml streptomycin (10,000 µg/ml)

Running buffer 1×PBS, 0.5% BSA, 2 mM EDTA

Rinsing buffer 1×PBS, 2 mM EDTA

Sorting buffer 1×PBS, 25 mM PH7.0 HEPES, 1% FBS, 100 U/ml penicillin (10,000U/ml), 100 µg/ml streptomycin (10,000 µg/ml)

Collection buffer 1×PBS, 10% FBS, 100 U/ml penicillin (10,000 U/ml), 100 µg/ml streptomycin (10,000 µg/ml)

14.3.2 Procedure

14.3.2.1 Preparation of Epidermal Sheets

Each mouse is sacrificed with CO_2 or through another ethical method. Hair from dorsal skin is removed with forceps by plucking against the direction of hair growth. The entire mouse body is washed thoroughly with 70% alcohol for 1 min and then rinsed with 1×PBS to remove the alcohol. The mouse body is then placed in a petri dish, and the skin is cut with scissors as shown in Fig. 14.9 a, b. Sheets of skin are rinsed with 70% alcohol for 1 min and then rinsed with 1×PBS again. Whole sheets of skin are placed in a petri dish, dermal side up, and the subcutaneous fat is scraped off with a blade. Skin sheets are sterilized in 75% alcohol for 5–10 s and washed in 1×PBS for about 0.5 min in culture hood. The specimens are each cut into four parts (equal size), and then placed, dermal side down, in a 60×15 mm tissue culture dish containing 10 ml of 0.25–0.5% Dispase enzyme solution. After incubation at 37 °C (5% CO_2) for 1 h, the epidermis is peeled off with a glass slide as shown in Fig. 14.9c.

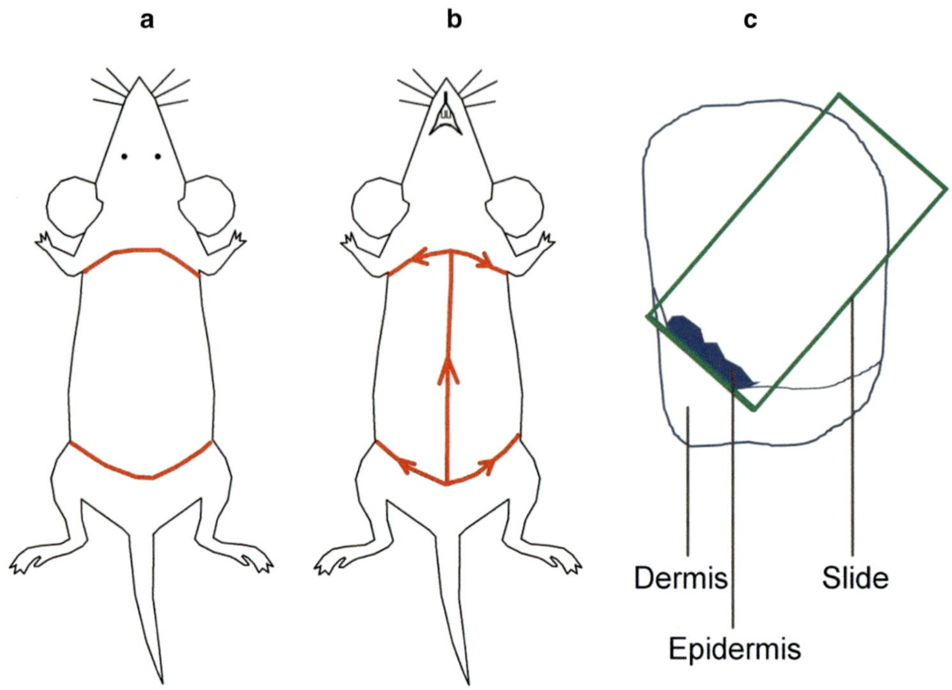

Fig. 14.9 (**a**) Dorsal side of the mouse. (**b**) Ventral side of the mouse. Red line and arrows show the direction when cutting the skin with scissors. (**c**) The epidermis is peeled from dermis with a glass slide after Dispase digestion

14.3.2.2 Epidermal Single Cell Suspension Preparation

Epidermal sheets are cut into 5×5 mm pieces, and then placed and shaken in trypsin–DNase solution (1.5 ml 0.25 % Trypsin–EDTA and 1 ml DNase I in 5 ml 1×DPBS) in the water bath for 15 min at 37 °C. Immediately afterwards, Complete Medium (CM: RPMI 1640 with L-glutamine, 10 % heat-inactivated FBS, 5×105 M 2-mercaptoethanol (1×1000), 0.15 % sodium bicarbonate (7.5 %), 1 mM MEM sodium pyruvate (100 mM), 1× nonessential amino acids (1×100), 100 U/ml penicillin (10,000 U/ml), 100 μg/ml streptomycin (10,000 μg/ml)) is added to stop the digestion. The remaining epidermal pieces and cell suspension are pipetted vigorously and filtered through a 100 μm nylon mesh into a 15 ml tube. The cells are spun at 450×g for 5 min at 4 °C. The supernatant is discarded, and the cells are resuspended in 5 ml 1×PBS with 1% FBS. The cells are filtered through a 40 μm cell strainer into a new tube. This step is then repeated. Afterwards, the cells are spun at 450×g for 5 min at 4 °C. This step is then repeated. The cells are resuspended in 2 ml CM, and the cells are counted using a hemocytometer.

> **Note**
> The typical yield of total single cell number after DNase digestion from the epidermis of a 4–6 weeks mouse is about 8–12×10^6 cells. Cell viability is about 85 %. Cells may go directly into culture for special purposes. If LCs are required in the culture, GM-CSF should be added into CM. It is important to use CM to stop the trypsin activity; otherwise, the skin pieces might be digested further in subsequent procedures.

14.3.2.3 Magnetic Cell Sorting of KCs, LCs, and gdT Cells

For further isolation and enrichment, a single cell suspension is centrifuged at 450×g for 5 min at 4 °C. 10 μl of FcR blocking reagent per 107 cells is added, mixed well, and incubated for 10 min at 4 °C. According to the total cell number, cell pellets are resuspended with “running” buffer (1×PBS, 0.5 % BSA, 2 mM EDTA). In brief, with fewer than 10^7 cells, 100 μl running buffer is required, and usually 10 μl running buffer/10^6 cells is recommended. Cells are then stained with PE-conjugated or Cy7-conjugated CD45.2 antibody (10 μl antibody/107 cells) according to the manufacturer’s instructions. The cells are mixed well and incubated for 10 min in the dark at 4 °C. The cells are washed by adding 5 ml running buffer and centrifuged at 450×g for 10 min. This step is repeated. The supernatant is discarded completely, and the cell pellet is resuspended in 80 μl of running buffer and 20 μl anti-PE microbeads/10^7 cells. They are mixed thoroughly and incubated for 15 min in the dark at 4 °C (agitated every 5 min). Cells are washed twice by adding 5 ml of running buffer, followed by centrifugation at

450×g for 5 min. In principle, 500 μl of running buffer is required to resuspend 10^8 cells. Given the size of the cell body, large cell columns are suggested. Place the column in the magnetic field and apply cell suspension onto the column as per manufacturer's protocol. Collect unlabeled KCs that pass through the column into the collection tube 1, in which more than 99 % are keratinocytes. After washing three times with 3 ml 1×PBS with 1 % FBS, the cells from collection tube 1 (KCs) are ready for use. Remove the column from the separator and place it on a suitable collection tube 2. Pipette 5 ml of buffer into the column. Immediately flush out the magnetically labeled cells by firmly pushing the plunger into the column. In collection tube 2, LCs, gdTs, and KCs will be found. Usually, LCs contribute roughly 25–35 %, and gdTs 30–50 %.

14.3.2.4 FACS Analysis and Sorting

For further enrichment of LCs and gdTs, FACS sorting is required. Spin the cells in collection tube 2 at 450×g for 5 min at 4 °C. Wash twice by adding 5 ml of precooled 1×PBS. Count cell numbers, and accordingly adjust the cell suspension to 10^6 cells/100 μl 1×PBS. Stain the cells with 1 μl APC (the fluorescence other than PE) conjugated anti-MHC class II antibody, so that the flow cytometer can distinguish the three populations of KCs, LCs, and gdTs. After incubation for 30 min in the dark at 4 °C, the cells are centrifuged at 450×g for 5 min at 4 °C. Set up the sorter according to the manufacturer's protocol. Label appropriate collection tubes and load cells onto FACS sorter. Gate and collect MHC $II^+CD45.2^+$ LCs and MHC $II^-CD45.2^+$ gdTs populations, respectively.

> **Note**
>
> The typical yield of Langerhans cells from the epidermis of a 4–6 week mouse is about (1.5–2)×10^5 cells per mouse.

14.4 Techniques for Acquisition and Manipulation of Dermal Dendritic Cells

Jang-June Park

14.4.1 Introduction

The dermis is a layer of skin between the epidermis and subcutaneous tissue, which consists of connective tissue and protects the body from physical and immunological stress and strain. The dermis is further divided into two layers, the superficial area adjacent to the epidermis as the papillary dermis and a deep thicker area as the reticular dermis [67]. The dermis is tightly connected to the epidermis through a basement membrane. Structural components of the dermis are collagen, elastic fibers, and extrafebrile matrix [68]. It also contains mechanoreceptors that provide the sense of touch and heat, hair, sweat glands, sebaceous glands, apocrine glands, lymphatic vessels, and blood vessels. Those blood vessels deliver nourishment to and remove waste from both dermal and epidermal cells. In the steady state, many types of immune cells are found in the dermis including memory T cells, mast cells, and dermal dendritic cells (dDCs) [69].

In the skin, Langerhans cells (LCs) were considered for a long time as the only antigen-presenting cells (APCs) that monitor pathogens penetrating the cutaneous barrier. Langerin, a hallmark of LCs, was thought to be a specific marker of LCs for a period of time [70]. There have been great advances in understanding skin immunology. Following detection of antigens in the skin, LCs mature and present antigens to T cells in cutaneous lymph nodes (LNs) [71, 72]. Recent reports showed that dermal DCs (dDCs) as well as LCs are major APCs in the skin immune response. Both dDCs and LCs in the dermis and epidermis migrate to cutaneous LNs and serve as direct precursors of the migratory dDCs and migratory LCs in cutaneous LNs, respectively (Fig. 14.10). In contact hypersensitivity (CHS) mouse model, $Langerin^+$ dDCs as well as $Langerin^-$ dDCs acquire antigens in dermis on Day 0. Then they migrate to LNs and cross-present antigens to CD8 T cells and present antigens to CD4 helper T cells on Days 1–2 [73]. LCs migrate to LNs on Day 3 and produce IL-10 and other unknown factors inhibiting antigen-specific effector CD4 and CD8 T cells that have been stimulated and expanded by $Langerin^+$ dDCs (Fig. 14.10).

The dDCs can be further divided into subsets as $Langerin^+$ dDC and $Langerin^-$ dDC. In contrast to migratory LCs, $Langerin^+$ dDCs express lower levels of Langerin and lack Birbeck granules, suggesting that these cells are not originated from LCs [74]. Therefore, in skin-draining LNs, Langerin + cells are thought to include $Langerin^{lo}$ blood-derived dDCs and $Langerin^{hi}$ LCs (Table 14.3).

Recently, a new DC subset expressing Langerin, the $Langerin^+CD103^+$ dermal dendritic cells (dDCs), was found in the skin immune system. They showed distinct expression of surface markers and differential function from migratory LCs [75–78]. Furthermore, it was shown that LCs and $Langerin^+CD103^+$ dDCs promote opposite T cell responses of Th17 and Th1, respectively [79, 80]. This suggests that different skin DC subsets have been developed for distinct roles in skin immunity.

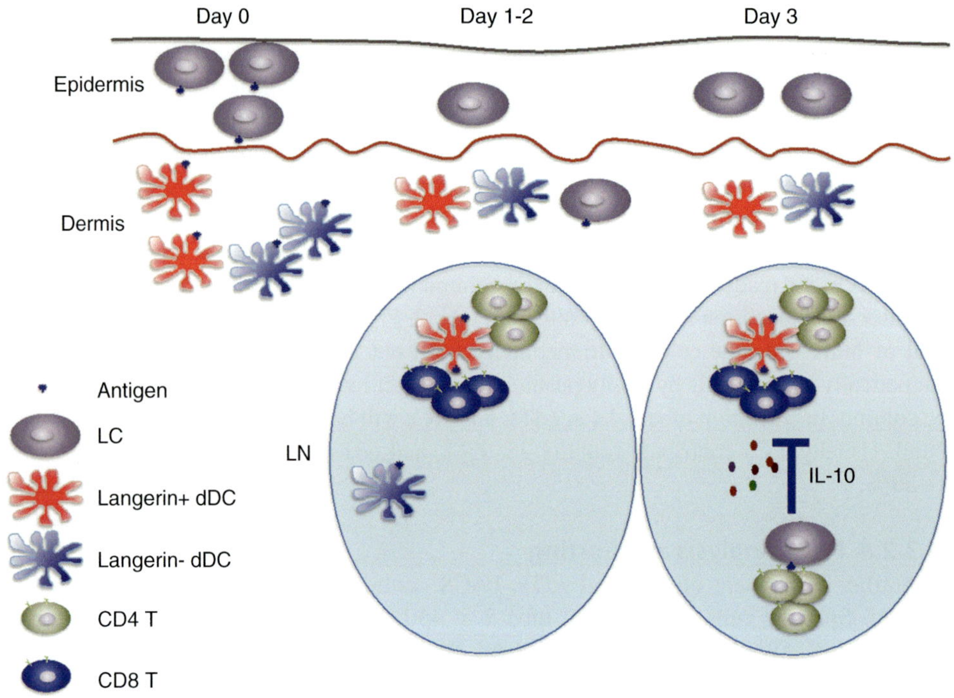

Fig. 14.10 Different skin DC subsets and T cells during contact hypersensitivity (CHS). Antigens are uptaken and presented by LCs in epidermis, Langerin⁺dDC and Langerin⁻ dDC in dermis. On day 1–2, Langerin⁺ dDCs cross-present antigens to CD8 T cells while presenting to CD4 T helper cells in skin draining LN. The role of Langerin⁻ dDCs in LNs remains elusive. On day 3, LCs produce IL-10 and other unknown suppressive factors to inhibit effector CD4 T and CD8 T cells

Table 14.3 Comparison of DC subsets in the skin

	LC	Dermal Langerin + DCs	Dermal Langerin – DCs
Tissue	Epidermis	Dermis	Dermis
Langerin (CD207)	+++	+	–
CD103	–	±	–
CD11b	+	–	±
Ep-Cam (CD326)	+	–	–

14.4.2 Procedure

The following protocol describes the dermal DCs in contact hypersensitivity (CHS) experiment that is an experimental mouse model of allergic contact dermatitis (ACD). In order to describe dermal DCs (dDCs), CHS is chosen because it provides the option of studying not only dermal immunology but also in vivo whole basic skin immunological mechanisms. Of note, this protocol shows how to purify dDCs and LCs for phenotyping them based on the markers in Table 14.3.

Mice Five-week-old male or female of BALB/c or C57BL/6 mice are fed and housed under specific pathogen-free (SPF) conditions.

Sensitization for CHS BALB/c or C57BL/6 mice are painted with 200 ml of 0.5 % (w/v) fluorescein isothiocyanate (FITC) in atopic dermatitis, a 1:1 mixture of acetone and dibutylphthalate, on shaved ears.

Dermal tissue processing and flow cytometry For dermal preparations, ears are split into dorsal and ventral halves with forceps. Epidermal and dermal sheets are then washed extensively in PBS before first digestion for 90 min at 37 °C with 5 U/ml Dispase I in PBS (BD Biosciences), which allows separation of the epidermis and dermis. After epidermal separation, dermal halves are then digested for 45 min at 37 °C in 2–5 mg/ml collagenase type IV in PBS. Tissues are filtered through a 70-μm nylon cell strainer (BD Falcon) to obtain single-cell suspensions. Cells are washed in running buffer (5 % FCS and 20 mM EDTA in PBS) and counted volumetrically with AccuCount beads (Spherotech). Positive staining is compared with that of fluorescence-minus-one controls. Cells are analyzed on a FACSCanto (BD) or LSR II (BD). Flow cytometry data are analyzed with FlowJo software (Tree Star).

Preparation of LN cells Brachial, axillary, and inguinal LNs are obtained from BALB/c mice under a naïve state or 1 day after sensitization for CHS. Draining brachial and axillary LNs are obtained from BALB/c or C57BL/6 mice 1 day after CHS elicitation when mice are sensitized with FITC$^+$ dDCs by footpad injection. LNs are minced and digested with 1 mg/ml collagenase from *Clostridium histolyticum* (Sigma) in RPMI1640 medium supplemented with 10 % FCS for 25 min at 37 °C. Digested cells are transferred to a new tube through nylon mesh and washed with PBS containing 0.5 % BSA and 2 mM EDTA.

Antibodies Fluorochrome-conjugated antibodies to the following cell-surface molecules are used: CD3, CD4, CD8, CD11b, CD11c, MHC class II, Langerin (CD207), CD103, and Ep-Cam (CD326).

Flow cytometry analysis Cells isolated from mouse tissues and primary cultured cells are incubated with antimouse CD16/CD32 mAb (1/100 dilution of ammonium sulfate-precipitated hybridoma culture supernatant; the 2.4G2 hybridoma is purchased from ATCC) to reduce nonspecific binding 5 min before the addition of the first antibodies. Cells are then incubated with biotin-, FITC-, PE-, PE-Cy7-, Percp-Cy5.5, PacBlue, APC-H7, and/or APC-conjugated antibodies for 30 min. Biotin-conjugated antibodies are visualized with PE-Cy7- or APC-labeled streptavidin. To exclude dead cells, except for intracellularly stained cells, all cells are resuspended in flow cytometry buffer (FCM) (PBS containing 5 % FCS, 2 mM EDTA, and 0.02 % sodium azide) containing 7-amino-actinomycin D (7-AAD) (eBioscience). To stain intracellular molecules, cells are fixed and permeabilized with BD Cytofix/Cytoperm (BD Biosciences, Franklin Lakes, NJ), according to the manufacturer's protocol. All procedures are performed on ice. Antibodies and reagents are diluted in FCM buffer. The cells are rinsed once with FCM buffer at the end of each incubation period. Samples are analyzed on a FACS Aria cell sorter (BD). Data are analyzed using FlowJo software (Tree Star, Ashland, OR).

14.5 Techniques for Acquisition and Manipulation of Melanocytes

Leihong Xiang

14.5.1 Introduction

Human epidermis is described as a stratified squamous epithelium which is mainly consisted of keratinocytes. However, there are also several types of nonkeratinocytes taking part in the physiology of skin, particularly prominent among which are the melanocytes. Not only does the melanocyte reside in the basal layer of the epidermis, it can also be seen in the basal layer of the hair matrix and the outer root sheath of hair follicles, thus accounting for the pigmentation of skin and hair. With a variety of pigmentation disorders unsolved, for example, vitiligo, melasma, postinflammatory pigmentation,etc., there has been a growing awareness of the necessity to study the biochemical and phenotypical characteristics of melanocytes by in vitro method. In this chapter, we will briefly outline the principles and procedures for the isolation, culture, and identification of human melanocytes.

Although methods have been achieved to isolate outer root sheath melanocytes (ORSM) successfully [81], epidermal melanocytes are still the routine sources for the large-scale propagation of pure cultures. The density of melanogenically active (dopa-positive) epidermal melanocyte populations varies between anatomical sites, with the highest in the face and genitals (~2000 mm^{-2} in male genitalia) [88]. Donors' age is also a critical factor affecting the proliferation and propagation of melanocytes [82], in that the populations of dopa-positive epidermal melanocytes decline steadily with advancing age [83]. As a result, neonatal foreskin would be the best source for human melanocyte isolation and culture.

Human melanocyte culture used to be a great challenge, for they do not grow or even survive in medium for fibroblasts, melanoma, or keratinocytes [88]. In addition, their small population in the epidermis leads to the distinct growth advantage of other resident cells while cultured in vitro. In 1982, challenges were overcome by the discovery that a phorbol ester acting in synergy with cholera toxin could establish pure pigment cell populations [84]. Phorbol ester enables selective proliferation of normal human melanocytes via protein kinase C (PKC) signaling cascade, while cholera toxin potently raises intracellular levels of cAMP, stimulating growth of melanocytes and extending their life span in vitro [84]. These discoveries suggested that the survival and proliferation of melanocytes are mainly medi ated by two distinct signaling pathways, which led to an intensive search and testing of melanocyte mitogens among those known growth factors. Subsequent identification of natural growth factors included basic fibroblast growth factor (bFGF, currently termed FGF2), mast cell growth factor/stem cell factor (M/SCF), endothelins (ET-1 to ET-3), hepatocyte growth factor (HGF), and melanocyte-stimulating hormone (MSH) [85]. Myriad studies have indicated that only by combination of those synergistic mitogens can the quiescent melanocytes in culture be released into cycling mode.

Cultured melanocytes can be easily distinguished by their bipolar or polydendritite morphology, while keratinocytes and fibroblasts grow with cobblestone or spindle appearance, respectively. In the meantime, series of methods have been developed so far to identify melanocytes in vitro, including $_L$-Dihydroxyphenylalanine (DOPA) staining, melanin-bleaching technique, and immunohistochemical staining. Details of the procedures will be demonstrated later in this chapter.

14.5.2 Materials

Reagents	Anti-S100 antibody
PBS	DAPI
Culture medium (see Reagent Setup)	**Equipment**
Penicillin–Streptomycin	Laminar flow hood
70 % ethanol, 75 % ethanol	Set of forceps and scissors
FBS	Sterile culture dishes, 100 mm
Dispase (Dispase® II, Roche)	4 °C refrigerator
DMEM (HYCLONE)	37 °C, 5 % CO_2 incubator
HMGSII (Invitrogen)	Cell strainer, 100 μm
M254 (Invitrogen)	Centrifuge
0.25 % Trypsin–EDTA	Inverted microscope
4 % paraformaldehyde	Fluorescence microscope
L-dihydroxyphenylalanine (DOPA)	Humidified chamber
Potassium chloride	6/24-well plates
Concentrated hydrochloric acid	T25 flasks
Potassium permanganate	Pipettes
Oxalic acid	Sterile centrifuge tubes, 15 ml, 50 ml
Chromic acid	**Reagent setup**
Calcium chloride	*Skin-transporting medium*: ice-cold 1 % penicillin–streptomycin 1×PBS
Perchlorate	
Hydrogen peroxide	*Epidermal isolation solution*: 0.25 % Dispase in DMEM with 1 % penicillin–streptomycin
Triton X-100	
BSA	*Melanocyte growth medium*: 1 % HMGSII in M254 with 1 % penicillin–streptomycin
PBST	
Anti-Mitf antibody	*DOPA solution*: 0.1 % DOPA in 1×PBS
Anti-TYRP1 antibody	Cells and sources
Anti-DCT antibody	Neonatal/adult human foreskin

14.5.3 Procedures

14.5.3.1 Melanocyte Isolation

The harvested fresh neonatal or adult human foreskin is preserved in skin-transporting medium at 4 °C before the procedure starts. Specimen should be processed within the first 6 h. Three to four sterile 100-mm culture dishes, one for 10 ml of 75 % ethanol and others for 10 ml of 1× PBS, are prepared in a laminar flow hood. Soak the human foreskin in 75 % ethanol for 1 min, and rinse it in dishes containing 1× PBS for at least three times. The skin ring is then cut open, trimmed off most of the fat and subcutaneous tissue with curved scissors, and then cut into small pieces (approximately 5×5 mm^2). Transfer the skin pieces into a 50-ml sterile centrifuge tube containing 10 ml epidermal isolation solution. Incubate the tube in the refrigerator at 4 °C for 18–24 h.

After incubation, 10 ml DMEM with 10 % FBS is added to deactivate the Dispase enzyme. Pour the tissue into an empty sterile 100-mm culture dish. With the help of forceps, epidermis (thin, brownish, translucent layer) can be gently torn apart from the dermis (thick, pink to white, opaque layer). While the dermis is discarded, each piece of epidermal tissue is rinsed with 1× PBS (twice at least), drained, and then collected into an empty culture dish. Chop them with scissors until the tissue becomes mash-like substances. Transfer them to a 50-ml tube with 5 ml of 0.25 % trypsin–EDTA and incubate them at 37 °C for 10 min.

5 ml DMEM with 10 % FBS is added to the tube while the incubation ended. Gently mince and pipette the epidermal tissue for 3–5 min with the tip side of a 10 ml pipette. Dilute the mixture with additional 20 ml of 1× PBS and then filter the mixture through a 100 μm cell strainer, generating a single-cell suspension with a translucent appearance. Spin cells down at 1200 rpm for 5 min. Discard the supernatant and resuspend the pellets in 5 ml of melanocyte growth medium at 5×10^5 per T25 flask. Incubate the cells at 37 °C and 5 % CO_2.

14.5.3.2 Melanocyte Culture

Cell attachment of both melanocytes and keratinocytes can be observed within the first 72 h in culture, with a predominance of the melanocytes (Fig.14.11). Change the medium with fresh melanocyte growth medium every 3 days until cells reach a confluence of 70–80 % (Fig. 14.11). Discard the medium and treat the cells with 0.25 % trypsin–EDTA at 37 °C for 3–5 min, in the condition of which melanocytes become preferentially detached compared with keratinocytes. Deactivate the trypsin with DMEM containing 10 % FBS. Mix the cell suspension by gently agitating and then pellet the cells by centrifugation at 1200 rpm for 5 min. Collected cells should be resuspended at 5×10^5 per T25

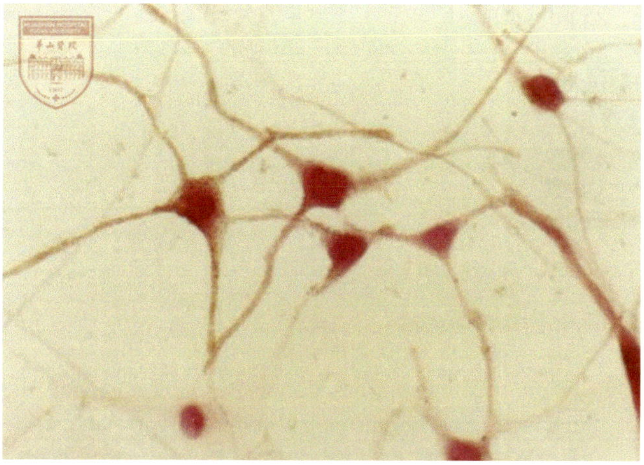

Fig. 14.11 Melanocytes Dopa staning(+).

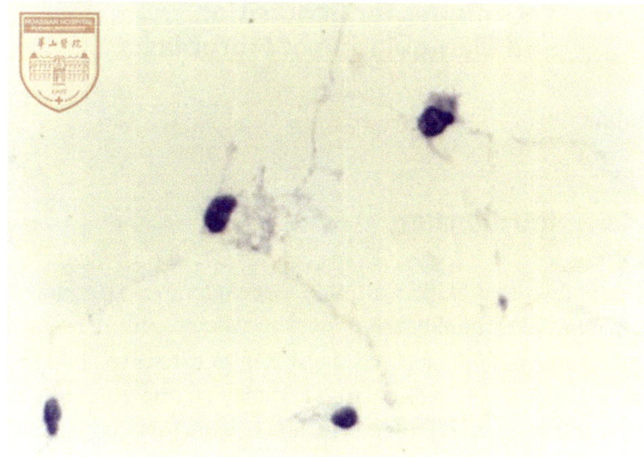

Fig. 14.12 Melanocytes melanin bleaching.

flask. In general, relatively pure melanocyte cultures can be obtained within two passages.

【Figures of melanocyte culture for day 1, 5,14…..】

14.5.4 Melanocyte Identification

14.5.4.1 L-Dihydroxyphenylalanine (DOPA) Staining

This classic method refers to a process in which the tyrosinase of melanocytes oxidizes dopa into dopa-melanin, which subsequently remains in or on the cells, coloring the reacting cells black [86].

Melanocytes are plated at a density of 5×10^5/ml in 24-well plate and cultured at 37 °C, 5 % CO_2 for 24 h. Cells are rinsed twice with PBS and then fixed in 4 % paraformaldehyde for 30 min at room temperature. Rinse the melanocytes again for three times. Treat the cells with freshly prepared 0.1 % DOPA at 37 °C for 4 h, during which DOPA solution should be changed once. After the incubation, rinse the cells three times and fix them with 4 % paraformaldehyde for another 20 min. Rinse the cells again before observing them under the bright field of inverted microscope (Fig. 14.11).

14.5.4.2 Melanin-bleaching Technique

The chemical structure of melanin, unlike other cell components, can be destroyed by potent oxidizing agents, resulting in the depigmentation of melanocytes while being stained. Therefore, melanin-bleaching techniques can be used as an aid to avoid false-positive staining caused by other factors [87].

Melanocytes are plated onto gelatin-coated chamber slides cultured at 37 °C, 5 % CO_2 for 24 h. Treat the cells with 1 g potassium chloride, 50 ml 70 % ethanol, and 1 ml concentrated hydrochloric acid for 2–3 h, followed by 0.1 %–0.25 % potassium permanganate for 2–4 h. Wash off the agents and bleach the cells with 1 % oxalic acid. The cells are rinsed again and then treated with freshly prepared mixture of 25 ml 1 % chromic acid solution and 25 ml 5 % calcium chloride solution for 8–10 h. Treatments of 40 % perchlorate solution for 2–16 h, 10 % hydrogen peroxide solution for 24–48 h, and 1 % bromine solution for 12–24 h are also given in order. Carefully wash the slides for 5–10 min. Routine staining for melanin is processed after this complete bleaching procedure, the results of which should be negative (Fig. 14.12).

14.5.4.3 Immunofluorescent Staining

Several melanocytic markers can be utilized to identify melanocytes, typically including Mitf (Microphthalmia-associated transcription factor), TYRP1 (Tyrosinase-related protein 1), DCT (DOPAchrome tautomerase, also known as TRP-2), and S100. Mitf is a cell type-specific regulator that is required for the development and/or survival of pigment cells, while the tyrosinase family is directly involved in melanin pigment production. S100 is normally present in cells derived from the neural crest, demonstrating the source of melanocytes. In the meantime, HMB45, a specific marker for malignant melanoma, can also be used as a negative control.

Melanocytes are plated onto gelatin-coated chamber slides cultured at 37 °C, 5 % CO_2 for 24 h. Cells are fixed in ice-cold 4 % paraformaldehyde in PBS for 15 min at room temperature, followed by the permeabilization of the samples for 10 min incubation with PBS containing 0.25 % Triton X-100. Unspecific binding of the antibodies within cells should be blocked with 1 % BSA in PBST for 30 min. Then, melanocytes are incubated overnight at 4 °C with diluted antibodies (e.g. Mitf, TYRP1, DCT, S100). After several washes with PBS, diluted second antibodies were added and incubated for 1 h at 37 °C in dark. The nuclei are counterstained with 4,6-diamidino-2-phenylinodole (DAPI). Slides are mounted and observed under fluorescence microscope.

14.6 Techniques for Acquisition and Manipulation of Fibroblasts

Yuling Shi

14.6.1 Introduction

It is known that skin is a tissue that undergoes continuous self-renewal throughout the lifetime of an organism and also has an extensive ability to repair wounds [89]. Fibroblasts (FB) play an important role in the repair process. Fibroblasts mainly exist in loose connective tissue. Collagens, the vital function of which is to keep elasticity and resilience of human skin, are compounded and secreted by FB. Necrosis and degeneration of cells that are caused by trauma like empyrosis and evulsion are common in daily life. Cell hyperplasia and formation of extracellular matrix are needed in tissue repair [90]. During the process of skin renovation, the participation of autologous/allosome can vastly promote the migration and multiplication of epidermal cells, which also can make the structural dermis more viable, which leads to a rapid repair of damaged tissue, as well as in the aging skin renovation [91]. Moreover, human fibroblasts (HFBs) play a significant role in testing novel ophthalmological drugs [92].

However, the checkpoint of in vitro culture of HFBs is that the capacity of cell multiplication decreases as the frequency of subculture increases. So, it is vital to find out a stable and efficient way to isolate and culture HFBs [93].

Explant outgrowth and mechanical as well as enzymatic disaggregation procedures are regularly used for HFBs isolation, but the former is relatively inefficient. Only a minority of cells grow out from the explants. So, here we describe one technique–enzymatic disaggregation, which is more efficient and permits a substantial increase in the number of human skin fibroblasts that can be obtained from human skin tissue explants [94].

14.6.2 Reagents

- Fetal bovine serum (FBS)
- High-glucose DMEM
- EDTA
- PBS without calcium and magnesium
- Type II collagenase
- Trypsin
- Paraformaldehyde

14.6.3 Equipments

- Forceps
- Scalpels
- 25 ml petri dish
- Scissors
- Incubator
- Pipette
- Microscope
- Tubes
- Centrifuge

14.6.4 Procedures

1. Obtain specimens from donors who have signed the informed consents, usually through surgery, and make sure donors have no history of SLE, scleroderma, psoriasis, or any other connective tissue diseases, as well as empyrosis, traumatic, and scar tissues.
2. Wash the obtained samples with the solution consisting of PBS (without calcium ion and magnesium ion) and penicillin and streptomycin. Gently remove all the subcutaneous tissue.
3. Cut the skin specimens into approximately 0.5–1 cm^2 pieces. Place explants into tubes containing trypsin made up in F-12 medium without FBS and leave overnight (about 18 h) at 4 °C.
4. The second day, use scalpels and forceps to separate the epidermis from the dermis. *Note that the dermis is very durable and cannot be easily disrupted by scraping.* Then, briefly mince the largest pieces of tissue.
5. Transfer minced dermis into the tubes containing 2.5 g/L trypsin and leave to digest for 15 min (or solution made up of 0.25 % pancreatin and 0.02 % EDTA for 2–3 min).
6. Transfer dermis into medium containing high-glucose DMEM and 10 %–15 % FBS to terminate digestion.
7. Centrifuge for 3–10 min, at 1000 rpm.
8. After centrifugation, transfer the residual tissue into 25 ml petri flask, and add little FBS and DMEM; *note that NOT to float the tissue.*
9. Place the petri flask into humidified incubator at 37 °C and 5 % CO_2 in air, and start incubation; supplement culture solution the next day.
10. The first outgrowth of the explants is usually heterogeneous, comprising skin keratinocytes and HFBs, The second and subsequent transfers are performed every 2–3 weeks, when sufficient cells had migrated from the explants. Obtain the cells every day under microscope; second culture can be performed when the quantity of the first outgrowth reaches 70 %.
11. Use 1.25 g/L trypsin to digest for 30 s; the retraction of cell body can be observed under microscope. Terminate digestion with DMEM supplemented with 10 % FBS.
12. Gently blow the cells with pipette, and centrifuge for 3–10 min, at 1000 rpm. Abandon the top fluid, Then the second transfer can be performed.

13. Skin explants can be transferred until the desired amount of HFBs are obtained or until no further outgrowth can be observed.
14. Remove the remaining HFBs in the original dish from the first outgrowth by trypsinization, which can be used to determine the life span.

14.6.5 Notes

- Donors of young age are preferred to obtain tissue from, because the cells are more active.
- Wash specimens sufficiently.
- Use plastic containers until all of these compounds adhere to glass.
- It is essential to remove all of the fats attached to the dermis in order for trypsin to easily penetrate the tissue and dissociate cells.
- Do not add too much fluid in step 8, not to float the tissues.

Immunofluorescence assay can be used for the identification of HFBs: Take the fifth generation and transplant into a six-well plate, the cover glass of which has been sterilized, and make the cell grow on the glass slides; the optimum quantity is 3.5×10^4. Take out the slides after 4 days; wash with PBS for three times; fix the cells with 40 g/L paraformaldehyde (pH 7.2) for 30 min; then wash with PBS three times again. Add anti-Vimentin antibody in the concentration of 1:100 as the first antibody, and IgG-FITC in the concentration of 1:200 as the second antibody; re-stain the nucleus with DAPi, and observe cells under fluorescence microscope. Set samples without anti-Vimentin antibody as negative control.

14.7 Isolation and Manipulation of Resident T Cells in Skin

Matthew Weiland and Ruiqun Qi

14.7.1 Abstract

The skin provides the host with a durable barrier against continuous environmental and pathogenic assaults. In the event of injury or invasion of pathogen, the epidermis and dermis contain distinct resident T cells, effective at wound repair and defense against foreign pathogens. Skin T cell subsets expressing both αβ and γδ TCR have distinct immunological roles. Skin γδ T cells are located in both the epidermal and dermal layers. γδ T cells in the epidermis, referred to as dendritic epidermal T cells, are a majority of the epidermal T cells in mouse; yet, they represent a smaller portion of T cells in human epidermis. Epidermal γδ T cells contribute to wound healing, inflammation, and both steady-state and tumor surveillance. Dermal γδ T cells are an important T cell subset and display characteristics that differ from their epidermal counterparts. Dermal γδ T cells are involved in antigen-specific $CD4^+$ T cell responses and also perform immunosurveillance. Skin αβ T cells are found in large numbers compared to blood, and almost all display a memory phenotype. These tissue-resident memory T cells express $CD4^+$, $CD8^+$, and include a T_{reg} subset. Skin $CD8^+$ T cells are restricted to the epidermis, whereas memory $CD4^+$ T cells are located in the dermis, while both recruit memory cells from circulation and control recurrent infections. Resident $CD4^+$ $Foxp3^+$ T cells are involved in the tight control of unnecessary activation of effector T cells present in skin. The skin has a variety of cells present in considerable numbers that contribute to immune response in the skin. In this chapter, we will provide an overview of the resident T cell subsets.

14.7.2 Epidermis

T cells resident to epidermis provide local protection at the sites of infection, coordinate successful wound repair, regulate inflammation, participate in tumor immunity, and carry long lasting memory phenotypes against foreign pathogens [95, 96]. There are two distinct T cell subsets in the epidermis, the γδ TCR expressing dendritic epidermal T cell (DETC) and the αβ TCR expressing $CD8^+$ resident memory T cell (T_{RM}). The function of DETC has not been fully elucidated; however, accumulating data has shown that skin γδ T cells play important roles in pathogen defense and steady-state surveillance [97–99]. $CD8^+$ T_{RM} controls infection by providing long-lasting immune defense to recurrent infection in the epidermis [96, 100]. Both cell types are present in significant numbers during the steady state and remain relatively fixed in position within the epidermis.

14.7.2.1 γδ T Cell-Dendritic Epidermal T Cells

As their name suggests, epidermal γδ TCR DETC have a dendritic-like morphology in the steady state and are in essence fixed in position and are characterized by the surface phenotype $Thy\text{-}1^+$ $CD45^+$ $CD69^+$ $MHCII^-$ (Table 14.4) [101, 102]. Their dendritic morphology enables close interaction with surrounding cells and continuous monitoring and maintenance of epidermal homeostasis [103]. Epidermal resident γδ T cells have a restricted TCR specific to skin in mouse; human DETC subsets have been identified, but are present in much smaller numbers, yet still contribute to successful wound healing [95, 104]. Mouse DETC support epidermal homeostasis through

Table 14.4 T cells resident in skin

T cell subset	T cell receptor	Phenotype	Location	Function
DETC (γδ T cell)	γδ TCR (Vγ5 Vδ1)	$CD45^+$ $MHCII^-$ $Thy\text{-}1^+$ $CD69^+$ CD25-	Epidermis	Wound healing, inflammation, immunosurveillance and tumor surveillance
Dermal γδ T cell	γδ TCR ($V\gamma5^-V\gamma4^+$)	$CD45^+$ $MHCII^-$ $CD69^+$ $CD25^{low}$	Dermis	Regulate $CD4^+$ T cell immunity, immunosurveillance
$CD8^+$ T_{RM} cell[a]	αβ TCR (diverse)	CD8+ $CD69^+$ $CD103^+$ $CD49a^+$ CLA^+ $CCR7^-$	Epidermis	Infection control, recruitment
$CD4^+$ T_{RM} cell[a]	αβ TCR (diverse)	$CD4^+$ $CD69^+$ $CD103^+$ CLA^+ CCR7-	Dermis	Infection control, recruitment
$CD4^+$ T_{reg} cell	αβ TCR (diverse)	$CD4^+$ $CD25^+$ $Foxp3^+$ $CD127^-$	Dermis	Control of effector T cells

[a]Resident after successful clearance of infection

direct interaction with keratinocytes, regulate inflammation by secreting chemokines and cytokines, respond rapidly to infection at local sites in epidermis, promote wound healing by secretion of growth factors, and promote tumor immunity through direct lysis of cancer cells and presumably through cytokine secretion [101]. Not only do DETC act as a first line of defense against foreign antigen, they perform a continuous immunosurveillance of the skin barrier. DETC perform this surveillance in the absence of foreign antigen and monitor local epidermis through recognition of a self-expressed ligand, all during the steady state [102, 105]. During the immunosurveillance of the epidermis, DETC participate in tumor immunity and destruction of tumor cells by recognition of ligands expressed by malignant cells [106].

14.7.2.2 CD8⁺ Resident Memory T Cells

$CD8^+$ T_{RM} cells can be characterized by the surface phenotype $CD8^+$ $CD69^+$ $CD103^+$ $CD49a^+$ CLA^+ $CCR7^-$ (Table 14.4) [96, 107, 108]. These resident T cells were first characterized in psoriatic lesions generated following grafts of prepsoriatic skin as a result of the presence of resident T cells [95, 109]. In addition, resident skin T cells were confirmed in human skin when distinct subsets of memory T cells were detected in skin tissue following T cell depletion with anti-CD52 [110]. $CD8^+$ T_{RM} cells are generated post-infection [100] and are present in large numbers [108] at original sites of infection. These memory cells offer immunity at sites of infection by initiating and maintaining immune defense [108]. $CD8^+$ T_{RM} cells reside in the epidermis and are mostly confined to the original infection sites [111]. Unlike their circulating counterparts, these resident T cells are nonmigratory due to the lack of chemokine receptors necessary for recirculation [95, 107, 112]. The memory phenotype of $CD8^+$ T_{RM} cells has been demonstrated in the rapid control of new infection with the same invading pathogen [96]. As a whole, they express genes characteristic of T cell activation and antiviral activity and function through cytolysis and secretion of antiviral cytokines [112, 113] making these $CD8^+$ T_{RM} cells potent effector cells superior to circulating memory T cells in providing fast and long-lasting immune defense against recurrent infections of the skin [100]. In addition to populating the original sites of infection, repeated pathogen invasion also leads to continuing increases of T_{RM} in the skin as a whole [100]. In addition to these contact-dependent functions of immune defense, it has been reported that skin T_{RM} cells survey skin, and, upon recognition of recurrent antigen, signal for a rapid response of circulating $CD8^+$ memory T cell populations to migrate to skin circumventing the delay in antigen exposure of circulating memory cells [113]. Taken together, resident memory T cells are not strictly confined to fighting pathogens alone; they coordinate recruitment of other memory T cells for control of infection.

14.7.3 Dermis

The dermis contains important cell types of both adaptive and innate cell types that are involved in the immune defense of the skin. Similar to the epidermis, the dermis has resident T cell subsets expressing γδ TCR and αβ TCR. Dermal γδ T cells appear to mediate $CD4^+$ T cells by secretion of IL-17, which may also contribute to skin-associated disease. The αβ T cell subsets present in the dermis are the $CD4^+$ T_{RM} cells and the $CD4^+$ regulatory T cells (T_{reg}). Memory $CD4^+$ T cells are located in the dermis and are capable of recruiting memory cells from circulation and controlling recurrent infections in the skin [95]. Resident $CD4^+$ $Foxp3^+$ T cells are involved in the tight control of unnecessary activation of effector T cells present in skin [114]. All three cell types make up a part of a network capable of controlling pathogens.

14.7.3.1 Dermal γδ T Cells

γδ T cells are a prominent population of resident T cells present in both mouse and human dermis. Similar to DETC, dermal γδ T cells have a surface phenotype of $CD45^+$ $CD69^+$ $MHCII^-$ $CD25^{low}$ (Table 14.4) [115]. In addition, dermal γδ T cells are $CCR6^+$ and do not express CD27 [116]. In comparison to their epidermal counterparts, dermal γδ T cells differ in TCR usage, phenotypic profile, survival requirements, and migratory behavior [115]. Dermal γδ T cells have a TCR population less restricted than DETC; yet, are mostly $V\gamma5^-V\gamma4^+$ [95, 115]. For survival and development, dermal γδ T cells are in part dependent on IL-7, whereas DETC are dependent on IL-15 [115]. Dermal γδ T cells are the principal cells in the dermis that mediate cutaneous inflammation during some types of infection through the production of IL-17 [115, 116]. Dermal γδ T cells are involved in antigen-specific $CD4^+$ T cell responses to some infections [117] most likely due to neutrophil recruitment through IL-17 secretion [95, 115]. Resident dermal γδ T cells also contribute to the immunosurveillance of skin. However, unlike αβ T cells, γδ T cells recognize antigens without the requirement for antigen processing and presentation by classical MHC molecules [115]. The importance of not being restricted to antigen presentation in the classical sense is that surveillance is not compatible with delays tied to cell expansion; response to exposure of foreign pathogen requires an immediate immune defense by dermal γδ T cells [117].

14.7.3.2 $CD4^+$ Resident Memory T Cells

$CD4^+$ T_{RM} cells are present in the dermis and maintain the surface phenotype of $CD4^+$ $CD69^+$ $CD103^+$ CLA^+ $CCR7^-$ (Table 14.4) [107, 112]. $CD4^+$ T_{RM} cells lack expression of the lymph node homing receptor CCR7, restricting their ability to migrate to draining lymph nodes [110]. Although widespread immune surveillance of dermal T_{RM} is constrained, they offer rapid immune protection to reinfection at local sites [96]. This is reflected in the fact that T cells resident at the site of repeated virus challenge in skin offer superior immune protection [110]. Stimulated $CD4^+$ T cells in the dermis demonstrated a prevalence of cells secreting the cytokines IFN-γ and IL-2, signaling that $CD4^+$ T_{RM} cells are bent toward a Th1 response [108]. The function of $CD4^+$ T_{RM} cells has not been fully elucidated; however, the importance of these cells is highlighted in the fact that patients with depletion of T cells from circulation still have intact immune responses [110].

14.7.3.3 $CD4^+$ T_{reg} Cell

Although they represent a minor subset of skin-resident memory T cells, $CD4^+$ T cells expressing Foxp3 consist of approximately 10% of all $CD4^+$ $CD8^+$ T_{RM} [114]. These T cells present in skin have a surface phenotype characteristic of T_{regs} of $CD4^+$ $CD25^+$ $Foxp3^+$ $CD127^-$ (Table 14.4) [108, 116]. Resident $CD4^+$ $Foxp3^+$ T cells are involved in the tight control of unnecessary activation of effector T cells present in skin. In fact, it has been demonstrated that skin-resident T_{reg} cells can block proliferation of self-reacting skin-resident T effector memory cells; yet, this blockage is discontinued when foreign antigens are encountered [114]. It is not surprising that a functional subset of T_{reg} cells is present in skin, given the large numbers of T cells that reside in the epidermis and dermis.

14.7.4 Concluding Comments

The immune cells found in the epidermis and dermis offer the most protection against foreign antigens encountered through breach of the skin. From the restrictive TCR of γδ T cells to the diverse TCR repertoires of the αβ T cells, there is a network of resident skin immune cells that survey and respond in specialized ways to control pathogens. The number of αβ T cells in skin is striking; there is an estimated 2×10^{10} T cells present in normal skin, which is nearly double the T cells found in blood, and practically all carry a memory phenotype [108]. The αβ memory T cells present in skin are restricted from migrating out of the epidermis or dermis and function by responding and recruiting immune functions necessary for the clearance of infection. As research continues and our understanding of the methods by which signaling of skin-resident T cells occurs and the self-antigens that stimulate γδ T cells grows, there will be opportunities to explore methods of producing desired immune responses through therapies or vaccinations in order to prevent skin-related disease and increasing protection against invading pathogens.

14.7.5 Materials

Reagents	Reagents setup
RPMI 1640 with L-glutamine	*Dermis digestion solution* RPMI 1640 with L-glutamine, 300 µg/ml hyaluronidase (3 mg/ml), 100 µg/ml DNase (1 mg/ml), 2.5 mg/ml collagenase XI (25 mg/ml), 10 mM HEPES (1 M)
Hyaluronidase (3 mg/ml)	
DNase (1 mg/ml)	
Collagenase XI (25 mg/ml)	
HEPES (1 M)	

Note: For the details on the other materials and tools that need to be prepared ahead of time, please refer to the chapter of "Isolation of cells in the epidermis: keratinocyte, Langerhans cells, and gamma/delta T cells"

14.7.6 Procedure

14.7.6.1 Preparation of Dermal Single Cell Suspension

For the procedure to get and separate skin epidermis and dermis tissues, please refer to the chapter of "Isolation of cells in the epidermis: keratinocyte, Langerhans cells and gamma/delta T cells." Once dermis tissue is obtained, the whole tissue needs first to be cut into small pieces. Size of the fragments is better if smaller than 1 × 1 mm. All tissue pieces are collected and put into 7 ml "dermis digestion solution" in a 6-cm size petri dish, and incubated at 37 °C in a shaking water bath, with 25 times/min shake, for 2 h. Cell suspension is collected and allowed to pass through a 40 µm nylon mesh strainer. Wash three times by using 5–10 ml 1 × PBS with 1% FBS in a 15 ml tube. Discard the supernatant and resuspend in a 500 µl 1 × PBS with 1% FBS for subsequent procedure.

> **Note**
> The typical yield of total skin dermal cells is approximately of 2×10^6 cells per mouse.

14.7.6.2 Magnetic Cell Sorting of Epidermal T Cells

For epidermal T cells isolation, first refer to the protocol in the chapter of "Isolation of cells in the epidermis: keratinocyte, Langerhans cells and gamma/delta T cells," to get total epidermal single cell suspension. Cells are then stained with PE- or Cy7-conjugated CD3 antibody (10 µl antibody/107 cells) according to the manufacturer's instructions. Mix well and incubate for 10 min in dark at 4 °C. Wash cells by adding 5 ml running buffer and centrifuge at 450 × g for 10 min. Repeat washing one more time. Discard supernatant completely and resuspend cell pellet in 80 µl of running buffer and 20 µl anti-PE microbeads/10^7 cells. Mix thoroughly and incubate for 15 min in dark at 4 °C (agitate every 5 min). Wash cells twice by adding 5 ml running buffer and centrifuge at 450 × g for 5 min. Principally, 500 µl running buffer is required for resuspension of 10^8 cells. Given the size of the cell body, large cell columns are suggested. Place the column in the magnetic field and apply cell suspension onto the column per manufacturer's protocol. Pipette 5 ml of buffer onto the column. Immediately flush out the magnetically labeled cells by firmly pushing the plunger into the column. In collection tube 2, all T cells are included. Cells are adjusted into 1×10^6 cells/100 µl and stained with anti-alpha/beta or anti-gamma/delta antibodies. Then, go to next FACS sorting.

14.7.6.3 FACS Analysis and Sorting of Dermal T Cells

For further enrichment of dermal T cells, FACS sorting is needed. The above prepared dermal total cells are stained with appropriate fluorescence-conjugated T cell specific antibodies. After incubation for 30 min in dark at 4 °C, cells are centrifuged with 450 × g for 5 min at 4 °C. Set up the sorter according to manufacturer's protocol. Label appropriate collection tubes and loading cells onto FACS sorter. Gate and collect specific T cell populations, respectively.

> **Note**
> Given very tiny amounts of total dermal cells and the small percentage of T cell subtype population, to get more T cells for further analysis or subsequent experiment, multiple mice to be sacrificed are suggested.

References

Immunohistochemistry

1. Emoto K, Yamashita S, Okada Y. Mechanisms of heat-induced antigen retrieval: does pH or ionic strength of the solution play a role for refolding antigens? J Histochem Cytochem: Off J Histochem Soc. 2005;53(11):1311–21.
2. Shi SR, Imam SA, Young L, Cote RJ, Taylor CR. Antigen retrieval immunohistochemistry under the influence of pH using

monoclonal antibodies. J Histochem Cytochem: Off J Histochem Soc. 1995;43(2):193–201.
3. Ramos-Vara JA. Technical aspects of immunohistochemistry. Vet Pathol. 2005;42(4):405–26.
4. Williamson JD, Colome MI, Sahin A, Ayala AG, Medeiros LJ. Pagetoid Bowen disease: a report of 2 cases that express cytokeratin 7. Arch Pathol Lab Med. 2000;124(3):427–30.
5. Clarke LE, Conway AB, Warner NM, Barnwell PN. Sceppa J, Helm KF. Expression of CK7, cam 5.2 and ber-Ep4 in cutaneous squamous cell carcinoma. J Cutan Pathol. 2013;40(7):646–50.
6. Sellheyer K, Krahl D. Ber-EP4 enhances the differential diagnostic accuracy of cytokeratin 7 in pagetoid cutaneous neoplasms. J Cutan Pathol. 2008;35(4):366–72.
7. De Nisi MC, D'Amuri A, Toscano M, Lalinga AV, Pirtoli L, Miracco C. Usefulness of CDX2 in the diagnosis of extramammary Paget disease associated with malignancies of intestinal type. Br J Dermatol. 2005;153(3):677–9.
8. Costache M, Bresch M, Boer A. Desmoplastic trichoepithelioma versus morphoeic basal cell carcinoma: a critical reappraisal of histomorphological and immunohistochemical criteria for differentiation. Histopathology. 2008;52(7):865–76.
9. Katona TM, Perkins SM, Billings SD. Does the panel of cytokeratin 20 and androgen receptor antibodies differentiate desmoplastic trichoepithelioma from morpheaform/infiltrative basal cell carcinoma? J Cutan Pathol. 2008;35(2):174–9.
10. Sellheyer K, Nelson P. Follicular stem cell marker PHLDA1 (TDAG51) is superior to cytokeratin-20 in differentiating between trichoepithelioma and basal cell carcinoma in small biopsy specimens. J Cutan Pathol. 2011;38(7):542–50.
11. Jensen K, Wilkinson B, Wines N, Kossard S. Procollagen 1 expression in atypical fibroxanthoma and other tumors. J Cutan Pathol. 2004;31(1):57–61.
12. Leinweber B, Hofmann-Wellenhof R, Kaddu S, McCalmont TH. Procollagen 1 and Melan-A expression in desmoplastic melanomas. Am J Dermatopathol. 2009;31(2):173.
13. Fullen DR, Garrisi AJ, Sanders D, Thomas D. Expression of S100A6 protein in a broad spectrum of cutaneous tumors using tissue microarrays. J Cutan Pathol. 2008;35(Suppl s2):28–34.
14. Wieland CN, Dyck R, Weenig RH, Comfere NI. The role of CD10 in distinguishing atypical fibroxanthoma from sarcomatoid (spindle cell) squamous cell carcinoma. J Cutan Pathol. 2011;38(11):884–8.
15. Longacre TA, Egbert BM, Rouse RV. Desmoplastic and spindle-cell malignant melanoma. an immunohistochemical study. Am J Surg Pathol. 1996;20(12):1489–500.
16. Palla B, Su A, Binder S, Dry S. SOX10 expression distinguishes desmoplastic melanoma from its histologic mimics. Am J Dermatopathol. 2013;35(5):576–81.
17. Folpe AL, Cooper K. Best practices in diagnostic immunohistochemistry: pleomorphic cutaneous spindle cell tumors. Arch Pathol Lab Med. 2007;131(10):1517–24.
18. Dotto JE, Glusac EJ. p63 is a useful marker for cutaneous spindle cell squamous cell carcinoma. J Cutan Pathol. 2006;33(6):413–7.
19. Kanner WA, Brill LB, Patterson JW, Wick MR. CD10, p63 and CD99 expression in the differential diagnosis of atypical fibroxanthoma, spindle cell squamous cell carcinoma and desmoplastic melanoma. J Cutan Pathol. 2010;37(7):744.
20. Sakamoto A, Oda Y, Yamamoto H, et al. Calponin and h-caldesmon expression in atypical fibroxanthoma and superficial leiomyosarcoma. Virchows Arch. 2002;440(4):404–9.
21. Rodig SJ, Cheng J, Wardzala J, et al. Improved detection suggests all Merkel cell carcinomas harbor Merkel polyomavirus. J Clin Invest. 2012;122(12):4645–53.
22. Nicholson SA, McDermott MB, Swanson PE, Wick MR. CD99 and cytokeratin-20 in small-cell and basaloid tumors of the skin. Appl Immunohistochem Mol Morphol. 2000;8(1):37–41.
23. Rossi S, Orvieto E, Furlanetto A, Laurino L, Ninfo V, Dei Tos AP. Utility of the immunohistochemical detection of FLI-1 expression in round cell and vascular neoplasm using a monoclonal antibody. Mod Pathol. 2004;17(5):547–52.
24. Cribier B, Noacco G, Peltre B, Grosshans E. Stromelysin 3 expression: a useful marker for the differential diagnosis dermatofibroma versus dermatofibrosarcoma protuberans. J Am Acad Dermatol. 2002;46(3):408–13.
25. Mori T, Misago N, Yamamoto O, Toda S, Narisawa Y. Expression of nestin in dermatofibrosarcoma protuberans in comparison to dermatofibroma. J Dermatol. 2008;35(7):419–25.
26. Chisholm C, Cockerell CJ. Functions and uses of immunohistochemical stains in cutaneous infiltrates of hematopoietic origin: a review for the practicing dermatologist. J Cutan Med Surg. 2011;15(2):65–83.
27. Pimpinelli N, Olsen EA, Santucci M, et al; International Society for Cutaneous Lymphoma. Defining early mycosis fungoides. J Am Acad Dermatol. 2005;53(6):1053–63.
28. Cho-Vega JH, Medeiros LJ, Prieto VG, Vega F. Leukemia cutis. Am J Clin Pathol. 2008;129(1):130–42.
29. Ostler DA, Prieto VG, Reed JA, Deavers MT, Lazar AJ, Ivan D. Adipophilin expression in sebaceous tumors and other cutaneous lesions with clear cell histology: an immunohistochemical study of 117 cases. Mod Pathol. 2010;23(4):567–73.
30. Mulay K, White VA, Shah SJ, Honavar SG. Sebaceous carcinoma: clinicopathologic features and diagnostic role of immunohistochemistry (including androgen receptor). Can J Ophthalmol. 2014;49(4):326–32.
31. Chhibber V, Dresser K, Mahalingam M. MSH-6: Extending the reliability of immunohistochemistry as a screening tool in muirtorre syndrome. Mod Pathol. 2008;21(2):159–64.
32. Mahalingam M, Nguyen LP, Richards JE, Muzikansky A, Hoang MP. The diagnostic utility of immunohistochemistry in distinguishing primary skin adnexal carcinomas from metastatic adenocarcinoma to skin: an immunohistochemical reappraisal using cytokeratin 15, nestin, p63, D2-40, and calretinin. Mod Pathol. 2010;23(5):713–9.
33. Alcaraz I, Cerroni L, Rütten A, Kutzner H, Requena L. Cutaneous metastases from internal malignancies. Am J Dermatopathol. 2012;34(4):347–93.
34. McKay KM, Doyle LA, Lazar AJ, Hornick JL. Expression of ERG, an Ets family transcription factor, distinguishes cutaneous angiosarcoma from histological mimics. Histopathology. 2012;61(5):989–91.
35. Le Huu AR, Jokinen CH, Rubin BP, Mihm MC, Weiss SW, North PE, Dadras SS. Expression of prox1, lymphatic endothelial nuclear transcription factor, in Kaposiform hemangioendothelioma and tufted angioma. Am J Surg Pathol. 2010;34(11): 1563–73.
36. Trindade F, Tellechea Ó, Torrelo A, Requena L, Colmenero I. Wilms tumor 1 expression in vascular neoplasms and vascular malformations. Am J Dermatopathol. 2011;33(6):569–72.
37. Fernandez AP, Sun Y, Tubbs RR, Goldblum JR, Billings SD. FISH for MYC amplification and anti-MYC immunohistochemistry: useful diagnostic tools in the assessment of secondary angiosarcoma and atypical vascular proliferations. J Cutan Pathol. 2012;39(2):234–42.
38. Kamino H, Tam ST. Immunoperoxidase technique modified by counterstain with azure B as a diagnostic aid in evaluating heavily pigmented melanocytic neoplasms. J Cutan Pathol. 1991;18(6):436–9.
39. Beltraminelli H, Shabrawi-Caelen LE, Kerl H, Cerroni L. Melan-a-positive "pseudomelanocytic nests": A pitfall in the histopathologic and immunohistochemical diagnosis of pigmented lesions on sun-damaged skin. Am J Dermatopathol. 2009;31(3):305–8.

40. Ramos-Herberth FI, Karamchandani J, Kim J, Dadras SS. SOX10 immunostaining distinguishes desmoplastic melanoma from excision scar. J Cutan Pathol. 2010;37(9):944–52.
41. Vollmer RT. Use of bayes rule and MIB-1 proliferation index to discriminate spitz nevus from malignant melanoma. Am J Clin Pathol. 2004;122(4):499–505.
42. George E, Polissar NL, Wick M. Immunohistochemical evaluation of p16INK4A, E-cadherin, and cyclin D1 expression in melanoma and spitz tumors. Am J Clin Pathol. 2010;133(3): 370–9.
43. Ribe A, McNutt NS. S100A6 protein expression is different in spitz nevi and melanomas. Mod Pathol. 2003;16(5):505–11.
44. Ordóñez NG. Value of SOX10 immunostaining in tumor diagnosis. Adv Anat Pathol. 2013;20(4):275–83.
45. Rose AE, Christos PJ, Lackaye D, et al. Clinical relevance of detection of lymphovascular invasion in primary melanoma using endothelial markers D2-40 and CD34. Am J Surg Pathol. 2011;35(10):1441–9.
46. Tetzlaff MT, Curry JL, Ivan D, et al. Immunodetection of phosphohistone H3 as a surrogate of mitotic figure count and clinical outcome in cutaneous melanoma. Mod Pathol. 2013;26(9): 1153–60.
47. Long GV, Wilmott JS, Capper D, et al. Immunohistochemistry is highly sensitive and specific for the detection of V600E BRAF mutation in melanoma. Am J Surg Pathol. 2013;37(1):61–5.

Techniques for Acquisition and Manipulation of Skin Cells

48. Poumay Y, Boucher F, Degen A, et al. Inhibition of basal cell proliferation during storage of detached cultured epidermis keratinocyte sheet. Acta Derm Venereol. 1991;71(3):195–8.
49. Zheng-hong D, Xiao-dong S, Wang Y-k, et al. Serum-free primary culture of human skin keratinocyte. J China Med Univ. 2010;39(12):1037–40.
50. Coolen NA, Verkerk M, Reijnen L, et al. Culture of keratinocytes for transplantation without the need of feeder layer cells. Cell Transplant. 2007;16(6):649–61.
51. Barlow Y, Pye RJ. Keratinocyte culture: Basic cell culture protocols. Methods Mol Biol. 1997;75:117–29.
52. Micallef L, Belaubre F, Pinon A, et al. Effects of extracellular calcium on the growth-differentiation switch in immortalized keratinocyte HaCaT cells compared with normal hunman keratinocytes. Exp Dermatol. 2009;18(2):143–51.

Isolation of Epidermal Cells

53. Xu YP, et al. Aging affects epidermal Langerhans cell development and function and alters their miRNA gene expression profile. Aging (Albany NY). 2012;4(11):742–54.
54. James W, Berger T, Elston D. Andrews' diseases of the skin: clinical dermatology. 10th ed, vol. 8. Saunders, UK; 2005. p. e74019.
55. Schuler G, et al. Murine epidermal Langerhans cells as a model to study tissue dendritic cells. Adv Exp Med Biol. 1993;329: 243–9.
56. Merad M, et al. Langerhans cells renew in the skin throughout life under steady-state conditions. Nat Immunol. 2002;3(12): 1135–41.
57. Kaplan DH, Kissenpfennig A, Clausen BE. Insights into Langerhans cell function from Langerhans cell ablation models. Eur J Immunol. 2008;38(9):2369–76.
58. Chorro L, Geissmann F. Development and homeostasis of 'resident' myeloid cells: the case of the Langerhans cell. Trends Immunol. 2010;31(12):438–45.
59. Gatzka M, et al. Reduction of CD18 promotes expansion of inflammatory gammadelta T cells collaborating with CD4+ T cells in chronic murine psoriasiform dermatitis. J Immunol. 2013;191(11):5477–88.
60. Ishida M, et al. Primary cutaneous B-cell lymphoma with abundant reactive gamma/delta T-cells within the skin lesion and peripheral blood. Int J Clin Exp Pathol. 2014;7(3):1193–9.
61. Nakamura K, et al. Differential requirement for CCR4 in the maintenance but not establishment of the invariant Vgamma5(+) dendritic epidermal T-cell pool. PLoS One. 2013;8(9):e74019.
62. Valladeau J, et al. Langerin, a novel C-type lectin specific to Langerhans cells, is an endocytic receptor that induces the formation of Birbeck granules. Immunity. 2000;12(1):71–81.
63. Stoitzner P, et al. Migratory Langerhans cells in mouse lymph nodes in steady state and inflammation. J Invest Dermatol. 2005;125(1):116–25.
64. Qi R, et al. Histone deacetylase activity is required for skin Langerhans cell maturation and phagocytosis. J Dermatol Sci. 2012;65(2):152–5.
65. Zaba LC, et al. Normal human dermis contains distinct populations of CD11c+BDCA-1+ dendritic cells and CD163+FXIIIA+ macrophages. J Clin Invest. 2007;117(9):2517–25.
66. Ebner S, et al. Expression of C-type lectin receptors by subsets of dendritic cells in human skin. Int Immunol. 2004;16(6):877–87.

Techniques for Acquisition and Manipulation of Melanocytes

67. James WD, Berger TG, Elston DM, Odom RB. Andrews' diseases of the skin: clinical dermatology. Philadelphia: Saunders Elsevier; 2006. p. 961.
68. Marks JG, Miller JJ, Lookingbill DP, Lookingbill DP. Lookingbill and Marks' principles of dermatology. Philadelphia: Saunders Elsevier; 2006. p. 331.
69. Kalesnikoff J, Galli SJ. New developments in mast cell biology. Nat Immunol. 2008;9:1215–23.
70. Stoitzner P, Holzmann S, McLellan AD, Ivarsson L, Stossel H, et al. Visualization and characterization of migratory Langerhans cells in murine skin and lymph nodes by antibodies against Langerin/CD207. J Invest Dermatol. 2003;120:266–74.
71. Steinman RM, Nussenzweig MC. Avoiding horror autotoxicus: the importance of dendritic cells in peripheral T cell tolerance. Proc Natl Acad Sci U S A. 2002;99:351–8.
72. Larregina AT, Falo Jr LD. Changing paradigms in cutaneous immunology: adapting with dendritic cells. J Invest Dermatol. 2005;124:1–12.
73. Wang L, Bursch LS, Kissenpfennig A, Malissen B, Jameson SC, et al. Langerin expressing cells promote skin immune responses under defined conditions. J Immunol. 2008;180:4722–7.
74. Douillard P, Stoitzner P, Tripp CH, Clair-Moninot V, Ait-Yahia S, et al. Mouse lymphoid tissue contains distinct subsets of langerin/CD207 dendritic cells, only one of which represents epidermal-derived Langerhans cells. J Invest Dermatol. 2005;125:983–94.
75. Bursch LS, Wang L, Igyarto B, Kissenpfennig A, Malissen B, et al. Identification of a novel population of Langerin+dendritic cells. J Exp Med. 2007;204:3147–56.
76. Poulin LF, Henri S, de Bovis B, Devilard E, Kissenpfennig A, et al. The dermis contains langerin+dendritic cells that develop

and function independently of epidermal Langerhans cells. J Exp Med. 2007;204:3119–31.
77. Ginhoux F, Collin MP, Bogunovic M, Abel M, Leboeuf M, et al. Blood-derived dermal langerin+dendritic cells survey the skin in the steady state. J Exp Med. 2007;204:3133–46.
78. Nagao K, Ginhoux F, Leitner WW, Motegi S, Bennett CL, et al. Murine epidermal Langerhans cells and langerin-expressing dermal dendritic cells are unrelated and exhibit distinct functions. Proc Natl Acad Sci U S A. 2009;106:3312–7.
79. Igyarto BZ, Haley K, Ortner D, Bobr A, Gerami-Nejad M, et al. Skin-resident murine dendritic cell subsets promote distinct and opposing antigen-specific T helper cell responses. Immunity. 2011;35:260–72.
80. Kaplan DH, Igyarto BZ, Gaspari AA. Early immune events in the induction of allergic contact dermatitis. Nat Rev Immunol. 2012;12:114–24.

Techniques for Acquisition and Manipulation of Melanocytes

81. Na GY, et al. Isolation and characterization of outer root sheath melanocytes of human hair follicles. Br J Dermatol. 2006;155(5):902–9.
82. Abdel-Malek ZA, et al. Proliferation and propagation of human melanocytes in vitro are affected by donor age and anatomical site. Pigment Cell Res. 1994;7(2):116–22.
83. Quevedo WC, Szabo G, Virks J. Influence of age and UV on the populations of dopa-positive melanocytes in human skin. J Invest Dermatol. 1969;52(3):287–90.
84. Eisinger M, Marko O. Selective proliferation of normal human melanocytes in vitro in the presence of phorbol ester and cholera toxin. Proc Natl Acad Sci U S A. 1982;79(6):2018–22.
85. Halaban R. The regulation of normal melanocyte proliferation. Pigment Cell Res. 2000;13(1):4–14.
86. Laidlaw GF. Melanoma studies: I. The dopa reaction in general pathology. Am J Pathol. 1932;8(5):477–90. 9.
87. Xiang LH, et al. The identification of biological characteristics of cultured melanocytes in vitro. J Clin Dermatol. 2001;30(3):166–7.
88. Nordlund JJ, et al. The Pigmentary system: physiology and pathophysiology. 2nd ed. Blackwell Publishing; 2006. p. 67, 446.

Techniques for Acquisition and Manipulation of Fibroblasts

89. Nowak JA, Fuchs E. Isolation and culture of epithelial stem cells. Methods Mol Biol. 2009;482:215–32.
90. Wu G, Zhou Y, Wensong T, et al. Growth and matabolism of human dermal fibroblasts in two-dimensional and three-dimenstional culture systems. J Clin Rehabil Tissue Eng Res. 2007;11(1):74–7.
91. Liu A, Jin J. Enhanced isolation and culture and authenticate of human fibroblasts. Guangdong Med J. 2008;12(29):1969–70.
92. De Falco E, Scafetta G, Napoletano C, et al. A standardized laboratory and surgical method for in vitro culture isolation and expansion of primary human Tenon's fibroblasts. Cell Tissue Bank. 2013;14(2):277–87.
93. Zhiru G, Kyle D, Stephen L. Isolation and culture of adult epithelial stem cells from human skin. J Vis Exp. 2011;31(49):pii: 2561. doi:10.3791/2561.
94. Huschtscha LO, Napier CE, Noble JR, et al. Enhanced isolation of fibroblasts from human skin explants. Biotechniques. 2012;53(4): 239–44.

Isolation and Manipulation of Resident T Cells in Skin

95. Heath WR, Carbone FR. The skin-resident and migratory immune system in steady state and memory: innate lymphocytes, dendritic cells and T cells. Nat Immunol. 2013;14(10):978–85. doi:10.1038/ni.2680.
96. Gebhardt T, Wakim LM, Eidsmo L, Reading PC, Heath WR, Carbone FR. Memory T cells in nonlymphoid tissue that provide enhanced local immunity during infection with herpes simplex virus. Nat Immunol. 2009;10(5):524–30. doi:10.1038/ni.1718.
97. Gatzka M, Hainzl A, Peters T, Singh K, Tasdogan A, Wlaschek M, Scharffetter-Kochanek K. Reduction of CD18 promotes expansion of inflammatory gammadelta T cells collaborating with CD4+ T cells in chronic murine psoriasiform dermatitis. J Immunol. 2013;191(11):5477–88. doi:10.4049/jimmunol.1300976.
98. Ishida M, Iwai M, Yoshida K, Kagotani A, Okabe H. Primary cutaneous B-cell lymphoma with abundant reactive gamma/delta T-cells within the skin lesion and peripheral blood. Int J Clin Exp Pathol. 2014;7(3):1193–9.
99. Nakamura K, White AJ, Parnell SM, Lane PJ, Jenkinson EJ, Jenkinson WE, Anderson G. Differential requirement for CCR4 in the maintenance but not establishment of the invariant Vgamma5(+) dendritic epidermal T-cell pool. PLoS One. 2013;8(9):e74019. doi:10.1371/journal.pone.0074019.
100. Jiang X, Clark RA, Liu L, Wagers AJ, Fuhlbrigge RC, Kupper TS. Skin infection generates non-migratory memory CD8+ T(RM) cells providing global skin immunity. Nature. 2012;483(7388):227–31. doi:10.1038/nature10851.
101. Macleod AS, Havran WL. Functions of skin-resident gammadelta T cells. Cell Mol Life Sci: CMLS. 2011;68(14):2399–408. doi:10.1007/s00018-011-0702-x.
102. Chodaczek G, Papanna V, Zal MA, Zal T. Body-barrier surveillance by epidermal gammadelta TCRs. Nat Immunol. 2012;13(3):272–82. doi:10.1038/ni.2240.
103. Havran WL, Jameson JM. Epidermal T cells and wound healing. J Immunol. 2010;184(10):5423–8. doi:10.4049/jimmunol.0902733.
104. Toulon A, Breton L, Taylor KR, Tenenhaus M, Bhavsar D, Lanigan C, Rudolph R, Jameson J, Havran WL. A role for human skin-resident T cells in wound healing. J Exp Med. 2009,206(4).743–50. doi:10.1084/jem.20081787.
105. Havran WL, Chien YH, Allison JP. Recognition of self antigens by skin-derived T cells with invariant gamma delta antigen receptors. Science. 1991;252(5011):1430–2.
106. Girardi M, Oppenheim DE, Steele CR, Lewis JM, Glusac E, Filler R, Hobby P, Sutton B, Tigelaar RE, Hayday AC. Regulation of cutaneous malignancy by gammadelta T cells. Science. 2001;294(5542):605–9. doi:10.1126/science.1063916.
107. Bromley SK, Yan S, Tomura M, Kanagawa O, Luster AD. Recirculating memory T cells are a unique subset of CD4+ T cells with a distinct phenotype and migratory pattern. J Immunol. 2013;190(3):970–6. doi:10.4049/jimmunol.1202805.
108. Clark RA, Chong B, Mirchandani N, Brinster NK, Yamanaka K, Dowgiert RK, Kupper TS. The vast majority of CLA+ T cells are resident in normal skin. J Immunol. 2006;176(7):4431–9.
109. Boyman O, Hefti HP, Conrad C, Nickoloff BJ, Suter M, Nestle FO. Spontaneous development of psoriasis in a new animal model shows an essential role for resident T cells and tumor necrosis factor-alpha. J Exp Med. 2004;199(5):731–6. doi:10.1084/jem.20031482.
110. Clark RA, Watanabe R, Teague JE, Schlapbach C, Tawa MC, Adams N, Dorosario AA, Chaney KS, Cutler CS, Leboeuf NR, Carter JB, Fisher DC, Kupper TS. Skin effector memory T cells do

not recirculate and provide immune protection in alemtuzumab-treated CTCL patients. Sci Transl Med. 2012;4(117):117ra117. doi:10.1126/scitranslmed.3003008.

111. Gebhardt T, Whitney PG, Zaid A, Mackay LK, Brooks AG, Heath WR, Carbone FR, Mueller SN. Different patterns of peripheral migration by memory CD4+ and CD8+ T cells. Nature. 2011;477(7363):216–9. doi:10.1038/nature10339.
112. Zhu J, Peng T, Johnston C, Phasouk K, Kask AS, Klock A, Jin L, Diem K, Koelle DM, Wald A, Robins H, Corey L. Immune surveillance by CD8alphaalpha+skin-resident T cells in human herpes virus infection. Nature. 2013;497(7450):494–7. doi:10.1038/nature12110.
113. Schenkel JM, Fraser KA, Vezys V, Masopust D. Sensing and alarm function of resident memory CD8(+) T cells. Nat Immunol. 2013;14(5):509–13. doi:10.1038/ni.2568.
114. Seneschal J, Clark RA, Gehad A, Baecher-Allan CM, Kupper TS. Human epidermal Langerhans cells maintain immune homeostasis in skin by activating skin resident regulatory T cells. Immunity. 2012;36(5):873–84. doi:10.1016/j.immuni.2012.03.018.
115. Sumaria N, Roediger B, Ng LG, Qin J, Pinto R, Cavanagh LL, Shklovskaya E, Fazekas de St Groth B, Triccas JA, Weninger W. Cutaneous immunosurveillance by self-renewing dermal gammadelta T cells. J Exp Med. 2011;208(3):505–18. doi:10.1084/jem.20101824.
116. Cai Y, Shen X, Ding C, Qi C, Li K, Li X, Jala VR, Zhang HG, Wang T, Zheng J, Yan J. Pivotal role of dermal IL-17-producing gammadelta T cells in skin inflammation. Immunity. 2011;35(4):596–610. doi:10.1016/j.immuni.2011.08.001.
117. Hayday AC. Gammadelta T cells and the lymphoid stress-surveillance response. Immunity. 2009;31(2):184–96. doi:10.1016/j.immuni.2009.08.006.

Immunotherapy

15

Sebastian Volc, Kamran Ghoreschi, and Hui Shen

Contents

S. Volc • K. Ghoreschi (✉)
Department of Dermatology, University Medical Center, Eberhard Karls University Tübingen, Liebermeisterstr. 25, 72076 Tübingen, Germany
e-mail: kamran.ghoreschi@med.uni-tuebingen.de

H. Shen (✉)
Department of Rheumatology, No.1 Hospital of China Medical University, Shenyang, China
e-mail: shenhuicam@sohu.com

15.1 Immunobiologics for Psoriasis

Sebastian Volc and Kamran Ghoreschi

15.1.1 Introduction

Psoriasis is a chronic inflammatory disease of the skin and joints, mediated by the immune system with an underlying polygenic predisposition. The disease affects 0.5–1 % of children and 2–3 % of adults and is associated with environmental triggers. Although psoriasis is considered as a T cell-mediated autoimmune disease, no autoantigen has yet been identified.

Psoriasis pathogenesis is characterized by infiltrating immune cells and their interaction with keratinocytes and endothelial cells [1, 2]. Historically, psoriasis was thought to be an epidermal disorder with a shortened epidermal turnover due to increased keratinocyte proliferation. Recent experimental data also reported that alterations in keratinocyte signaling pathways like epidermal deletion of JunB/c-Jun, deficiency in IκBα, or over-expression of constitutively active STAT3 in keratinocytes induce psoriasis-like skin inflammation in mice. However, there is overwhelming data favoring certain T cell subsets as central players in psoriasis pathogenesis.

The concept of psoriasis as a T cell-mediated disease was initially created based on observations with patients undergoing bone marrow transplantation for hematological malignancies. While in some patients psoriasis developed de novo after receiving bone marrow from psoriasis-positive donors, in others preexisting psoriasis disappeared after bone marrow transplantation from psoriasis-negative donors [3, 4]. Further, T cell depletion by monoclonal anti-CD4 antibodies or an IL-2 fusion toxin (DAB_{389}IL-2) have been reported to clear psoriasis in humans. The role of T cells in psoriasis was further confirmed by clinical responses to therapies affecting T cells such as alefacept and efalizumab.

X.-H. Gao, H.-D. Chen (eds.), *Practical Immunodermatology*, DOI 10.1007/978-94-024-0902-4_15

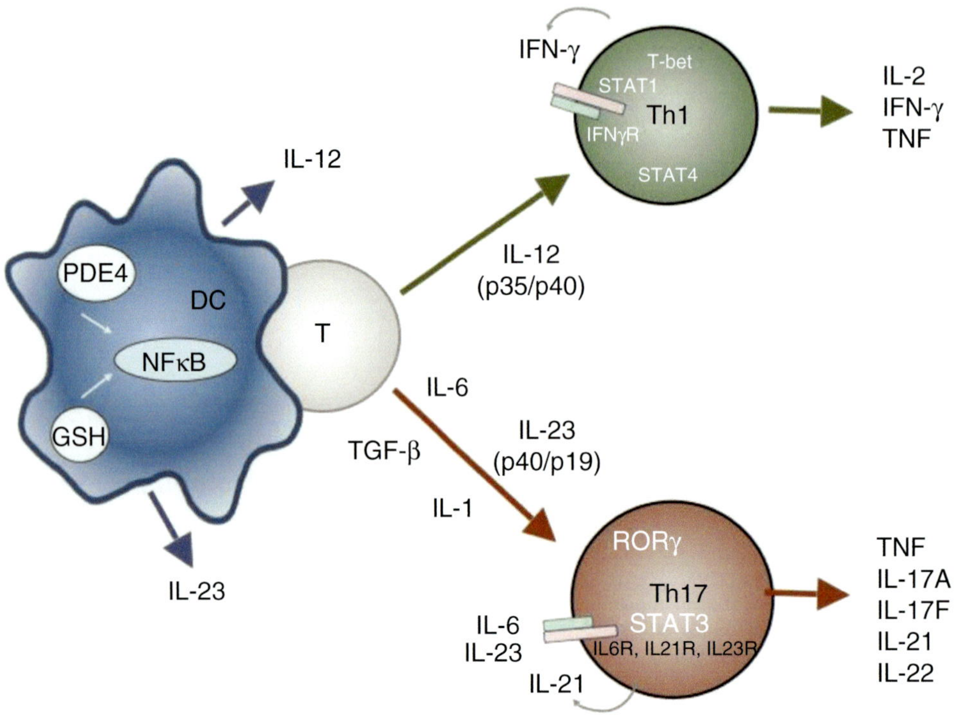

Fig. 15.1 Phenotype of DC and T cells in psoriasis pathogenesis Innate immune signals secreted from keratinocytes and innate immune cells activate dendritic cells (DC) like dermal DC to mature and to produce cytokines like IL-12 and IL-23. The activated DC interact with naïve T cells within the skin and skin-draining lymph nodes. Upon activation naïve T cells differentiate into Th1 and Th17 cells. While Th1 differentiation depends on IL-12, Th17 differentiation requires multiple signals including IL-6, IL-1, TGF-β and IL-23. Th1 and Th17 cell subsets produce the cytokines driving psoriatic inflammation (e.g. TNF, IL-17A, IL-22). The most relevant cytokines in psoriasis pathogenesis are TNF, IL-17A and IL-23. This immune response is regulated by the interaction of intracellular proteins (glutathione, GSH; phosphodiesterase 4, PDE4) and transcription factors (NFkappaB, STAT1, STAT3, RORgamma, T-bet) (Adapted from Belge et al. [21])

15.1.2 Role of T Helper Cells in Psoriasis Pathogenesis

Today, a number of cells and mediators that are relevant in psoriasis are described. Most likely, early psoriasis of the skin is initiated by the release of innate immune signals secreted from either stressed keratinocytes or skin-resident dendritic cells (DC) [2]. The mediators expressed in early psoriatic skin lesions include interleukin (IL-)1 family members, interferons (IFNs), IL-6 and tumor necrosis factor (TNF). The production of IFN-α by plasmacytoid DC together with other stimuli activate myeloid DCs in the skin to produce IL-12 and IL-23.

Subsequently, these DCs activate T cells like CD4$^+$ T helper (Th) cells and CD8$^+$ T cells and promote their proliferation and differentiation. Several reports demonstrated the clonal expansion of T cells in psoriatic skin lesions. Psoriasis pathogenesis is dominated by IL-17A-producing Th17 cells that also produce IL-17F, IL-21, IL-22, and TNF. Further, IFN-γ-producing Th1 cells that also express IL-2 and TNF are found in psoriatic skin. The cytokines involved in Th17 cell differentiation are IL-6, IL-1, TGF-β, and IL-23 [5]. In contrast, Th1 cell differentiation depends on IL-12 (Fig. 15.1). Both Th cell subsets interact with immune cells, keratinocytes, and endothelial cells and amplify the inflammatory cascade. Especially Th17 cell cytokines are involved in the proliferation of keratinocytes, the release of antimicrobial peptides, and the recruitment of neutrophils. The interaction between inflammatory immune cells, keratinocytes, endothelial cells, and fibroblasts causes psoriatic tissue reorganization characterized by the hyperproliferation of keratinocytes and endothelial cells [6].

A number of genetic susceptibilities has been described to be associated with the risk for psoriasis. Despite certain human leukocyte antigens (HLAs) like HLA-Cw6 and the classical psoriasis susceptibility loci like *PSORS1*, some other genetic alterations have been described to be linked to psoriasis. In some cohorts of patients with psoriasis, mutations within the *CARD14* gene or the *IL36RN* gene have been found [7]. Genome-wide studies also revealed single nucleotide polymorphisms in gene loci associated with the immune response including *IL23A*, *IL23R*, *IL4*, *RUNX3*, *REL*, *STAT3*, and *TYK2* [8].

15.1.3 A Model Disease for Th17-Mediated Inflammation

The fact that psoriasis heals without scar formation, together with the accessibility of skin biopsies and the amount of data

Table 15.1 Classical oral immunotherapies and modern small molecules

Immunotherapies	Legal status for psoriasis	Mode of action
Cyclosporine A	Approved in 1993	Inhibits T cell activation and cytokine secretion
DMF	Phase 3 (Tecfidera®, approved for MS in 2013)	GSH conjugation, Nrf2 activation, inhibition of IL-12 and IL-23, induction of IL-10 and Th2
FAE (Fumaderm®)	Approved in 1995 (only in Germany)	GSH conjugation, changes in DC cytokine production, Th2 induction
Methotrexate	Approved in 1972	Folic acid antagonist; inhibits T cell activation
JAKi (Tofacitinib – Xeljanz®)	Phase 3 (Xeljanz® approved in 2012 for RA in selected countries)	JAK inhibitor silencing cytokine receptor signaling, inhibiting Th1 and Th17 responses
PDE4i (Apremilast – Otezla®)	Approved in 2014	PDE4 inhibitor, increase of cAMP, inhibition of IL-12, IL-23, TNF, and IFN-γ, induction of IL-10
Retinoids (Acitretin)	Approved in 1992	Vitamin A analogs inhibiting epidermal proliferation and differentiation

The table includes compounds that are at least in phase 3 in international studies

available on psoriasis pathogenesis, makes this human disease an interesting model when studying mechanisms of chronic inflammation. It is also an increasingly frequent target for proof-of-principle studies dedicated to new therapies with antibodies, cytokines, and small molecules.

For a long period of time, inflammatory organ-specific autoimmune diseases were thought to be mediated by Th1 cells. A major shift in the Th1/Th2 dogma occurred in the beginning of this millennium, when IL-23 and Th17 cells were found to dominate the pathology in organ-specific autoimmune disease models [9]. IL-23 and Th17 immune responses were found to be pathogenic in experimental autoimmune encephalomyelitis in mice, a well established model of multiple sclerosis. These findings suggested that Th17 cells might be the pathogenic drivers in some T cell dependent autoimmune diseases including psoriasis [1, 2, 10]. Finally, data from recent clinical trials using antibodies targeting IL-23, IL-17, or the IL-17 receptor illustrated the functional importance of IL 23 and Th17 cell pathology in psoriasis [11–14].

Moderate to severe psoriasis is treated with systemic therapies, such as methotrexate, cyclosporine, or retinoids. Since 2000, modern systemic therapies such as biologics and immunotherapies with small molecules have been tested and approved. These targeted therapies have not only improved the skin condition of patients and their quality of life, but have also offered new key insights into the immunopathogenesis of psoriasis. Patients with psoriasis also suffer for a number of comorbidities, which may also be affected by therapeutic dampening of systemic inflammation. In the following, we will summarize the different categories of systemic antipsoriatics.

15.1.4 Immunotherapies with Oral Compounds

In psoriasis, traditional immunosuppressive compounds like methotrexate (MTX) and cyclosporine (CSA) are used for quite some time (Table 15.1). Acitretin is a second-generation, mono-aromatic retinoid and also used in psoriasis, especially in combination with phototherapy. The antiproliferative properties of retinoids are beneficial in patients with palmoplantar psoriasis. Fumaric acid esters (FAE) containing dimethyl fumarate (DMF) as main component are used for the treatment of psoriasis of the skin as approved in Germany. They inhibit proinflammatory cytokine production in DC (inhibition of IL-12 and IL-23), impair the development of Th1 and Th17 responses, and instead induce Th2 cells. In the meanwhile, DMF as single therapeutic agent has been approved for multiple sclerosis and is also under clinical investigation for psoriasis (Table 15.1).

More recently, novel anti-inflammatory oral compounds have been studied in phase 3 trials for psoriasis including a Janus kinase (JAK) inhibitor and a phosphodiesterase 4 (PDE4) inhibitor (Table 15.1). JAKs consist of a group of intracellular tyrosine kinases that are involved in the transmission of signals from cytokine receptors on the cellular membrane to the nucleus [15]. Upon activation, JAKs associate with the receptor and activate signal transducers and activators of transcription (STATs) proteins, a group of transcription factors that regulate gene expression. Several JAK inhibitors are under clinical investigation for the treatment of psoriasis and psoriatic arthritis. The clinically most advanced JAK inhibitor for psoriasis is tofacitinib and currently in phase 3 as oral compound [16]. Some other oral inhibitors with slightly distinct selectivities for the group of JAKs are currently under clinical investigation for psoriasis. JAK inhibitors like tofacitinib and ruxolitinib are also tested as topical formulations for psoriasis of the skin.

A different way to regulate inflammation is by blocking PDE4, which results in increased intracellular cAMP levels, affects PKA, CREB, and the activity of other transcription factors like NFκB. The first PDE4 inhibitor approved for the treatment of chronic plaque psoriasis and psoriatic arthritis is apremilast (FDA 2014, EMA 2014) [17].

15.1.5 Immunotherapies with Biologics

15.1.5.1 Terminology of Antipsoriatic Biologics

Antipsoriatic biologics can be divided into antibodies and fusion proteins. In order to provide some clarity in the terminology of antipsoriatic biologics, we first explain the wording of biologics used in this chapter. The suffix *-mab* stands for monoclonal antibody, while the suffix *-cept* represents fusion proteins. The *-mab* suffix is preceded by the letters *-xi-* in case of chimeric antibodies, by *-zu-* in case of humanized antibodies, or by *-u-* in case of fully human antibodies. In addition, antibodies targeting interleukins contain *-k(i)-* or *-ki(n)-* and immunomodulatory antibodies contain *-l(i)-* or *-li(m)-*. The attachment of polyethylene glycol is marked by *-pegol*. This modification is done to slow down enzyme-related degradation and to decrease the antibody's immunogenicity. To give one example, the name of the TNF antagonist ada-*lim-u-mab* points out that this is an immune system-targeting (*−lim-*) human (*−u-*) monoclonal antibody (*−mab*).

15.1.5.2 Antipsoriatic Biologics Targeting Cell Surface Receptors

The first developed antipsoriatic biologics with action on the immune system targeted cell surface receptors. One of the first targets in treating psoriasis and also rheumatoid arthritis with biologics was CD4. The rationale of this therapy was to deplete disease-inducing Th cells. In early 1990s, a few patients were treated with anti-CD4 antibodies and showed moderate to good efficacy. However, the strategy of CD4 depletion was not further pursued and anti-CD4 antibodies have not been approved for psoriasis.

In contrast, antipsoriatic biologics interfering with T cell activation and migration have been used in the clinics. Among the first biologics approved for psoriasis was efalizumab, a humanized antibody directed against CD11a (subunit of human leukocyte function antigen (LFA-)1) [18]. This antibody prevents the binding of LFA-1 to ICAM-1 and thereby the adhesion of leukocytes like T cells to other cell types including endothelial cells. Thus, efalizumab inhibits the transmigration of activated lymphocytes into the tissue like the skin. Although efalizumab was an effective therapy, this biologic had to be withdrawn from the market in 2009 due to fatal cases of progressive multifocal leukoencephalopathy (PML) associated with John Cunningham (JC)-virus (three confirmed PML cases reported).

Alefacept is a fusion protein of extracellular CD2-binding portion of LFA-3 and Fc-IgG1 [19]. It blocks the interaction between CD2 on activated T cells and LFA-3 on antigen presenting cells. Alefacept inhibits the activation of T cells and induces apoptosis in memory T cells. It was approved by the FDA in 2001, but was withdrawn from the US market in 2011 due to supply disruption according to the manufacturer.

A novel biologic targeting a T cell surface marker is itolizumab. This humanized monoclonal antibody is directed against CD6, a T cell marker involved in lymphocyte stimulation. Efficacy and safety of itolizumab has been shown in a phase 3 trial for psoriasis and a first approval has been filed in India in 2013 [20]. These three antibodies are listed in Table 15.2.

15.1.5.3 Antipsoriatic Biologics Targeting Cytokines or Their Receptors

An increasing number of antibodies and fusion proteins has been established to treat psoriasis and psoriatic arthritis by targeting cytokines rather than blocking immune cells through surface receptors. A group of TNF antagonists is widely established in the treatment of psoriasis. TNF is a critical cytokine in psoriasis pathogenesis and secreted by many cells including Th17 cells, Th1 cells, mast cells, DC, and also nonimmune cells. Blocking TNF with a fusion protein (etanercept) or with monoclonal antibodies (adalimumab, infliximab, golimumab, certolizumab pegol) has revolutionized the therapy of psoriasis and psoriatic arthritis (summarized in [21]). The use of TNF antagonists can be combined with methotrexate and shows excellent response rates for psoriasis of the skin and joints.

More recently, antibodies have been developed that interfere directly with the Th17 response by either neutralizing IL-23 or IL-17. IL-23 is the key cytokine in the generation of pathogenic Th17 cells [5], while IL-17 is secreted by Th17 cells. The first biologic directly interfering with the Th17 pathway, ustekinumab, is already in use for treating psoriasis and psoriatic arthritis [11]. Ustekinumab binds the p40 subunit shared by IL-23 and IL-12. Thus, this antibody neutralizes two cytokine pathways, which are involved in the activation of Th17 cells (via IL-23) and Th1 cells (via IL-12). The simultaneous

Table 15.2 Immunobiologics targeting cell surface receptors

Biologics	Trade name	Legal status	Target	Mode of action
Alefacept	Amevive®	Approved in 2001 (FDA only); discontinued 2011	CD2	Fusion protein of extracellular CD2-binding portion of LFA-3 and Fc-IgG1; inhibition of T cell activation
Efalizumab	Raptiva®	Approved in 2002; discontinued 2009	CD11a	Humanized antibody binding to CD11a subunit of LFA1; inhibition of leukocyte migration
Itolizumab	Alzumab®	Approved in India 2013	CD6	Humanized antibody against CD6, impairs T cell activation

blockade of IL-23 and IL-12 may be responsible for the excellent efficacy of ustekinumab in psoriasis. However, the selected neutralization of IL-23 may also be effective and safe in psoriasis. Therefore, two novel antibodies (guselkumab and tildrakizumab) selectively targeting the p19 unit, which is part of IL-23 but not IL-12, are in phase 3 development [22].

Instead of interfering with IL-23 one can directly block IL-17A, the lineage-defining cytokine of Th17 cells or its receptor (IL-17RA). Two monoclonal antibodies, secukinumab and ixekizumab, directed against IL-17A and one monoclonal antibody, brodalumab, directed against IL-17RA are now tested for efficacy and safety in psoriasis [14, 23, 24]. In the treatment of psoriasis, this new generation of biologics has demonstrated excellent efficacy in first trials as published. Table 15.3 provides an overview of these cytokine-targeting antibodies.

Our patients with psoriasis benefit tremendously from the efficacy of modern oral drugs and biologics. Yet, there are still certain hurdles including safety issues and the high therapy costs. We expect that in the future the drug spectrum for treating psoriasis with immunobiologics will be extended. There are further antipsoriatic biologics in development that target cytokines other than TNF, IL-23, or IL-17, but also small molecules and biosimilars, the generic-equivalents for immunobiologics. We have learned a lot about the pathogenesis of psoriasis by using targeted therapies. These immunobiologics will also help us to better understand the pathogenesis of other inflammatory (auto)immune diseases of the skin and internal organs. Similarities and differences in the relevance of cytokine neutralization are already visible when treating patients with distinct autoimmune diseases such as psoriasis, rheumatoid arthritis, Crohn's disease, or multiple sclerosis. Moreover, immunobiologics open a new chance in the treatment of patients with metastasized melanoma. Thus, immunobiologics have gained an exceptionally important status in dermatology.

15.2 Immunobiologics for Lupus

Hui Shen

Systemic lupus erythematosus (SLE) is a chronic autoimmune disease affecting multiple organs and systems. Lupus nephritis (LN) is a severe complication of SLE, leading to proteinuria and finally chronic renal failure. Traditional treatments for SLE include antimalarial drugs, glucocorticoids, and immunosuppressive and cytotoxic agents (such as cyclophosphamide, mycophenolate mofetil, cyclosporine, and azathioprine). Corticosteroids and immunosuppressive agents are effective in SLE therapy, especially for LN, but these drugs have considerable side effects and low complete remission rate. Thus we need new drugs or to discover specific biologics that can offer better therapeutic benefits and lower side effects with a selective target.

During the past 50 years, significant progresses have been made in understanding the immunopathogenesis of SLE. Several important biologics have been discovered and used in the treatment of SLE, especially LN. However, the clinical trials of these novel therapies to date in general have not been proved successful. Trial failures can be attributed to multiple reasons, including the inappropriate study end points and the limitations of studies design in which only specific populations were involved.

Despite the negative results from the clinical trials, the US Food and Drug Administration (FDA) had approved biological (belimumab) for SLE therapy in over 50 years. This chapter will focus on biologics for lupus, especially the only one FDA approved biological (belimumab), as well as the currently available biologics for off label use in SLE (rituximab), and the new experimental strategies which are still in clinical trials. Therapeutics are summarized in Table 15.4 and discussed in detail next.

Table 15.3 Immunobiologics targeting cytokines and their receptors

Biologics	Trade name	Legal status	Mode of action
Adalimumab	Humira®	Approved in 2004	Human antibody neutralizing TNF
Brodalumab	*TBA*	Phase 3	Human antibody binding IL-17 receptor A (IL-17RA)
Certolizumab pegol	Cimzia®	Approved in 2009 for PsA	Humanized antibody neutralizing TNF, PEGylated
Etanercept	Enbrel®	Approved in 2000	Fusion protein of TNFR and Fc-IgG1; blocks TNF
Golimumab	Simponi®	Approved in 2009 for PsA	Human antibody neutralizing TNF
Guselkumab	*TBA*	Phase 3	Human antibody neutralizing IL-23p19
Infliximab	Remicade®	Approved in 2000	Chimeric antibody neutralizing TNF
Ixekizumab	*TBA*	Phase 3	Humanized antibody neutralizing IL-17A
Secukinumab	Cosentyx®	Approved in 2014	Human antibody neutralizing IL-17A
Tildrakizumab	*TBA*	Phase 3	Humanized antibody neutralizing IL-23p19
Ustekinumab	Stelara®	Approved in 2009	Human antibody neutralizing IL-12/IL-23p40

The table includes biologics that are at least in phase 3 development. *TBA* to be announced

Table 15.4 Novel therapies for systemic lupus erythematosus

Biologics	Company	Mechanism of action	Molecule type
Belimumab	GSK	Anti-sBLYS	Monoclonal antibody
Rituximab	Roche	CD20 (B cells)	Monoclonal antibody
Ocrelizumab	Roche	CD20 (B cells)	Monoclonal antibody
Atacicept	Merck Serono	Anti-BLYS& APRIL	Recombinant protein
Epratuzumab	UCB/Immunomedics	Anti-CD22	Monoclonal antibody
Tabalumab	Eli Lilly	Anti-s&mBLYS	Monoclonal antibody
Blisibimod	Anthera	Anti-s&mBLYS	Recombinant protein
Sirolimus	Pfizer	mTOR inhibitor	Recombinant protein
Antroquinonol	Golden Biotech	T cells	Small molecule
Y 27		Treg cells	Small molecule
Laquinimod	Teva/Active Biotech	Immunomodulator	Small molecule
Abatacept (Orencia)	Bristol-Myers	CTLA4-B7	Recombinant protein
Toculizumab	Roche	IL-6 receptor	Monoclonal antibody
Sirukumab	Johnson & GSK	Anti-IL-6	Monoclonal antibody
B-N10		Anti-IL-10	Monoclonal antibody
Rontalizumab	Genentech/Roche	Anti-IFN a	Monoclonal antibody
Sifalimumab	MedImmune	Anti-IFN a	Monoclonal antibody
Infliximab	Johnson	Anti-TNFa	Monoclonal antibody
BIIB-023	Biogen Idec	Anti-TWEAK	Monoclonal antibody
Eculizumab	Alexion	Complement C5	Monoclonal antibody
CR2-Crry		Complement C3	Recombinant protein
IRS 954 and IRS 661	Invivogen	TLR	Synthetic peptide
Spiegelmer	NOXXON Pharma	CCL2	Synthetic peptide
Bortezomib	Gene Operation	Proteasome	Small molecule
Delanzomib	MedChem Express	Proteasome	Small molecule
R788 (Fostamatinib)	Rigel Pharma	Syk	Small molecule
SB203580	MedChem Express	P38MAPK	Small molecule

15.2.1 Targeting B Cells Therapy

B cells have an important role in the pathogenesis of SLE. B cells mediate tissue damage by secreting autoantibodies and also present autoantigens to T cells by acting as APCs [25]. In the past decade, targeted B cells therapy has been developing fast [26–29].

CD20 is a specific surface antigen for B lymphocytes, which is expressed only on B cells but not plasma cells. Anti-CD20 antibodies were the first uncovered biologicals targeting B cells. B cell activating factor (BAFF), also known as B-lymphocyte stimulator (BLyS), is essential for survival, proliferation, and differentiation of B cells. In patients with SLE, BAFF is overexpressed and causes autoimmune B cell proliferation and survival. Studies [30] indicate that selective blockade of BAFF alone was sufficient to prevent and treat LN. As belimumab (target BAFF) was the only biologic drug approved by FDA for treatment of lupus for the last 50 years, we will discuss this drug first.

15.2.1.1 Belimumab

Origin

Belimumab (Benlysta; GlaxoSmithKline), is a fully human IgG1λ monoclonal antibody against soluble BAFF (sBAFF).

Mechanism of Action

Belimumab is a human monoclonal antibody that inhibits sBAFF and blocks the binding of sBAFF to its receptors [31].

Indications

It was the first drug approved to treat SLE by the FDA for over 50 years. The European Medicines Agency (EMA) licensed the use of belimumab to treat SLE in 2011.

The efficacy and superiority of belimumab was demonstrated by two large multinational, randomized, double-blind, phase III studies – the BLISS-52 and BLISS-76 trials [32, 33]. The two studies included 1684 patients, with scores of SLEDAI ≥6. However, the cases with severe kidney and central nervous system lupus were excluded from the trials.

In both trials, belimumab treatment improved symptoms of musculoskeletal and mucocutaneous organs in SLE patients. Subset analysis suggests that belimumab has greater therapeutic benefit than standard therapy alone in patients with higher disease activity as well as greater serologic activity (e.g., anti-DNA positivity and hypocomplementemia) [34, 35]. Improvement was observed in the hematological and renal domains [36]. Moreover, belimumab significantly reduced SLE flare rates and corticosteroid use in BLISS-52.

However, these two trials excluded patients with active nephritis or central nervous system disease, so its effectiveness has not been demonstrated in those cases. A phase III study for SLE patients with kidney disease is now recruiting. Although subgroup analysis of patients with mild-to-moderate kidney involvement enrolled in phase III trials suggested a potential renal benefit [37], a belimumab renal response outcomes trial is expected to be completed by 2017 [38].

In summary, intravenous belimumab is approved by the FDA as an add-on therapy in adults with active, antinuclear antibody-positive or anti-double-stranded DNA-positive SLE with a high degree of disease activity. EMA also licensed belimumab in adult patients with active, autoantibody-positive SLE with a high degree of disease activity (e.g., positive anti-dsDNA and low complement). Belimumab can also be used in cutaneous lupus. However, owing to lack of studies, it is not recommended for use in severe LN or CNS lupus, or in combination with other B cell-targeted therapy or intravenous cyclophosphamide.

Dosage

Belimumab is administered intravenously at 10 mg/kg initially every 2 weeks for the first three doses, and then it is given every 4 weeks. The efficacy of belimumab varies from patient to patient, and the action of the drug can take as long as 6–12 weeks. The therapy should be reconsidered if there is lack of improvement within 6 months. Belimumab is very expensive, costing about $28,000 for the first year.

Adverse Effects

In general, belimumab is well tolerated and not associated with a high rate of adverse events while compared with placebo. The most frequently reported adverse events include headache, nausea, diarrhea, fever, fatigue, as well as hypersensitivity and infusion-site reactions [39]. Data showed that infusion reactions were reported in 16.8 % of belimumab therapy compared with 14.7 % of placebo recipients, but this difference was not statistically significant [40]. Most infusion reactions were mild to moderate and occurred during the first or second infusion. It is suggested that patients be treated with an antihistamine prior to a belimumab infusion.

15.2.1.2 Rituximab

Origin

Rituximab (Rituxan; Roche) is a humanized/mouse chimeric monoclonal antibody specific for human CD20, which is primarily found on the surface of B cells.

Mechanism of Action

Rituximab targets human CD20 receptor on B cells and achieved significant depletion of B cells.

Indications

Studies have showed the efficacy of rituximab in the treatment of SLE patients who have failed to respond to the standard therapy [41–43]. It is reported that rituximab improved articular, cutaneous, renal, and hematological manifestations of SLE patients with satisfactory safety. A meta-analysis showed that rituximab therapy decreased disease activity and antibody and autoantibody levels and reduction in steroid use [44, 45].

However, these results were not confirmed by two rituximab phase III multicentre randomized placebo-controlled trials, known as the exploratory phase II/III SLE evaluation of rituximab (EXPLORER) trial in active SLE and the LN Assessment with Rituximab (LUNAR) trial in LN [46, 47]. Although statistically significant improvements in serum complement C3, C4, and anti-dsDNA levels were observed in the rituximab treated group, the 2 trials failed to find a benefit of rituximab in renal or nonrenal lupus when added to standard-of-care treatment [47, 48].

Interestingly, several open label studies, in contrast to controlled trials, have shown a beneficial effect of rituximab in patients with LN not responding to standard treatments or in patients with refractory diseases [49–51]. Studies have shown that rituximab is a treatment option with a lot of potential and seems to be much less toxic in comparison to cyclophosphamide [52–55].

In summary, rituximab is not approved but is widely off-label used to treat difficult cases of SLE. Despite the negative EXPLORER and LUNAR studies, rituximab is currently the option for nonrenal lupus if standard care has failed. Rituximab might also be considered in patients with refractory disease and cutaneous lupus erythematosus.

Dosage

Rituximab is commonly administered as an infusion once per week for 4 weeks at a dose of 375 mg/m^2 body surface area, in combination with corticosteroids and other immunosuppressive agents. An alternative regimen of 1 g doses on day 1 and 15, and at the same interval 6 months later, was used in the EXPLORER trial.

Adverse Effects
The most frequent adverse effects of rituximab in patients with SLE are mild infusion reactions [56]. Neutropenia and severe infections were reported in up to 10 % of the rituximab-treated patients. Infections include hepatitis B reactivation, other viral infections, and progressive multifocal leukoencephalopathy (PML).

15.2.1.3 Ocrelizumab
Ocrelizumab (Roche) is a humanized anti-CD20 monoclonal antibody and targets mature B lymphocytes. It had reached phase III clinical trials for SLE. BELONG trial aimed at demonstrating the efficacy and safety of Ocrelizumab in SLE. In March 2010, Roche announced the suspension of clinical trials in lupus for excess deaths due to opportunistic infections. Thus, serious infections, that is, requiring IV antibiotics, were twice in the 400 mg Ocrelizumab group compared to the placebo.

15.2.1.4 Atacicept
Atacicept (Merck Serono) is a recombinant humanized fusion protein that blocks activation of B cells by blocking the binding of BLyS and a proliferation-inducing ligand (APRIL). Atacicept is selectively effective on mature B cells and plasma cells. Studies have looked at atacicept in animal models of SLE. Unfortunately, a phase II/III trial of atacicept in LN had to be terminated due to the occurrence of extremely low immunoglobulin levels and pneumonia in some patients. At this moment, a safe efficacious dose for atacicept has yet to be established.

15.2.1.5 Epratuzumab
Epratuzumab (LymphoCide, UCB/Immunomedics) is a humanized IgG1 monoclonal antibody that binds to the glycoprotein CD22 of mature and malignant B cells. It modulates B cell function and migration. Treatment with epratuzumab improved lupus disease activity compared with placebo in a phase II study [57]. Clinical trials showed success in early SLE patients and the drug is in phase III clinical trials. EMBLEM and ALLEVIA clinical trials tested epratuzumab on lupus patients with moderate to severe nonrenal disease in combination with standard treatment. However, the data is still not solid, and the effect on LN has not been addressed yet.

15.2.1.6 Tabalumab and Blisibimod
Tabalumab (Eli Lilly) and Blisibimod (Anthera) are anti-BLYS biologics. Unlike belimumab, tabalumab and blisibimod are inhibitors of both soluble and membrane bound BAFF. The benefits and safety of the tabalumab and blisibimod in SLE were in phase III clinical trials and are currently unavailable. Hopefully, it can demonstrate superior benefits to belimumab as it blocks both soluble and membrane bound BAFF.

15.2.2 Targeting T Cells Therapy

T cells play multiple roles in the pathogenesis of SLE. They regulate B cell responses for production of autoantibodies and modulate T helper and effector function and expansion. T cells infiltrate the kidney to injure renal parenchyma cells directly via cytotoxicity or indirectly via activation and recruitment of macrophages and NK cells.

15.2.2.1 Sirolimus
Sirolimus (Rapamune, Pfizer), also known as rapamycin, is a macrolide (one of a group of drugs containing a macrolide ring) produced by the bacteria *Streptomyces hygroscopicus*. The immunosuppressive effect of sirolimus is to bind the cytosolic protein FK-binding protein 12 (FKBP12). The sirolimus-FKBP12 complex inhibits the mTOR, necessary for the proliferation and clonal expansion of activated T cells. Treatment of NZB/WF 1 mice with sirolimus inhibited the production of autoantibodies and the development of proteinuria and glomerular deposits of Ig [58, 59]. Sirolimus administration improved disease activity and dependence on prednisone in SLE patients resistant or intolerant to immunosuppressant medications. Prospective clinical trial in SLE patients with sirolimus is ongoing. The most serious complication is lung toxicity.

15.2.2.2 Antroquinonol
Antroquinonol is an antrodia camphorate extract which modulates T cell activity and reduces the production of IL-18. Trials in NZB/WF 1 mice showed that it could protect the kidney from immunologic damage by blocking a TNF- and IL-1-mediated inflammatory process [60].

15.2.2.3 Y27
Regulatory T cells (Treg) is a new subset of helper T (Th) cells. Treg cells suppress the autoimmune reaction and play a protection role in SLE and other autoimmune diseases. Studies in patients with LN show that $CD4^+CD25^+$ Treg numbers and suppressive functions are reduced. Y27 is a novel 4-hydroxyquinoline-3-formamide derivative primarily derived from H1521, which could enhance suppressive capacity of $CD4^+CD25^+$ Tregs. Y27 treatment effectively ameliorated autoimmune syndromes in MRL/lpr mice and BDF1 mice and ameliorate glomerular injury [61].

15.2.2.4 Laquinimod
Laquinimod (Teva/Active Biotech) is a small-molecule derivative of quinolone-3-carboxamide. Laquinimod appears to modulate the inflammatory environment by polarizing T cells toward Tregs and away from TH1 and TH17 phenotypes [62]. It has been studied and just completed a phase 2 trial in LN.

15.2.3 Targeting Cytotoxic T-Lymphocyte Antigen 4 (CTLA4) Therapy

Costimulation is a critical step in driving expansion of autoreactive T cells. Engagement of CD28 on naive T cells by either B7-1 or B7-2 ligands on APCs provides a potent costimulatory signal to T cells. Trials in organ transplantation animal models showed that blockade of CD28 costimulation can prevent the induction of pathogenic T cell responses and allowing for prolonged acceptance of allografts [63, 64]. CTLA4 is a homolog of CD28, but it exerts an inhibitory signal. CTLA4 binds to B7-1 or B7-2 molecules with much higher avidity, rendering T cells less sensitive to stimulation by APCs and limiting their proliferative responses.

15.2.3.1 Abatacept

Origin
Abatacept (Orencia; Bristol-Myers Squibb) (also called CTLA4-Ig) is a soluble glycosylated fusion protein which links the extracellular domain of human of CTLA4 and the Fc portion of human IgG1.

Mechanism of Action
Abatacept is the first in a new class of drugs known as selective costimulation modulators. It targets T cell costimulation modulator that binds to B7 and thereby blocks its interaction with CD28, expressed on T cells, preventing the activation of T cell.

Indications
Abatacept was tested both in SLE and in LN patients. Earlier studies have demonstrated the efficacy and safety of abatacept in SLE. Merrill et al. reported a flare rate following 12 months of treatment with abatacept versus placebo in nonrenal SLE patients [65, 66]. The other study examined the efficacy and safety of combination therapy of abatacept and mycophenolate, compared to mycophenolate alone, in LN [66]. Unfortunately, none of the clinical trials so far have met their predetermined defined complete renal response rates for efficacy [67], much like the case of rituximab in SLE.

In contrast, re-analysis of the results of the trial using different outcome definitions reached opposite conclusions [68]. The results of the ACCESS (Abatacept and Cyclophosphamide Combination Therapy for Lupus Nephritis) trial, aimed at comparing abatacept to "placebo" on a cyclophosphamide regime background of LN patients, should soon become available. Another data showed that abatacept as an add-on treatment to immunosuppressive and steroid therapy gave the probability of achieving complete renal response at 12 months.

However, future studies must take into consideration the appropriate definitions of response, degree of background treatments, and patients included in order to develop the optimal treatment strategies for patients.

In summary, abatacept is a prescription medicine that reduces signs and symptoms in adults with moderate to severe rheumatoid arthritis (RA). Currently, abatacept remains a possible therapeutic option as an off-label therapy in SLE.

Adverse Effects
Most common adverse events (≥10%) are headache, upper respiratory tract infection, nasopharyngitis, and nausea.

15.2.4 Targeting IL-6 Therapy

IL-6 is a proinflammatory cytokine produced by activated lymphocytes that stimulate T, B cell differentiation and autoantibody secretion [69]. IL-6 has effects on B cells, it is necessary for its stimulation and promotes Ig secretion by plasma cells, and on T cells promotes the differentiation of Th17 cells and inhibits the differentiation of Tregs by suppressing the transcription of Foxp3. High serum levels of IL-6 were found in patients with active SLE.

15.2.4.1 Toculizumab

Toculizumab (Roche) is a humanized monoclonal antihuman IL-6 receptor antibody that blocks IL-6 from binding to its receptor. Study showed that toculizumab is very effective in patients with rheumatoid arthritis and is currently in preliminary trials in patients with SLE.

A phase 1 clinical trial of toculizumab in SLE demonstrated safety and tolerability of renal and nonrenal lupus patients. IL-6 receptor blockade has been shown to reduce immunoglobulin levels and produce small decreases in anti-dsDNA levels, as well as improvement in disease activity scores. Toculizumab can also benefit serositis with pericardial effusion, autoimmune hemolytic anemia, and cutaneous lesion in SLE patients [70–72].

15.2.4.2 Sirukumab

Sirukumab (Johnson & Johnson/GlaxoSmithKline) is a humanized monoclonal antibody against IL-6 and presently is undergoing a phase 2 clinical trial to assess its safety and efficacy in LN.

15.2.5 Anti-IL-10 Therapy

IL-10 is a multifunctional cytokine that has a complex role in SLE. It is mainly produced by Treg cells and inhibits Th1 cell and macrophage activation [73]. On the other hand, it promotes activation and differentiation of B lymphocytes and the production of IgG. High serum levels of IL-10 are found in SLE patients and correlate with disease activity.

15.2.5.1 B-N10

B-N10 is an anti-IL-10 murine mAb. In the absence of a humanized mAb to IL-10, the murine anti-IL-10 mAb (B-N10) was used. One study evaluated the safety and clinical efficacy of administering B-N10 to SLE patients with active and steroid-dependent disease [73]. Cutaneous lesions and joint symptoms improved in all patients and the SLE Disease Activity Index decreased. Prednisone administration was also decreased.

15.2.6 Anti-IL-17 Therapy

IL-17 is a family of six related cytokines (IL-17A, B, C, D, E, F) that functions in host defense against extracellular bacterial and fungal infections and contributes to the pathogenesis of autoimmune inflammatory diseases. IL-17 influences B cell survival, proliferation, and differentiation [74]. They showed that IL-17 was as efficient as BAFF in protecting B cells from apoptosis. Some studies demonstrate the role of IL-17 in lupus disease [75]. $CD4^+$ Th17 cells (IL-17 producing cells) appear to mediate pathogenesis in some lupus mouse models. High levels of IL-17 have been reported in SLE patients [76]. It may be possible that Th17 cells play a role in lupus pathogenesis and that anti-IL-17 therapy may be helpful specifically in those patients.

15.2.7 Anti-interferon (IFN) Therapy

Type-I IFNs contribute to the differentiation and activation of DCs, as well as the activation, proliferation, and survival of T and B cells, and to autoantibody production. Increased circulating levels of IFN-α were detected in SLE patients, which correlate with both disease activity and severity.

15.2.7.1 Rontalizumab

Rontalizumab (Genentech/Roche), a humanized IgG1 monoclonal antibody that neutralizes IFNα, were assessed in a phase I dose-escalation study of single and repeat doses of rontalizumab in adults with mildly active SLE.

15.2.7.2 Sifalimumab

Sifalimumab (MedImmune) are humanized antibodies that target IFN-a. No statistically significant differences in clinical activity (SLEDAI) between sifalimumab and placebo were observed. However, a trend toward normal complement C3 or C4 level at week 26 was seen in the sifalimumab groups compared with baseline [77].

15.2.8 Antitumour Necrosis Factor Alpha (TNF-α) Therapy

TNF-α is a cytokine produced mainly by activated monocytes, macrophages, T and NK cells. TNF-α induces the expression of other proinflammatory cytokines, such as IL-1 and IL-6. Data on increased TNF-α levels in serum, kidney, and skin samples of SLE patients as well as results in other mouse models of the disease point to an inflammatory role of TNF in SLE. It seemed that anti-TNF-α treatment will benefit SLE patients. However, it appeared that levels of ANA and dsDNA antibodies increased, as well as occasionally drug induced lupus during TNF blockade. Despite the controversial results regarding the treatment, anti-TNF therapy has been tried for several years.

15.2.8.1 Infliximab

Infliximab (Remicade, Johnson) is a chimeric monoclonal antibody against TNF-α. Clinical trials showed that infliximab therapy may lead to long-term remission in patients with LN, hemophagocytic syndrome, and interstitial lung disease. Patients with LN often respond to infliximab but symptoms recur after cessation of therapy, necessitating longer term therapy, which is more risky than short term treatment. However, the most serious adverse effects were infections [78, 79]. In the study, autoantibody production and systemic immune activation were not inhibited. These findings support use of infliximab for induction treatment but not for maintenance given the concern for drug-induced toxicity over time.

15.2.9 Antitumour Necrosis Factor-Like Weak Inducer of Apoptosis (TWEAK) Therapy

TWEAK is a member of the TNF superfamily. TWEAK can stimulate many cytokines, chemokines, and cell adhesion molecules [80] and participates in tissue inflammation in many diseases, including SLE [81]. Anti-TWEAK currently is being evaluated in a phase 3 LN trial. ATLAS (Anti-TWEAK in lupus nephritis patients) is exploring kidney protection in LN afforded by neutralizing anti-TWEAK antibodies when conventional immunosuppressive therapy does not result in complete remission within a reasonable period of time [82].

15.2.9.1 BIIB-023

BIIB-023 (Biogen Idec) is a TWEAK-specific mAb. A multicenter, randomized, double blind, placebo controlled study was conducted to evaluate the efficacy, safety, and tolerability of BIIB023 in subjects with IN.

15.2.10 Anticomplement Therapy

Complement appears to play a dual role in the progression of SLE, serving a beneficial role in enhancing immune complex clearance, while serving a pathogenic role in inducing local inflammation. Complement modulates the adaptive immune response through modification of T cell immunity, development of natural antibodies, and regulation of autoreactive B cells. It has become increasingly recognized that the complement system was a potential therapeutic target in SLE.

15.2.10.1 Eculizimab

Eculizumab (Alexion Pharmaceuticals) is a recombinant humanized monoclonal IgG2/4 κ antibody produced by murine myeloma cells directed at human complement component C5. Eculizumab inhibits the conversion of C5 to C5a and C5b, thus preventing formation of the membrane attack complex (C5b-9) and the chemotactic fragment C5a [83]. It is conceivable that in LN, eculizumab could prevent direct complement-mediated injury to intrinsic glomerular cells and attenuate kidney inflammation by reducing renal leukocyte recruitment [84]. A phase I clinical trial showed that the adverse events were mild and there was no dose-dependent trend in adverse events. Infection-related adverse events were similar between eculizumab and placebo.

15.2.10.2 CR2-Crry

CR2-Crry is a targeted inhibitor of mouse C3. Administration of CR2-Crry in animal model was associated with a significant survival benefit, improved kidney function, and a significant reduction in autoantibody production, glomeru lonephritis, and renal vasculitis reduction. The presence of skin lesions was also dramatically reduced by CR2 Crry treatment [85].

15.2.11 Anti-TLR Therapy

TLR family has critical roles in the induction of innate immune responses to pathogens by recognition of numerous microbial products, including LPS (TLR4). TLRs can also upregulate the expression of MHCII and costimulatory molecules. Moreover TLR induces the production of IL-6, IL-12, TNF, and IFN.

15.2.11.1 IRS 954

Immunoregulatory sequence (IRS) 954 is a specific inhibitor of TLR7 and TLR9. Recent findings in both human and mouse models suggest that TLR7 and TLR9 may play a central role in SLE by promoting elevated IFN-a levels from pDC and by activating B cells to produce autoantibodies. A study showed that IRS 954 can prevent progression of disease when injected in the lupus prone (NZBxNZW) F1 and MRL/lpr mice. IRS 954 significantly reduced serum levels of nucleic acid-specific autoantibodies as well as decreased proteinuria, reduced glomerulonephritis, end-organ damage and increased survival rate [86, 87].

15.2.11.2 IRS 661

IRS 661 specifically blocks signaling via TLR-7. Pawar et al. evaluated the specific inhibition of TLR7 with IRS 661, and only IRS 661 significantly reduced serum levels of IL-12p40, anti-dsDNA IgG2a, IgG2b, and anti-Sm IgG [87].

15.2.12 Antichemokine Therapy

The monocyte chemoattractant protein CCL2 is crucial for monocyte and T cell recruitment from the vascular to the extravascular compartment at sites of inflammation. There is strong evidence that CCL2, and its receptor CCR2, has a crucial role in SLE. CCL2 is expressed in human LN and was shown to mediate experimental lupus. Therefore, CCL2 antagonists may be beneficial for therapy.

15.2.12.1 Spiegelmer

Spiegelmer (the l-enantiomeric RNA oligonucleotide mNOX-E36) binds murine CCL2 with high affinity and neutralizes its action in vitro and in vivo.

Autoimmune-prone MRL/lpr mice treated with spiegelmer showed prolonged survival and improvement of lupus nephritis and peribronchial inflammation and lupus-like inflammatory skin lesions. Thus, inhibition of CCL2 represents a novel strategy for the treatment of LN [88].

15.2.13 Proteasome Inhibitors Therapy

The proteasome is a multienzymatic protein complex that can regulate the expression of gene and cytokine by activation of NF-kB.

15.2.13.1 Bortezomib

Bortezomib is a proteasome inhibitor. Studies showed that it can improve renal pathology and survival of experimental LN in NZB/WF 1 mice [89] or MRL/lpr mice [89, 90].

15.2.13.2 Delanzomib

Delanzomib is an orally active inhibitor of the chymotrypsin-like activity of proteasome. MRL/lpr or NZB/WF 1 mice with fatal LN were treated with delanzomib. Reductions in antichromatin, anti-Smad dsDNA antibody-secreting cells, and serum proinflammatory cytokines were observed. Delanzomib treatment also suppressed the development and progression of renal tissue damage and extended the survival of ill mice by decreased proteinuria and improved renal histopathology types [91].

15.2.14 Kinase Inhibitors Therapy

In LN, T cell activation is associated with an increase of the phosphorylation of activation signal transduction molecules, including tyrosine kinase Syk and MAPK. MAPKs are responsible for the synthesis and release of several cytokines and chemokines such as IL-1, IL-6, MCP1, and CCR5, among others.

15.2.14.1 R788 (Fostamatinib)

Fostamatinib is administered orally as a disodium salt, which is a small molecule inhibitor of the enzyme spleen tyrosine kinase (Syk). Treatment of NZB/WF 1 mice with fostamatinib delayed the onset of proteinuria and azotemia, reduced renal pathology and kidney infiltrates, and significantly prolonged survival of these lupus-prone NZB/NZW mice [92].

15.2.14.2 SB203580

SB203580, a specific inhibitor of p38 MAPK, can ameliorate renal function by decreasing the levels of proteinuria and serum BUN, decreasing renal pathologic changes, and reducing Ig and C3 deposits in the kidney when administered to MRL/lpr mouse model of SLE [93].

In summary, for the better understanding of the benefits and adverse effects of new biologics in SLE, it will be necessary to standardize clinical trial end points and make sure the clinical trial include all kinds of patients. This is a beginning to develop through working groups such as the Lupus Nephritis Trials Network. Hopefully, after belimumab, next approved biologic for lupus will be uncovered soon.

Glossary

APC	Antigen presenting cell
CD8⁺	CD8-positive (cytotoxic T cell)
CSA	Cyclosporine A
DC	Dendritic cell
DMF	Dimethyl fumarate
EAE	Experimental allergic encephalomyelitis
EMA	European Medicines Agency
FAE	Fumaric esters
FDA	Federal Drug Administration (USA)
GSH	Glutathione
IBD	Inflammatory bowel disease
IFN-γ	Interferon γ
IL	Interleukin
JAK	Janus kinase
JC virus	John Cunningham virus; human polyomavirus; associated with PML
LFA1, 3	Lymphocyte function associated antigen 1, 3
-mab	Monoclonal antibody
MS	Multiple sclerosis
MTX	Methotrexate
NFκB	Nuclear factor "kappa-light-chain-enhancer" of activated B cells
PDE4	Phosphodiesterase 4
PML	Progressive multifocal leukoencephalopathy
PsA	Psoriatic arthritis
PSO	Psoriasis
RA	Rheumatoid arthritis
STAT	Signal transducers and activators of transcription
TBA	To be announced
TGF-β	Transforming growth factor-β
Th	T helper cell
TNF	Tumor necrosis factor

References

Immunobiologics for Psoriasis

1. Ghoreschi K, Weigert C, Röcken M. Immunopathogenesis and role of T cells in psoriasis. Clin Dermatol. 2007;25(6):574–80.
2. Lowes MA, Suárez-Fariñas M, Krueger JG. Immunology of psoriasis. Annu Rev Immunol. 2014;32(1):227–55.
3. Snowden JA, Heaton DC. Development of psoriasis after syngeneic bone marrow transplant from psoriatic donor: further evidence for adoptive autoimmunity. Br J Dermatol. 1997;137(1):130–2.
4. Kanamori H, Tanaka M, Kawaguchi H, Yamaji S, Fujimaki K, Tomita N, et al. Resolution of psoriasis following allogeneic bone marrow transplantation for chronic myelogenous leukemia: case report and review of the literature. Am J Hematol. 2002;71(1): 41–4.
5. Ghoreschi K, Laurence A, Yang XP, Tato CM. Generation of pathogenic TH17 cells in the absence of TGF-[bgr] signalling. Nature. 2010;467(7318):967–71.
6. Bolognia JL, Jorizzo JL,Schaffer JV. Dermatology. 3rd ed. Elsevier Saunders: London; 2012.
7. Marrakchi S, Guigue P, Renshaw BR, Puel A, Pei X-Y, Fraitag S, et al. Interleukin-36-receptor antagonist deficiency and generalized pustular psoriasis. N Engl J Med. 2011;365(7):620–8.
8. Tsoi LC, Spain SL, Knight J, Ellinghaus E, Stuart PE, Capon F, et al. Identification of 15 new psoriasis susceptibility loci highlights the role of innate immunity. Nat Genet. 2012;44(12):1341–8.
9. Bettelli E, Korn T, Kuchroo VK. Th17: the third member of the effector T cell trilogy. Curr Opin Immunol. 2007;19(6):652–7.
10. Nestle FO, Kaplan DH, Barker J. Psoriasis. N Engl J Med. 2009;361(5):496–509.
11. Leonardi CL, Kimball AB, Papp KA, Yeilding N, Guzzo C, Wang Y, et al. Efficacy and safety of ustekinumab, a human interleukin-12/23 monoclonal antibody, in patients with psoriasis: 76-week results from a randomised, double-blind, placebo-controlled trial (PHOENIX 1). Lancet. 2008;371(9625):1665–74.
12. Leonardi C, Matheson R, Zachariae C, Cameron G, Li L, Edson-Heredia E, et al. Anti–interleukin-17 monoclonal antibody ixekizumab in chronic plaque psoriasis. N Engl J Med. 2012;366(13): 1190–9.

13. Papp KA, Leonardi C, Menter A, Ortonne J-P, Krueger JG, Kricorian G, et al. Brodalumab, an anti–interleukin-17–receptor antibody for psoriasis. N Engl J Med. 2012;366(13):1181–9.
14. Langley RG, Elewski BE, Lebwohl M, Reich K, Griffiths CEM, Papp K, et al. Secukinumab in plaque psoriasis – results of two phase 3 trials. N Engl J Med. 2014;371(4):326–38.
15. Ghoreschi K, Laurence A, O'Shea JJ. Janus kinases in immune cell signaling. Immunol Rev. 2009;228(1):273–87.
16. Bissonnette R, Iversen L, Sofen H, Griffiths CEM, Foley P, Romiti R, et al. Tofacitinib withdrawal and re-treatment in moderate-to-severe chronic plaque psoriasis: a randomised controlled trial. Br J Dermatol. 2014;172(5):1395–406.
17. Papp K, Cather JC, Rosoph L, Sofen H, Langley RG, Matheson RT, et al. Efficacy of apremilast in the treatment of moderate to severe psoriasis: a randomised controlled trial. Lancet. 2012;380(9843):738–46.
18. Lebwohl M, Tyring SK, Hamilton TK, Toth D, Glazer S, Tawfik NH, et al. A novel targeted T-cell modulator, efalizumab, for plaque psoriasis. N Engl J Med. 2003;349(21):2004–13.
19. Ellis CN, Krueger GG, Alefacept Clinical Study Group. Treatment of chronic plaque psoriasis by selective targeting of memory effector T lymphocytes. N Engl J Med. 2001;345(4):248–55.
20. Krupashankar DS, Dogra S, Kura M, Saraswat A, Budamakuntla L, Sumathy TK, et al. Efficacy and safety of itolizumab, a novel anti-CD6 monoclonal antibody, in patients with moderate to severe chronic plaque psoriasis: results of a double-blind, randomized, placebo-controlled, phase-III study. J Am Acad Dermatol. 2014;71(3):484–92. Elsevier.
21. Belge K, Brück J, Ghoreschi K. Advances in treating psoriasis. F1000Prime Rep. 2014;6(4):4.
22. Sofen H, Smith S, Matheson RT, Leonardi CL, Calderon C, Brodmerkel C, et al. Guselkumab (an IL-23-specific mAb) demonstrates clinical and molecular response in patients with moderate-to-severe psoriasis. J Allergy Clin Immunol. 2014;133(4):1032–40.
23. Gordon KB, Leonardi CL, Lebwohl M, Blauvelt A, Cameron GS, Braun D, et al. A 52-week, open-label study of the efficacy and safety of ixekizumab, an anti-interleukin-17A monoclonal antibody, in patients with chronic plaque psoriasis. J Am Acad Dermatol. 2014;71(6):1176–82. Elsevier.
24. Papp K, Leonardi C, Menter A, Thompson EHZ, Milmont CE, Kricorian G, et al. Safety and efficacy of brodalumab for psoriasis after 120 weeks of treatment. J Am Acad Dermatol. 2014;71(6):1183–90. Elsevier.

Immunobiologics for Lupus

25. Tsokos GC. Systemic lupus erythematosus. N Engl J Med. 2011;365(22):2110–21.
26. Xiong W, Lahita RG. Novel treatments for systemic lupus erythematosus. Ther Adv Musculoskelet Dis. 2011;3(5):255–66. Pubmed Central PMCID: 3383530.
27. Yoo DH. Anticytokine therapy in systemic lupus erythematosus. Lupus. 2010;19(12):1460–7.
28. Yildirim-Toruner C, Diamond B. Current and novel therapeutics in the treatment of systemic lupus erythematosus. J Allergy Clin Immunol. 2011;127(2):303–12; quiz 13–4. Pubmed Central PMCID: 3053574.
29. Bezalel S, Asher I, Elbirt D, Sthoeger ZM. Novel biological treatments for systemic lupus erythematosus: current and future modalities. Isr Med Assoc J. 2012;14(8):508–14.
30. Ding H, Wang L, Wu X, Yan J, He Y, Ni B, et al. Blockade of B-cell-activating factor suppresses lupus-like syndrome in autoimmune BXSB mice. J Cell Mol Med. 2010;14(6B):1717–25.
31. Baker KP, Edwards BM, Main SH, Choi GH, Wager RE, Halpern WG, et al. Generation and characterization of LymphoStat-B, a human monoclonal antibody that antagonizes the bioactivities of B lymphocyte stimulator. Arthritis Rheum. 2003;48(11):3253–65.
32. Navarra SV, Guzman RM, Gallacher AE, Hall S, Levy RA, Jimenez RE, et al. Efficacy and safety of belimumab in patients with active systemic lupus erythematosus: a randomised, placebo-controlled, phase 3 trial. Lancet. 2011;377(9767):721–31.
33. Furie R, Petri M, Zamani O, Cervera R, Wallace DJ, Tegzova D, et al. A phase III, randomized, placebo-controlled study of belimumab, a monoclonal antibody that inhibits B lymphocyte stimulator, in patients with systemic lupus erythematosus. Arthritis Rheum. 2011;63(12):3918–30.
34. Stohl W, Hiepe F, Latinis KM, Thomas M, Scheinberg MA, Clarke A, et al. Belimumab reduces autoantibodies, normalizes low complement levels, and reduces select B cell populations in patients with systemic lupus erythematosus. Arthritis Rheum. 2012;64(7):2328–37. Pubmed Central PMCID: 3350827.
35. van Vollenhoven RF, Petri MA, Cervera R, Roth DA, Ji BN, Kleoudis CS, et al. Belimumab in the treatment of systemic lupus erythematosus: high disease activity predictors of response. Ann Rheum Dis. 2012;71(8):1343–9. Pubmed Central PMCID: 3396451.
36. Manzi S, Sanchez-Guerrero J, Merrill JT, Furie R, Gladman D, Navarra SV, et al. Effects of belimumab, a B lymphocyte stimulator-specific inhibitor, on disease activity across multiple organ domains in patients with systemic lupus erythematosus: combined results from two phase III trials. Ann Rheum Dis. 2012;71(11):1833–8. Pubmed Central PMCID: 3465857.
37. Dooley MA, Houssiau F, Aranow C, D'Cruz DP, Askanase A, Roth DA, et al. Effect of belimumab treatment on renal outcomes: results from the phase 3 belimumab clinical trials in patients with SLE. Lupus. 2013;22(1):63–72.
38. Runkel L, Stacey J. Lupus clinical development: will belimumab's approval catalyse a new paradigm for SLE drug development? Expert Opin Biol Ther. 2014;14(4):491–501.
39. Ramos-Casals M, Sanz I, Bosch X, Stone JH, Khamashta MA. B-cell-depleting therapy in systemic lupus erythematosus. Am J Med. 2012;125(4):327–36. Pubmed Central PMCID: 3925418.
40. Wallace DJ, Navarra S, Petri MA, Gallacher A, Thomas M, Furie R, et al. Safety profile of belimumab: pooled data from placebo-controlled phase 2 and 3 studies in patients with systemic lupus erythematosus. Lupus. 2013;22(2):144–54.
41. Lu TY, Ng KP, Cambridge G, Leandro MJ, Edwards JC, Ehrenstein M, et al. A retrospective seven-year analysis of the use of B cell depletion therapy in systemic lupus erythematosus at University College London Hospital: the first fifty patients. Arthritis Rheum. 2009;61(4):482–7.
42. Ramos-Casals M, Soto MJ, Cuadrado MJ, Khamashta MA. Rituximab in systemic lupus erythematosus: a systematic review of off-label use in 188 cases. Lupus. 2009;18(9):767–76.
43. Turner-Stokes T, Lu TY, Ehrenstein MR, Giles I, Rahman A, Isenberg DA. The efficacy of repeated treatment with B-cell depletion therapy in systemic lupus erythematosus: an evaluation. Rheumatology. 2011;50(8):1401–8.
44. Gunnarsson I, Jonsdottir T. Rituximab treatment in lupus nephritis – where do we stand? Lupus. 2013;22(4):381–9.
45. Ahuja A, Shupe J, Dunn R, Kashgarian M, Kehry MR, Shlomchik MJ. Depletion of B cells in murine lupus: efficacy and resistance. J Immunol. 2007;179(5):3351–61.
46. Merrill JT, Neuwelt CM, Wallace DJ, Shanahan JC, Latinis KM, Oates JC, et al. Efficacy and safety of rituximab in moderately-to-severely active systemic lupus erythematosus: the randomized, double-blind, phase II/III systemic lupus erythematosus evaluation of rituximab trial. Arthritis Rheum. 2010;62(1):222–33.
47. Rovin BH, Furie R, Latinis K, Looney RJ, Fervenza FC, Sanchez-Guerrero J, et al. Efficacy and safety of rituximab in patients with

active proliferative lupus nephritis: the Lupus Nephritis Assessment with Rituximab study. Arthritis Rheum. 2012;64(4):1215–26.
48. Bacconnier L, Combe B, Canaud B, Morel J. Efficacy of rituximab in a patient with lupus nephritis despite low levels of CD19. Rheumatology. 2010;49(12):2452–3.
49. Jonsdottir T, Zickert A, Sundelin B, Henriksson EW, van Vollenhoven RF, Gunnarsson I. Long-term follow-up in lupus nephritis patients treated with rituximab – clinical and histopathological response. Rheumatology. 2013;52(5):847–55.
50. Davies RJ, Sangle SR, Jordan NP, Aslam L, Lewis MJ, Wedgwood R, et al. Rituximab in the treatment of resistant lupus nephritis: therapy failure in rapidly progressive crescentic lupus nephritis. Lupus. 2013;22(6):574–82.
51. Lightstone L. The landscape after LUNAR: rituximab's crater-filled path. Arthritis Rheum. 2012;64(4):962–5.
52. Appel GB. New and future therapies for lupus nephritis. Cleve Clin J Med. 2012;79(2):134–40.
53. Jonsdottir T, Sundelin B, Welin Henriksson E, van Vollenhoven RF, Gunnarsson I. Rituximab-treated membranous lupus nephritis: clinical outcome and effects on electron dense deposits. Ann Rheum Dis. 2011;70(6):1172–3.
54. Bertsias G, Boumpas DT. Update on the management of lupus nephritis: let the treatment fit the patient. Nat Clin Pract Rheumatol. 2008;4(9):464–72.
55. Tesar V, Hruskova Z. Treatment of proliferative lupus nephritis: a slowly changing landscape. Nat Rev Nephrol. 2011;7(2):96–109.
56. Terrier B, Amoura Z, Ravaud P, Hachulla E, Jouenne R, Combe B, et al. Safety and efficacy of rituximab in systemic lupus erythematosus: results from 136 patients from the French AutoImmunity and Rituximab registry. Arthritis Rheum. 2010;62(8):2458–66.
57. Wallace DJ, Kalunian K, Petri MA, Strand V, Houssiau FA, Pike M, et al. Efficacy and safety of epratuzumab in patients with moderate/severe active systemic lupus erythematosus: results from EMBLEM, a phase IIb, randomised, double-blind, placebo-controlled, multicentre study. Ann Rheum Dis. 2014;73(1):183–90. Pubmed Central PMCID: 3888603.
58. Ramos-Barron A, Pinera-Haces C, Gomez-Alamillo C, Santiuste-Torcida I, Ruiz JC, Buelta-Carrillo L, et al. Prevention of murine lupus disease in (NZBxNZW)F1 mice by sirolimus treatment. Lupus. 2007;16(10):775–81.
59. Alperovich G, Rama I, Lloberas N, Franquesa M, Poveda R, Goma M, et al. New immunosuppresor strategies in the treatment of murine lupus nephritis. Lupus. 2007;16(1):18–24.
60. Tsai PY, Ka SM, Chang JM, Lai JH, Dai MS, Jheng HL, et al. Antroquinonol differentially modulates T cell activity and reduces interleukin-18 production, but enhances Nrf2 activation, in murine accelerated severe lupus nephritis. Arthritis Rheum. 2012;64(1):232–42.
61. Xiao ZY, Chen SH, Cheng JP, Zhou WX, Zhang YX, Yang RF, et al. Y27, a novel derivative of 4-hydroxyquinoline-3-formamide, prevents the development of murine systemic lupus erythematosus-like diseases in MRL/lpr autoimmune mice and BDF1 hybrid mice. Arthritis Res Ther. 2012;14(6):R235. Pubmed Central PMCID: 3674632.
62. Jolivel V, Luessi F, Masri J, Kraus SH, Hubo M, Poisa-Beiro L, et al. Modulation of dendritic cell properties by laquinimod as a mechanism for modulating multiple sclerosis. Brain. 2013;136(Pt 4):1048–66.
63. Salomon B, Bluestone JA. Complexities of CD28/B7: CTLA-4 costimulatory pathways in autoimmunity and transplantation. Annu Rev Immunol. 2001;19:225–52.
64. Greenfield EA, Nguyen KA, Kuchroo VK. CD28/B7 costimulation: a review. Crit Rev Immunol. 1998;18(5):389–418.
65. Linsley PS, Brady W, Urnes M, Grosmaire LS, Damle NK, Ledbetter JA. CTLA-4 is a second receptor for the B cell activation antigen B7. J Exp Med. 1991;174(3):561–9. Pubmed Central PMCID: 2118936.
66. Merrill JT, Burgos-Vargas R, Westhovens R, Chalmers A, D'Cruz D, Wallace DJ, et al. The efficacy and safety of abatacept in patients with non-life-threatening manifestations of systemic lupus erythematosus: results of a twelve-month, multicenter, exploratory, phase IIb, randomized, double-blind, placebo-controlled trial. Arthritis Rheum. 2010;62(10):3077–87.
67. Wofsy D, Hillson JL, Diamond B. Abatacept for lupus nephritis: alternative definitions of complete response support conflicting conclusions. Arthritis Rheum. 2012;64(11):3660–5.
68. Wofsy D, Hillson JL, Diamond B. Comparison of alternative primary outcome measures for use in lupus nephritis clinical trials. Arthritis Rheum. 2013;65(6):1586–91.
69. Kitani A, Hara M, Hirose T, Harigai M, Suzuki K, Kawakami M, et al. Autostimulatory effects of IL-6 on excessive B cell differentiation in patients with systemic lupus erythematosus: analysis of IL-6 production and IL-6R expression. Clin Exp Immunol. 1992;88(1):75–83. Pubmed Central PMCID: 1554365.
70. Kamata Y, Minota S. Successful treatment of massive intractable pericardial effusion in a patient with systemic lupus erythematosus with tocilizumab. BMJ Case Rep. 2012;2012:pii: bcr2012007834.
71. Alten R, Maleitzke T. Tocilizumab: a novel humanized anti-interleukin 6 (IL-6) receptor antibody for the treatment of patients with non-RA systemic, inflammatory rheumatic diseases. Ann Med. 2013;45(4):357–63.
72. Garcia-Hernandez FJ, Gonzalez-Leon R, Castillo-Palma MJ, Ocana-Medina C, Sanchez-Roman J. Tocilizumab for treating refractory haemolytic anaemia in a patient with systemic lupus erythematosus. Rheumatology. 2012;51(10):1918–9.
73. Llorente L, Richaud-Patin Y, Garcia-Padilla C, Claret E, Jakez-Ocampo J, Cardiel MH, et al. Clinical and biologic effects of anti-interleukin-10 monoclonal antibody administration in systemic lupus erythematosus. Arthritis Rheum. 2000;43(8):1790–800.
74. Doreau A, Belot A, Bastid J, Riche B, Trescol-Biemont MC, Ranchin B, et al. Interleukin 17 acts in synergy with B cell-activating factor to influence B cell biology and the pathophysiology of systemic lupus erythematosus. Nat Immunol. 2009;10(7):778–85.
75. Hsu HC, Yang P, Wang J, Wu Q, Myers R, Chen J, et al. Interleukin 17-producing T helper cells and interleukin 17 orchestrate autoreactive germinal center development in autoimmune BXD2 mice. Nat Immunol. 2008;9(2):166–75.
76. Wong CK, Lit LC, Tam LS, Li EK, Wong PT, Lam CW. Hyperproduction of IL-23 and IL-17 in patients with systemic lupus erythematosus: implications for Th17-mediated inflammation in auto-immunity. Clin Immunol. 2008;127(3):385–93.
77. Petri M, Wallace DJ, Spindler A, Chindalore V, Kalunian K, Mysler E, et al. Sifalimumab, a human anti-interferon-alpha monoclonal antibody, in systemic lupus erythematosus: a phase I randomized, controlled, dose-escalation study. Arthritis Rheum. 2013;65(4):1011–21. Pubmed Central PMCID: 3654174.
78. Bethunaickan R, Sahu R, Liu Z, Tang YT, Huang W, Edegbe O, et al. Anti-tumor necrosis factor alpha treatment of interferon-alpha-induced murine lupus nephritis reduces the renal macrophage response but does not alter glomerular immune complex formation. Arthritis Rheum. 2012;64(10):3399–408. Pubmed Central PMCID: 3443508.
79. Aringer M, Smolen JS. Therapeutic blockade of TNF in patients with SLE-promising or crazy? Autoimmun Rev. 2012;11(5):321–5.
80. Gao HX, Campbell SR, Burkly LC, Jakubowski A, Jarchum I, Banas B, et al. TNF-like weak inducer of apoptosis (TWEAK) induces inflammatory and proliferative effects in human kidney cells. Cytokine. 2009;46(1):24–35.

81. Winkles JA. The TWEAK-Fn14 cytokine-receptor axis: discovery, biology and therapeutic targeting. Nat Rev Drug Discov. 2008;7(5):411–25. Pubmed Central PMCID: 3018765.
82. Ruiz-Ortega M, Ortiz A, Ramos AM. Tumor necrosis factor-like weak inducer of apoptosis (TWEAK) and kidney disease. Curr Opin Nephrol Hypertens. 2014;23(1):93–100.
83. Sekine H, Ruiz P, Gilkeson GS, Tomlinson S. The dual role of complement in the progression of renal disease in NZB/W F(1) mice and alternative pathway inhibition. Mol Immunol. 2011;49(1–2): 317–23.
84. Barilla-Labarca ML, Toder K, Furie R. Targeting the complement system in systemic lupus erythematosus and other diseases. Clin Immunol. 2013;148(3):313–21.
85. Atkinson C, Qiao F, Song H, Gilkeson GS, Tomlinson S. Low-dose targeted complement inhibition protects against renal disease and other manifestations of autoimmune disease in MRL/lpr mice. J Immunol. 2008;180(2):1231–8.
86. Barrat FJ, Meeker T, Chan JH, Guiducci C, Coffman RL. Treatment of lupus-prone mice with a dual inhibitor of TLR7 and TLR9 leads to reduction of autoantibody production and amelioration of disease symptoms. Eur J Immunol. 2007;37(12):3582–6.
87. Pawar RD, Ramanjaneyulu A, Kulkarni OP, Lech M, Segerer S, Anders HJ. Inhibition of Toll-like receptor-7 (TLR-7) or TLR-7 plus TLR-9 attenuates glomerulonephritis and lung injury in experimental lupus. J Am Soc Nephrol. 2007;18(6):1721–31.
88. Kulkarni O, Pawar RD, Purschke W, Eulberg D, Selve N, Buchner K, et al. Spiegelmer inhibition of CCL2/MCP-1 ameliorates lupus nephritis in MRL-(Fas)lpr mice. J Am Soc Nephrol. 2007;18(8): 2350–8.
89. Hainz N, Thomas S, Neubert K, Meister S, Benz K, Rauh M, et al. The proteasome inhibitor bortezomib prevents lupus nephritis in the NZB/W F1 mouse model by preservation of glomerular and tubulointerstitial architecture. Nephron Exp Nephrol. 2012;120(2):e47–58.
90. Ichikawa HT, Conley T, Muchamuel T, Jiang J, Lee S, Owen T, et al. Beneficial effect of novel proteasome inhibitors in murine lupus via dual inhibition of type I interferon and autoantibody-secreting cells. Arthritis Rheum. 2012;64(2):493–503.
91. Seavey MM, Lu LD, Stump KL, Wallace NH, Ruggeri BA. Novel, orally active, proteasome inhibitor, delanzomib (CEP-18770), ameliorates disease symptoms and glomerulonephritis in two preclinical mouse models of SLE. Int Immunopharmacol. 2012;12(1): 257–70.
92. Bahjat FR, Pine PR, Reitsma A, Cassafer G, Baluom M, Grillo S, et al. An orally bioavailable spleen tyrosine kinase inhibitor delays disease progression and prolongs survival in murine lupus. Arthritis Rheum. 2008;58(5):1433–44.
93. Jin N, Wang Q, Zhang X, Jiang D, Cheng H, Zhu K. The selective p38 mitogen-activated protein kinase inhibitor, SB203580, improves renal disease in MRL/lpr mouse model of systemic lupus. Int Immunopharmacol. 2011;11(9):1319–26.

Erratum to: Immnopathology

Cheng Sun, Haoyu Sun, and Zhigang Tian

Erratum to:
Chapter 5 in: X.-H. Gao, H.-D. Chen (eds.), *Practical Immunodermatology*, DOI 10.1007/978-94-024-0902-4_5

The original version of this chapter unfortunately contained a mistake. The presentation of Fig. 5.2 was incorrect. Please refer next page (E2) for the corrected image.

The updated online version of the original chapter can be found under DOI 10.1007/978-94-024-0902-4_5

C. Sun • H. Sun
Institute of Immunology, School of Life Sciences and Medical Center, University of Science and Technology of China, Hefei, China

Z. Tian (✉)
Institute of Immunology, School of Life Sciences and Medical Center, University of Science and Technology of China, Hefei, China
e-mail: tzg@ustc.edu.cn

X.-H. Gao, H.-D. Chen (eds.), *Practical Immunodermatology*, DOI 10.1007/978-94-024-0902-4_16

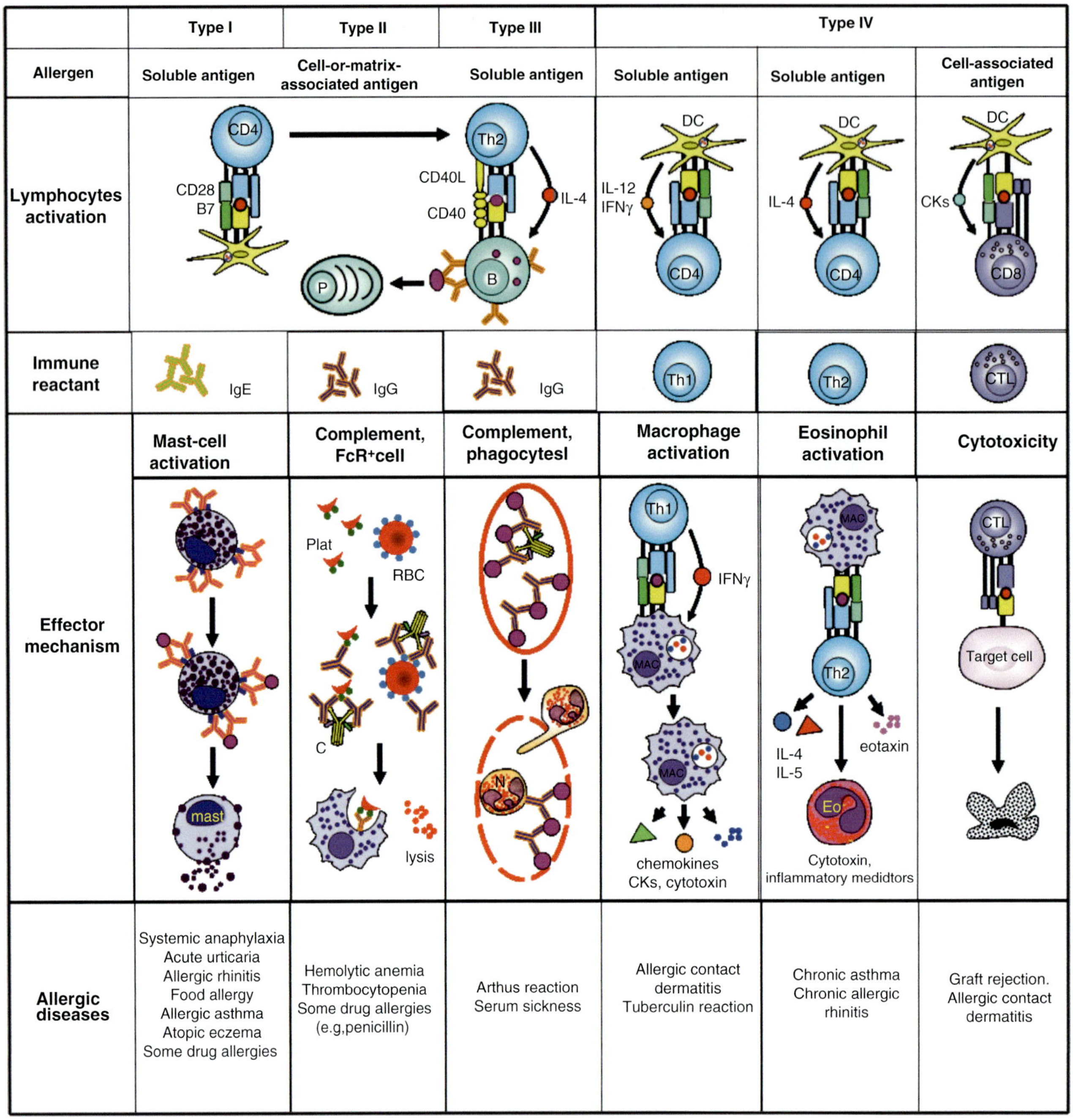

The original chapter has been corrected.

Index

X.-H. Gao, H.-D. Chen (eds.), *Practical Immunodermatology*, DOI 10.1007/978-94-024-0902-4

MIX
Papier aus verantwortungsvollen Quellen
Paper from responsible sources
FSC® C105338

If you have any concerns about our products,
you can contact us on
ProductSafety@springernature.com

In case Publisher is established outside the EU,
the EU authorized representative is:
Springer Nature Customer Service Center GmbH
Europaplatz 3, 69115 Heidelberg, Germany

Printed by Libri Plureos GmbH
in Hamburg, Germany